AF739016

PREFACE

The complexity and significance of the insulin-like growth factor (IGF) system is staggering. From conception through postnatal growth, development, reproduction, and aging, in health and disease, the IGF axis orchestrates critical aspects of metabolism and physiology. The IGF proteins and their cell receptors are widely expressed in the body and many important functions of IGF system are rapidly being discovered. The impact of nutrition as a fundamental influence on anabolism, growth, and in some instances pathology, is intertwined with IGF in ways that are only just beginning to be appreciated. Nutritional state is one of the most potent regulators of IGFs. Understanding the interactions among nutrition and the IGF axis is critical to understanding the role of these growth factors in normal growth and development and in pathological states. Conversely, IGFs are key mediators by which growth, cell differentiation, and division is influenced by nutrient availability. This volume is the first comprehensive review of nutrition and the IGF system in health and disease. It brings together internationally known and distinguished researchers, physicians, and professors of biology, medicine, nutrition, molecular biology, physiology, biochemistry, animal science, and endocrinology. Inclusion of the most recent basic, clinical, and epidemiological data, across all phases of the life span, as well as perspectives from multiple disciplines, is a major aim of this volume.

IGF encompasses a complex system that includes two proteins (IGF-I and IGF-II), at least six distinct carrier proteins (IGFBP-1–6) that have unique roles in modulating IGF bioactivity as well as independent actions, and two major cellular receptors (IGFR-I and IGFR-II) with significant cross-reactivity with the insulin receptor. Many excellent reviews of the IGF system, chronicling their initial characterization 40–50 yr ago, and ongoing delineation of their roles are available (Appendix A). Virtually all cells and tissues in the body are affected by IGFs in some fashion. As endocrine factors, the IGFs were first recognized as "sulfation factors" that mediated the effects of growth hormone (GH) on cartilage growth and were named "somatomedins" as their critical role in somatic growth during pre- and postnatal life became apparent. In a larger context, IGF actions are part of the hypothalamic–pituitary axis and inseparable from GH. In addition, as the nomenclature suggests, the overlap between IGFs and insulin in terms of structural homology and biological properties is significant. IGFs have rapid insulin-like metabolic actions as well as more long-term growth-promoting activities. There is significant cross-reactivity between IGF-I and the insulin receptor at the cellular level. The importance of the IGF system, in relation to nutrition in the pathogenesis, prevention, and treatment of insulin resistance and diabetes mellitus and their related complications is being actively investigated (Chapter 14).

In addition to the endocrine activity, the pleiotropic effects of the IGFs are related to their local paracrine and autocrine production and activity. Cell differentiation, DNA and protein synthesis, and cell survival are examples of the potent effects of the IGFs in various tissues and organ systems. The specific roles and relative activities of the IGF proteins vary by tissues. The complexity and importance of the IGF system as it is interrelated with nutrition and metabolic status is approached from many perspectives and in the context of a variety of conditions under normal and pathological circumstances in the present volume. The essential components and molecular aspects of the IGF system and some of the newer concepts in the insulin/IGF signaling pathways lay the groundwork (Chapter 1) for discussion of the direct effects of nutrient availability on the IGF system in Part II. The remaining sections of this volume describe IGF and nutrition in major organ systems and their roles in pathological conditions. Resources related to IGF and nutrition, including the professional societies, organizations, and journals are provided in Appendix B.

Fasting, starvation, and nutritional imbalances have profound effects on the IGFs that are independent of pituitary GH secretion and actions. Protein and energy availability, and micronutrients such as zinc (Chapters 2 and 5), regulate IGF-I gene expression as well as circulating levels of the IGFs, and ultimately the biological activity of IGFs in growth and development. Much of bone health and disease involves some aspect of the IGF system (Chapter 10). Calcium, vitamin D, and protein intakes exert strong influences on bone metabolism that are mediated in part by IGF activity. Observational and interventional studies in the elderly provide strong evidence for the relationship among protein intake, IGF-I, and osteoporosis.

The loss of normal anabolic response to IGFs occurs in malnutrition, but also in catabolic states brought about by metabolic and physical stresses such as infection, injury, and organ failure. The conflicting, competing or perhaps overlapping influences of nutrition and catabolic stress on IGF function during critical illness are considered from a number of perspectives (Chapters 2, 3, 11, and 16).

Many chronic diseases cause profound metabolic changes that lead to catabolism and unintentional weight loss. Persistent inflammation and other anti-anabolic factors in chronic disease can lead to the loss of energy and protein reserves and protein energy malnutrition that cannot be explained nor reversed by altered dietary intake (Chapter 3). The imbalance of anabolic and catabolic signals provides the underlying mechanisms for the wasting (cachexia) and malnutrition of chronic diseases. Understanding the specific role of IGF in the prolonged catabolism of conditions such as heart failure (Chapter 17), chronic critical illness (Chapters 2, 11, 16), inflammatory bowel disease (Chapter 15), and chronic renal failure (Chapter 13) is important to minimizing the malnutrition, morbidity, and mortality of chronic diseases.

Malnutrition is reflected in altered circulating levels of IGF-I and some of the IGFBPs, particularly IGFBP-1, in the blood. This ability of IGF-I to serve as a marker of the adequacy of nutrient intake has been recognized since early research in animals. The possibility of assessing nutritional status with a marker such as IGF-I that is itself a potent anabolic agent is appealing (Chapter 4). Understanding the impact of nutrition support modalities such as parenteral nutrition is furthered by understanding its direct effects on the IGF system (Chapter 15). In addition, the acuity and sensitivity of serum IGF-I concentrations to nutrient adequacy is particularly vital in situations of acute catabolic stress such as critical illness where existing markers of nutrition are limited and when starvation, but also avoidance of overfeeding, is of paramount importance.

The regulation of IGF by nutritional status has many implications across the life span. The IGF–GH axis is a critical component in the orchestration of normal prenatal and postnatal growth (Chapters 6 and 7), and reproduction (Chapter 8). Compromises in normal growth, reproductive function, and IGF activity by malnutrition have been demonstrated in animal models, but the specific sites of nutritional regulation and the implications for human growth and development remain to be elucidated. Many age-related disabilities in older years are believed to be tied to changes in the IGF proteins (Chapter 9). Circulating levels of IGF-I, IGFBP-1, and perhaps other IGFs, are nutritionally regulated throughout life.

The IGF system is integrally involved in such diverse tissues as skeletal muscle (Chapter 11), the nervous system (Chapter 12), the heart (Chapter 17), the gastrointestinal system (Chapter 15), and the kidneys (Chapter 13). The IGFs offer promising therapies for many debilitating conditions such as multiple sclerosis, Alzheimer's disease, ALS, kidney failure, heart failure, diabetic neuropathy, stroke, and traumatic injury. The interaction of IGF and nutrition in normal functioning as well as disease development and therapy is just beginning.

In cancer research, there has been tremendous interest in the IGF proteins because of their critical role in apoptosis, cell division, and differentiation. The impact of biologically active components in food, overall nutritional state, and possible interactions with IGF are relevant to our understanding of the fundamental mechanisms of tumorigenesis and how the environment and thus potentially modifiable factors can induce or prevent cancer (Chapters 6 and 18).

We are a long way from fully understanding the relationships between the IGF system and nutritional state, but the potential interactions and impact on health and disease are profound and compelling. Understanding the interplay between nutrition and the IGFs has tremendous implications for understanding fundamental biological processes, disease prevention, therapy, and health. Ultimately, it is hoped that this volume introduces and/or expands knowledge for researchers, health professionals and students, but also fosters continued exploration of these two vitally important and intertwined fields of study. The editors thank all of the contributors, who despite being incredibly busy, gave up their time to make this volume come together. The authors acknowledge the technical assistance of Jessica Jannicelli, Nicole Furia, and the staff at Humana Press. In addition, the authors express their sincere appreciation to Paul Dolgert, Editorial Director, Humana Press, and Adrianne Bendich, Series Editor of the *Nutrition and Health* series.

M. Sue Houston, PhD, RD
Jeffrey M. P. Holly, PhD
Eva L. Feldman, MD, PhD

CONTENTS

Contributors

MARTIN L. ADAMO, PhD • *Department of Biochemistry, The University of Texas Health Science Center at San Antonio, San Antonio, TX*

PATRICK AMMANN, MD • *Division of Bone Diseases [WHO Collaborating Center for Osteoporosis Prevention], Department of Internal Medicine, University Hospital, Geneva, Switzerland*

VÉRONIQUE BEAULOYE, MD, PhD • *Unité de Diabétologie et Nutrition, School of Medicine, Université Catholique de Louvain, Brussels, Belgium*

DALIT BEN-YOSEF, PhD • *Section on Cellular and Molecular Physiology, Clinical Endocrinology Branch, National Institute of Diabetes and Digestive and Kidney Diseases, National Institute of Health, Bethesda, MD*

BRUCE R. BISTRIAN, MD, PhD • *Division of Clinical Nutrition, Department of Medicine, Beth Israel Deaconess Medical Center, Harvard Medical School, Boston, MA*

CYNTHIA L. BLANCO, MD • *Division of Neonatology, Department of Pediatrics, The University of Texas Health Science Center at San Antonio, San Antonio, TX*

JASON L. BLUM, MS • *Interdisciplinary Program for Biomedical Research, Department of Pharmacology, University of Florida, Gainesville, FL*

APARNA BOLE, BA • *Department of Neurology, University of Michigan, Ann Arbor, MI*

JEAN-PHILIPPE BONJOUR, MD • *Division of Bone Diseases [WHO Collaborating Center for Osteoporosis Prevention], Department of Internal Medicine, University Hospital, Geneva, Switzerland*

MARIJKE BRINK, PhD • *Division of Cardiology, Fondation pour Recherches Médicales, Genève, Switzerland*

KERSTIN BRISMAR, MD, PhD • *Department of Molecular Medicine, Karolinska Institutet, Stockholm, Sweden*

THIERRY CHEVALLEY, MD • *Division of Bone Diseases [WHO Collaborating Center for Osteoporosis Prevention], Department of Internal Medicine, University Hospital, Geneva, Switzerland*

PATRICE DELAFONTAINE, MD, FACC, FAHA, FACP • *Section of Cardiology, Tulane University Health Sciences Center, New Orleans, LA*

EVA L. FELDMAN, MD, PhD • *JDRF Center for the Study of Complications in Diabetes, Department of Neurology, University of Michigan, Ann Arbor, MI*

ROBERT J. FERRY, JR., MD • *Division of Endocrinology & Diabetes, Departments of Pediatrics, Cellular & Structural Biology and Medical Reserve Corps, Texas Medical Rangers, Texas State Guard, The University of Texas Health Science Center at San Antonio, San Antonio, TX*

ROBERT A. FROST, PhD • *Department of Cellular and Molecular Physiology, Pennsylvania State University, College of Medicine, Hershey, PA*

STEVEN S. GUEST, MD • *Department of Medicine, Stanford University, Santa Clara Valley Medical Center, Palo Alto, CA*

KERSTIN HALL, MD, PhD • *Department of Molecular Medicine, Karolinska Institutet, Stockholm, Sweden*
LISA HERON, PhD • *Section on Cellular and Molecular Physiology, Clinical Endocrinology Branch, National Institute of Diabetes and Digestive and Kidney Diseases, National Institute of Health, Bethesda,* MD
JEFFREY M. P. HOLLY, PhD • *Division of Surgery, Department of Hospital Medicine, Bristol Royal Infirmary, Bristol, UK*
M. SUE HOUSTON, PhD, RD • *Food and Nutrition Program, School of Family and Consumer Sciences, Bowling Green State University, Bowling Green, OH*
JEAN-MARIE KETELSLEGERS, MD, PhD • *Unité de Diabétologie et Nutrition, School of Medicine, Université Catholique de Louvain, Brussels, Belgium*
INSEOK KWAK, PhD • *Department of Molecular & Cellular Biology, Baylor College of Medicine, Houston, TX*
CHARLES H. LANG, PhD • *Department of Cellular and Molecular Physiology, Pennsylvania State University, College of Medicine, Hershey, PA*
DEREK LE ROITH, MD, PhD • *Section on Cellular and Molecular Physiology, Clinical Endocrinology Branch, National Institute of Diabetes and Digestive and Kidney Diseases, National Institute of Health, Bethesda, MD*
MOIRA S. LEWITT, MD, PhD • *Department of Molecular Medicine, Karolinska Institutet, Stockholm, Sweden*
PEI-RA LING, MD, PhD • *Division of Clinical Nutrition, Department of Medicine, Beth Israel Deaconess Medical Center, Harvard Medical School, Boston, MA*
RUTH S. MACDONALD, PhD, RD • *Departments of Food Science and Nutritional Sciences, University of Missouri, Columbia, MO*
GARY MEYER, PhD • *Department of Neurology, University of Michigan, Ann Arbor, MI*
DENISE M. NEY, PhD • *Department of Nutritional Sciences, University of Wisconsin-Madison, Madison, WI*
CLAIRE M. PERKS, PhD • *Division of Surgery, Department of Hospital Medicine, Bristol Royal Infirmary, Bristol, UK*
RALPH RABKIN, MD • *Department of Medicine, Stanford University and Veterans Affairs Palo Alto Health Care System, Palo Alto, CA*
RENÉ RIZZOLI, MD • *Division of Bone Diseases, Department of Internal Medicine, University Hospital, Geneva, Switzerland*
CHARLES T. ROBERTS, JR., PhD • *Department of Pediatrics, Oregon Health and Science University, Portland, OR*
FRANZ SCHAEFER, MD • *Division of Pediatric Nephrology, University Children's Hospital, Heidelberg, Germany*
FRANK A. SIMMEN, PhD • *Arkansas Children's Nutrition Center and Department of Physiology and Biophysics, University of Arkansas for Medical Sciences, Little Rock, AR*
ROSALIA C. M. SIMMEN, PhD • *Arkansas Children's Nutrition Center and Department of Physiology and Biophysics, University of Arkansas for Medical Sciences, Little Rock, AR*
YAO-HUA SONG, MD, PhD • *Section of Cardiology, Tulane University Health Science Center, New Orleans, LA*

JEAN-PAUL THISSEN, MD, PhD • *Unité de Diabétologie et Nutrition, School of Medicine, Université Catholique de Louvain, Brussels, Belgium*
LOUIS E. UNDERWOOD, MD, PhD • *Division of Pediatric Endocrinology, University of North Carolina, Chapel Hill, NC*
GRETA VAN DEN BERGHE, MD, PhD • *Department of Intensive Care Medicine, University Hospital Gasthuisberg, University of Leuven, Leuven, Belgium*
LAI WANG, PhD • *Department of Biochemistry, The University of Texas Health Science Center at San Antonio, San Antonio, TX*
HONG ZHAO, MD, PhD • *Section on Cellular and Molecular Physiology, Clinical Endocrinology Branch, National Institute of Diabetes and Digestive and Kidney Diseases, National Institute of Health, Bethesda, MD*

I Overview

1 Overview and Molecular Aspects of the Insulin-Like Growth Factor System

Martin L. Adamo, Lai Wang, Lisa Heron, Dalit Ben-Yosef, Hong Zhao, and Derek Le Roith

KEY POINTS

- The IGF system consists of two ligands, IGF-I and IGF-II, and several receptors: the IGF-I receptor, the insulin receptor, and the IGF-II/mannose-6-phosphate receptor. There are also six IGF-binding proteins.
- IGF-I is a circulating growth factor and also is produced by many tissues to act as an autocrine/paracrine factor. IGF-I stimulates cellular proliferation, differentiation, and survival.
- IGF-I and IGF-II expression are regulated by many hormonal and nutritional factors in a manner consistent with the effect of these factors on growth, differentiation, and metabolism.
- IGF-I and IGF-II act through the IGF-I receptor, which is a tyrosine kinase that activates a number of intracellular signaling pathways.
- Insulin acts through the insulin receptor, which is similar to the IGF-I receptor. IGF-II can also bind to an alternative form of the insulin receptor. The IGF-II/mannose-6-phosphate receptor clears IGF-II, thereby decreasing its levels.
- IGF-binding proteins protect IGFs in the serum and act at the local level to either inhibit or enhance IGF action. Some IGFBPs have IGF-independent actions on cell growth and survival.
- Recent studies indicate that despite the apparent similarity of IGF-I and insulin receptors, activation of the receptors results in inherently distinct effects on cellular gene expression. and function. IGF-I primarily stimulates growth and cell survival, whereas insulin regulates metabolism.
- The insulin/IGF receptors and intracellular signaling systems are conserved in invertebrates, where they regulate lifespan, growth, and metabolism.

1. INTRODUCTION

The insulin-like growth factor (IGF) system includes three ligands (insulin, IGF-I, and IGF-II), three receptors (the insulin receptor [IR], the IGF-I receptor [IGF-IR], and the mannose-6-phosphate [M6P/IGF-II receptor]), as well as six IGF binding proteins (IGF

From: *IGF and Nutrition in Health and Disease*
Edited by: M. S. Houston, J. M. P. Holly, and E. L. Feldman © Humana Press Inc., Totowa, NJ

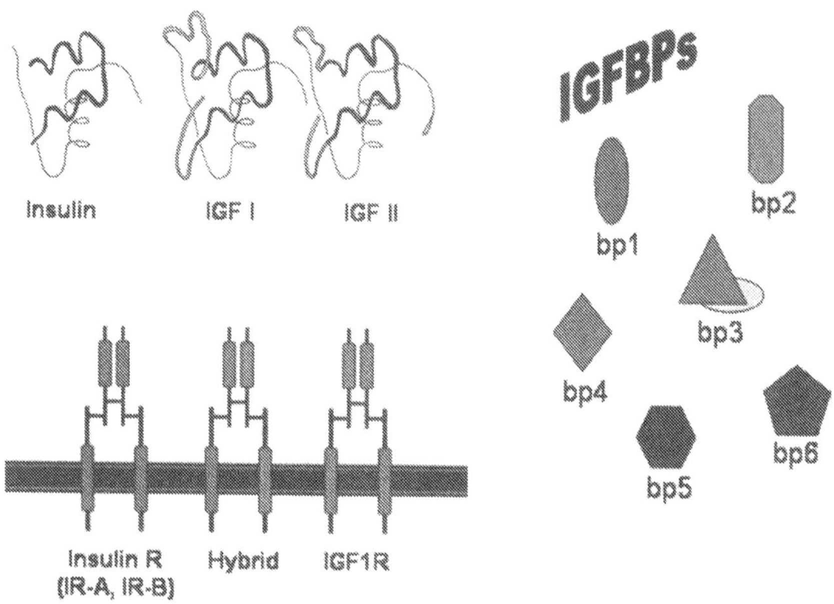

Fig. 1. Components of the IGF system include ligands (insulin, IGF-I and IGF-II), binding proteins (bp 1–6), as well as the receptors.

BPs). This family of growth factors has been extensively studied because of its critical role in both normal physiology and in various disease states, such as cancer, diabetes, and malnutrition. The various components of the IGF family are widely expressed and, therefore, other important functions are rapidly being discovered.

This chapter presents an overview of the IGF system (Fig. 1), including the biological functions of its various components and how the expression of these components is controlled, and will focus on more recent findings because many excellent reviews already have covered the well-known aspects of the IGF system *(1–3)*.

2. LIGANDS

2.1. IGF-I

IGF-I is a 70-amino acid residue single-chain polypeptide with four domains, which are designated as B, C, A, and D. In comparison, proinsulin includes the B, C, and A domains, whereas mature insulin includes only the B and A domains. Circulating "endocrine" IGF-I is synthesized and released primarily in the liver *(4)*, although most tissues of the body synthesize IGF-I to serve as an autocrine/paracine factor.

The major factors that regulate hepatic IGF-I biosynthesis are growth hormone (GH), insulin, and nutritional status (reviewed in Chapter 2). GH stimulates transcription of IGF-I in the liver. This is associated with chromatin rearrangements in the second intron of the *IGF-I* gene *(5)*. Hypophysectomized mice with a targeted deletion of the Stat-5b transcription factor fail to respond to GH with the characteristic increase in hepatic IGF-I mRNA *(6)*. GH also activates the Stat-5a and Stat-3 transcription factors *(7,8)*. Stat-5a-deficient mice exhibit reduced levels of IGF-I mRNA expression in liver *(9)*. Recently, GH was shown to stimulate transcription of the *IGF-I* gene by promoting Stat 5b binding to two growth hormone response elements within the second intron *(10)*.

2.1.1. IGF-I IN HEPATIC TISSUES

Insulin stimulates transcription of the *IGF-I* gene in a phosphatidyl inositol 3′-kinase (PI3 kinase)-dependent manner in the liver. This is mediated through a novel insulin response element (IRE), which is located within the transcribed portion of exon 1 *(11,12)*. The Sp1 transcription factor acts synergistically with an as-yet-unidentified IRE binding protein in this insulin-stimulated transcriptional activation. In contrast, nutritional deprivation, including fasting and protein restriction, reduce hepatic IGF-I mRNA through a posttranscriptional mechanism *(13,14)*. Because alteration of amino acids and glucose in cultured hepatocytes also regulates IGF-I mRNA posttranscriptionally *(14,15)*, it is possible that specific macronutrients and micronutrients, such as zinc (reviewed in Chapter 5) directly contribute to the effects of altered nutritional status on regulation of the IGF family of genes.

2.1.2. IGF-1 IN EXTRA-HEPATIC TISSUES

GH also stimulates IGF-I biosynthesis in several extra-hepatic tissues, except for those in the female reproductive tract *(16–19)*. GH increases IGF-I transcription in a preadipocyte cell line *(20)*, resulting in increased levels of an alternatively spliced form of IGF-I mRNA that is translated more efficiently *(21)*. GH also increases IGF-I mRNA in a cultured skeletal muscle cell line *(22)*. Finally, GH increases expression of a luciferase reporter gene driven by the IGF-I promoter in the brain of transgenic mice in vivo and in cultured brain cells from these animals in vitro *(23)*.

Although GH can clearly regulate IGF-I gene expression, IGF-I can also be regulated independently of GH in several extra-hepatic tissues. Prostaglandin E2 (PGE2) and parathyroid hormone (PTH) increased IGF-I mRNA in cultured osteoblasts, whereas GH had little effect *(24)*. More recently, studies have shown that cyclic adenosine monophosphate (cAMP) stimulates transcription of IGF-I in osteoblasts via a mechanism that involves protein kinase A (PKA)-dependent nuclear translocation and retention of the C/EBP-δ transcription factor *(25,26)*. It also has been demonstrated that PTH fails to promote bone formation in IGF-I-deficient mice *(27)*. This is consistent with the important physiological role of PTH and locally produced PGE2 in facilitating bone repair and supporting growth in an IGF-I-dependent but GH-independent manner *(28)*. Estradiol also increases the expression of IGF-I in osteoblasts *(29)*, although the precise mechanism of action and its physiological significance are unclear. Estradiol had no effect on activity of the proximal IGF-I promoter in osteoblastic cells *(30)*. In that study, estradiol actually inhibited cAMP-stimulated transactivation of the IGF-I promoter, and this was associated with diminished binding of C/EBP-δ to the IGF-I promoter. More recently, a so-called "antiestrogen" that may have bone-specific trophic effects transactivated the IGF-I promoter in Hep3B cells via the estrogen receptor ER-α *(31)*. This effect was antagonized by estradiol *(31)*.

Thyroid-stimulating hormone (TSH) increases IGF-I mRNA in thyroid cells *(32)*. This is proposed to be important in the interaction between TSH and IGF-I in promoting thyroid growth and function *(33)*. Although gonadotrophins stimulate IGF-I mRNA in cultured granulosa cells *(34)*, there is currently no evidence that follicle-stimulating hormone (FSH) regulates IGF-I expression in vivo *(19)*. Rather, estrogen may be an important local regulator of IGF-I in ovary and uterus *(35,36)*.

Other examples of local control of IGF-I expression include angiotensin II stimulation of IGF-I production in the cardiovascular system *(37)*, the induction of IGF-I expression in compensatory renal growth *(38)*, and in skeletal muscle growth and repair (reviewed in ref. *39*). However, in these latter two cases, the specific factors that induce IGF-I mRNA are not known. In addition, the marked tissue-specific regulation of IGF-I mRNA that occurs during muscle development is probably not dependent on GH *(40)*. In liver, GH does not appear to initiate the postnatal induction of exon 1 transcripts, although it may contribute to this process. GH may play a more important role in the induction of exon 2 transcripts *(41)*. In addition, liver-specific transcription factors, such as hepatic nuclear factor (HNF)-1α, are important in hepatic IGF-I expression *(42)*. Subsequent chapters (i.e., Chapter 8, reproduction; Chapter 10, bone; Chapter 11, muscle; Chapter 12, neurological; chapter 13, renal ; Chapter 15, gastrointestinal, and Chapter 17, cardiovascular) will review the function and regulation of IGF proteins and their relation to nutrition in extra-hepatic tissues.

2.1.3. IGF-I in Growth and Development

Total deletion of the *IGF-I* gene leads to prenatal and postnatal growth retardation in mice, particularly during the peri-pubertal growth spurt *(2,43,44)*. The growth of certain soft tissues is relatively unaffected in these animals *(45,46)*, indicating that IGF-I plays a role largely in musculoskeletal growth. However, other defects in IGF-I knockout mice, including hypomyelination *(47)* and sterility because of deficiencies in gonadal differentiation and function *(16,19)*, indicate that soft tissues are indeed dependent on IGF-I from either serum or local production for normal growth and development. The role of IGF proteins in postnatal growth and development is discussed extensively in Chapter 3 and 6.

To further characterize the endocrine vs the autocrine/paracrine roles of IGF-I in growth and development, liver IGF-I-deficient (LID) mice were generated *(4)*. The LID mice grew and developed normally despite a 75% reduction in serum IGF-I levels *(4)*. Tissue-specific deletion of the IGF-I gene in the liver did not affect postnatal growth and development, possibly because these mice maintained sufficient circulating levels of IGF-I during early postnatal growth. The acid labile subunit (ALS) is a protein that binds to the IGF/IGFBP-3 binary complex, primarily in serum. Association with ALS prolongs the half-life ($t_{1/2}$) of IGFs in serum and facilitates their endocrine actions. When LID mice were crossed with mice carrying the null ALS allele, circulating IGF-I levels were significantly reduced and the double-knockout mice exhibited significant postnatal growth retardation *(48)*. Thus, circulating IGF-I plays an important role in growth.

Although circulating IGF-I clearly plays a critical physiological role, autocrine/paracrine expression of IGF-I is also important. Follicular expression of IGF-I correlated precisely with FSH receptor expression and FSH receptor levels were decreased in IGF-I knockout mice *(19)*. Exogenous replacement of IGF-I restored FSH receptor levels to normal. Although the latter result does not rule out an effect of circulating IGF-I on follicular function, cell culture studies showed that neutralization of endogenous IGF-I inhibited FSH action in granulosa cells *(49)*. Calvariae cultured in vitro from IGF-I knockout mice exhibited reduced collagen synthesis and, as was described previously, in vivo bone growth was unable to respond optimally to PTH in IGF-I knockout mice.

Recently, it has been shown that tissue-specific promoter-driven expression of IGF-I transgenes stimulates growth and development in a number of tissues, including bone *(50)*, thyroid gland *(33)*, and skeletal muscle *(51)*. Use of the muscle-specific IGF-I transgene has been proposed to be superior to systemic administration of IGF-I in maintaining muscle cell function, because it avoids increased serum IGF-I and potential cancer risk *(51)*. However, transgenic expression of IGF-I in epidermal basal cells using the keratin 5 promoter increased tumor formation *(52)*.

To determine the effects of protein calorie malnutrition on extra-hepatic tissues, liver-specific IGF-I-deficient mice were assigned to one of four isocaloric diets that differed in the protein content (20, 12, 4, and 0%), for a period of 10 d. A low protein intake decreased the nonhepatic IGF-I secretion into the circulation, whereas it caused an increase in the level of circulating GH. The lack of dietary protein led to an up-regulation of GH and IGF-I receptor expression in the spleen, whereas the IGF-I mRNA remained unchanged. Upregulation of IGF-binding protein-3 mRNA levels was also observed and suggests that the protein deprivation may lead to an increased sequestration of circulating or locally synthesized IGF-I *(53)*.

2.2. IGF-II

The role of IGF-II in growth and development was clearly demonstrated by the dramatic effects seen when the IGF-II gene was ablated in mice *(43)*. From embryonic d 11 onward there was proportionate growth retardation. There were no further postnatal effects on growth in these mice, because IGF-II expression and circulating levels decrease dramatically after birth in rodents. Expression of IGF-II in cultured cells is regulated by various agents, including FSH, chorionic gonadotrophin and cAMP in ovarian cells, adrenocorticotropic hormone (ACTH) and cAMP in fetal adrenal cells, glucocorticoid and thyroid hormone in hepatic cells, and glucose in a pancreatic beta cell line *(54)*. IGF-II is also increased in response to glucose in fetal hepatocytes *(15)*, and plays an important autocrine/paracrine role in skeletal muscle myoblast differentiation in vitro *(55)*. In the circulation, IGF-II is a 67-amino acid, single-chain polypeptide. However, patients with certain types of tumors occasionally release "big-IGF-II," a larger precursor form with a 21 amino-acid extension (E-peptide). Big-IGF-II may cause hypoglycemia by interfering with the normal effect of the IGFBPs on neutralizing circulating IGFs, thereby enabling big-IGF-II to interact with insulin receptors *(56)*.

3. RECEPTORS

3.1. The Insulin-Like Growth Factor-1 Receptor

The insulin-like growth factor-1 receptor (IGF-IR) is the product of a single gene that spans more than 100 kilobases and contains 21 exons. The receptor is organized into functional domains that resemble those found in the insulin receptor (IR), a closely related membrane spanning tyrosine kinase receptor *(57-59)*. The mature receptor is expressed in an $\alpha 2\beta 2$-configuration (Fig. 2), where two α chains are joined by disulfide bonds. The α-subunit lies entirely in the extracellular region and contains a cysteine-rich domain that forms the primary binding site for IGFs. The βsubunit includes a 24-amino acid residue hydrophobic transmembrane domain, a short extracellular region, and a large cytoplasmic region that includes a tyrosine kinase domain. The

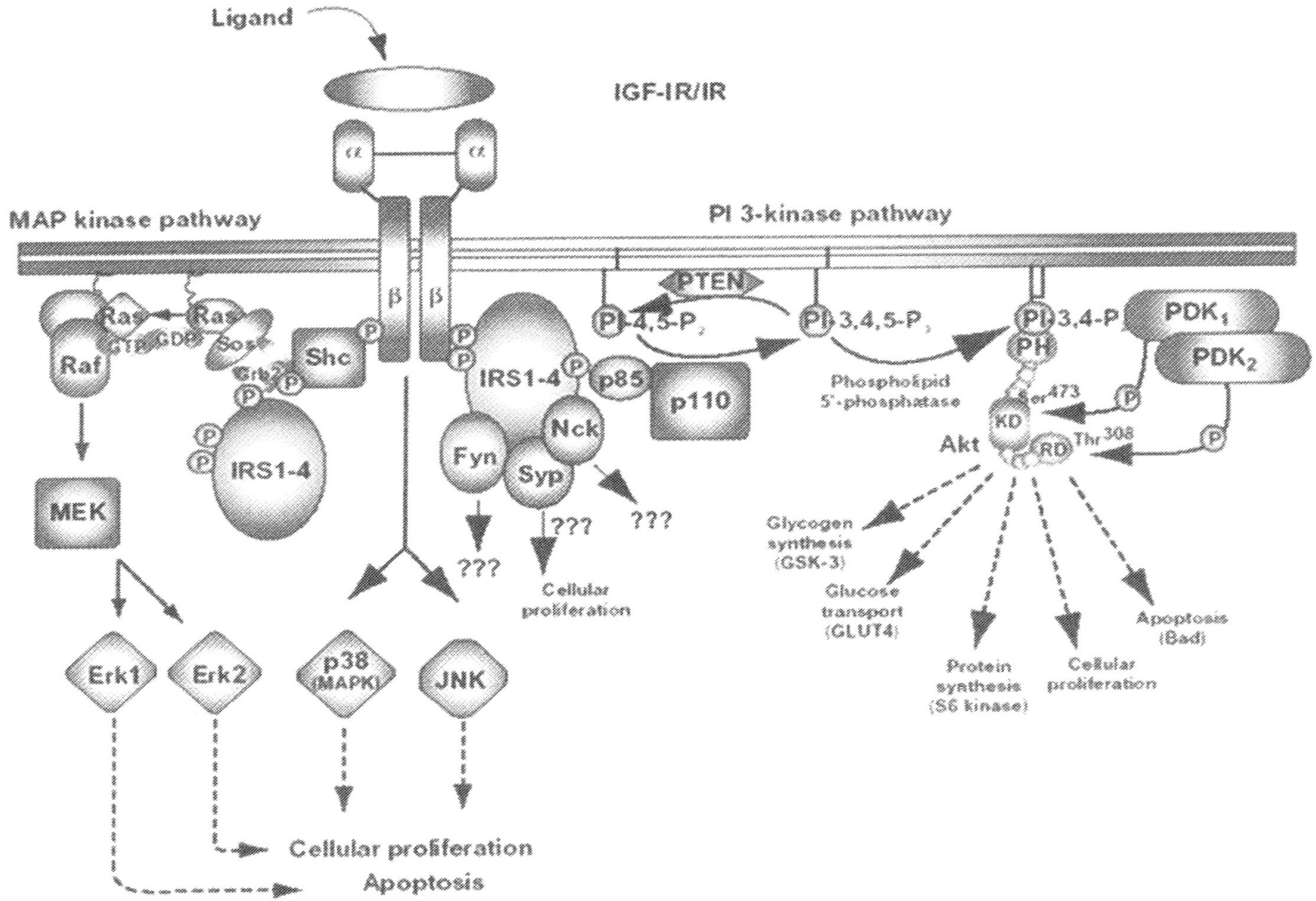

Fig. 2. Postreceptor mechanisms are shown in this figure and include a large array of substrates and enzymes for a large number of biological actions.

tyrosine kinase region is highly conserved between the IGF-IR and the IR, which share approx 84% similarity at the amino acid level. The juxtamembrane region contains motifs that are also found in the IR and bind to important intracellular substrates. The most divergent region between the two receptors is the cytoplasmic carboxyl-terminus domain.

3.1.1. IGF-IR Functioning

Like the IR, IGF-IRs are internalized following ligand binding and activation. Activation of the IGF-IR enhances the association of EHD1 with the IGF-IR and SNAP29, a synaptosome-associated protein. EHD1 belongs to a family of proteins that contain Eps15 homology (EH) domain-containing proteins and are involved in forming protein complexes that promote clathrin-coated vesicles and are involved in endocytosis. Overexpression of EHD1 in NIH-3T3 fibroblasts inhibits IGF-I signaling and supports the hypothesis that endocytosis may be a mechanism whereby the IGF-IR signal is abrogated *(60)*.

Genetic disruption of the IGF-IR results in fetal growth retardation and is invariably lethal at birth, or shortly thereafter *(44)*. More recently, a cre-lox approach was used to generate mice with a spectrum of IGF-I receptor deficiencies *(61)*. Mice exhibited reduced growth from the age of 3 wk and were markedly deficient in adipose tissue stores. Interestingly, this defect was primarily owing to decreased mitogenesis in adipose tissue. IGF-IR-deficient mice had lower numbers of adipocytes, but each adipocyte was larger. This finding somewhat modifies the current thinking about IGF-I and fat cell differentiation, and suggests that the IGF-I receptor may principally transmit a mitogenic or survival signal to preadipocytes.

3.1.2. Postreceptor Pathways

Binding of IGFs to the IGF-IR results in receptor autophosphorylation of the β-subunit and activation of its tyrosine kinase. After receptor activation, various IR substrates (IRS1-4) bind to the juxtamembrane region of the receptor, become phosphorylated on tyrosine residues, and thereby act as docking proteins for SH2 domain-containing substrates, including Grb2, Shc and PI3K *(57,62)*, as shown in Fig. 2. The adapter protein Grb2 links activated growth factor receptors with the Ras/Raf/mitogen-activated protein (MAP) kinase pathway.

MAP kinase, also termed extracellular signal regulated protein kinase (ERK), and PI3K are important regulators of cellular proliferation and survival. With respect to cell cycle control, IGF-I stabilizes cyclin D1 mRNA via a PI3K-dependent mechanism. Cyclin E is also increased by IGF-I *(63)*. In addition, IGF-I regulates certain cyclin-dependent kinase inhibitors, thereby regulating cyclin dependent kinase(cdk) activity. It has been shown that exposure to IGF-I decreases p27 protein levels at a posttranscriptional level and via a PI3K-dependent mechanism *(63,64)*. Activation of PI3K can inhibit translation of p27 mRNA, increase the degradation of p27 protein *(65)*, and inhibit p27 gene transcription through the forkhead transcription factor *(66)*. The degradation of p27 can also be increased by ERK. This may explain why an inhibitor of MEK, the upstream activator of ERK, blocks IGF-I-stimulated increases in cdk-2 activity *(67)*. The IGF-I mediated increases in cyclin D1, cyclin E, and cdk2 and the IGF-I-induced decrease in p27 can speed the transition from G1 to S in the cell cycle.

In contrast, p21, a cdk inhibitor is actually increased by IGFs in some cells *(63,67,68)*. This has been shown to occur through both ERK and PI3K pathways and may serve to induce differentiation of myocytes or to promote cell survival. IGF-I can also increase cyclin B and cdc2 levels, which is associated with increased entry into M phase and with increased ERK activity *(69)*.

Promotion of cell survival is one of the major effects of IGF-I. Several mechanisms for the molecular basis of IGF-I-mediated cell survival have been described, including PI3K/Akt, MAP kinase, and 14-3-3 proteins, all of which are associated with increases in the phosphorylation of BAD *(70)*. In neuronal cells, IGF-I promoted phosphorylation of the forkhead transcription factor via PI3K/Akt, thereby inhibiting apoptosis *(71)*. Furthermore, IGF-I promotes transcription of the antiapoptotic bcl-2 gene, by promoting cAMP response element binding site (CREB) phosphorylation via both the p38 stress-activated protein kinase and PI3K/Akt pathways *(72,73)*.

Activation of the PI3K pathway has also been shown to mediate certain IGF-I-induced changes in gene expression and differentiation *(74)*. The induction of uncoupling protein expression and glucose transport protein-4 expression in brown adipose cells by IGF-I are dependent on both PI3K and ERK, respectively *(75)*. The activation of the osteocalcin promoter in osteoblasts by IGF-I was blocked by an inhibitor of protein kinase C (PKC). Because certain PKC isotypes have recently been shown to be activated by PI3K, this effect of IGF-I could well be mediated through PI3K. More recently, IGF-I was found to stimulate muscle growth (ordered proliferation followed by differentiation) through the calcineurin signaling pathway, although other pathways, including PI3K, may be able to relay IGF-I signals *(51)*.

Protein tyrosine phosphatases can also mediate signaling through the IGF-IR. Interestingly, one tyrosine phosphatase, SHP-2, binds directly to the IGF-IR and enhances its signaling *(76)*. In contrast, other protein tyrosine phosphatases generally negatively regulate growth factor receptor signal transduction *(77)*. In addition, insulin-stimulated cell proliferation and survival, but not glycogen and protein synthesis, were recently found to depend on a PI3K-dependent activation of MAP kinase phosphatase-1 (MKP-1), thereby leading to dephosphorylation and inactivation of cJun-N-terminal kinase *(77b)*. It is not clear whether this result is relevant to IGF-I, because IGF-I activates c-Jun N-terminal kinase in MCF-7 cells in a growth stimulatory mechanism *(78)*.

Overexpression of IGF-IRs in NIH 3T3 cells has been shown to induce activation of Janus kinase (JAK)-1 and JAK-2. JAK-1 was recruited to the IGF-IR and was able to phosphorylate IRS-1 *(79)*. Interestingly, a more recent study in cardiomyocytes showed that IGF-I can activate JAK-1 and induce phosphorylation of Stat-1 and Stat-2 on both tyrosine and serine residues. The authors implied that activation of the JAK-STAT pathway played a role in IGF-I-stimulated growth and function of cardiomyocytes *(80)*.

3.2. Insulin Receptor Splicing Variants

The IR closely resembles the IGF-IR but is generally considered to have much lower affinities for the IGFs, especially IGF-I, than for insulin. Indeed, IGF-I binds the IR with an affinity 100- to 1000-fold lower than that for insulin. Interestingly, the affinity of the IR for IGF-II is generally much higher, being only 10- to 100-fold lower than that for insulin *(57)*. Indeed there are a number of examples where the function of IGF-II may be predominantly mediated via the IR. Dwarf mice with a disruption in the IGFII gene are more growth retarded than mice in which the IGFR gene has been deleted, suggesting that another receptor must be involved. This receptor was identified as the IR in further genetic analyses *(44,81)*. IGF-II can also stimulate the IR in fibroblasts that are deficient in IGF-IRs *(82)*.

The IR exists in two isoforms as a result of alternative splicing of exon II, which encodes 12 amino acids. In isoform A (IR-A), exon 11 is deleted, whereas IR-B includes exon 11 *(82)*. IR-A is expressed in the central nervous system, hemopoeitic cells, fetal cells and in certain cancers *(83)*. IR-B, however, is localized specifically in insulin-sensitive, highly metabolic tissues, such as adipose tissue, muscle, and liver *(84)*. The two isoforms have slightly altered binding affinities for insulin and exhibit different levels of responses. Most interestingly, IGF-II binds to IR-A with high affinity, but it does not bind to the IR-B isoform. IGF-II activates IR-A and effectively stimulates the Akt/Glycogen synthase kinase 3 (GSK3) pathway, as well as promotes progression from the G0/G1 to the S and G2/M phases of the cell cycle. Thus, IGF-II may exert some of its mitogenic effects via the IR as well as through the IGF-IR. This feature is of particular importance because IGF-II is frequently expressed in cancer cells and can act as an autocrine/paracrine growth factor; some of these cancers, breast cancers in particular, express significant levels of IRs *(85)*. The roles of IGF proteins in cancer are discussed further in Chapters 6 and 18.

3.3. Mannose-6-Phosphate/IGF-II Receptor

This receptor is primarily involved in targeting newly synthesized lysosomal enzymes from the Golgi to lysosomes and in delivering extracellular lysosomal enzymes to the appropriate cellular compartment. This receptor binds mannose-6 phosphate (M6P) residues of these enzymes as well as those on IGFs (not insulin). Its affinity for IGF-II is much greater than for IGF-I *(86)*, and the receptor is considered to be an important pathway for the internalization and degradation of IGF-II. Indeed, M6P/IGF-II receptor gene-deleted mice are larger than controls *(87)*. Furthermore, these results support the idea that this receptor does not have any major signaling functions in vivo. On the other hand, the M6P/IGF-II receptor may play a significant role as a tumor suppressor, as it initiates the degradation of IGF-II and activates transforming growth factor (TGF)-β1 from a precursor molecule *(88)*. Interestingly, microsatellite instability in the M6P/IGF-II receptor gene has been described in various cancers, including stomach, colon, and endometrium *(89)*.

4. INSULIN-LIKE GROWTH FACTOR BINDING PROTEINS

To date, six IGFBPs have been described that have high affinity for the IGFs *(90,91)*. These proteins are characterized by their well-conserved amino and carboxyl terminal domains that contain several highly conserved cysteine residues. IGFBPs are found in the circulation and are also expressed at the local tissue level. In the circulation, IGFBPs act as "transport proteins" for the IGFs, but at the local level they act as modulators of IGF activity *(90)*. In the circulation, the major proportion of IGF is bound to a 150 kD complex that includes IGFBP-3 and ALS, which protects the IGFs from proteases and prolongs their circulating half-life *(91)*. IGFBPs may also function as carrier proteins, since other IGFBPs may be part of a 50-kDa circulating complex that facilitates the transfer of IGFs from the circulation to target cells.

At the target cell level, the IGFBPs have multiple roles; some IGFBPs modulate the effects of the IGFs and others act independently from the IGFs and the IGF-IR *(92)*.

Inhibition of IGF-I action depends on the ability of IGFBPs to prevent the interaction of IGFs with the IGF-IR *(93,94)*. However, the binding affinities of IGFBPs are altered by various modifications, including phosphorylation, partial proteolysis, and attachment to the cell surface or extracellular matrix (ECM). For example, dephosphorylation of IGFBP-1 lowers its affinity for IGFs. Attachment of IGFBP-3 to the cell surface or IGFBP-5 to the ECM lowers their respective affinities for IGFs. All of these actions are proposed to enhance the delivery of IGFs to the IGF-IR.

IGF-independent actions have been reported for IGFBP-1. When the RGD sequence was prevented from interacting with the integrin $\alpha5\beta1$ receptor, IGFBP-1 was prevented from stimulating cell migration *(95)*. In breast cancer cells, cell surface binding of IGFBP-1 to integrin resulted in dephosphorylation of FAK, detachment from the ECM, and cellular apoptosis *(96)*.

It has been suggested that IGF-independent actions of IGFBP-3 inhibit cellular proliferation via the type V TGF-β receptor, but not through Smad signaling *(97)* or the type II TGF-β receptor *(98)*. However, there is some question as to whether the latter effect is truly IGF-independent. A proapoptotic action of IGFBP-3 was also reported to be independent of IGF and p53 *(99)*. This is somewhat surprising, because p53 has been shown to induce IGFBP-3 *(100)*. Although it is not entirely clear if these effects are totally independent of IGF, IGFBP-3 has been shown to increase the bax/bcl-2 ratio in p53-deficient breast cancer cells and to promote apoptosis induced by ionizing radiation *(101)*. Other proapoptotic actions of IGFBP-3 have been reported *(102,103)*. A number of potential IGF-independent survival effects of IGFBP-4 and IGFBP-5 have been reported; however, the mechanisms underlying these effects are not known *(102)*. Finally, IGFBP-3 and IGFBP-5 are translocated into the nucleus via the importin 5 subunit *(104,105)*. The consequences of these actions are not known. Taken together, these results suggest that multiple novel and IGF-I-independent actions of IGFBPs can regulate growth and survival.

5. INSULIN VS IGF ACTION

Insulin classically controls carbohydrate, lipid, and protein metabolism in mammals, whereas the IGFs promote cell growth, survival, and differentiation. Because their cognate receptors are so similar in structure and function and share many common signaling pathways, a vexing question remains: do differences in receptor distribution or post-receptor signaling determine the specificity of insulin vs IGF actions in the whole animal *(106)*? A number of intracellular substrate molecules have been identified that mediate specific effects of one or the other of these two receptors. pp120, a plasma membrane glycoprotein, plays a specific role in the actions of insulin. pp120 is a substrate of the IR that becomes tyrosine phosphorylated upon activation of the receptor, and is involved in the endocytosis of the insulin/IR complex *(107)*. Apparently, pp120-induced internalization of the IR complex reduces the cellular mitogenic response to insulin in certain cells. Conversely, in the absence of pp120, mitogenic responses to insulin may be artificially enhanced *(108)*. The tyrosine phosphorylation of pp120 is essential for receptor endocytosis, as mutant forms of pp120 failed to become phosphorylated and did not induce endocytosis of the IR. The activated IR is capable of phosphorylating tyrosine residues on pp120, whereas the IGF-IR is not. Thus, pp120 appears to be an important endogenous substrate that is specific for the IR.

To investigate the signaling specificity of the IR and IGF-IR, Siddle and coworkers performed a number of elegant studies where they generated various chimeric receptors *(109)*. These chimeras consisted of an extracellular portion of the neurotrophin receptor TrkC fused to the intracellular portion of either the IR or IGF-IR. Constructs encoding these chimeric receptors were stably transfected into 3T3-L1 adipocytes. Because these cells do not express endogenous TrkC receptors, exposing cells to neurotrophin-3 specifically activated the intracellular tyrosine kinase domain of each receptor. This approach has the advantage of eliminating potential complications from regulation of endogenous receptors. These studies revealed that activation of the TrkC-IR tyrosine kinase resulted in higher level of IRS-1 phosphorylation, a significantly greater association of IRS-1 with PI3K, and an increase in translocation of glucose transport protein-4, as compared with the cells expressing the TrkC–IGF–IR chimera. In contrast, cells expressing the TrkC–IGF–IR chimera displayed a higher level of Shc phosphorylation, increased association of Shc with Grb2, and increased activation of ERK, as compared to cells expressing TrkC–IR. Thus, the IR was found to have a greater role in stimulating metabolic effects in these cells, whereas the IGF-IR was found to have a greater effect on mitogenic pathways, as has been previously postulated *(110)*. Similarly, Accili and coworkers demonstrated that the IR more effectively stimulates glycogen synthesis in hepatocytes and 3T3-L1 adipocytes than does the IGF-IR *(111)*. The precise molecular basis for the different functional specificities between the IR and IGF-IR remains speculative, although a number of possibilities have been suggested. One such possibility is that the divergent carboxyl terminal domains of these two receptors may interact with different substrates. Another possibility is the differences in endocytosis and subsequent cellular trafficking of the IR and IGF-IR may result in specific cellular localizations of the two receptor subtypes.

5.1. Differentiation of Insulin and IGF Actions by cDNA Microarray Analysis

To further define the differential effects of insulin and IGF-I receptors, NIH-3T3 fibroblasts were stably transfected with cDNAs encoding either the IR or the IGF-IR. Cells overexpressing either the IR or the IGF-IR and corresponding control cells were stimulated with insulin or IGF-I, respectively. mRNA was isolated from these cells 90 min later and control vs insulin- or IGF-I-treated samples were subjected to microarray analysis using mouse arrays with 3899 genes. Fibroblasts generally exhibit proliferative responses, but little in the way of metabolic responses. Thus, if the IR and IGF-IR signaling pathways are truly separate, differential gene expression should be exhibited. Expression levels of 30 genes were significantly increased in IGF-IR-overexpressing cells treated with IGF-I that were not induced in response to insulin stimulation of the IR-overexpressing cells (Table 1). Conversely, insulin specifically induced the expression of 10 genes that were not induced by IGF-I. Most of the genes induced by IGF-I corresponded to ones previously known to be involved in mitogenesis and/or differentiation. The conclusion from these studies was that IGF-I is a more potent activator of the mitogenic pathway than is insulin in mouse fibroblast NIH-3T3 cells *(112)*.

Table 1
Genes Upregulated by IGF-I and Not by Insulin

	IGF-1	*Insulin*
Mitogenesis and differentiation		
IL-3 receptor, α-chain	5.32	1.23
Colony-stimulating factor, macrophage	4.12	1.32
Glial cell line-derived neurotrophic factor	3.96	0.80
Integrin-5 (fibronectin receptor)	3.55	0.94
Early growth response-1	3.65	0.58
Jun oncogene	3.01	1.11
Twist gene	2.95	1.54
Forkhead homolog 14	2.91	1.08
Wee 1-like protein kinase	2.75	1.95
IGF binding protein 10	2.48	1.48
SRY box-containing gene 2	2.39	0.59
IL-4 receptor α	2.30	0.80
DNA-binding protein A	2.29	1.65
MAK16	2.27	1.70
Nerve growth factor-induced clone A-binding protein 2	2.31	1.25
Mothers against decapetalegic-5	2.24	1.49
Early development regulator	2.22	1.67
Ets variant gene 6 (*TEL* oncogene)	2.21	0.97
Apoptosis		
T-cell death-associated gene 51	9.00	1.52
Fas-binding protein (Daxx)	5.99	1.55
Cellular processes		
Variant histone H3.3	3.30	1.39
Kinesin heavy-chain member 1A	2.83	0.67
Chromatin nonhistone high-mobility group protein	2.64	1.15
Eukaryote release factor 1	2.34	1.19
Aspartate-glutamate-alanine-aspartate (DEAD) box polypeptide 5	2.22	1.24
Splicing factor, arginine/serine 3	2.41	1.69
Metabolism		
Gibbon ape leukemia virus receptor-1	4.88	1.20
Glycerol phosphate dehydrogenase 1, mitochondrial	2.74	0.91
Others		
Nuclear factor erythroid-derived 2, -like 2	2.90	0.86
Immediate early protein Gly96	2.46	1.13

Numbers represent the fold increase (or decrease) above unity.

6. EVOLUTIONARY ASPECTS OF INSULIN AND IGF-I SIGNALING

An insulin/IGF-I signaling cascade has been identified in both *Caenorhabditis elegans* and *Drosophila melanogaster (113,114)*, as shown in Fig. 3. Mutations of the IR/IGF-IR ortholog Daf-2 in *C. elegans* give rise to dauer larvae, which have a prolonged lifespan and reduced metabolic activity. This mutation enhances survival during periods of food deprivation and other environmental stresses. Similar effects are exhib-

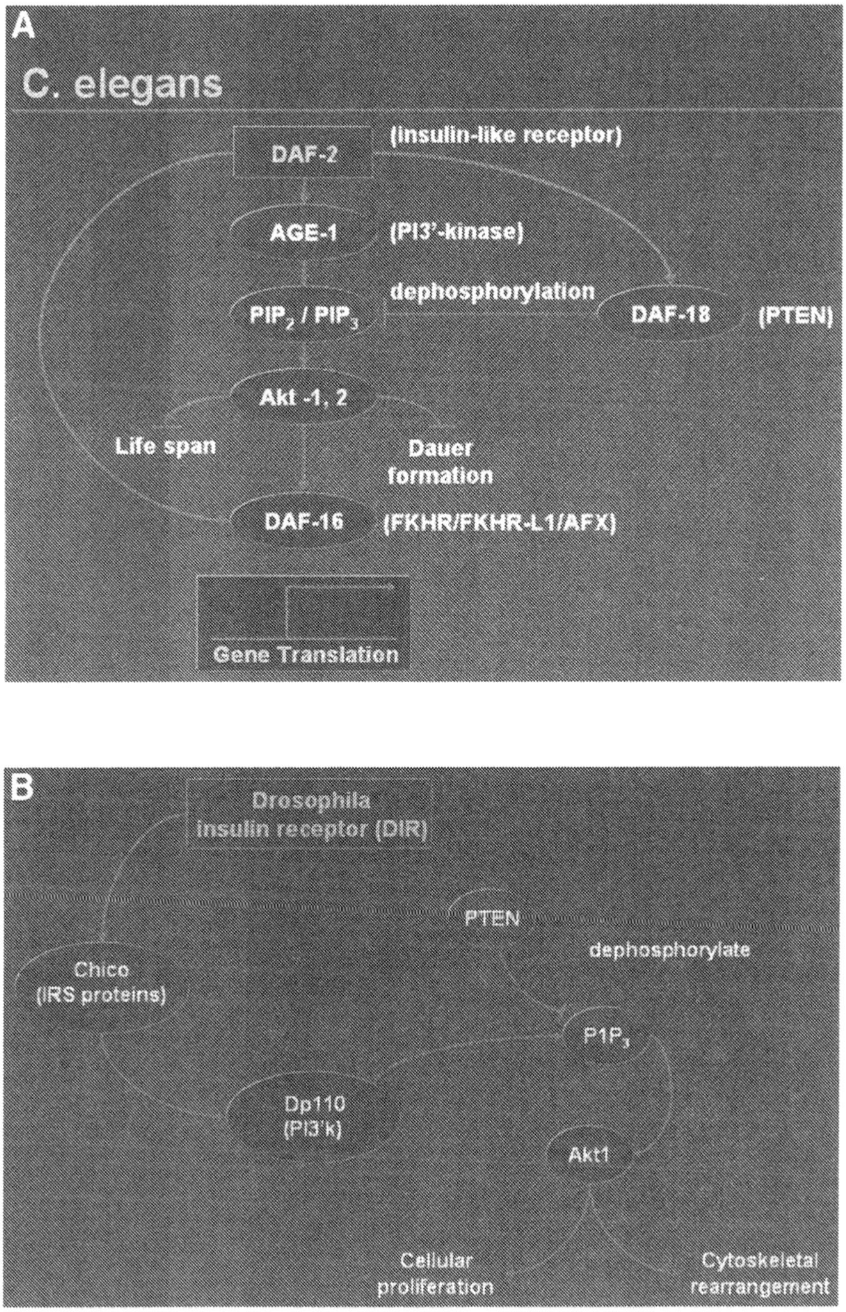

Fig. 3. Insulin/IGF-related system in *C. elegans* (**A**) and *Drosophila melanogaster* (**B**).

ited with mutations of PI3K and Akt *(114,115)*. Mutations of other substrates and signaling proteins, include Daf-16 (a homolog of the mammalian FOXO forkhead transcription factors) and Daf-19 (a homolog of the mammalian phosphoinositide phosphatase (PTEN), which inhibits P13K) can negate the effect of the Daf-2 mutation *(116,117)*. These studies have shed new light on the role of the insulin/IGF signaling pathways in more primitive organisms. Furthermore, they suggest an intriguing mechanism whereby enhanced caloric intake may shorten lifespan by increasing insulin/IGF signaling and, conversely, lifespan may be lengthened by caloric restriction. This hypothesis has further been substantiated in GH receptor knockout mice, which exhibit reduced levels of circulating IGF-I and lifespans that are 65% longer than normal *(118)*.

In *D. melanogaster*, the IR homolog (DIR) differs substantially from the mammalian IR and IGF-IR, as DIR itself binds directly to many of its downstream signaling substrates via its carboxyl-terminal extension *(119)*. In contrast, the mammalian IR and IGF-IR use the IRS family of docking proteins to link insulin and IGF-I signaling to downstream substrate molecules. The *Drosophila* homolog of the IRS family of molecules, known as CHICO, has been shown to play an important role in cell proliferation and overall body growth *(120)*.

7. SUMMARY AND CONCLUSIONS

This brief introductory chapter has outlined the essential components of the IGF system and has described some newer concepts in the insulin/IGF signaling pathways. These include various evolutionary aspects, divergences in the two signaling pathways, and effects on gene expression. Many of these aspects are relevant to the subsequent chapters, including those related to nutrition, therapeutic aspects of IGF-I and insulin, and even cancer.

REFERENCES

1. Clemmons DR. Use of mutagenesis to probe IGF-binding protein structure/function relationships. Endocr Rev 2001;22:800–817.
2. Le Roith D, Bondy C, Yakar S, Liu JL, Butler A. The somatomedin hypothesis: 2001. Endocr Rev 2001;22:53–74.
3. Van Obberghen E, Baron V, Delahaye L, et al. Surfing the insulin signaling web. Eur J Clin Invest 2001;31:966–977.
4. Yakar S, Liu JL, Stannard B, et al. Normal growth and development in the absence of hepatic insulin-like growth factor I. Proc Natl Acad Sci USA 1999;96:7324–7329.
5. Bichell DP, Kikuchi K, Rotwein P. Growth hormone rapidly activates insulin-like growth factor I gene transcription in vivo. Mol Endocrinol 1992;6:1899–1908.
6. Davey HW, Xie T, McLachlan MJ, Wilkins RJ, Waxman DJ, Grattan DR. STAT5b is required for GH-induced liver IGF-I gene expression. Endocrinology 2001;142:3836–3841.
7. Gronowski AM, Zhong Z, Wen Z, Thomas MJ, Darnell JE, Jr., Rotwein P. In vivo growth hormone treatment rapidly stimulates the tyrosine phosphorylation and activation of Stat3. Mol Endocrinol 1995;9:171–177.
8. Herrington J, Smit LS, Schwartz J, Carter-Su C. The role of STAT proteins in growth hormone signaling. Oncogene 2000;19:2585–2597.
9. Teglund S, McKay C, Schuetz E, et al. Stat5a and Stat5b proteins have essential and nonessential, or redundant, roles in cytokine responses. Cell 1998;93:841–850.
10. Woefle J, Chia DJ, Rotwein P. Mechanism of growth hormone (GH) action. Identification of conserved stat5 binding sites that mediate GH-induced insulin-like growth factor-I gene activation. J Biol Chem 2003;278:51261–51266.
11. Kaytor EN, Zhu JL, Pao CI, Phillips LS. Physiological concentrations of insulin promote binding of nuclear proteins to the insulin-like growth factor I gene. Endocrinology 2001;142:1041–1049.
12. Kaytor EN, Zhu JL, Pao CI, Phillips LS. Insulin-responsive nuclear proteins facilitate Sp1 interactions with the insulin-like growth factor-I gene. J Biol Chem 2001;276:36896–6901.

13. Hayden JM, Straus DS. IGF-I and serine protease inhibitor 2.1 nuclear transcript abundance in rat liver during protein restriction. J Endocrinol 1995;145:397–407.
14. Zhang J, Chrysis D, Underwood LE. Reduction of hepatic insulin-like growth factor I (IGF-I) messenger ribonucleic acid (mRNA) during fasting is associated with diminished splicing of IGF-I premRNA and decreased stability of cytoplasmic IGF-I mRNA. Endocrinology 1998;139:4523–4530.
15. Goya L, de la Puente A, Ramos S, Martin MA, Escriva F, Pascual-Leone AM. Regulation of insulinlike growth factor-I and -II by glucose in primary cultures of fetal rat hepatocytes. J Biol Chem 1999;274:24633–24640.
16. Baker J, Hardy MP, Zhou J, et al. Effects of an Igf1 gene null mutation on mouse reproduction. Mol Endocrinol 1996;10:903–918.
17. Murphy LJ, Bell GI, Duckworth ML, Friesen HG. Identification, characterization, and regulation of a rat complementary deoxyribonucleic acid which encodes insulin-like growth factor-I. Endocrinology 1987;121:684–691.
18. Peter MA, Winterhalter KH, Boni-Schnetzler M, Froesch ER, Zapf J. Regulation of insulin-like growth factor-I (IGF-I) and IGF-binding proteins by growth hormone in rat white adipose tissue. Endocrinology 1993;133:2624–2631.
19. Zhou J, Kumar TR, Matzuk MM, Bondy C. Insulin-like growth factor I regulates gonadotropin responsiveness in the murine ovary. Mol Endocrinol 1997;11:1924–1933.
20. Doglio A, Dani C, Fredrikson G, Grimaldi P, Ailhaud G. Acute regulation of insulin-like growth factor-I gene expression by growth hormone during adipose cell differentiation. Embo J 1987;6:4011–4016.
21. Kamai Y, Mikawa S, Endo K, Sakai H, Komano T. Regulation of insulin-like growth factor-I expression in mouse preadipocyte Ob1771 cells. J Biol Chem 1996;271:9883–9886.
22. Sadowski CL, Wheeler TT, Wang LH, Sadowski HB. GH regulation of IGF-I and suppressor of cytokine signaling gene expression in C2C12 skeletal muscle cells. Endocrinology 2001;142:3890–3900.
23. Ye P, Umayahara Y, Ritter D, et al. Regulation of insulin-like growth factor I (IGF-I) gene expression in brain of transgenic mice expressing an IGF-I-luciferase fusion gene. Endocrinology 1997;138:5466–5475.
24. Bichell DP, Rotwein P, McCarthy TL. Prostaglandin E2 rapidly stimulates insulin-like growth factor-I gene expression in primary rat osteoblast cultures: evidence for transcriptional control. Endocrinology 1993;133:1020–1028.
25. Billiard J, Umayahara Y, Wiren K, Centrella M, McCarthy TL, Rotwein P. Regulated nuclear-cytoplasmic localization of CCAAT/enhancer-binding protein delta in osteoblasts. J Biol Chem 2001;276:15354–15361.
26. Billiard J, Grewal SS, Lukaesko L, Stork PJ, Rotwein P. Hormonal control of insulin-like growth factor I gene transcription in human osteoblasts: dual actions of cAMP-dependent protein kinase on CCAAT/enhancer-binding protein delta. J Biol Chem 2001;276:31238–31246.
27. Miyakoshi N, Kasukawa Y, Linkhart TA, Baylink DJ, Mohan S. Evidence that anabolic effects of PTH on bone require IGF-I in growing mice. Endocrinology 2001;142:4349–4356.
28. Edwall D, Prisell PT, Levinovitz A, Jennische E, Norstedt G. Expression of insulin-like growth factor I messenger ribonucleic acid in regenerating bone after fracture: influence of indomethacin. J Bone Miner Res 1992;7:207–213.
29. Ernst M, Rodan GA. Estradiol regulation of insulin-like growth factor-I expression in osteoblastic cells: evidence for transcriptional control. Mol Endocrinol 1991;5:1081–1089.
30. McCarthy TL, Ji C, Shu H, et al. 17beta-estradiol potently suppresses cAMP-induced insulin-like growth factor-I gene activation in primary rat osteoblast cultures. J Biol Chem 1997;272: 18132–18139.
31. Fournier B, Gutzwiller S, Dittmar T, Matthias G, Steenbergh P, Matthias P. Estrogen receptor (ER)-alpha, but not ER-beta, mediates regulation of the insulin-like growth factor I gene by antiestrogens. J Biol Chem 2001;276:35444–35449.
32. Hofbauer LC, Rafferzeder M, Janssen OE, Gartner R. Insulin-like growth factor I messenger ribonucleic acid expression in porcine thyroid follicles is regulated by thyrotropin and iodine. Eur J Endocrinol 1995;132:605–610.

33. Clement S, Refetoff S, Robaye B, Dumont JE, Schurmans S. Low TSH requirement and goiter in transgenic mice overexpressing IGF-I and IGF-Ir receptor in the thyroid gland. Endocrinology 2001;142:5131–5139.
34. Hatey F, Langlois I, Mulsant P, Bonnet A, Benne F, Gasser F. Gonadotropins induce accumulation of insulin-like growth factor I mRNA in pig granulosa cells in vitro. Mol Cell Endocrinol 1992;86:205–211.
35. Hernandez ER, Roberts CT, Jr., LeRoith D, Adashi EY. Rat ovarian insulin-like growth factor I (IGF-I) gene expression is granulosa cell-selective: 5'-untranslated mRNA variant representation and hormonal regulation. Endocrinology 1989;125:572–574.
36. Murphy LJ, Friesen HG. Differential effects of estrogen and growth hormone on uterine and hepatic insulin-like growth factor I gene expression in the ovariectomized hypophysectomized rat. Endocrinology 1988;122:325–332.
37. Brink M, Chrast J, Price SR, Mitch WE, Delafontaine P. Angiotensin II stimulates gene expression of cardiac insulin-like growth factor I and its receptor through effects on blood pressure and food intake. Hypertension 1999;34:1053–1059.
38. Mulroney SE, Lumpkin MD, Roberts CT, Jr., LeRoith D, Haramati A. Effect of a growth hormone-releasing factor antagonist on compensatory renal growth, insulin-like growth factor-I (IGF-I), and IGF-I receptor gene expression after unilateral nephrectomy in immature rats. Endocrinology 1992;130:2697–2702.
39. Florini JR, Ewton DZ, Coolican SA. Growth hormone and the insulin-like growth factor system in myogenesis. Endocr Rev 1996;17:481–517.
40. Shoba L, An MR, Frank SJ, Lowe WL, Jr. Developmental regulation of insulin-like growth factor-I and growth hormone receptor gene expression. Mol Cell Endocrinol 1999;152:125–136.
41. Kikuchi K, Bichell DP, Rotwein P. Chromatin changes accompany the developmental activation of insulin- like growth factor I gene transcription. J Biol Chem 1992;267:21505–21511.
42. Lee YH, Sauer B, Gonzalez FJ. Laron dwarfism and non-insulin-dependent diabetes mellitus in the Hnf- 1alpha knockout mouse. Mol Cell Biol 1998;18:3059–3068.
43. Baker J, Liu JP, Robertson EJ, Efstratiadis A. Role of insulin-like growth factors in embryonic and postnatal growth. Cell 1993;75:73–82.
44. Liu JP, Baker J, Perkins AS, Robertson EJ, Efstratiadis A. Mice carrying null mutations of the genes encoding insulin-like growth factor I (Igf-1) and type 1 IGF receptor (Igf1r). Cell 1993;75:59–72.
45. Liu JL, LeRoith D. Insulin-like growth factor I is essential for postnatal growth in response to growth hormone. Endocrinology 1999;140:5178–5184.
46. Wang J, Zhou J, Powell-Braxton L, Bondy C. Effects of Igf1 gene deletion on postnatal growth patterns. Endocrinology 1999;140:3391–3394.
47. Beck KD, Powell-Braxton L, Widmer HR, Valverde J, Hefti F. Igf1 gene disruption results in reduced brain size, CNS hypomyelination, and loss of hippocampal granule and striatal parvalbumin-containing neurons. Neuron 1995;14:717–730.
48. Yakar S, Rosen CJ, Beamer WG, et al. Circulating levels of IGF-1 directly regulate bone growth and density. J Clin Invest 2002;110:771–781.
49. Li D, Kubo T, Kim H, Shimasaki S, Erickson GF. Endogenous insulin-like growth factor-I is obligatory for stimulation of rat inhibin alpha-subunit expression by follicle-stimulating hormone. Biol Reprod 1998;58:219–225.
50. Zhao G, Monier-Faugere MC, Langub MC, et al. Targeted overexpression of insulin-like growth factor I to osteoblasts of transgenic mice: increased trabecular bone volume without increased osteoblast proliferation. Endocrinology 2000;141:2674–2682.
51. Musaro A, McCullagh K, Paul A, et al. Localized Igf-1 transgene expression sustains hypertrophy and regeneration in senescent skeletal muscle. Nat Genet 2001;27:195–200.
52. DiGiovanni J, Bol DK, Wilker E, et al. Constitutive expression of insulin-like growth factor-1 in epidermal basal cells of transgenic mice leads to spontaneous tumor promotion. Cancer Res 2000;60:1561–1570.
53. Naranjo WM, Yakar S, Sanchez-Gomez M, Perez AU, Setser J, D LE. Protein calorie restriction affects nonhepatic IGF-I production and the lymphoid system: studies using the liver-specific IGF-I gene-deleted mouse model. Endocrinology 2002;143:2233–2241.

54. Lu F, Han VK, Milne WK, et al. Regulation of insulin-like growth factor-II gene expression in the ovine fetal adrenal gland by adrenocorticotropic hormone and cortisol. Endocrinology 1994;134:2628–2635.
55. Stewart CE, Rotwein P. Growth, differentiation, and survival: multiple physiological functions for insulin-like growth factors. Physiol Rev 1996;76:1005–1026.
56. Daughaday WH, Emanuele MA, Brooks MH, Barbato AL, Kapadia M, Rotwein P. Synthesis and secretion of insulin-like growth factor II by a leiomyosarcoma with associated hypoglycemia. N Engl J Med 1988;319:1434–1440.
57. LeRoith D, Werner H, Beitner-Johnson D, Roberts CT, Jr. Molecular and cellular aspects of the insulin-like growth factor I receptor. Endocr Rev 1995;16:143–163.
58. Ullrich A, Bell JR, Chen EY, et al. Human insulin receptor and its relationship to the tyrosine kinase family of oncogenes. Nature 1985;313:756–761.
59. Ullrich A, Gray A, Tam AW, et al. Insulin-like growth factor I receptor primary structure: comparison with insulin receptor suggests structural determinants that define functional specificity. EMBO J 1986;5:2503–2512.
60. Rotem-Yehudar R, Galperin E, Horowitz M. Association of insulin-like growth factor 1 receptor with ehd1 and snap29. J Biol Chem 2001;276:33054–33060.
61. Holzenberger M, Hamard G, Zaoui R, et al. Experimental IGF-I receptor deficiency generates a sexually dimorphic pattern of organ-specific growth deficits in mice, affecting fat tissue in particular. Endocrinology 2001;142:4469–4478.
62. De Meyts P, Wallach B, Christoffersen CT, et al. The insulin-like growth factor-I receptor. Structure, ligand-binding mechanism and signal transduction. Horm Res 1994;42:152–169.
63. Dupont J, Karas M, LeRoith D. The potentiation of estrogen on insulin-like growth factor I action in MCF-7 human breast cancer cells includes cell cycle components. J Biol Chem 2000;275:35893–35901.
64. Chakravarthy MV, Abraha TW, Schwartz RJ, Fiorotto ML, Booth FW. Insulin-like growth factor-I extends in vitro replicative life span of skeletal muscle satellite cells by enhancing G1/S cell cycle progression via the activation of phosphatidylinositol 3'-kinase/Akt signaling pathway. J Biol Chem 2000;275:35942–35952.
65. Takuwa N, Takuwa Y. Ras activity late in G1 phase required for p27kip1 downregulation, passage through the restriction point, and entry into S phase in growth factor-stimulated NIH 3T3 fibroblasts. Mol Cell Biol 1997;17:5348–5358.
66. Dijkers PF, Medema RH, Pals C, et al. Forkhead transcription factor FKHR-L1 modulates cytokine-dependent transcriptional regulation of p27(KIP1). Mol Cell Biol 2000;20:9138–9148.
67. Zhang W, Lee JC, Kumar S, Gowen M. ERK pathway mediates the activation of Cdk2 in IGF-1-induced proliferation of human osteosarcoma MG-63 cells. J Bone Miner Res 1999;14:528–535.
68. Lawlor MA, Rotwein P. Insulin-like growth factor-mediated muscle cell survival: central roles for Akt and cyclin-dependent kinase inhibitor p21. Mol Cell Biol 2000;20:8983–8995.
69. Reiss K, Valentinis B, Tu X, Xu SQ, Baserga R. Molecular markers of IGF-I-mediated mitogenesis. Exp Cell Res 1998;242:361–372.
70. Peruzzi F, Prisco M, Dews M, et al. Multiple signaling pathways of the insulin-like growth factor 1 receptor in protection from apoptosis. Mol Cell Biol 1999;19:7203–7215.
71. Zheng WH, Kar S, Quirion R. Insulin-like growth factor-1-induced phosphorylation of the forkhead family transcription factor FKHRL1 is mediated by Akt kinase in PC12 cells. J Biol Chem 2000;275:39152–39158.
72. Pugazhenthi S, Miller E, Sable C, et al. Insulin-like growth factor-I induces bcl-2 promoter through the transcription factor cAMP-response element-binding protein. J Biol Chem 1999;274:27529–27535.
73. Pugazhenthi S, Nesterova A, Sable C, et al. Akt/protein kinase B up-regulates Bcl-2 expression through cAMP- response element-binding protein. J Biol Chem 2000;275:10761–10766.
74. Singleton JR, Feldman EL. Insulin-like growth factor-I in muscle metabolism and myotherapies. Neurobiol Dis 2001;8:541–554.
75. Valverde AM, Navarro P, Teruel T, Conejo R, Benito M, Lorenzo M. Insulin and insulin-like growth factor I up-regulate GLUT4 gene expression in fetal brown adipocytes, in a phosphoinositide 3-kinase- dependent manner. Biochem J 1999;337:397–405.
76. Xiao S, Rose DW, Sasaoka T, et al. Syp (SH-PTP2) is a positive mediator of growth factor-stimulated mitogenic signal transduction. J Biol Chem 1994;269:21244–21248.

77. Tonks NK, Neel BG. Combinatorial control of the specificity of protein tyrosine phosphatases. Curr Opin Cell Biol 2001;13:182–195.
77b. Desbois-Mouthon C, Cadoret A, Eggelpoel M-J B-V, et al. Insulin-mediated cell proliferation and survival involve inhibition of C-Jun N-terminal kinases through a phosphatidyl inositol 3-kinase and mitogen-actuated protein kinase phosphatase-1-dependent pathway. Endocrinol 2000;141:922–931.
78. Monno S, Newman MV, Cook M, Lowe WL, Jr. Insulin-like growth factor I activates c-Jun N-terminal kinase in MCF-7 breast cancer cells. Endocrinology 2000;141:544–550.
79. Esposito DL, Blakesley VA, Koval AP, Scrimgeour AG, LeRoith D. Tyrosine residues in the C-terminal domain of the insulin-like growth factor-I receptor mediate mitogenic and tumorigenic signals. Endocrinology 1997;138:2979–2988.
80. Takahashi T, Fukuda K, Pan J, et al. Characterization of insulin-like growth factor-1-induced activation of the JAK/STAT pathway in rat cardiomyocytes. Circ Res 1999;85:884–891.
81. Louvi A, Accili D, Efstratiadis A. Growth-promoting interaction of IGF-II with the insulin receptor during mouse embryonic development. Dev Biol 1997;189:33–48.
82. Morrione A, Valentinis B, Xu SQ, et al. Insulin-like growth factor II stimulates cell proliferation through the insulin receptor. Proc Natl Acad Sci USA 1997;94:3777–3782.
83. Frasca F, Pandini G, Scalia P, et al. Insulin receptor isoform A, a newly recognized, high-affinity insulin- like growth factor II receptor in fetal and cancer cells. Mol Cell Biol 1999;19:3278–3288.
84. Mosthaf L, Grako K, Dull TJ, Coussens L, Ullrich A, McClain DA. Functionally distinct insulin receptors generated by tissue-specific alternative splicing. EMBO J 1990;9:2409–2413.
85. Sciacca L, Costantino A, Pandini G, et al. Insulin receptor activation by IGF-II in breast cancers: evidence for a new autocrine/paracrine mechanism. Oncogene 1999;18:2471–2479.
86. Rechler MM, Nissley SP. The nature and regulation of the receptors for insulin-like growth factors. Annu Rev Physiol 1985;47:425–442.
87. Wang ZQ, Fung MR, Barlow DP, Wagner EF. Regulation of embryonic growth and lysosomal targeting by the imprinted Igf2/Mpr gene. Nature 1994;372:464–467.
88. Kovacina KS, Steele-Perkins G, Purchio AF, et al. Interactions of recombinant and platelet transforming growth factor- beta 1 precursor with the insulin-like growth factor II/mannose 6- phosphate receptor. Biochem Biophys Res Commun 1989;160:393–403.
89. Souza RF, Appel R, Yin J, et al. Microsatellite instability in the insulin-like growth factor II receptor gene in gastrointestinal tumours. Nat Genet 1996;14:255–257.
90. Zapf J. Physiological role of the insulin-like growth factor binding proteins. Eur J Endocrinol 1995;132:645–654.
91. Rajaram S, Baylink DJ, Mohan S. Insulin-like growth factor-binding proteins in serum and other biological fluids: regulation and functions. Endocr Rev 1997;18:801–831.
92. Lalou C, Lassarre C, Binoux M. A proteolytic fragment of insulin-like growth factor (IGF) binding protein-3 that fails to bind IGFs inhibits the mitogenic effects of IGF- I and insulin. Endocrinology 1996;137:3206–3212.
93. Baxter RC. Insulin-like growth factor (IGF)-binding proteins: interactions with IGFs and intrinsic bioactivities. Am J Physiol Endocrinol Metab 2000;278:E967–E976.
94. Jones JI, Clemmons DR. Insulin-like growth factors and their binding proteins: biological actions. Endocr Rev 1995;16:3–34.
95. Jones JI, Gockerman A, Busby WH, Jr., Wright G, Clemmons DR. Insulin-like growth factor binding protein 1 stimulates cell migration and binds to the alpha 5 beta 1 integrin by means of its Arg-Gly-Asp sequence. Proc Natl Acad Sci USA 1993;90:10553–10557.
96. Perks CM, Newcomb PV, Norman MR, Holly JM. Effect of insulin-like growth factor binding protein-1 on integrin signalling and the induction of apoptosis in human breast cancer cells. J Mol Endocrinol 1999;22:141–150.
97. Leal SM, Huang SS, Huang JS. Interactions of high affinity insulin-like growth factor-binding proteins with the type V transforming growth factor-beta receptor in mink lung epithelial cells. J Biol Chem 1999;274:6711–6717.
98. Fanayan S, Firth SM, Butt AJ, Baxter RC. Growth inhibition by insulin-like growth factor-binding protein-3 in T47D breast cancer cells requires transforming growth factor-beta (TGF- beta) and the type II TGF-beta receptor. J Biol Chem 2000;275:39146–39151.

99. Rajah R, Valentinis B, Cohen P. Insulin-like growth factor (IGF)-binding protein-3 induces apoptosis and mediates the effects of transforming growth factor-beta1 on programmed cell death through a p53- and IGF-independent mechanism. J Biol Chem 1997;272:12181–12188.
100. Buckbinder L, Talbott R, Velasco-Miguel S, et al. Induction of the growth inhibitor IGF-binding protein 3 by p53. Nature 1995;377:646–649.
101. Butt AJ, Firth SM, King MA, Baxter RC. Insulin-like growth factor-binding protein-3 modulates expression of Bax and Bcl-2 and potentiates p53-independent radiation-induced apoptosis in human breast cancer cells. J Biol Chem 2000;275:39174–39181.
102. Perks CM, Bowen S, Gill ZP, Newcomb PV, Holly JM. Differential IGF-independent effects of insulin-like growth factor binding proteins (1–6) on apoptosis of breast epithelial cells. J Cell Biochem 1999;75:652–664.
103. Maile LA, Gill ZP, Perks CM, Holly JM. The role of cell surface attachment and proteolysis in the insulin-like growth factor (IGF)-independent effects of IGF-binding protein-3 on apoptosis in breast epithelial cells. Endocrinology 1999;140:4040–4045.
104. Schedlich LJ, Young TF, Firth SM, Baxter RC. Insulin-like growth factor-binding protein (IGFBP)-3 and IGFBP-5 share a common nuclear transport pathway in T47D human breast carcinoma cells. J Biol Chem 1998;273:18347–18352.
105. Schedlich LJ, Le Page SL, Firth SM, Briggs LJ, Jans DA, Baxter RC. Nuclear import of insulin-like growth factor-binding protein-3 and -5 is mediated by the importin beta subunit. J Biol Chem 2000;275:23462–23470.
106. Dupont J, LeRoith D. Insulin and IGF-I Receptors: Similarities and Differences. Hormone Research 2001;55:22–26.
107. Najjar SM, Blakesley VA, Li Calzi S, Kato H, LeRoith D, Choice CV. Differential phosphorylation of pp120 by insulin and insulin-like growth factor-1 receptors: role for the C-terminal domain of the beta- subunit. Biochemistry 1997;36:6827–68234.
108. Formisano P, Najjar SM, Gross CN, et al. Receptor-mediated internalization of insulin. Potential role of pp120/HA4, a substrate of the insulin receptor kinase. J Biol Chem 1995;270:24073–24077.
109. Urso B, Cope DL, Kalloo-Hosein HE, et al. Differences in signaling properties of the cytoplasmic domains of the insulin receptor and insulin-like growth factor receptor in 3T3-L1 adipocytes. J Biol Chem 1999;274:30864–30873.
110. Blakesley VA, Kalebic T, Helman LJ, et al. Tumorigenic and mitogenic capacities are reduced in transfected fibroblasts expressing mutant insulin-like growth factor (IGF)-I receptors. The role of tyrosine residues 1250, 1251, and 1316 in the carboxy-terminus of the IGF-I receptor. Endocrinology 1996;137:410–417.
111. Park BC, Kido Y, Accili D. Differential signaling of insulin and IGF-1 receptors to glycogen synthesis in murine hepatocytes. Biochemistry 1999;38:7517–7523.
112. Dupont J, Khan J, Qu BH, Metzler P, Helman L, LeRoith D. Insulin and IGF-1 Induce Different Patterns of Gene Expression in Mouse fibroblast NIH-3T3 cells: identification by cDNA microarray analysis. Endocrinology 2001;142:4969–4975.
113. Petruzzelli L, Herrera R, Arenas-Garcia R, Fernandez R, Birnbaum MJ, Rosen OM. Isolation of a Drosophila genomic sequence homologous to the kinase domain of the human insulin receptor and detection of the phosphorylated Drosophila receptor with an anti-peptide antibody. Proc Natl Acad Sci USA 1986;83:4710–4714.
114. Tissenbaum HA, Ruvkun G. An insulin-like signaling pathway affects both longevity and reproduction in Caenorhabditis elegans. Genetics 1998;148:703–717.
115. Kimura KD, Tissenbaum HA, Liu Y, Ruvkun G. daf-2, an insulin receptor-like gene that regulates longevity and diapause in Caenorhabditis elegans. Science 1997;277:942–946.
116. Ogg S, Paradis S, Gottlieb S, et al. The Fork head transcription factor DAF-16 transduces insulin-like metabolic and longevity signals in C. elegans. Nature 1997;389:994–999.
117. Ogg S, Ruvkun G. The C. elegans PTEN homolog, DAF-18, acts in the insulin receptor-like metabolic signaling pathway. Mol Cell 1998;2:887–893.
118. Bartke A, Coschigano K, Kopchick J, et al. Genes that prolong life: relationships of growth hormone and growth to aging and life span. J Gerontol A Biol Sci Med Sci 2001;56:B340–B349.

119. Marin-Hincapie M, Garofalo RS. The carboxyl terminal extension of the Drosophila insulin receptor homologue binds IRS-1 and influences cell survival. J Biol Chem 1999;274:24987–24994.
120. Bohni R, Riesgo-Escovar J, Oldham S, et al. Autonomous control of cell and organ size by CHICO, a Drosophila homolog of vertebrate IRS1–4. Cell 1999;97:865–875.

II IGF and Nutritional Status

2 Regulation of Insulin-Like Growth Factor-I by Nutrition

Jean-Paul Thissen, Véronique Beauloye, Jean-Marie Ketelslegers, and Louis E. Underwood

KEY POINTS

- Nutrition is one of the principal regulators of circulating IGF-I. Many mechanisms are involved in the nutritional regulation of IGF-I.
- Both energy and protein are critical to the regulation of serum IGF-I concentrations. After fasting, adequate energy and protein are necessary for restoration of serum IGF-I, but energy may be somewhat more important than protein. While a low intake of protein is able to increase IGF-I in the presence of adequate energy, there is a threshold requirement of energy below which optimal protein intake fails to raise IGF-I after fasting.
- The decline of serum IGF-I during dietary restriction is independent of diet-induced alterations in pituitary GH secretion. In severe dietary restriction (fasting), a marked decrease in the number of liver somatogenic receptors suggests that a GH receptor defect is involved in the decline of serum IGF-I. In protein restriction, the decline of serum IGF-I results from a postreceptor defect in GH action at the hepatic level.
- Nutritional deprivation decreases hepatic IGF-I production by diminishing IGF-I gene expression. Decline in IGF-I gene expression results from both transcriptional and post-transcription mechanisms.
- Diet restriction also increases the clearance and degradation of serum IGF-I through changes in the levels of circulating IGFBPs.
- The molecular mechanisms leading to the decline of IGF-I in catabolic stress seem to be similar to those operational in food deprivation.
- Nutrients may also control the biological action of IGF-I, either directly or indirectly, through changes in IGFBPs.

1. INTRODUCTION

Starvation causes growth arrest and decreases body cell mass. Although secondary changes in the hormonal milieu play a major role, the mechanisms by which insufficient nutrition cause growth retardation are not well elucidated. Given its stimulatory

From: *IGF and Nutrition in Health and Disease*
Edited by: M. S. Houston, J. M. P. Holly, and E. L. Feldman © Humana Press Inc., Totowa, NJ

effect on cell proliferation and differentiation and its anabolic effect on protein metabolism *(1)*, the decline in insulin-like growth factor (IGF)-I in states of undernutrition likely contributes to the observed growth arrest and loss of cell mass observed. In this chapter, we will review the mechanisms responsible for the decrease of IGF-I in response to fasting and food deprivation and compare the responses to insufficient nutrition to those that occur during critical illness *(2)*.

2. EVIDENCE FOR THE NUTRITIONAL REGULATION OF IGF-I IN HUMANS

2.1. Fasting and Malnutrition

Fasting among normal volunteers causes serum IGF-I to begin to decline within 24 h and to reach 20% of prefast values by 10 d *(3)*. Changes in serum IGF-I concentrations parallel changes in nitrogen balance, suggesting that decreased IGF-I might mediate a decline in protein synthesis or an increase in protein breakdown. Decreased serum IGF-I is not restricted to fasting but also is observed in protein calorie malnutrition (marasmus, kwashiorkor, anorexia nervosa, celiac disease, AIDS, inflammatory bowel diseases) *(4)*. In general, the magnitude of IGF-I reduction relates to the severity of the nutritional insult as reflected by serum albumin concentrations, weight deficit, or loss of body cell mass. The sensitivity of serum IGF-I to nutrient deprivation and repletion makes it a useful marker of nutritional status (reviewed in Chapter 4). Growth hormone (GH) secretion often is increased in malnourished patients, suggesting that they have resistance to the action of GH *(5)*. The injection of pharmacological doses of GH, however, may still increase IGF-I and cause nitrogen retention in some malnourished patients *(6)*.

Serious illness is also associated with low circulating concentrations of IGF-I despite augmented GH concentrations *(7)*. This rise in GH secretion persists despite the calorie and protein supply afforded by artificial feeding, indicating that nutrient deprivation is not always responsible for the GH resistance observed in such patients.

2.2. Respective Roles of Energy and Protein Intake

Both energy and protein are important in regulating IGF-I because each is essential for restoration of serum IGF-I concentrations after fasting. Refeeding a diet sufficient in calories and protein raises IGF-I to nearly 70% of the basal prefast values within 5 d, whereas refeeding a protein-deficient isocaloric diet results in a 2-d delay in the upward inflection of IGF-I and increases IGF-I to only 50% of control prefast values. In contrast, refeeding a diet deficient in both protein and energy results in a further decrease of IGF-I in serum *(8)*. The importance of energy intake in regulating IGF-I is supported by the observation that there is a threshold energy requirement (similar or equal to 11 kcal/kg/d) below which optimal protein intake fails to raise IGF-I during fasting *(9)*. The source of energy also might be critical for the regulation of serum IGF-I because the carbohydrate content of the diet appears to be a major determinant of the response of IGF-I to GH when energy intake is severely restricted *(10)*. The role of protein intake in the regulation of IGF-I is illustrated by the observation that the increase in IGF-I after fasting is proportional to the protein content of the refeeding diet. The quality of dietary protein is also important because IGF-I concentrations after fasting are restored more readily by a protein-restricted diet rich in essential amino acids than by one that is rich in nonessential amino acids *(11)*.

Energy and amino acid deprivation do not appear to play a major role in the decline of IGF-I observed in critically ill patients. Evidence obtained mainly from animal models suggests that factors, such as cytokines, glucocorticoids, and acidosis, are important in this regard.

3. MECHANISMS INVOLVED IN THE NUTRITIONAL REGULATION OF IGF-I PRODUCTION

3.1. Role of GH Secretion

Because GH is the principal hormonal stimulus of IGF-I production, impaired GH secretion may cause decreased IGF-I concentrations when food intake decreases (Fig. 1). In rats, the pulsatile secretion of GH is markedly attenuated by decreased availability of nutrients *(12)*, and this could result in the decline of serum IGF-I. Unlike rats, however, humans *(13)* and other species have increased GH secretion when food intake is decreased. Fasting for 5 d increases the 24-h integrated GH concentration and the maximum amplitude and pulse frequency of GH *(13)*. These observations suggest that impaired GH secretion is not responsible for decreased serum IGF-I concentrations in food-restricted humans.

Decreased GH secretion in starved rats could result from increased somatostatin, somatotropin-releasing inhibitory hormone (SRIH), tone or from reduced growth hormone-releasing hormone (GHRH) stimulation of somatotroph cells *(14)*. The involvement of SRIH is suggested by in vivo immunoneutralization studies in which GH secretion is restored in fasted rats after intravenous injection of antiserum to SRIH *(15)*. Increased SRIH observed in the peripheral circulation of fasted rats likely originates more probably from peripheral sources (gastrointestinal tract and pancreas) and not the hypothalamus *(12,16,17)*. These observations suggest that a relative or absolute excess of SRIH is involved in fasting-induced inhibition of GH secretion. The decline in GH secretion during fasting could also result from diminished GHRH secretion because levels of GHRH mRNA in the hypothalamus are decreased markedly after 72 h of fasting *(16)*. This decrease, however, is not associated with a reduction in hypothalamic GHRH peptide content, suggesting that release of peptide may be decreased in parallel with the reduction in mRNA. Given the evidence for an inhibitory effect of SRIH on GHRH release *(18)*, the imbalance between GHRH mRNA and peptide in the hypothalamus might be secondary to high SRIH tone. Lack of dietary protein blunts spontaneous GH secretion *(19)*. The protein content of the diet seems to be critical for the regulation of hypothalamic GHRH gene expression *(20)*. Furthermore, dietary protein restriction attenuates GH responsiveness to GHRH and reduces pituitary size and GH content.

Several extrahypothalamic hormones are also implicated in the regulation of GH secretion and might be involved in nutrition-induced alterations in GH secretion. Leptin, a product of adipose tissue, is capable of entering the brain to inhibit food intake and increase energy expenditure. Because administration of leptin antiserum to rats causes a marked decrease in GH secretion *(21)* and leptin levels are reduced by fasting in rats as in humans *(22–24)*, it has been suggested that leptin may be an integrative

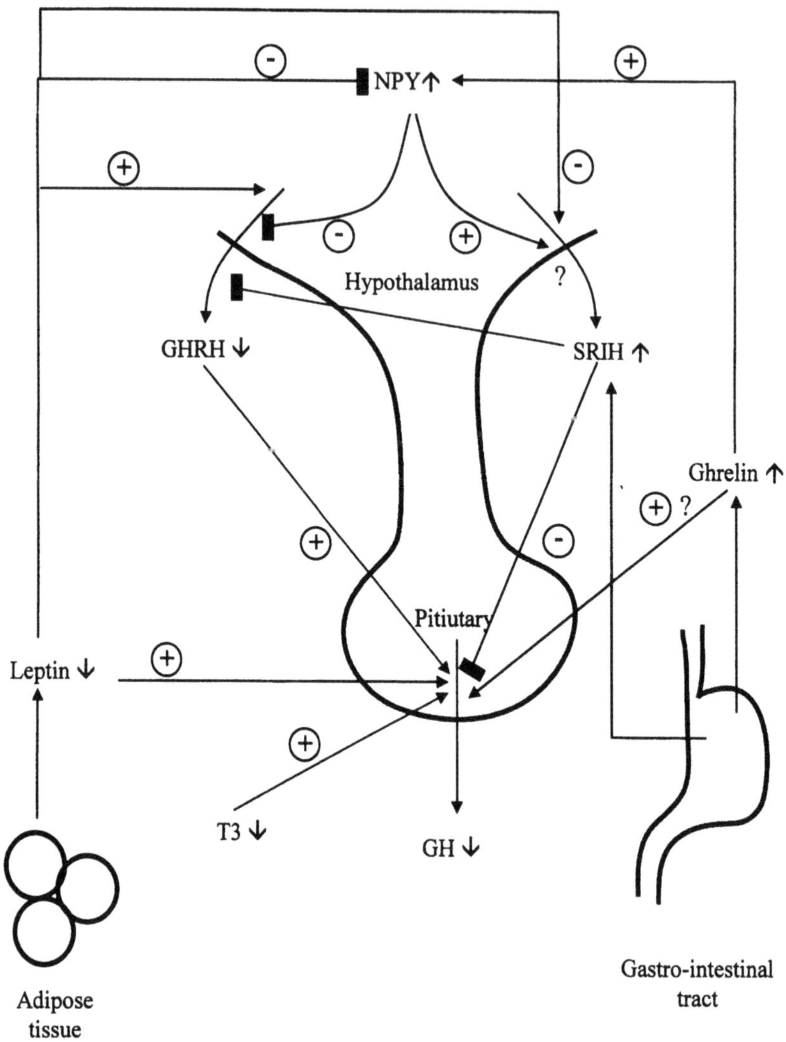

Fig. 1. Regulation of GH secretion by fasting in the rat. GH, growth hormone; SRIH, somatotropin-releasing inhibitory hormone; GHRH, growth hormone-releasing hormone; NPY, neuropeptide Y; T3, triiodothyronine.

signal for coordinating growth with nutritional status. This is supported by the observation that exogenous leptin prevents the fasting-induced fall of serum GH in rats *(25–27)*. Despite its stimulatory effect on GH secretion, exogenous leptin does not restore serum IGF-I in fasted animals to normal. The effect of leptin on GH secretion in rats appears to be exerted at the hypothalamic level by regulating neurons that produce GHRH, SRIH, and neuropeptide Y (NPY). The rescue of GH secretion by leptin may be mediated by preventing decline of GHRH mRNA, and induction of NPY mRNA in fasted rats *(26)*. Alternatively, the GH-releasing activity of leptin may be mediated in part by inhibition of SRIH *(28)*, as suggested by the ability of leptin to decrease SRIH mRNA and secretion in vitro *(29)*. Finally, leptin may stimulate GH secretion directly, as illustrated by in vitro experiments *(30)*. The effects of leptin on GH secretion in humans remain to be clarified.

Ghrelin, an important regulator of GH secretion and energy homeostasis *(31)* produced mainly by the stomach, is regulated by nutrient intake *(32)* and promotes GH release at both the hypothalamic and pituitary levels *(33)*. Although both GH and ghrelin increase during fasting in humans, no correlations seem to exist between plasma ghrelin and GH or IGF-I concentrations. Further investigation is needed to delineate the role of ghrelin in enhancing GH secretion in fasting humans. Thyroid hormones stimulate the production of growth hormone in cultures of GH1 pituitary cells *(34)*, and decreased plasma triiodothyronine (T3) in fasted rats has been implicated in the decrease of GH mRNA in the pituitary during fasting *(35)*. Moreover, retinoic acid, acting in synergy with thyroid hormones, stimulates production of growth hormone in cultured pituitary cells *(36,37)*. We speculate that the stunted growth accompanying vitamin A deficiency might be mediated by decreased GH production.

GH secretion of rats is impaired in several other models of dietary manipulation that are accompanied by growth retardation and low serum IGF-I concentrations (lysine deficiency, potassium deficiency, zinc deficiency and selenium excess) as well as in response to stressful stimuli such as sepsis *(38)*.

3.2. Role of GH Receptor and Postreceptor Defects

It is unlikely that impaired GH secretion alone causes the decrease in IGF-I observed in nutritionally restricted rats because the administration of GH to fasted or protein-restricted rats does not produce a normal increase of IGF-I in blood *(39–43)*. Also, protein energy malnutrition in humans is accompanied by high circulating concentrations of GH that fail to maintain IGF-I in the normal range *(44,45)*. These observations suggest that GH resistance accompanies nutritional deprivation. Because the liver is a principal site for production of IGF-I *(46,47)*, reduction of GH binding by the liver could impair production of IGF-I. Rats that are fasted exhibit parallel decline in serum IGF-I concentrations and in somatogenic (GH) binding capacity in liver *(48)*.

Changes in hepatic GH receptors (GHR) caused by dietary restriction of rats are paralleled by changes in concentrations of GH binding protein (GHBP) in serum *(49)*. In humans, GHBP decreases in parallel with serum IGF-I concentrations during severe dietary restriction *(50)*. However, the consequences of changes in circulating GHBP in the control of GH action are disputed.

Regulation of the GHR by fasting occurs at the level of gene expression *(51)*. GH receptor mRNA is reduced by fasting *(52,53)*, and the magnitude and time-course of this decline is similar to the decline in liver IGF-I mRNA, suggesting that there may be a causal relationship between the two. This decline in GHR mRNA may be driven in part by nutritionally induced changes in hormones, such as glucocorticoids, thyroid hormones, and insulin, or in metabolites such as glucose. Glucocorticoids in excess *(54,55)*, insufficient thyroid hormones *(56–58)* or insulin *(59–61)*, and reduced supply of glucose *(62,63)* that occur in response to food deprivation are associated with low liver GHR binding and mRNA. Decreased liver GHR mRNA occurs in humans who have GH resistance caused by malnutrition *(64)* or postoperative catabolism *(65)*. GH resistance associated with decreased liver GHR mRNA and binding is also present in

Table 1
Effect of Fasting, Sepsis, and Chronic Renal Failure on GH-Induced JAK-2, GHR, STAT-5 Phosphorylation, and on SOCS-3 Gene Expression

	Fasting	*Sepsis*	*Chronic renal failure*
P-JAK-2/JAK-2	↘	↘	↘
P-GHR/GHR	↘	ND	ND
P-STAT-5/STAT-5	↘	↘	↘
SOCS-3 mRNA	↗↗	↗↗	↗↗

P, phosphorylated; JAK, Janus kinase; STAT, signal transducers and activators of transcription; SOCS, suppressors of cytokine signaling; GHR, growth hormone receptor; ND, not determined.

other dietary models of malnutrition, such as zinc deficiency *(66)* and in catabolic conditions, such as chronic renal failure *(67)* and sepsis *(68)*.

In contrast to fasting, the role of the liver GH receptors in the decline of serum IGF-I in protein restriction is more questionable. Although protein restriction in young rats results in a dramatic decline of serum IGF-I, liver GH binding sites decrease only modestly. In older animals, protein restriction also causes a decline in serum IGF-I but does not reduce GH binding to liver membranes *(69)* or to freshly isolated hepatocytes *(70)*. Also, no changes in serum GHBP are observed *(71)*. Serum IGF-I responses to a single injection of GH in hypophysectomized protein-restricted animals are severely blunted *(42)*. Despite the fact that continuous infusion of GH into protein-restricted rats increases liver GH binding to the level of control-fed rats, serum IGF-I is not increased *(43)*. Taken together, these studies suggest that a postreceptor defect in GH action may participate in the GH resistance observed in protein restriction.

Intracellular defects in GH action could be a direct effect of limited nutrients or could result from secondary hormonal changes. Although it is not clear whether this postreceptor defect is specific to GH or is one that limits the synthesis of IGF-I regardless of the stimulus, the latter alternative seems the more likely. In hepatocyte primary cultures, the stimulation of IGF-I gene expression by insulin *(72)* as well as by GH *(73)* is blunted by a reduction in the concentration of amino acids in the medium.

3.3. Role of GH Transduction Pathways

Although the decrease in liver GH binding associated with fasting is well established, the consequences of this decline on the GH transduction pathway are less clear (Table 1). To investigate the effect of fasting on the liver GH transduction pathway, Beauloye et al. assessed the activation of the Janus kinase-signal transducers and activators of transcription (JAK-STAT) pathway in response to GH injected in the portal vein of fasted and fed rats *(74)*. Although GH stimulated the phosphorylation of JAK-2, GHR, and STAT-5 in fed animals, the phosphorylation of these molecules was blunted markedly in the fasted animals. The inhibitory effect of fasting on these GH signaling molecules occurred without any changes in their protein content. The effect of fasting on GH-induced GHR and STAT-5 phosphorylation was detectable as early as 3 min after GH treatment and persisted at least until 30 min after GH injection. These findings suggest that the effects of fasting on the GHR signaling pathway are not caused by delayed GH activation. The observation that the phosphorylation of STAT-5 by JAK-2 is required for GH to stimulate IGF-I expression *(75)* supports the role of the alterations caused by fasting in the decrease of liver IGF-I production.

Although the mechanisms by which fasting alters the JAK-STAT pathway remains to be determined, it is likely that this defect results mainly from decreased liver GH binding sites. Another mechanism might be the superinduction of an intracellular negative feedback loop mediated by suppressors of cytokine signaling (SOCS) proteins. The ability of overexpressed SOCS-3 to blunt JAK-STAT activation in transfected cells *(76,77)* and the increased SOCS-3 expression by fasting *(74)* suggest a role for SOCS-3 in the fasting-induced JAK-STAT alterations. Impaired JAK-STAT signal transduction, possibly mediated through decreased GH receptors and SOCS proteins overexpression, may also contribute to the GH resistance observed in chronic renal failure *(78)* and in sepsis *(79)*.

3.4. Role of Hormones in the Nutritional Regulation of IGF-I

3.4.1. Insulin

Dietary restriction causes serum insulin concentrations to decline. Insulin-deficient diabetic rats have low serum IGF-I and decreased liver GH binding *(60,80,81)*. Replacement of insulin restores both to normal. Insulin, therefore, might regulate serum IGF-I concentrations through changes in liver GH binding *(82)*. The addition of insulin to hepatocytes in culture increases GHR mRNA and GH binding *(61,83)*. Recent onset or mild streptozotocin-induced diabetes in rats, however, can be accompanied by low serum IGF-I without change in hepatic GH binding *(84)*. In this situation, the decline of IGF-I is attributed to a postreceptor defect, likely related to the insulin deficiency directly, or less likely to metabolic abnormalities caused by insulin deficiency. In primary cultures of hepatocytes, insulin stimulates the accumulation of IGF-I mRNA in the absence of GH *(85,86)*. Insulin also potentiates the stimulatory effect of GH and amino acids on IGF-I production *(72,85,87)*. Although its exact mechanism of action is not known, the stimulatory effect of insulin seems to result from an enhanced rate of IGF-I gene transcription (Fig. 2) in adult hepatocytes *(88)* and from enhanced IGF-I mRNA stability in fetal hepatocytes *(89)*. Despite insulin's stimulatory role on IGF-I production, protein restriction (and perhaps decreased availability of specific amino acids) may be more important mechanistically than decline in serum insulin concentrations for the decreased circulating IGF-I in protein-restricted rats *(90)*. In rats made diabetic with streptozotocin who are treated with insulin and then submitted to a low- or normal protein diet, the diet decline in IGF-I persists despite high circulating insulin (two to three times normal values). This suggests that dietary protein restriction decreases serum IGF-I independent of insulin and that protein restriction by itself is the major cause of reduced serum IGF-I in this model.

3.4.2. Thyroid Hormones

The involvement of the thyroid hormones in the nutritional regulation of IGF-I is suggested by the close relationship between the decline of circulating IGF-I and of thyroxine (T3) in fasted humans *(91)* and rats *(92)*. Low serum IGF-I in hypothyroid animals reinforces the possibility of thyroid hormone regulation of IGF-I *(93)*. It is possible, however, that the major effect of thyroid hormones on IGF-I synthesis is

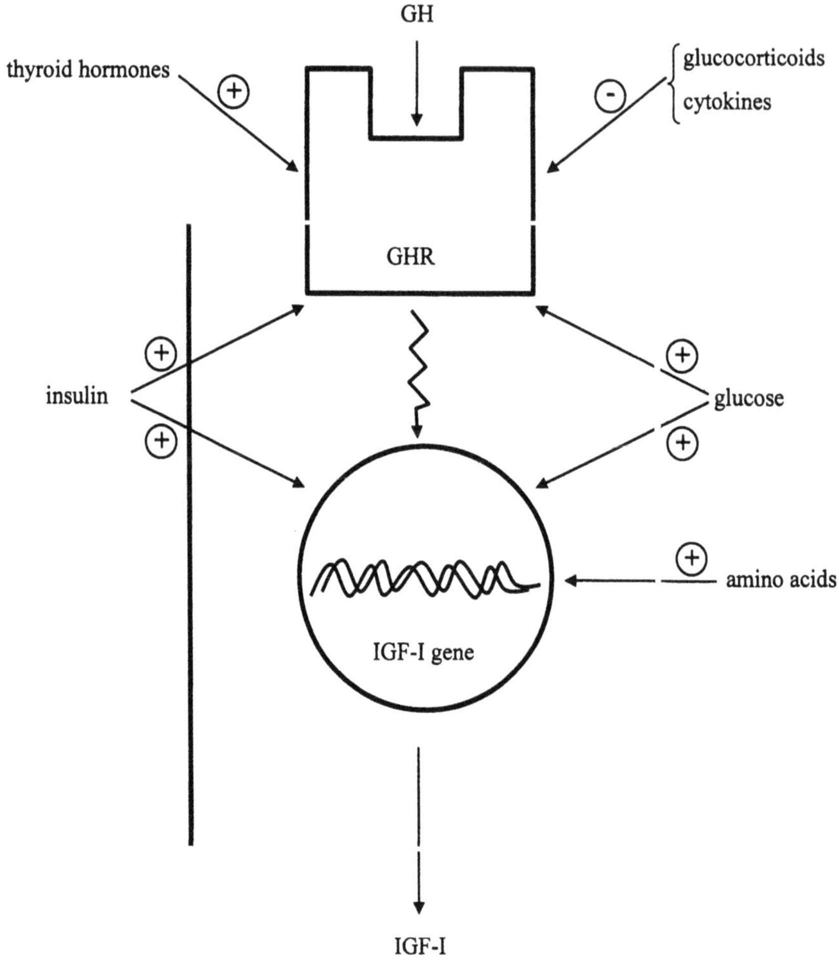

Fig. 2. Role of hormonal changes and nutrient availability in the regulation of IGF-I production by liver in response to food deprivation. GH, growth hormone; GHR, growth hormone receptor.

exerted on the pituitary *(94)*, where thyroid hormones regulate GH gene expression *(95)*. Hypothyroidism is not only accompanied by a decline in GH secretion but is also associated with blunted IGF-I production in response to GH and resistance to the growth-promoting effect of GH *(93)*. This suggests that thyroid hormones participate in IGF-I production by the liver. Studies show that thyroid hormones potentiate hepatic IGF-I synthesis in response to GH both in vivo and in vitro *(83,96)*. Hepatic GH binding is upregulated by thyroid hormones. This supports the role of thyroid hormones in the potentiation of GH induction of IGF-I. Low serum T3 concentrations might play a role in the decline in GH and serum IGF-I concentrations in fasted rats because treatment of fasted rats with T3 seems to attenuate the decline in serum IGF-I *(97)*.

3.4.3. Glucocorticoids and Proinflammatory Cytokines

A role for glucocorticoids in the GH resistance caused by food deprivation is suggested by their inhibitory effect on GH-induced IGF-I production in vivo *(98)* and in vitro *(55,99)* concurrent with their increased circulating concentrations during fasting. Part of the GH resistance caused by excess glucocorticoids might be caused by their capacity to inhibit GHR mRNA and GH binding to hepatocytes *(54,55)* and to other cell types *(99,100)*. In diabetic rats, which have increased glucocorticoids and GH resistance, adrenalectomy restores the GH-induced IGF-I response *(101,102)*. In contrast with diabetic rats, however, adrenalectomy of fasted animals failed to reverse the fasting-induced inhibition of the early steps of the liver GH receptor-signaling pathway *(74)*. In addition to inhibit IGF-I production, glucocorticoids may also impair growth by induction of IGFBP-1 and reduction of free IGF-I *(103)* in the circulation.

In severe catabolic states such as sepsis, proinflammatory cytokines, namely tumor necrosis factor-α, interleukin-1β, and interleukin-6 are implicated in the development of GH resistance and the decrease in circulating IGF-I (refs. *104–106*; see also chapter 16). As reviewed in Chapter 3, metabolic acidosis, as in renal failure, also has been shown to cause resistance to GH *(107)* and to decrease circulating IGF-I *(108)*.

3.5. The Role of Nutrient Availability in the Nutritional Regulation of IGF-I

Evidence for a direct role of amino acid availability in regulating IGF-I comes from experiments using primary cultures of rat hepatocytes *(109)*. In this model, amino acid deprivation causes a rapid and progressive decline in IGF-I mRNA and IGF-I peptide production, whereas amino acid excess causes an increase *(73,88)*. Among the amino acids, tryptophan seems to be the most critical in regulating IGF-I, as its removal from the medium for 48h causes a dramatic decline in IGF-I mRNA and in IGF-I release. Across a broad range of amino acid concentrations, GH and insulin raised IGF-I mRNA levels in proportion to the amino acid concentration *(110)*. Taken together, these observations suggest that GH, insulin and amino acids can regulate hepatic production of IGF-I independently.

It is not known, however, whether amino acids, insulin and GH control IGF-I synthesis at the same point. Whereas insulin and GH are believed to act at the transcriptional level, decreased IGF-I mRNA in amino acid-deprived cultured hepatocytes results from decreased transcription rate *(88)* and enhanced degradation *(111)*. An amino-responsive element has been described in the IGF-I gene *(112)*. It does not seem, however, to share common features with the one characterized in the *CHOP* and *asparagine synthase* genes, two genes induced by amino acid deprivation *(113)*. Several transcription factors appear to be affected by dietary protein/amino acid availability, but it remains to be determined whether these are involved in the observed effects of amino acids on IGF-I transcription. Restriction of amino acids leads to accumulation of uncharged transfer RNA, which could impair gene expression by altering the rate of transcription *(114)*.

In parallel with inhibition of IGF-I, amino acid deficiency stimulates the in vitro expression and release of IGFBP-1, a binding protein considered to inhibit the actions of IGF-I. Limitation in any one of the essential amino acids causes strong induction of IGFBP-1 *(73,115)*. However, restriction in vivo of single essential amino acids is not sufficient to induce IGFBP-1, and general amino acid depletion is necessary *(116)*. The direct effect of amino acid deprivation on IGFBP-1 explains why higher levels of IGFBP-1 are observed in protein-restricted rats than in starved rats.

IGF-I gene expression also may be regulated by glucose in hepatocytes, particularly those of fetal origin *(63,117)*. In this model, glucose stimulates IGF-I mRNA and peptide secretion. Experiments with analogs suggest that glucose-6 phosphate is necessary for the induction of IGF-I mRNA. A similar observation was made for IGF-II. The glucose-induced rise in IGF-II mRNA was mediated by stimulation of gene transcription and increased transcript stability. This effect was observed in the absence of GH, indicating that it did not result from the potentiation of the GH action on IGF-I *(63)*.

Although reduced amino acid availability is thought to be responsible for the decrease of liver IGF-I mRNA in response to protein restriction, such a direct mechanism does not seem to be the rule for all nutrients. For example, chelation-induced depletion of zinc in rat hepatocytes does not cause IGF-I gene expression to decline, despite the clear inhibition of the metallothionein mRNA *(118)*.

3.6. Role of Changes in IGF-I Gene Expression

Decreased serum IGF-I in dietary energy or protein restriction correlates with reduced steady-state levels of hepatic IGF-I mRNA *(119–122)*, suggesting that nutritional regulation of IGF-I gene expression takes place at a pretranslational level. In fasted animals, the levels of IGF-I mRNAs with different 5′ untranslated regions (class 1 and class 2 transcripts) appear to be coordinately decreased *(123,124)*. However, although the levels of IGF-IB mRNA declined markedly, IGF-IA mRNA was not altered significantly *(125)*. Despite this preferential decrease in IGF-IB mRNA, fasting caused both propeptides IGF-IA and IGF-IB to decrease *(123,125)*. All size-class transcripts (0.8–1.2, 1.7, 4.7, and 7.5 kb) are proportionately reduced by fasting *(53)*. Dietary protein restriction, however, caused a greater decrease of the 7.5 kb IGF-I mRNA than the other size-classes *(122,126)*.

Based on nuclear run-off studies *(53,111,125)* and analysis of nuclear transcripts *(127,128)*, both transcriptional and posttranscriptional mechanisms may mediate the decrease in IGF-I expression observed in fasted as well as protein-restricted animals.

The weight of evidence suggests that transcription is the major locus for nutritional regulation of IGF-I. The co-ordinate decrease in transcription of nutritionally sensitive genes, such as albumin, transthyretin, and IGF-I in protein-restricted rats might result from altered activity of transcription factors. The DNA binding activity of factors involved in the expression of the IGF-I gene in liver (hepatocyte nuclear factor [HNF]-1α, HNF-3, HNF-4, CCAAT/enhancer binding protein [C/EBP], Sp1) is altered in response to protein restriction *(129)*. The transcriptional activity of HNF-1α is reduced in hepatocytes exposed to medium deficient in amino acids *(130)*. In contrast, C/EBP homologous protein (the CHOP transcription factor) is stimulated in these conditions *(131,132)*. The induction of CHOP is of interest as increased levels of CHOP could interfere with C/EBP binding *(133)*. Although the role of HNF-1α and C/EBPα in the stimulation of basal expression of IGF-I in liver is well established *(134,135)*, their contribution to reduced IGF-I gene expression in the liver of protein-restricted rats is unsettled. Other transcription factors involved in the transcriptional regulation of IGF-I, such as Sp1 *(136)*, might also direct the response to nutrient availability *(137)*.

Nutritional regulation also seems to take place at the nuclear RNA splicing step. The observation that IGF-IA and IGF-IB mRNAs result from alternative splicing after transcription of a single gene, yet only IGF-IB mRNA levels are decreased by fasting suggests that the decrease in liver total IGF-I mRNA might also involve regulation of the pre-mRNA processing *(111)*.

Protein restriction may result in decreased stability of the IGF-I mRNA, in particular for the 7.5-kb transcript *(122,126)*. Reduction of the 7.5-kb transcript in protein restricted rats is confirmed by the observation that IGF-I mRNA stability in vitro is decreased in hepatocytes exposed to amino acid deprivation *(111)*. In this model, the 7.5-kb mRNA is degraded faster than the two smaller IGF-I mRNA species. Differential regulation of the 7.5-kb IGF-I mRNA might be related to its 3′-untranslated region, which contains several AU-rich sequences *(138)*. Such sequences in other genes are known to interact with cytosolic RNA-binding proteins and to be involved in the regulation of the stability and/or translation of the mRNA *(139)*.

Regulation of IGF-I synthesis by nutrients also may be under translational control because discrepancies have been observed between serum IGF-I peptide concentrations and liver IGF-I mRNA levels *(122,140–142)*. In protein-restricted rats, injections of high doses of GH for 1 wk restores liver IGF-I mRNA abundance to normal without normalization of liver or serum IGF-I concentrations *(122)*. This divergent response to GH is not the result of a secretory defect of IGF-I because there was no accumulation of IGF-I in liver. It also seems unlikely that tissues other than liver might make significant contributions to the IGF-I released into the serum, given the observation that 80–90% of circulating IGF-I is produced by the liver *(47)*. The mechanisms responsible for this presumed impairment of the translation of IGF-I mRNA are not known. It appears, however, that all IGF-I mRNA size-classes are associated with polysomes, even in the liver of protein-restricted rats *(143)*, suggesting that they have the capacity to engage in IGF-I synthesis.

In addition to liver, reduced IGF-I mRNA during diet restriction is observed in most other organs *(52,123)*. The decrement in IGF-I gene expression, however, is most dramatic in the liver. Fasting of young rats for 48 h decreases IGF-I mRNA levels by 80% in liver and lung, by 60% in kidney and muscle, and by only 30% in stomach, brain, and testes. No changes are observed in the heart. In a different study, prolongation of fasting for 3 d caused IGF-I mRNA in heart muscle to decrease but caused no change in the brain *(52)*. Protein restriction for 1 wk, however, does not seem to reduce IGF-I mRNA in tissues (kidney, heart, diaphragm, brain, and aorta) other than liver *(52)* and muscle *(144)*. The decline of circulating IGF-I in mice in whom the ability of liver to produce IGF-I has been knocked out indicates that the decline of circulating IGF-I during protein restriction originates from nonhepatic as well *(145)*.

4. MECHANISMS INVOLVED IN THE NUTRITIONAL REGULATION OF IGF-I ACTION

4.1. Role of IGF Binding Proteins

Among the proposed functions of the IGF binding proteins (IGFBPs) are the prolongation of the plasma half-life of IGF-I and IGF-II, control of the rate of IGF transport from the vascular compartment, and regulation of the interaction between IGF-I and the type 1 IGF receptor on the cell surface *(146–148)*. Because they control the bioavailability of IGF-I to tissues *(149)*, the IGFBPs are believed to exert both stimulatory *(150–152)* and inhibitory *(153–155)* effects on IGF-I actions (Table 2). IGF-I bioavailability may be controlled by posttranslational modifications of IGFBPs (partial proteolytic degradation by specific IGFBP proteases, selective dephosphorylation)

Table 2
Effect of Food Deprivation on Circulating IGF-I and IGFBP Levels and Their Hepatic Gene Expression

	Circulating levels	*Hepatic gene expression*
IGF-I	Total ↙	↙
	Free ↙	
IGFBP-1	↗	↗
IGFBP-2	↗	↗
IGFBP-3	↘	↘
ALS	↘	~
IGFBP-4	~	~

IGFBP, insulin-like growth factor binding protein; ALS, acid-labile subunit.

resulting in IGFBPs with reduced affinity for IGF-I. Less than 1% of IGF-I circulates as free peptide *(156)*, and most (>90%) is bound to the 150-kDa complex, which consists of IGF-I, IGFBP-3, or IGFBP-5 and an acid labile subunit (ALS). This complex is believed not to cross the capillary endothelium *(157)* and is credited with prolonging the half-life of IGF-I in the circulation. The complex has a relatively long half-life of 3–6 h in rats *(158)* and 12–15 h in humans *(159)*, whereas free IGF-I disappears with an apparent half-life of 14 min *(160)*. IGFBP-3 probably serves as a storage pool for IGF-I. IGFBP-1, IGFBP-2, and IGFBP-4 are associated with IGF-I in smaller complexes (30–40 kDa) that can cross the capillary endothelium *(161)*. IGFBP-1 and IGFBP-2 contain RGD sequences (Arg-Gly-Asp) *(149)* that may allow attachment to cell surface integrin receptors. They may be involved in the delivery of IGF-I to tissues. Although serum concentrations of IGFBP-3 correlate positively with ALS and total IGF-I, IGFBP-1 and free IGF-I correlate inversely. It is hypothesized that IGFBP-1 is an important determinant of free IGF-I in vivo *(162,163)*. IGF-independent actions have been shown for IGFBP-1, -3, and -5 *(149)*. In particular, IGFBP-3 binds specifically and with high affinity to the cell surface of various cell types and inhibits monolayer cell growth, presumably by specific interaction with cell membrane proteins that function as IGFBP-3 receptors *(164)*. The functions and nutrition-related regulatory mechanisms of IGFBP-5, IGFBP-6, and IGFBP-related proteins (Mac25, CTGF, NOV, CYR61) *(165)* are largely unknown.

Nutrient intake is a major regulator of the plasma concentrations of the IGFBPs. Serum IGFBP-3 concentrations in humans are relatively constant throughout the day, and this is the likely mechanism for the stability of serum IGF-I concentrations *(166)*. In contrast, serum IGFBP-1 is markedly and rapidly suppressed by nutrient intake *(167,168)*. An effect mediated primarily by increased insulin *(169,170)*, glucose *(171,172)*, and probably by amino acid concentrations *(73,116)*. Insulin also may selectively stimulate the transport of IGFBP-1 to the extravascular space *(173)*, which might explain the rapidity of the insulin-induced fall in IGFBP-1. IGFBP-2 levels are more stable than IGFBP-1 and are not subject to postprandial changes *(174)*.

Dietary manipulations change the abundance of serum IGFBPs in humans and animals. In general, dietary restriction decreases serum IGFBP-3 and ALS concentrations while it increases serum IGFBP-1 and IGFBP-2 *(5)*. Fasting of rats for 24 h increases serum IGFBP-1 and -2 *(175,176)*, and produces parallel increases of liver IGFBP-1 and IGFBP-2 mRNA *(177)*. Likewise, 24-h fasting in humans causes a 4-fold increase of IGFBP-1 *(162,168)* whereas prolonged fasting for 9 d or protein restriction for 6 d is needed to cause an increase in plasma IGFBP-2 *(174,178)*. Maternal fasting also induces an increase of IGFBP-1 and IGFBP-2 in fetal serum *(179)*, thereby increasing the IGF binding capacity of serum. Free IGF-I changes in parallel with total IGF-I in fasted rats *(180)* and children *(162)*. Unlike IGFBP-1, fasting for 24 h does not affect serum IGFBP-3 *(181)* and ALS *(180)* in rats and humans. A decline of serum IGFBP-3 and ALS, however, occurs after fasting for 48–72 h *(179,180,182)*.

During more chronic dietary restriction, serum IGFBP-3 declines and a parallel change in the liver IGFBP-3 mRNA is observed *(180,183)*. Unlike other situations in which IGFBP-3 concentrations are low, that is, pregnancy *(184)*, after surgery *(185)*, and catabolic states *(186)*, the decline of IGFBP-3 in food-deprived rats and humans is not associated with proteolytic activity in serum *(187)*. In response to reduced nutrition, serum ALS levels also decline, but steady-state hepatic ALS mRNA levels are not changed, indicating that ALS synthesis in fasting is regulated primarily at the posttranscriptional level *(180,188–190)*. Because both IGFBP-3 and ALS production is stimulated by GH and insulin *(188,191,192)*, it is not clear whether their decrease in response to food deprivation is due to decreased GH secretion, to defects in the GH action pathway and/or to the lack of the stimulatory effect of insulin. IGFBP-3 and ALS genes are stimulated directly by insulin, even in the absence of GH *(192)*. The decline of IGFBP-3 may be related to decreased serum IGF-I itself, because IGF-I infusion in protein-restricted-rats normalizes serum IGFBP-3 *(193)*. The induction of IGFBP-3 by IGF-I provides a mechanism by which the concentrations of these two peptides could be regulated coordinately. As with fasting, an increase in liver IGFBP-1 and -2 mRNA and increased serum concentrations of IGFBP-1 and -2 occurs with chronic energy or protein restriction *(71,183,189,190,194)*.

Changes in IGFBPs similar to those produced by food deprivation have been observed in response to catabolic states. The most dramatic changes are an increase in circulating IGFBP-1 levels and the presence of an IGFBP-3 proteolytic activity. Proteolytic activity that degrades IGFBP-3 specifically appears in the circulation after major surgery *(185)* and in severe catabolic states *(186)*. The decreased affinity for IGF-I caused by the enzymatic alteration of IGFBP-3 is associated with increased free IGF-I *(195)*. This might increase the bioavailability of IGF-I for the tissues. Increases in IGFBP-2 and IGFBP-4 and decline in ALS levels are also observed *(186,196,197)*.

As a consequence of these changes, when the IGF binding by serum is evaluated by chromatography after the serum sample has been incubated with radiolabeled IGF-I, dietary restriction consistently causes a decrease in the 150-kDa complex and an increase in the small binding protein complex *(198,199)*. These changes might alter the transport of IGF-I across the endothelium and the bioavailability of IGF-I to the tissues.

4.2. Role of the Clearance of Circulating IGF-I

Because IGFBPs are responsible for transport of IGF-I in the circulation, nutrient-induced changes in the concentrations of the IGFBPs could alter the clearance of circulating IGF-I. Plasma IGF-I clearance is accelerated in situations where serum IGFBP-3 is decreased, for example, hypophysectomized *(200)* or pregnant rats *(184)*. By monitoring the decline of radioactivity in the circulation of rats injected with [^{125}I]-IGF-I, it has been shown that the clearance and the volume of distribution of [^{125}I]-IGF-I were increased in protein-restricted rats by 50% and 75%, respectively *(199)*. Pharmacokinetic analysis indicates that the accelerated clearance of IGF-I in protein-restricted rats is the result of more rapid distribution of IGF-I into tissues (shorter $t_{1/2}$) rather than a change in the elimination half-life ($t_{1/2}$). In fed rats, IGF-I is almost equally distributed between the 150-kDa and the 30-kDa binding protein complexes, whereas in protein-restricted rats, IGF-I is bound preferentially to IGFBPs in the 30-kDa complex *(199)*. Because the small IGFBP complexes are believed to facilitate the transport of IGF-I from serum to tissues, the preferential association of IGF-I with these IGFBPs in protein-restricted animals might allow faster transcapillary passage and distribution to tissues. Unlike the rat, clearance of radiolabeled IGF-I in fasted sheep is not enhanced. This could result from species differences, or it could indicate that only chronic or a more specific dietary restriction affect clearance and distribution of IGF-I. Despite the rapid decline in circulating IGF-I after LPS injection, pharmacokinetic analysis of blood [^{125}I]-IGF-I decay curves indicates that the half-time for whole blood clearance is not altered by LPS *(201)*.

4.3. Role of the Sensitivity to IGF-I

In addition to decreasing IGF-I production, dietary restriction impairs the anabolic actions of IGF-I. When protein restricted or zinc-deficient rats were infused with IGF-I by osmotic minipump, carcass growth (body weight and tibial epiphyseal plate) was not stimulated, despite the normalization of serum IGF-I *(193,202)*. In contrast, growth of the spleen and kidney was enhanced. Similarly, IGF-I failed to increase cancellous and periosteal bone formation in protein-restricted rats, while exogenous IGF-I increased the bone formation rate in well-fed rats *(203)*. In rats fed parenterally with a limited supply of amino acids, anabolic effects of IGF-I on carcass lean mass were not observed, in contrast to visceral tissues *(204)*. Treatment of neonatal protein energy-deprived rats with IGF-I does not stimulate somatic growth. In contrast, erythroid precursors in bone marrow are increased, suggesting that the actions of IGF-I on growth and erythropoiesis are unrelated *(205)*. These results suggest that, in addition to its effects on IGF-I gene expression and IGF binding proteins, food deprivation causes organ-specific resistance to the anabolic properties of exogenous IGF-I. These observations support the concept that nutrient insufficiency can block the anabolic properties of IGF-I, but do not block other properties *(206–208)*.

Resistance to IGF-I during food deprivation occurs despite increased binding of IGF-I by tissues. Rats that are fasted for 48 h have increased IGF-I binding to stomach, lung, testes, and kidney, as reflected by alterations in the IGF-I receptor number and/or affinity *(123)*. Change in the abundance of the type 1 IGF receptor mRNA parallels the change in binding. Protein restriction also is associated with an increase of IGF-I binding to muscle *(209)*.

That nutrients can control the response to IGF-I directly has been observed in fibroblast cultures where zinc depletion inhibits the mitogenic action of IGF-I *(210)*. Although the interaction between anabolic action of IGF-I and amino acid availability has not been studied at the cellular level, several pieces of evidence indicate that crosstalk between the pathways activated by these stimuli are likely. For example, induction of the transcription factor CHOP by amino acid depletion requires the presence of IGF-I *(132)*. In muscle cells, a target for IGF-I action, amino acids activate p70 S6 kinase, an intermediate in the initiation of protein synthesis, in synergy with insulin *(211)*. Furthermore, both insulin and amino acids are required to stimulate protein synthesis and to inhibit protein degradation in muscle tissue *(212)*. If these observations can be extended to IGF-I, they suggest that amino acids might modulate the anabolic action of IGF-I, at least on protein metabolism.

The possibility that nutrients and hormones modulate the anabolic action of IGF-I has been investigated in humans. In energy restricted obese subjects, exogenous GH produced a twofold increase in serum IGF-I, accompanied by attenuation of nitrogen loss *(213)*. After a few weeks, however, resistance to the anabolic properties of IGF-I occurred. In similar experiments, infusion of IGF-I for 1 wk increased serum IGF-I concentrations fourfold and produced marked attenuation of the nitrogen wasting *(214)*. In volunteers made catabolic by glucocorticoid treatment, IGF-I infusion did not produce any significant decrease of proteolysis, suggesting that the anabolic action of IGF-I in humans may depend on the hormonal and nutritional environment *(215)*. GH administered together with IGF-I appears to function in a complementary fashion to promote protein anabolism *(216)*. There are several ways by which GH could produce nitrogen retention that are not fully replicated by infusion of IGF-I. For example, GH may alter concentrations of IGFBPs and modify the metabolism of carbohydrate or fat to facilitate IGF-I action.

The loss of anabolic response to IGF-I has been described in catabolic states, such as AIDS *(217)*, sepsis *(218)*, and uremia *(219)*. In uremia, resistance is caused by a postreceptor defect characterized by inhibition of the autophosphorylation of the type 1 IGF receptor (IGF-1R) β-subunit and IRS-1 *(220)*. Although perturbed IGFBPs in chronic renal failure may play an important role in altering IGF-I storage and delivery to tissues, IGF-I analogs with low affinity to IGFBPs fail to obliterate this IGF-I resistance *(220)*. In addition, malnutrition and acidosis have been excluded as mediators of the IGF-I resistance of uremic rats *(220)*. In more severe catabolic states, such as sepsis, the anticatabolic action of IGF-I can also be blunted. In rats made septic by cecal ligature and puncture, IGF-I failed to inhibit muscle proteolysis, despite the suppression of the gene expression of several components of the ubiquitin-proteasome proteolytic pathway *(221)*. However, IGF-I retained its antiproteolytic action in burned rats *(222)*. Careful dissection of the factors controlling the anabolic actions of IGF-I will need to be performed.

5. SUMMARY AND CONCLUSIONS

Nutrition is one of the principal regulators of circulating IGF-I.

- In humans, serum IGF-I concentrations are markedly reduced by energy and/or protein deprivation.
- Both energy and proteins are critical in the regulation of serum IGF-I concentrations. After fasting, optimal intake of both energy and protein is necessary for the restoration of circulating IGF-I, but energy may be somewhat more important than protein in this regard. While a low intake of protein is able to increase IGF-I in presence of adequate

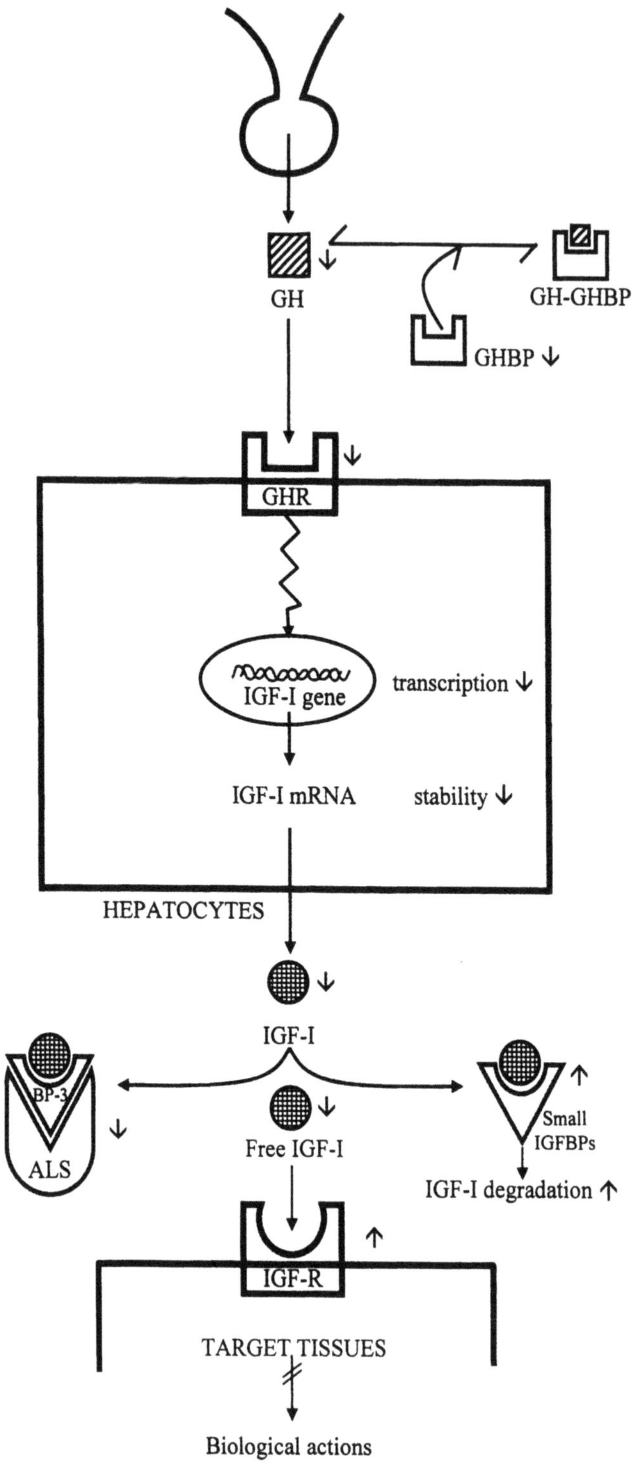

Fig. 3. Changes in IGF-I system induced by food deprivation. GH, growth hormone; GHBP, growth hormone binding protein; GHR, growth hormone receptor; ALS, acid-labile subunit; IGF-R, insulin-like growth factor receptors; IGFBP, IGF-binding proteins; BP-3, IGF-binding protein-3.

energy, there is a threshold requirement of energy below which optimal protein intake fails to raise IGF-I after fasting.

- When energy intake is severely reduced, the carbohydrate content of the diet is a major determinant of IGF-I responsiveness to GH.
- The content of essential amino acids in the diet is also critical for the optimal restoration of IGF-I after fasting.

Many mechanisms are involved in the nutritional regulation of IGF-I (Fig. 3).

- Decline of serum IGF-I during dietary restriction is independent of the diet-induced alterations in pituitary GH secretion.
- The role of liver GH receptors is dependent of the severity of the nutritional insult. In severe dietary restriction (fasting), a marked decrease of the number of somatogenic receptors suggests that a receptor defect is involved in the decline of circulating IGF-I. In contrast, in less severe forms of dietary restriction (protein restriction), the decline of IGF-I results from a postreceptor defect in GH action at the hepatic level.
- Nutritional deprivation decreases hepatic IGF-I production by diminishing IGF-I gene expression.
- Decline in IGF-I gene expression results from both transcriptional and post-transcriptional mechanisms.
- Decline in IGF-I gene expression is mainly caused by nutrient deficiency, and less importantly by nutritionally induced changes in hormones (insulin, T3).
- Diet restriction also increases the clearance and degradation of serum IGF-I through changes in the levels of circulating insulin-like growth factor-binding proteins (IGFBPs).
- Finally, nutrients may also control the biological action of IGF-I, either directly or indirectly through changes in IGFBPs.

GH resistance with decreased IGF-I production is also present in situations characterized by catabolic stress.

- Proinflammatory cytokines and glucocorticoids probably mediate the decreased IGF-I production in these situations.
- The molecular mechanisms leading to the decline of IGF-I seem to be similar to those operational in food deprivation.
- As with nutrients, these hormonal factors can control the anabolic action of IGF-I, in particular on skeletal muscle.

REFERENCES

1. Haymond MW, Mauras N. The rationale for the use of recombinant human growth hormone and insulin-like growth factor-I for catabolic conditions in humans. Horm Res 1996;46:202–207.
2. Frost RA, Fuhrer J, Steigbigel R, Mariuz P, Lang CH, Gelato MC. Wasting in the acquired immune deficiency syndrome is associated with multiple defects in the serum insulin-like growth factor system. Clin Endocrinol (Oxf) 1996;44:501–514.
3. Clemmons DR, Klibanski A, Underwood LE, McArthur JW, Ridgway EC, Beitins IZ, et al. Reduction of plasma immunoreactive somatomedin-C during fasting in humans. J Clin Endocrinol Metab 1981;53:1247–1250.
4. Thissen JP, Ketelslegers JM, Underwood LE. Nutritional regulation of the insulin-like growth factors. Endocr Rev 1994;15:80–101.
5. Argente J, Caballo N, Barrios V, Munoz MT, Pozo J, Chowen JA, et al. Multiple endocrine abnormalities of the growth hormone and insulin-like growth factor axis in patients with anorexia nervosa: effect of short- and long-term weight recuperation. J Clin Endocrinol Metab 1997;82:2084–2092.

6. Chu LW, Lam KSL, Tam SCF, Hu WJHC, Hui SL, Chiu A, et al. A randomized controlled trial of low-dose recombinant human growth hormone in the treatment of malnourished elderly medical patients. J Clin Endocrinol Metab 2001;86:1913–1920.
7. Ross R, Miell J, Freeman E, Jones J, Matthews D, Prece M, et al. Critically ill patients have high basal growth hormone levels with attenuated oscillatory activity associated with low levels of insulin-like growth factor-I. Clin Endocrinol (Oxf) 1991;35:47–54.
8. Isley WL, Underwood LE, Clemmons DR. Dietary components that regulate serum somatomedin-C concentrations in humans. J Clin Invest 1983;71:175–182.
9. Isley WL, Underwood LE, Clemmons DR. Changes in plasma somatomedin-C in reponse to ingestion of diets with variable protein and energy content. JPEN 1984;8:407–411.
10. Snyder DK, Clemmons DR, Underwood LE. Dietary carbohydrate content determines responsiveness to growth hormone in energy-restricted humans. J Clin Endocrinol Metab 1989;69:745–752.
11. Clemmons DR, Seek MM, Underwood LE. Supplemental essential aminoacids augment the somatomedin-C/insulin-like growth factor-I response to refeeding after fasting. Metabolism 1985;34:391–395.
12. Tannenbaum GS, Rorstad O, Brazeau P. Effects of prolonged food deprivation on the ultradian growth hormone rhythm and immunoreactive somatostatin tissue levels in the rat. Endocrinology 1979;104:1733–1738.
13. Ho KY, Veldhuis JD, Johnson ML, Furlanetto R, Evans WS, Alberti KGMM, et al. Fasting enhances growth hormone secretion and amplifies the complex rhythms of growth hormone secretion in man. J Clin Invest 1988;81:968–975.
14. Tannenbaum GS, Ling N. The interrelationship of growth hormone (GH)-releasing factor and somatostatin in generation of the ultradian rhythm of GH secretion. Endocrinology 1984;115:1952–1957.
15. Tannenbaum GS, Epelbaum J, Colle E, Brazeau P, Martin JB. Antiserum to somatostatin reverses starvation-induced inhibition of growth hormone but not insulin secretion. Endocrinology 1978;102:1909–1914.
16. Bruno JF, Olchovsky D, White JD, Leidy JW, Song J, Berelowitz M. Influence of food deprivation in rat on hypothalamic expression of growth hormone-releasing factor and somatostatin. Endocrinology 1990;127:2111–2116.
17. Wu V, Sumii K, Tari A, Sumii M, Walsh JH. Regulation of rat antral gastrin and somatostatin gene expression during starvation and after refeeeding. Gastroenterology 1991;101:1552–1558.
18. Katakami H, Downs TR, Frohman LA. Inhibitory effect of hypothalamic medial preoptic area somatostatin on growth hormone-releasing factor in the rat. Endocrinology 1988;123:1103–1109.
19. Harel Z, Tannenbaum GS. Dietary protein restriction impairs both spontaneous and growth hormone-releasing factor-stimulated growth hormone release in the rat. Endocrinology 1993;133:1035–1043.
20. Bruno JF, Song J, Berelowitz M. Regulation of rat hypothalamic preprogrowth hormone-releasing factor messenger ribonucleic acid by dietary protein. Endocrinology 1991;129:1226–1232.
21. Pombo M, Pombo CM, Astorga R, Cordido F , Popovic V, Garcia-Mayor RV, et al. Regulation of growth hormone secretion by signals produced by the adipose tissue. J Endocrinol Invest 1999;22(5 Suppl):22–26.
22. Palacio AC, Perez BF, Santos JL, Schlesinger L, Monckeberg F. Leptin levels and IgF-binding proteins in malnourished children: Effect of weight gain. Nutrition 2002;18:17–19.
23. Maccario M, Aimaretti G, Corneli G, Gauna C, Grottoli S, Bidlingmaier M et al. Short-term fasting abolishes the sex-related difference in GH and leptin secretion in humans. Am J Physiol Endocrinol Metab 2000;279:E411–E416.
24. Soliman AT, ElZalabany MM, Salama M, Ansari BM. Serum leptin concentrations during severe protein-energy malnutrition: correlation with growth parameters and endocrine function. Metabolism 2000;49:819–825.
25. Carro E, Se-aris R, Considine RV, Casanueva FF, Dieguez C. Regulation of in vivo growth hormone secretion by leptin. Endocrinology 1997;138:2203–2206.
26. Vuagnat BAM, Pierroz DD, Lalaoui M, Englaro P, Pralong FP, Blum WF, et al. Evidence for a leptin-neuropeptide Y axis for the regulation of growth hormone secretion in the rat. Neuroendocrinology 1998;67:291–300.
27. LaPaglia N, Steiner J, Kirsteins L, Emanuele M, Emanuele N. Leptin alters the response of the growth hormone releasing factor growth hormone insulin-like growth factor-I axis to fasting. J Endocrinol 1998;159:79–83.

28. Tannenbaum GS, Gurd W, Lapointe M. Leptin is a potent stimulator of spontaneous pulsatile growth hormone (GH) secretion and the GH response to GH-releasing hormone. Endocrinology 1998;139:3871–3875.
29. Quintela M, Senaris R, Heiman ML, Casanueva FF, Dieguez C. Leptin inhibits in vitro hypothalamic somatostatin secretion and somatostatin mRNA levels. Endocrinology 1997;138:5641–5644.
30. Baratta M, Saleri R, Mainardi GL, Valle D, Giustina A, Tamanini C. Leptin regulates GH gene expression and secretion and nitric oxide production in pig pituitary cells. Endocrinology 2002;143:551–557.
31. Horvath TL, Diano S, Sotonyi P, Heiman M, Tschöp M. Minireview: Ghrelin and the regulation of energy balance-A hypothalamic perspective. Endocrinology 2001;142:4163–4169.
32. Lee HM, Wang GY, Englander EW, Kojima M, Greeley GH, Jr. Ghrelin, a new gastrointestinal endocrine peptide that stimulates insulin secretion: enteric distribution, ontogeny, influence of endocrine, and dietary manipulations. Endocrinology 2002;143:185–190.
33. Kojima M, Hosoda H, Matsuo H, Kangawa K . Ghrelin: discovery of the natural endogenous ligand for the growth hormone secretagogue receptor. Trends in Endocrinology and Metabolism 2001;12:118–122.
34. Samuels HH, Horwitz ZD, Stanley F, Casanova J, Shapiro LE. Thyroid hormone controls glucocorticoid action in cultured GH1 cells. Nature 1977;268:254–257.
35. Yanagisawa M, Fukasawa N, Hase K, Sakurai S, Sakatsume Y, Iitaka M, et al. The effect of triiodothyronine replacement on the pituitary growth hormone gene expression in the fasting rat. 73th Endocrine Society Meeting abstract #202, 1991.
36. Bedo G, Santisteban P, Aranda A. Retinoic acid regulates growth hormone gene expression. Nature 1989;339:231–234.
37. Morita S, Fernandez-Mejia C, Melmed S. Retinoic acid selectively stimulates growth hormone secretion and messenger ribonucleic acid levels in rat pituitary cells. Endocrinology 1989;124:2052–2056.
38. Peisen JN, McDonnell KJ, Mulroney SE, Lumpkin MD. Endotoxin-induced suppression of the somatotropic axis is mediated by interleukin-1beta and corticotrophin-releasing factor in the juvenile rat. Endocrinology 1995;136:3378–3390.
39. Phillips LS, Young HS. Nutrition and somatomedin. I. Effect of fasting and refeeding on serum somatomedin activity and cartilage growth activity in rats. Endocrinology 1976;99:304–314.
40. Takano K, Hizuka N, Kawai K, Shizume K. Effect of growth hormone and nutrition on the level of somatomedin A in the rat. Acta Endocrinol (Copenh) 1978;87:485–494.
41. Shapiro B, Pimstone BL. Sulphation factor (somatomedin activity) in experimental protein malnutrition in the rat. J Endocrinol 1978;77:233–240.
42. Maes M, Amand Y, Underwood LE, Maiter D, Ketelslegers JM. Decreased serum insulin-like growth factor-I response to growth hormone in hypophysectomized rats fed a low protein diet: evidence for a postreceptor defect. Acta Endocrinol (Copenh) 1988;117:320–326.
43. Thissen JP, Triest S, Underwood LE, Maes M, Ketelslegers JM. Divergent responses of serum insulin-like growth factor-I and liver growth hormone (GH) receptors to exogenous GH in protein-restricted rats. Endocrinology 1990;126:908–913.
44. Grant DB, Hambley J, Becker D, Pimstone BL. Reduced sulphation factor in undernourished children. Arch Dis Child 1973;48:596–600.
45. Soliman AT, Hassan AEI, Aref MK, Hintz RL, Rosenfeld RG, Rogol AD. Serum Insulin-like growth factor I and II concentrations and growth hormone and insulin responses to arginine infusion in children with protein-energy malnutrition before and after nutritional rehabilitation. Pediatr Res 1986;20:1122–1130.
46. Schwander JC, Hauri C, Zapf J, Froesch ER. Synthesis and secretion of insulin-like growth factor and its binding protein by the perfused rat liver: dependence on growth hormone status. Endocrinology 1983;113:297–305.
47. Sjögren K, Liu JL, Blad K, Skrtic S, Vidal O, Wallenius V, et al. Liver-derived insulin-like growth factor I (IGF-I) is the principal source of IGF-I in blood but is not required for postnatal body growth in mice. Proc Natl Acad Sci USA 1999;96:7088–7092.
48. Maes M, Underwood LE, Ketelslegers JM. Plasma somatomedin-C in fasted and refed rats: close relationship with changes in liver somatogenic but not lactogenic binding sites. J Endocrinol 1983;97:243–252.
49. Mulumba N, Massa G, Ketelslegers JM, Maes M. Ontogeny and nutritional regulation of the serum growth hormone binding protein in the rat. Acta Endocrinol (Copenh) 1991;125:409–415.

50. Hochberg Z, Hertz P, Colin V, Ish-Shalom S, Yeshurun D, Youdim MBH et al. The distal axis of growth hormone (GH) in nutritional disorders: GH-binding protein, insulin-like growth factor-I (IGF-I), and IGF- I receptors in obesity and anorexia nervosa. Metabolism 1992;41:106–112.
51. Schwartzbauer G, Menon RK. Regulation of growth hormone receptor gene expression. Mol Genet Metab 1998;63:243–253.
52. Bornfeldt KE, Arnqvist HJ, Enberg B, Mathews LS, Norstedt G. Regulation of insulin-like growth factor-I and growth hormone receptor gene expression by diabetes and nutritional state in rat tissues. J Endocrinol 1989;122:651–656.
53. Straus DS, Takemoto CD. Effect of fasting on insulin-like growth factor-I and growth hormone receptor mRNA levels and IGF-I gene transcription in rat liver. Mol Endocrinol 1990;4:91–100.
54. Gabrielsson BG, Carmignac DF, Flavell DM, Robinson ICAF. Steroid regulation of growth hormone (GH) receptor and GH-binding protein messenger ribonucleic acids in the rat. Endocrinology 1995;136:209–217.
55. Beauloye V, Ketelslegers J-M, Moreau B, Thissen J-P. Dexamethasone inhibits both growth hormone (GH)-induction of insulin-like growth factor-I(IGF-I) mRNA and GH receptor (GHR) mRNA levels in rat primary cultured hepatocytes. Growth Hormone IGF Res 1999;9:205–211.
56. Dauncey MJ, Burton KA, White P, Harrison AP, Gilmour RS, Duchamp C et al. Nutritional regulation of growth hormone receptor gene expression. FASEB J 1994;8:81–88.
57. Romero GS, Stephan DA, Sperling MA, Menon RK. Distinct sexual dimorphism in the effect of hypothyroidism on the expression of the growth hormone receptor and growth hormone- binding protein gene in rat liver. Horm Res 1996;45:273–278.
58. Mullis PE, Eblé A, Marti U, Bürgi U, Postel-Vinay MC. Regulation of human growth hormone receptor gene transcription by triiodothyronine (T3). Mol Cell Endocrinol 1999;147:17–25.
59. Menon RK, Stephan DA, Rao RH, Shen-Orr Z, Downs LS, Jr., Roberts CT, Jr., et al. Tissue-specific regulation of the growth hormone receptor gene in streptozocin-induced diabetes in the rat. J Endocrinol 1994;142:453–462.
60. Maes M, Ketelslegers JM, Underwood LE. Low plasma somatomedin-C in streptozotocin-induced diabetes mellitus: correlation with changes in somatogenic and lactogenic liver binding sites. Diabetes 1983;32:1060–1069.
61. Leung KC, Doyle N, Ballesteros M, Waters MJ, Ho KKY. Insulin regulation of human hepatic growth hormone receptors: Divergent effects on biosynthesis and surface translocation. J Clin Endocrinol Metab 2000;85:4712–4720.
62. Niimi S, Hayakawa T, Tanaka A, Ichihara A. Glucose regulation of growth hormone receptors in primary cultured rat hepatocytes. Endocrinology 1991;129:2734–2739.
63. Brameld JM, Gilmour RS, Buttery PJ. Glucose and amino acids interact with hormones to control expression of insulin-like growth factor-I and growth hormone receptor mRNA in cultured pig hepatocytes. J Nutr 1999;129:1298–1306.
64. Shuto Y, Nakano T, Sanno N, Domoto H, Sugihara H, Wakabayashi I. Clinical case seminar—Reduced growth hormone receptor messenger ribonucleic acid in an aged man with chronic malnutrition and growth hormone resistance. J Clin Endocrinol Metab 1999;84:2320–2323.
65. Hermansson M, Wickelgren RB, Hammarqvist F, Bjarnason R, Wennström I, Carlsson B, et al. Measurement of human growth hormone receptor messenger ribonucleic acid by a quantitative polymerase chain reaction- based assay: Demonstration of reduced expression after elective surgery. J Clin Endocrinol Metab 1997;82:421–428.
66. Ninh NX, Maiter D, Lause P, Chrzanowska B, Underwood LE, Ketelslegers J-M et al. Continuous administration of growth hormone (GH) does not prevent the decrease of IGF-I gene expression in zinc-deprived rats despite normalization of liver GH binding. Growth Regul 1997;7:1–8.
67. Tonshoff B, Eden S, Weiser E, Carlsson B, Robinson IC, Blum WF et al. Reduced hepatic growth hormone (GH) receptor gene expression and increased plasma GH binding protein in experimental uremia. Kidney Int 1994;45:1085–1092.
68. Defalque D, Brandt N, Ketelslegers JM, Thissen JP. GH insensitivity induced by endotoxin injection is associated with decreased liver GH receptors. Am J Physiol 1999;276:E565–E572.
69. Fliesen T, Maiter D, Gerard G, Underwood LE, Maes M, Ketelslegers J-M. Reduction of serum insulin-like growth factor-I by dietary protein restriciton is age dependent. Pediatr Res 1989;26:415–419.

70. Thissen JP, Triest S, Maes M, Underwood LE, Ketelslegers JM. The decreased plasma concentrations of insulin-like growth factor-I in protein-restricted rats is not due to decreased number of growth hormone receptors on isolated hepatocytes. J Endocrinol 1990;124:159–165.
71. Oster MH, Fielder PJ, Levin N, Cronin MJ. Adaptation of the growth hormone and insulin-like growth factor- I axis to chronic and severe calorie or protein malnutrition. J Clin Invest 1995;95:2258–2265.
72. Phillips LS, Goldstein S, Pao CI. Nutrition and somatomedin XXVI. Molecular regulation of IGF-I by insulin in cultured rat hepatocytes. Diabetes 1991;40:1525–1530.
73. Thissen JP, Pucilowska J, Underwood LE. Differential regulation of IGF-I and IGFBP-1 mRNAs by amino acid availability and growth hormone in rat hepatocyte primary culture. Endocrinology 1994;134:1570–1576.
74. Beauloye V, Willems B, de C, V, Frank SJ, Edery M, Thissen JP. Impairment of liver GH receptor signaling by fasting. Endocrinology 2002;143:792–800.
75. Davey HW, Xie T, McLachlan MJ, Wilkins RJ, Waxman DJ, Grattan DR. STAT5b is required for GH-induced liver *Igf*-I gene expression. Endocrinology 2001;142:3836–3841.
76. Nicholson SE, Hilton DJ. The SOCS proteins: a new family of negative regulators of signal transduction. J Leukocyte Biol 1998;63:665–668.
77. Hansen JA, Lindberg K, Hilton DJ, Nielsen JH, Billestrup N. Mechanism of inhibition of growth hormone receptor signaling by suppressor of cytokine signaling proteins. Mol Endocrinol 1999;13:1832–1843.
78. Schaefer F, Chen Y, Tsao T, Nouri P, Rabkin R. Impaired JAK-STAT signal transduction contributes to growth hormone resistance in chronic uremia. J Clin Invest 2001;108:467–475.
79. Mao YL, Ling PR, Fitzgibbons TP, McCowen KC, Frick GP, Bistrian BR et al. Endotoxin-induced inhibition of growth hormone receptor signaling in rat liver in vivo. Endocrinology 1999;140:5505–5515.
80. Phillips LS, Young HS. Nutrition and somatomedin. II. Serum somatomedin activity and cartilage growth activity in streptozotocin-diabetic rats. Diabetes 1976;25:516–527.
81. Scott CD, Baxter RC. Production of insulin-like growth factor-I and its binding protein in rat hepatocytes cultured from diabetic and insulin- treated diabetic rats. Endocrinology 1986;119:2346–2352.
82. Baxter RC, Bryson JM, Turtle JR. Somatogenic receptors of rat liver: regulation by insulin. Endocrinology 1980;107:1176–1181.
83. Tollet P, Enberg B, Mode A. Growth hormone (GH) regulation of cytochrome P-450IIC12, Insulin-like growth factor-I (IGF-I), and GH receptor messenger RNA expression in primary rat hepatocytes: a hormonal interplay with insulin, IGF-I, and thyroid hormone. Mol Endocrinol 1990;4:1934–1942.
84. Maes M, Underwood LE, Ketelslegers J-M. Low serum somatomedin-C in insulin-dependent diabetes: evidence for a postreceptor mechanism. Endocrinology 1986;118:377–382.
85. Johnson TR, Blossey BK, Denko CW, Ilan J. Expression of insulin-like growth factor-I in cultured rat hepatocytes: effects of insulin and growth hormone. Mol Endocrinol 1989;3:580–587.
86. Boni-Schnetzler M, Schmid C, Meier PJ, Froesch ER. Insulin regulates insulin-like growth factor I mRNA in rat hepatocytes. Am J Physiol 1991;260:E846–E851.
87. Houston B, O'Neill IE. Insulin and growth hormone act synergistically to stimulate insulin-like growth factor-I production by cultured chicken hepatocytes. J Endocrinol 1991;128:389–393.
88. Pao CI, Farmer PK, Begovic S, Villafuerte BC, Wu G, Robertson DG, et al. Regulation of Insulin-like growth factor-I (IGF-I) and IGF- binding protein-1 gene transcription by hormones and amino acids in rat hepatocytes. Mol Endocrinol 1993;7:1561–1568.
89. Goya L, De la Puente A, Ramos S, Mart'n MA, Escrivá' F, Alvarez C, et al. Regulation of IGF-I and -II by insulin in primary cultures of fetal rat hepatocytes. Endocrinology 2001;142:5089–5096.
90. Maiter D, Fliesen T, Underwood LE, Maes M, Gerard G, Davenport ML, et al. Dietary protein restriction decreases insulin-like growth factor I independent of insulin and liver growth hormone binding. Endocrinology 1989;124:2604–2611.
91. Caufriez A, Golstein J, Lebrun P, Herchuelz A, Furlanetto R, Copinschi G. Relations between immunoreactive somatomedin-C, insulin and T3 patterns during fasting in obese subjects. Clin Endocrinol (Oxf) 1984;20:65–70.
92. Glas AR, Mellitt R, Burman KD, et al. Serum triiodothyronine in undernourished rats: dependence on dietary composition rather than total calorie or protein intake. Endocrinology 1978;102:1925–1928.

93. Burstein PJ, Draznin B, Johnson CJ, Schalch DS. The effect of hypothyroidism on growth, serum growth hormone, the growth hormone-dependent somatomedin, insulin-like growth factor, and its carrier protein in rats. Endocrinology 1979;104:1107–1111.
94. Harakawa S, Yamashita S, Tobinaga T, Matsuo K, Hirayu H, Izumi M, et al. In vivo regulation of hepatic insulin-like growth factor-I messenger ribonucleic acids with thyroid hormone. Endocrinol Japon 1990;37:205–211.
95. Evans RM, Birnberg NC, Rosenfeld MG. Glucocorticoid and thyroid hormones transcriptionally regulate growth hormone gene expression. Proc Natl Acad Sci USA 1982;79:7659–7663.
96. Wolf M, Ingbar SH, Moses AC. Thyroid hormone and growth hormone interact to regulate insulin-like growth factor-I messenger ribonucleic acid and circulating levels in the rat. Endocrinology 1989;125:2905–2914.
97. keda T, Fujiyama K, Hoshino T, Takeuchi T, Mashiba H, Tominaga M. Possible role of thyroid hormone in decreased somatomedin-C levels in diabetic and starved rats. Ann Nutr Metab 1990;34:8–12.
98. Luo J, Murphy LJ. Dexamethasone inhibits growth hormone induction of insulin-like growth factor-I messenger ribonucleic acid (mRNA) in hypophysectomized rats and reduces IGF-I mRNA abundance in the intact rat. Endocrinology 1989;125:165–171.
99. Jux C, Leiber K, Hügel U, Blum W, Ohlsson C, Klaus G, et al. Dexamethasone impairs growth hormone (GH)-stimulated growth by suppression of local insulin-like growth factor (IGF)-I production and expression of GH- and IGF-I-receptor in cultured rat chondrocytes. Endocrinology 1998;139:3296–3305.
100. King APJ, Carter-Su C. Dexamethasone-induced antagonism of growth hormone (GH) action by down-regulation of GH binding in 3T3–F442A fibroblasts. Endocrinology 1995;136:4796–4803.
101. Rodgers BD, Lau AOT, Nicoll CS. Hypophysectomy or adrenalectomy of rats with insulin-dependent diabetes mellitus partially restores their responsiveness to growth hormone. Proc Soc Exp Biol Med 1994;207:220–226.
102. Bryson JM, Baxter RC. Adrenal involvement in the diabetes-induced loss of Growth Hormone and Prolactin receptors in the livers of female rats. Diabetologia 1986;29:106–111.
103. Unterman TG, Jentel JJ, Oehler DT, Lacson RG, Hofert JF. Effects of glucocorticoids on circulating levels and hepatic expression of insulin-like growth factor (IGF)-binding proteins and IGF-I in the adrenalectomized streptozotocin-diabetic rat. Endocrinology 1993;133(6):2531–2539.
104. Fan J, Char D, Bagby GJ, Gelato MC, Lang CH. Regulation of insulin-like growth factor- I (IGF-I) and IGF binding proteins by tumor necrosis factor. Am J Physiol 1995;269:R1204–R1212.
105. Lang CH, Fan J, Cooney R, Vary TC. IL-1 receptor antagonist attenuates sepsis-induced alterations in the IGF system and protein synthesis. Am J Physiol Endocrinol Metab 1996;270:E430–E437.
106. Thissen JP, Verniers J. Inhibition by interleukin-1β and tumor necrosis factor-a of the insulin-like growth factor I messenger ribonucleic acid response to growth hormone in rat hepatocyte primary culture. Endocrinology 1997;138:1078–1084.
107. Maniar S, Kleinknecht C, Zhou X, Motel V, Yvert JP, Dechaux M. Growth hormone action is blunted by acidosis in experimental uremia or acid load. Clin Nephrol 1996;46:72–76.
108. Bereket A, Wilson TA, Kolasa AJ, Fan J, Lang CH. Regulation of the insulin-like growth factor system by acute acidosis. Endocrinology 1996;137:2238–2245.
109. Harp JB, Goldstein S, Phillips LS. Molecular regulation of IGF-I by amino acid availability in cultured hepatocytes. Diabetes 1991;40:95–101.
110. Wheelhouse NM, Stubbs AK, Lomax MA, MacRae JC, Hazlerigg DG. Growth hormone and amino acid supply interact synergistically to control insulin-like growth factor-I production and gene expression in cultured ovine hepatocytes. J Endocrinol 1999;163:353–361.
111. Zhang JH, Chrysis D, Underwood LE. Reduction of hepatic insulin-like growth factor I (IGF-I) messenger ribonucleic acid (mRNA) during fasting is associated with diminished splicing of IGF-I pre-mRNA and decreased stability of cytoplasmic IGF-I mRNA. Endocrinology 1998;139:4523–4530.
112. Phillips LS, Huang S. Identification of an amino acid responsive element in the rat IGF-I gene. 10th International Congress of Endocrinology, June 12–15, 1966, San Francisco, CA.
113. Fafournoux P, Bruhat A, Jousse C. Amino acid regulation of gene expression. Biochem J 2000;351:1–12.
114. Dudek SM, Semenkovich CF. Essential amino acids regulate fatty acid synthase expression through an uncharged transfer RNA-dependent mechanism. J Biol Chem 1995;270:29323–29329.

115. Jousse C, Bruhat A, Ferrara M, Fafournoux P. Physiological concentration of amino acids regulates insulin- like-growth-factor-binding protein 1 expression. Biochemical J 1998;334:147–153.
116. Takenaka A, Oki N, Takahashi SI, Noguchi T. Dietary restriction of single essential amino acids reduces plasma insulin-like growth factor-I (IGF-I) but does not affect plasma IGF-binding protein-1 in rats. J Nutr 2000;130:2910–2914.
117. Goya L, De la Puente A, Ramos S, Mart'n MA, Escrivá F, Pascual-Leone AM. Regulation of insulin-like growth factor-I and -II by glucose in primary cultures of fetal rat hepatocytes. J Biol Chem 1999;274:24633–24640.
118. Lefebvre D, Beckers F, Ketelslegers JM, Thissen JP. Zinc regulation of insulin-like growth factor-I (IGF-I), growth hormone receptor (GHR) and binding protein (GHBP) gene expression in rat cultured hepatocytes. Mol Cell Endocrinol 1998;138:127–136.
119. Emler CA, Schalch DS. Nutritionally-induced changes in hepatic insulin-like growth factor-I (IGF-I) gene expression in rats. Endocrinology 1987;120:832–834.
120. Moats-Staats BM, Brady JLJ, Underwood LE, D'Ercole AJ. Dietary protein restriction in artificially reared neonatal rats causes a reduction of insulin-like growth factor-I gene expression. Endocrinology 1989;125:2368–2374.
121. Straus DS, Takemoto CD. Specific decrease in liver insulin-like growth factor-I and brain insulin-like growth factor-II gene expression in energy- restricted rats. J Nutr 1991;121:1279–1286.
122. Thissen JP, Triest S, Moats-Staats BM, Underwood LE, Mauerhoff T, Maiter D et al. Evidence that pretranslational and translational defects decrease serum IGF-I concentrations during dietary protein restriction. Endocrinology 1991;129:429–435.
123. Lowe WL, Jr., Adamo M, Werner H, Roberts CT, Jr., LeRoith D. Regulation by fasting of rat insulin-like growth factor I and its receptor. Effects on gene expression and binding. J Clin Invest 1989;84:619–626.
124. Adamo M, Ben-Hur H, Roberts CT, Jr., LeRoith D. Regulation of start site usage in the leader exons of the rat insulin-like growth factor-I gene by development, fasting, and diabetes. Molecular Endocrinology 1991;5:1677–1686.
125. Zhang JH, Whitehead RE, Jr., Underwood LE. Effect of fasting on insulin-like growth factor (IGF)-IA and IGF-IB messenger ribonucleic acids and prehormones in rat liver. Endocrinology 1997;138:3112–3118.
126. Straus DS, Takemoto CD. Effect of dietary protein deprivation on insulin-like growth factor-I and -II, IGF binding protein-2, and serum albumin gene expression in rat. Endocrinology 1990;127:1849–1860.
127. Hayden JM, Marten NW, Burke EJ, Straus DS. The effect of fasting on insulin-like growth factor-I nuclear transcript abundance in rat liver. Endocrinology 1994;134:760–768.
128. Hayden JM, Straus DS. IGF-I and serine protease inhibitor 2.1 nuclear transcript abundance in rat liver during protein restriction. J Endocrinol 1995;145:397–407.
129. Marten NW, Sladek FM, Straus DS. Effect of dietary protein restriction on liver transcription factors. Biochem J 1996;317:361–370.
130. Marten NW, Hsiang CH, Yu L, Stollenwerk NS, Straus DS. Functional activity of hepatocyte nuclear factor-1 is specifically decreased in amino acid-limited hepatoma cells. Biochim Biophys Acta 1999;1447:160–174.
131. Marten NW, Burke EJ, Hayden JM, Straus DS. Effect of amino acid limitation on the expression of 19 genes in rat hepatoma cells. FASEB J 1994;8:538–544.
132. Entingh AJ, Law BK, Moses HL. Induction of the C/EBP homologous protein (CHOP) by amino acid deprivation requires insulin-like growth factor I, phosphatidylinositol 3-kinase, and mammalian target of rapamycin signaling. Endocrinology 2001;142:221–228.
133. Ron D, Habener JF. CHOP, a novel developmentally regulated nuclear protein that dimerizes with transcription factors C/EBP and LAP and functions as a dominant- negative inhibitor of gene transcription. Genes Dev 1992;6:439–453.
134. Nolten LA, van Schaik FM, Steenbergh PH, Sussenbach JS. Expression of the insulin-like growth factor I gene is stimulated by the liver-enriched transcription factors C/EBP alpha and LAP. Mol Endocrinol 1994;8:1636–1645.
135. Nolten LA, Steenbergh PH, Sussenbach JS. Hepatocyte nuclear factor 1 alpha activates promoter 1 of the human insulin-like growth factor I gene via two distinct binding sites. Mol Endocrinol 1995;9:1488–1499.

136. Zhu JL, Kaytor EN, Pao CI, Meng XP, Phillips LS. Involvement of Sp1 in the transcriptional regulation of the rat insulin- like growth factor-1 gene. Mol Cell Endocrinol 2000;164:205–218.
137. Leung-Pineda V, Kilberg MS. Role of Sp1 and Sp3 in the Nutrient-regulated Expression of the Human Asparagine Synthetase Gene. J Biol Chem 2002;277:16585–16591.
138. Hoyt EC, Hepler JE, Van Wyk JJ, Lund PK. Structural characterization of exon 6 of the rat IGF-I gene. DNA and cell biology 1992;11:433–441.
139. Klausner RD, Harford JB. Cis-trans models for post-transcriptional gene regulation. Science 1989;246:870–872.
140. Davenport ML, D'Ercole AJ, Underwood LE. Effect of maternal fasting on fetal growth, serum insulin-like growth factors (IGFs), and tissue IGF messenger ribonucleic acids. Endocrinology 1990;126:2062–2067.
141. Goldstein S, Harp JB, Phillips LS. Nutrition and Somatomedin XXII: molecular regulation of insulin-like growth factor-I during fasting and refeeding in rats. J Molecular Endocrinology 1991;6:33–43.
142. Katsumata M, Kawakami S, Kaji Y, Takada R, Dauncey MJ. Differential regulation of porcine hepatic IGF-I mRNA expression and plasma IGF-I concentration by a low lysine diet. J Nutr 2002;132:688–692.
143. Thissen JP, Underwood LE. Translational status of the Insulin-like growth factor-I mRNAS in liver of protein-restricted rats. J Endocrinol 1992;132:141–147.
144. VandeHaar M, Moats-Staats BM, Davenport ML, Walker JL, Ketelslegers JM, Sharma BK, et al. Reduced serum concentrations of insulin-like growth factor-I (IGF-I) in protein-restricted growing rats are accompanied by reduced IGF-I mRNA levels in liver and skeletal muscle. J Endocrinol 1991;130:305–312.
145. Naranjo WM, Yakar S, Sanchez-Gomez M, Perez AU, Setser J, LeRoith D. Protein calorie restriction affects nonhepatic igf-I production and the lymphoid system: studies using the liver-specific igf-I gene-deleted mouse model. Endocrinology 2002;143:2233–2241.
146. Hintz RL, Liu F. Demonstration of specific plasma protein binding for somatomedin. J Clin Endocrinol Metab 1977;45:988–995.
147. Kaufmann U, Zapf J, Torretti B, Froesch ER. Demonstration of a specific serum carrier protein of nonsuppressible insulin-like activity in vivo. J Clin Endocrinol Metab 1977;44:160–165.
148. Furlanetto RW, Underwood LE, Van Wyk JJ, D'Ercole AJ. Estimation of somatomedin-C levels in normals and patients with pituitary disease by radioimmunoassay. J Clin Invest 1977;60:648–657.
149. Jones JI, Clemmons DR. Insulin-like growth factors and their binding proteins: Biological actions. Endocr Rev 1995;16:3–34.
150. Elgin RG, Busby WHJ, Clemmons DR. An insulin-like growth factor (IGF) binding protein enhances the biologic response to IGF-I. Proc Natl Acad Sci USA 1987;84:3254–3258.
151. Blum WF, Jenne EW, Reppin F, Kietzmann K, Ranke MB, Bierich JR. Insulin-like growth factor I (IGF-I)-binding protein complex is a better mitogen than free IGF-I. Endocrinology 1989;125:766–772.
152. Ernst M, Rodan GA. Increased activity of insulin-like growth factor (IGF) in osteoblastic cells in the presence of growth hormone (GH): positive correlation with the presence of the GH-induced IGF-binding protein BP-3. Endocrinology 1990;127:807–814.
153. Burch WW, Correa J, Shively JE, Powell DR. The 25-kilodalton insulin-like growth factor (IGF)-binding protein inhibits both basal and IGF-I-mediated growth of chick embryo pelvic cartilage in vitro. J Clin Endocrinol Metab 1990;70:173–180.
154. Ross M, Francis GL, Szabo L, Wallace JC, Ballard FJ. Insulin-like growth factor (IGF)-binding proteins inhibit the biological activities of IGF-I and IGF-II but not des(1–3)IGF-I. Biochem J 1989;258:267–272.
155. De Mellow JS, Baxter RC. Growth hormone dependent insulin-like growth factor binding protein both inhibits and potentiates IGF-I stimulated DNA synthesis in skin fibroblasts. Biochem Biophys Res Commun 1988;156:199–204.
156. Frystyk J, Gronbæk H, Skjærbæk C, Flyvbjerg A, Orskov H, Baxter RC. Developmental changes in serum levels of free and total insulin- like growth factor I (IGF-I), IGF-Binding protein-1 and -3, and the acid-labile subunit in rats. Endocrinology 1998;139:4286–4292.
157. Binoux M, Hossenlopp P. Insulin-like growth factor (IGF) and IGF-binding proteins: comparison of human serum and lymph. J Clin Endocrinol Metab 1988;67:509–514.

158. Zapf J, Hauri C, Waldvogel M, Froesch ER. Acute metabolic effects and half-lives of intravenously administered insulinlike growth factors I and II in normal and hypophysectomized rats. J Clin Invest 1986;77:1768–1775.
159. Guler HP, Zapf J, Schmid C, Froesch ER . Insulin-like growth factor-I and II in healthy man. Acta Endocrinol (Copenh) 1989;121:753–758.
160. Frystyk J, Hussain M, Skjaerbaek C, Porksen N, Froesch ER, Orskov H. The pharmacokinetics of free insulin-like growth factor-I in healthy subjects. Growth Horm IGF Res 1999;9:150–156.
161. Bar RS, Clemmons DR, Boes M, Busby WH, Booth BA, Dake BL et al. Transcapillary permeability and subendothelial distribution of endothelial and amniotic fluid insulin-like growth factor binding proteins in the rat heart. Endocrinology 1990;127:1078–1086.
162. Katz LE, DeLeon DD, Zhao H, Jawad AF. Free and Total Insulin-Like Growth Factor (IGF)-I Levels Decline during Fasting: Relationships with Insulin and IGF-Binding Protein-1. J Clin Endocrinol Metab 2002;87:2978–2983.
163. Frystyk J, Grofte T, Skjaerbaek C, Orskov H. The effect of oral glucose on serum free insulin-like growth factor-I and -II in health adults. J Clin Endocrinol Metab 1997;82:3124–3127.
164. Oh Y, Muller HL, Pham H, Rosenfeld RG. Demonstration of receptors for insulin-like growth factor binding protein-3 on Hs578T human breast cancer cells. J Biol Chem 1993;268:26045–26048.
165. Hwa V, Oh Y, Rosenfeld RG. The insulin-like growth factor-binding protein (IGFBP) superfamily. Endocr Rev 1999;20:761–787.
166. Baxter RC, Martin JL. Radioimmunoassay of growth hormone-dependent insulinlike growth factor binding protein in human plasma. J Clin Invest 1986;78:1504–1512.
167. Baxter RC, Cowell CT. Diurnal rhythm of growth hormone-independent binding protein for insulin-like growth factors in human plasma. J Clin Endocrinol Metab 1987;65:432–440.
168. Busby WH, Snyder DK, Clemmons DR. Radioimmunoassay of a 26,000-dalton plasma insulin-like growth factor-binding protein: control by nutritional variables. J Clin Endocrinol Metab 1988;67:1225–1230.
169. Suikkari AM, Koivisto VA, Rutanen EM, Yki-Jarvinen H, Karonen SL, Seppala M. Insulin regulates the serum levels of low molecular weight insulin-like growth factor-binding protein. J Clin Endocrinol Metab 1988;66:266–272.
170. Conover CA, Butler PC, Wang M, Rizza RA, Lee PDK. Lack of growth hormone effect on insulin-associated suppression of insulin-like growth factor binding protein-1 in humans. Diabetes 1990;39:1251–1256.
171. Snyder DK, Clemmons DR. Insulin-dependent regulation of insulin-like growth factor- binding protein-1. J Clin Endocrinol Metab 1991;71:1632–1636.
172. Lewitt MS, Baxter RC. Inhibitors of glucose uptake stimulate the production of insulin- like growth factor-binding protein (IGFBP-1) by human fetal liver. Endocrinology 1990;126:1527–1533.
173. Bar RS, Boes M, Clemmons DR, Busby WH , Sandra A, Dake BL et al. Insulin differentially alters transcapillary movement of intravascular IGFBP-1, IGFBP-2 and endothelial cell IGF-binding proteins in the rat heart. Endocrinology 1990;127:497–499.
174. Clemmons DR, Snyder DK, Busby WH. Variables controlling the secretion of insulin-like growth factor binding protein-2 in normal human subjects. J Clin Endocrinol Metab 1991;73:727–733.
175. Orlowski CC, Brown AL, Ooi GT, Yang YWH, Tseng LYH, Rechler MM. Tissue, developmental, and metabolic regulation of messenger ribonucleic acid encoding a rat insulin-like growth factor-binding proteins. Endocrinology 1990;126:644–652.
176. Murphy LJ, Seneviratne C, Moreira P, Reid RE. Enhanced expression of insulin-like growth factor-binding protein-1 in the fasted rat: the effects of insulin and growth hormone administration. Endocrinology 1991;128:689–696.
177. Tseng LYH, Ooi GT, Brown AL, Straus DS, Rechler MM. Transcription of the insulin-like growth factor-binding protein-2 is increased in neonatal and fasted rat liver. Mol Endocrinol 1992;6:1195–1201.
178. Smith WJ, Underwood LE, Clemmons DR. Effects of caloric or protein restriction on insulin-like growth factor-I (IGF-I) and IGF-binding proteins in children and adults. J Clin Endocrinol Metab 1995;80:443–449.
179. Gallaher BW, Breier BH, Oliver MH, Harding JE, Gluckman PD. Ontogenic differences in the nutritional regulation of circulating IGF binding proteins in sheep plasma. Acta Endocrinol (Copenh) 1992;126:49–54.

180. Frystyk J, Delhanty PJD, Skjærbæk C, Baxter RC. Changes in the circulating IGF system during short-term fasting and refeeding in rats. Am J Physiol Endocrinol Metab 1999;277:E245–E252.
181. Baxter RC, Martin JL, Tyler MI, Howden MEH. Growth hormone-dependent insulin-like growth factor (IGF) binding protein from human plasma differs from other human IGF binding proteins. Biochem Biophys Res Commun 1986;139:1256–1261.
182. McCusker RH, Cohick WS, Busby WH, Clemmons DR. Evaluation of the developmental and nutritional changes in porcine IGFBP-1 and IGFBP-2 serum levels by immunoassay. Endocrinology 1991;129:2631–2638.
183. Donovan SM, Atilano LC, Hintz RL, Wilson DM, Rosenfeld RG. Differential regulation of the insulin-like growth factors (IGF- I and -II) and IGF binding proteins during malnutrition in the neonatal rat. Endocrinology 1991;129:149–157.
184. Davenport ML, Clemmons DR, Miles MV, Camacho-Hubner C, D'Ercole AJ, Underwood LE. Regulation of serum insulin-like growth factor I (IGF-I) and IGF binding proteins during rat pregnancy. Endocrinology 1990;127:1278–1286.
185. Davenport ML, Isley WL, Pucilowska JB, Pemberton LB, Lyman B, Underwood LE et al. Insulin-like growth factor binding protein-3 proteolytic activity is induced following elective surgery. J Clin Endocrinol Metab 1992;75:590–595.
186. Timmins AC, Cotterill AM, Hughes SCC, Holly JMP, Ross RJM, Blum W, et al. Critical illness is associated with low circulating concentrations of insulin-like growth factors-I and -II, alterations in insulin-like growth factor binding proteins, and induction of an insulin-like growth factor binding protein 3 protease. Crit Care Med 1996;24:1460–1466.
187. Stoving RK, Flyvbjerg A, Frystyk J, Fisker S, Hangaard J, Hansen-Nord M et al. Low serum levels of free and total insulin-like growth factor I (IGF-I) in patients with anorexia nervosa are not associated with increased IGF-binding protein-3 proteolysis. J Clin Endocrinol Metab 1999;84:1346–1350.
188. Dai J, Baxter RC. Regulation in vivo of the acid-labile subunit of the rat serum insulin-like growth factor-binding protein complex. Endocrinology 1994;135:2335–2341.
189. Oster MH, Levin N, Fielder PJ, Robinson ICAF, Baxter RC, Cronin MJ. Developmental differences in the IGF-I system response to severe and chronic calorie malnutrition. Am J Physiol Endocrinol Metab 1996;270:E646–E653.
190. Takenaka A, Mori M, Yamada S, Ohgane J , Takahashi SI, Noguchi T. Nutritional regulation of gene expression of insulin-like growth factor-binding proteins and the acid-labile subunit in various tissues of rats. J Endocrinol 1996;150:33–41.
191. Dai J, Scott CD, Baxter RC. Regulation of the acid-labile subunit of the insulin-like growth factor complex in cultured rat hepatocytes. Endocrinology 1994;135:1066–1072.
192. Bereket A, Wilson TA, Blethen SL, Sakurai Y, Herndon DN, Wolfe RR, et al. Regulation of the acid-labile subunit of the insulin-like growth factor ternary complex in patients with insulin-dependent diabetes mellitus and severe burns. Clin Endocrinol (Oxf) 1996;44:525–532.
193. Thissen JP, Underwood LE, Maiter D, Maes M, Clemmons DR, Ketelslegers JM. Failure of IGF-I infusion to promote growth in protein- restricted rats despite normalization of serum IGF-I concentrations. Endocrinology 1991;128:885–890.
194. Lemozy S, Pucilowska JB, Underwood LE. Reduction of insulin-like growth factor-I (IGF-I) in protein-restricted rats is associated with differential regulation of IGF- binding protein messenger ribonucleic acids in liver and kidney, and peptides in liver and serum. Endocrinology 1994;135:617–623.
195. Skjaerbaek C, Frystyk J, Orskov H, Kissmeyer-Nielsen P, Jensen MB, Laurberg S et al. Differential changes in free and total insulin-like growth factor I after major, elective abdominal surgery: the possible role of insulin- like growth factor-binding protein-3 proteolysis. J Clin Endocrinol Metab 1998;83:2445–2449.
196. Lang CH, Pollard V, Fan J, Traber LD, Traber DL, Frost RA, et al. Acute alterations in growth hormone insulin-like growth factor axis in humans injected with endotoxin. Am J Physiol Regul Integr Comp Physiol 1997;273:R371–R378.
197. Lang CH, Fan J, Frost RA, Gelato MC, Sakurai Y, Herndon DN et al. Regulation of the insulin-like growth factor system by insulin in burn patients. J Clin Endocrinol Metab 1996;81:2474–2480.
198. Takahashi S, Kajikawa M, Umezawa T, Takahashi SI, Kato H, Miura Y et al. Effect of dietary proteins on the plasma immunoreactive insulin- like growth factor-I/somatomedin-C concentrations in the rat. Br J Nutr 1990;63:521–534.

199. Thissen JP, Davenport ML, Pucilowska J, Miles MV, Underwood LE. Increased serum clearance and degradation of [125I]-labeled IGF- I in protein-restricted rats. Am J Physiol 1992;262:E406–E411.
200. Cohen KL, Nissley SP. The serum half-life of somatomedin activity: evidence for growth hormone dependence. Acta Endocrinol (Copenh) 1976;83:243–258.
201. Fan J, Char D, Kolasa AJ, Pan W, Maitra SR, Patlak CS et al. Alterations in hepatic production and peripheral clearance of IGF-I after endotoxin. Am J Physiol Endocrinol Metab 1995;269:E33–E42.
202. Ninh NX, Maiter D, Verniers J, Lause P , Ketelslegers JM, Thissen JP. Failure of exogenous IGF-I to restore normal growth in rats submitted to dietary zinc deprivation. J Endocrinol 1998;159:211–217.
203. Bourrin S, Ammann P, Bonjour JP, Rizzoli R. Dietary protein restriction lowers plasma insulin-like growth factor I (IGF-I), impairs cortical bone formation, and induces osteoblastic resistance to IGF-I in adult female rats. Endocrinology 2000;141:3149–3155.
204. Kee AJ, Baxter RC, Carlsson AR, Smith RC. Parenteral amino acid intake alters the anabolic actions of insulin- like growth factor I in rats. Am J Physiol 1999;277:E63–E72.
205. Philipps AF, Persson B, Hall K, Lake M , Skottner A, Sanengen T et al. The effects of biosynthetic insulin-like growth factor-I supplementation on somatic growth, maturation, and erythropoiesis on the neonatal rat. Pediatr Res 1988;23:298–305.
206. Hirschberg R, Kopple JD. Evidence that insulin-like growth factor-I increases renal plasma flow and glomerular filtration rate in fasted rats. J Clin Invest 1989;83:326–330.
207. Jacob R, Barrett E, Plewe G, Fagin KD, Sherwin RS. Acute effects of insulin-like growth factor-I on glucose and amino acid metabolism in the awake fasted rat. J Clin Invest 1989;83:1717–1723.
208. Tomas FM, Knowles SE, Owens PC, Read LC, Chandler CS, Gargowsky SE et al. Effects of full-length and truncated insulin-like growth factor- I on nitrogen balance and muscle protein metabolism in nitrogen- restricted rats. J Endocrinol 1991;128:97–105.
209. Dardevet D, Manin M, Balage M, Sornet C, Grizard J. Influence of low- and high-protein diets on insulin and insulin- like growth factor-I binding to skeletal muscle and liver in the growing rats. Br J Nutr 1991;65:47–60.
210. Lefebvre D, Boney CM, Ketelslegers JM, Thissen JP. Inhibition of insulin-like growth factor-I mitogenic action by zinc chelation is associated with a decreased mitogen-activated protein kinase activation in RAT-1 fibroblasts. FEBS Lett 1999;449:284–288.
211. Patti ME, Brambilla E, Luzi L, Landaker EJ, Kahn CR. Bidirectional modulation of insulin action by amino acids. J Clin Invest 1998;101:1519–1529.
212. Balage M, Sinaud S, Prod'homme M, Dardevet D, Vary TC, Kimball SR et al. Amino acids and insulin are both required to regulate assembly of the eIF4E.eIF4G complex in rat skeletal muscle. Am J Physiol Endocrinol Metab 2001;281:E565–E574.
213. Snyder DK, Clemmons DR, Underwood LE. Treatment of obese, diet-restricted subjects withg growth hormone for 11 weeks: effects of anabolism, lipolysis, and body composition. J Clin Endocrinol Metab 1988;67:54–61.
214. Clemmons DR, Smith-Banks A, Underwood LE. Reversal of diet-induced catabolism by infusion of recombinant Insulin-like growth factor-I (IGF-I) in humans. J Clin Endocrinol Metab 1992;75:234–238.
215. Mauras N, Beaufrere B. Recombinant human IGF-I enhances whole body protein anabolism and significantly diminishes the protein catabolic effect of prednisone in humans without a diabetogenic effect. J Clin Endocrinol Metab 1995;80:869–874.
216. Kupfer SR, Underwood LE, Baxter RC, Clemmons DR. Enhancement of the anabolic effects of growth hormone and insulin-like growth factor-I by use of both agent simultaneously. J Clin Invest 1993;91:391–396.
217. McNurlan MA, Garlick PJ, Steigbigel RT, DeCristofaro KA, Frost RA, Lang CH et al. Responsiveness of muscle protein synthesis to growth hormone administration in HIV-infected individuals declines with severity of disease. J Clin Invest 1997;100:2125–2132.
218. Vary TC, Dardevet D, Grizard J, Voisin L, Buffiere C, Denis P et al. Differential regulation of skeletal muscle protein turnover by insulin and IGF-I after bacteremia. Am J Physiol 1998;275:E584–E593.
219. Fouque D, Peng SC, Kopple JD. Impaired metabolic response to recombinant insulin-like growth factor-1 in dialysis patients. Kidney Int 1995;47:876–883.

220. Ding H, Gao XL, Hirschberg R, Vadgama JV, Kopple JD. Impaired actions of insulin-like growth factor 1 on protein Synthesis and degradation in skeletal muscle of rats with chronic renal failure. Evidence for a postreceptor defect. J Clin Invest 1996;97:1064–1075.
221. Fang CH, Li BG, Sun X, Hasselgren PO. Insulin-like growth factor I reduces ubiquitin and ubiquitin-conjugating enzyme gene expression but does not inhibit muscle proteolysis in septic rats. Endocrinology 2000;141:2743–2751.
222. Fang CH, Li BG, Wang JJ, Fischer JE, Hasselgren PO. Treatment of burned rats with insulin-like growth factor I inhibits the catabolic response in skeletal muscle. Am J Physiol Regul Integr Comp Physiol 1998;275:R1091–R1098.

3 Nutrition and IGF Proteins in Chronic Malnutrition and Critical Illness

Pei-Ra Ling and Bruce R. Bistrian

KEY POINTS

- The systemic inflammatory response found in severe stress, or its persistence as seen in chronic diseases, can cause a rapid or prolonged catabolic hypermetabolic condition leading to accelerated energy and nitrogen loss that cannot be compensated by dietary intake and results in protein energy malnutrition.
- The catabolic response to systemic inflammation is the consequence of multiple factors including increased levels of proinflammatory cytokines and catabolic hormones, decreased concentrations of anabolic hormones and growth factors such as IGFs, as well as tissue resistance to their effects. Although nutritional therapy has beneficial effects, adequate nutrition support alone cannot overcome the catabolic effects induced by severe illness.
- Cytokines reduce the levels of IGF-I and impair the action of IGF-I directly, as well as indirectly, by altering the IGFBPs.
- The most effective nutrition support for patients with conditions of acute or chronic systemic inflammation is actively being studied. Specific amino acids, omega-3-fatty acids, and antioxidant vitamins are examples of anabolic nutrition therapies that may, with anabolic hormone therapy, be effective in the management of disease-related malnutrition.

1. INTRODUCTION

Severe injury, infection, and other critical illnesses, such as AIDS, cancer, and many chronic diseases, cause profound metabolic changes in the host to support the injury response, generally characterized by increasing the catabolism of certain tissues such as muscle and fat to mobilize stored nutrients while decreasing nutrient availability for growth. Net loss of body protein and fat mass results in adults, and growth cessation occurs in children. During the acute phase of the systemic inflammatory response, enhanced catabolism of endogenous protein and fat serve to meet the suddenly increased energy and amino acid requirement that is vital for a successful outcome. However, the intensity of the systemic inflammatory response found in severe stress, or its persistence as seen in chronic diseases, can cause a rapid, or prolonged, catabolic and hypermetabolic condition, leading to the exhaustion of energy and protein reserves in both instances. If such accelerated energy and nitrogen loss cannot be compensated by enhanced dietary intake, protein energy malnutrition (PEM) results. It has been

From: *IGF and Nutrition in Health and Disease*
Edited by: M. S. Houston, J. M. P. Holly, and E. L. Feldman © Humana Press Inc., Totowa, NJ

reported that malnutrition is commonly observed both in hospitalized critically ill patients and patients with chronic diseases *(1–4)*. The unintentional loss of more than 10% of weight significantly contributes to the increased morbidity and mortality in critically ill patients *(5)*. Approximately two-thirds of patients who die with advanced cancer suffer from cancer cachexia. For this reason, investigations into nutritional and other anticatabolic therapy to blunt catabolism in such patients have been an important research interest for many years.

The catabolic response to severe illness is the consequence of multiple factors that arise as components of the systemic inflammatory response, including decreased nutrient intake, increased levels of cytokines and catabolic hormones, and decreased levels of anabolic hormones as well as tissue resistance to their effects. Although nutritional therapy has beneficial effects in these patients, adequate nutrition support alone cannot overcome the catabolic effects induced by severe illness *(6–8)*. The relative ineffectiveness of nutritional therapy under such conditions could be caused by the failure to modify the impact of endogenous catabolic and antianabolic factors associated with severe illness. New therapies, including anticytokine strategies and pharmacologic doses of anabolic hormones, particularly growth hormone, insulin-like growth factor, and anabolic steroids, are currently being investigated for their role in the prevention or amelioration of lean tissue loss during catabolic states. Previous chapters have extensively reviewed various aspects of IGF-I system under different physiological and pathological conditions. In this chapter, we will briefly review the mechanisms responsible for the development of protein energy malnutrition in critical illnesses, particularly the role of cytokines in protein malnutrition. Subsequently, attention will be focused on nutrition support in critical illness, including the optimal levels of energy and protein intake, the effects of omega-3 fatty acids, and the potential role of major anabolic hormones and vitamin and antioxidant supplementation for improvement in the efficacy of nutritional repletion in severe acute or chronic activation of the systemic inflammatory response.

2. CYTOKINES: MAJOR FACTORS CONTRIBUTING TO THE DEVELOPMENT OF MALNUTRITION

2.1. Effects of Cytokines on Protein Metabolism

It has been long appreciated that there is a catabolic nitrogen response to fever and infection *(9,10)*. Early studies demonstrated that factor(s) derived from white blood cells, originally termed leukocyte endogenous mediator, could be responsible for these responses *(11,12)*. Subsequently, a number of different peptides that share some of the actions under the general term leukocyte endogenous mediator have been identified. All of these proteins, a family with over 80 members and still growing, are called cytokines. Tumor necrosis factor (TNF), interleukin (IL)-1, and IL-6 are postulated as the three major cytokines responsible for wasting during critical illness *(13,14)*.

Over the past several years, evidence has accumulated that the levels of circulating TNF-α, IL-1, and IL-6 are elevated in critically burned patients and in patients with septic shock or severe sepsis *(15–18)*. The increased serum levels of these cytokines, particularly IL-6, can be a sensitive predictor of mortality in patients with septic shock *(19–23)*, cancer *(24)*, and some chronic diseases *(25,26)*, suggesting that these cytokines are major contributors to wasting in critical illness. In many chronic illnesses the evidence for the presence of a systemic inflammatory response often require the use of more sensitive measures such as serum levels of soluble TNF receptors *(27)* or acute phase proteins like C-reactive protein *(28,29)* because of the lower intensity of inflammation

Advances in recombinant technology have made it possible to investigate the roles of individual cytokine in wasting. In our laboratory, major proximal cytokines in recombinant form, IL-1β and TNF-α, alone and in combination, have been investigated for their effects on protein metabolism *(30)*. Studies using both acute and chronic infusion of IL-1β into rats and matched pair-fed controls demonstrated that IL-1 infusion at 20 μg/kg/d for 6 d caused weight loss and urinary nitrogen loss, reduction of plasma zinc concentration and increased energy expenditure *(31)*. In this study, dynamic protein metabolism was assessed by the continuous infusion of tracer. At a steady state, estimates of protein synthesis were calculated based on the incorporation of the tracer from the tissue free amino acid pool into the protein bound pool *(32–34)*. Protein breakdown was determined from the dilution of specific radioactivity in the tissue free amino acid pool relative to the plasma pool *(35,36)*. The algebraic sum of these isotopic estimates of protein synthesis and breakdown rates was in general agreement with independent assessment of tissue growth. The results showed that IL-1 significantly decreased the rate of protein synthesis in muscle and increased leucine release from skeletal muscle tissue as compared to control (saline infusion). Moreover, IL-1 significantly increased urinary 3-methylhistidine excretion, reflecting skeletal muscle protein catabolism *(31)*. Using the same tracer model, the effects of TNF (100 μg/kg/d) and IL-1 (20 μg/kg/d), either alone or in combination, on protein metabolism were also compared in rats after 6 d of infusion *(37)*. Both TNF and IL-1 significantly reduced food intake and caused weight loss, net nitrogen loss and skeletal muscle catabolism, whereas liver weight was increased. Isotopic study also showed that the significant changes in skeletal muscle and whole body protein catabolism were greater for both cytokine groups containing TNF (i.e., TNF and IL/TNF) compared with IL-1. Although both IL-1 and TNF have been demonstrated to participate in protein catabolism through decreases in expression of eukaryotic initiation factor-2 Bε (eIF-2Bε) *(38–40)*, these results suggest that there are different mechanisms for host wasting in response to IL-1 and TNF. For instance, it has been demonstrated that glucocorticoids *(41)*, and nuclear factor-kappaB (NF-κB) activation *(42)* are essential to mediate TNF-induced catabolism but not IL-1. However, both IL-1 and TNF induce anorexia, and the reduced food intake in human and animals will decrease the rate of protein synthesis and muscle growth. Therefore, by having a semistarved control group in both our studies, the effects of cytokines and/or food restriction on nitrogen loss and protein metabolism at the whole body level and in muscle could be identified. Our data showed that the effects of cytokines were independent from and additive to those resulting from semistarvation *(31,37)*. Other studies also demonstrated that pretreatment of rats with IL-6 for 6 h induced fever and increased the release of tyrosine and 3-methylhistidine in incubated extensor digitorum muscle in an ex vivo system, suggesting that IL-6 also augments muscle proteolysis *(43)*. However, it is not clear whether the proteolytic-inducing effects of IL-6 are direct or require the release of other mediators, such as TNF and IL-1.

The role of cytokines in wasting in critical illnesses is also confirmed by modifying the release and/or biological activity of cytokines using anticytokine antibodies or cytokine receptor antagonists. Blockade of IL-1 action by administration of IL-1 receptor antagonist (IL-1ra) to experimental animals prevents muscle proteolysis in response to endotoxin *(44)*. However, anticytokine antibodies and receptor antagonists are specific for an individual cytokine. Infusion of a single cytokine can stimulate the production of other cytokines in vivo whereas endotoxin or disease elicits the production of many cytokines. Thus, one single anticytokine antibody may not efficiently limit muscle wasting, particularly if given post exposure. Moreover, it also is difficult to know whether the effect of anti-cytokine antibodies to reverse catabolism is a direct or indirect effect. For instance, the administration of IL-1ra significantly inhibits the neutrophilia and the induction of corticosterone secretion by IL-1, the latter action being anti-catabolic. Mice with deletions for IL-1, TNF, or IL-6 genes can specifically define which cytokine knockout mice express physiological deficits. In IL-6 gene-deficient mice, for example, anorexia, cachexia, and lethargy in response to administration of LPS and turpentine are suppressed *(45,46)*, suggesting IL-6 contributes to the development of wasting during critical illnesses. All these experimental data provide strong evidence that cytokines do play unique and important roles in wasting.

2.2. *Effects of Cytokines on Anabolic Hormone Actions*

2.2.1. Insulin

It has been recognized that resistance to the actions of anabolic hormones, including insulin, growth hormone, and IGF-I, appears to be a significant contributing factor to the catabolic response during severe stressful illness, advanced HIV infection and cancer. Evidence suggests that the resistance to anabolic hormones is related to the release of cytokines during critical illness.

We conducted a study *(47)* to characterize the effects of endotoxin, TNF, and IL-1 on the glucoregulatory action of insulin in the rat using the euglycemic hyperinsulinemic clamp technique. Results showed that the glucose infusion rate necessary to maintain similar glucose levels at similar hyperinsulinemic conditions varied significantly according to treatment. Animals receiving saline infusion required 4.2 ± 2.5 mmol glucose/kg.h to maintain normoglycemia, which was the highest level among the five groups. Animals that received IL-1 infusion required slightly but not significantly less glucose, 3.4 ± 0.3 mmol glucose/kg/h, as compared with saline infusion. With TNF infusion, the requirement for maintenance of normoglycemia was 2.3 ± 0.5 mmol glucose/kg/h. Animals receiving endotoxin infusion required only 1.9 ± 0.5 mmol glucose/kg/h. Animals treated with the combination of TNF and IL-1 required the lowest amount of glucose, 1.0 ± 0.3 mmol glucose/kg/h. Thus these data suggested that endotoxin, TNF, and possibly IL-1 can rapidly induce a state of insulin resistance. However, the loss of insulin sensitivity is tissue specific in these animals. It has been noted that under certain conditions, such as in patients with HIV lipodystrophy *(48)*, the state of insulin resistance is more pronounced in skeletal muscle than in liver or fat. Similarly, the resistance to elevated insulin may only be present in non-tumor tissues in patients with cancer *(49)*.

TNF significantly decreases insulin receptor autophosphorylation, tyrosine phosphorylation of endogenous IRS-1, and kinase activity *(50)*, which may provide the molecular mechanisms to explain insulin resistance that develops under conditions of excess cytokine production. Endotoxin, for example, markedly diminished insulin-stimulated insulin receptor and IRS-1 tyrosine phosphorylation *(51–53)*. Using the pair-feeding method, we also found that endotoxin inhibited insulin-stimulated tyrosine phosphorylation of insulin receptor (50%), IRS-1 (62%), and IRS-2 (approx 100%) in muscle tissue as compared with pair-fed controls *(54)*. Because the nutritional conditions in both groups were controlled at a similar level, our results further suggest that cytokines released during endotoxin infusion induce insulin resistance through defects at many steps in the insulin signaling pathway, and that such effects are direct and independent from the malnutrition induced by food restriction.

Cytokine-induced stress hormones, such as glucocorticoids and epinephrine, also contribute to anabolic hormone resistance in critical illness. Glucocorticoids are known to impair insulin-mediated glucose uptake in skeletal muscle by inhibiting translocation of the Glut4 glucose transporter *(55)*. Infusion of epinephrine in the absence of other hormones impairs insulin-mediated glucose uptake *(56)*. Under experimental conditions in which critical illness was mimicked by the infusion of multiple stress hormones, discontinuation of epinephrine infusion while maintaining other hormones resulted in a rise in plasma insulin, improvement of insulin sensitivity and reduction of free fatty acid levels *(57)*.

2.2.2. Growth Hormone–IGF Axis

Growth hormone resistance is also a common feature of critical illness, characterized by growth hormone hypersecretion and very low IGF-I levels as a result of acquired peripheral growth hormone resistance and malnutrition. In catabolic states, it is thought that the decreased tissue abundance of growth hormone receptor in liver and muscle contributes at least in part to GH resistance *(58,59)*. After endotoxin administration into the rat (4 h after 1 mg/kg of endotoxin), we further found there was a marked decrease in GH-stimulated receptor tyrosine phosphorylation (70%), phosphorylation/Jak2 (50%) and STAT5 phosphorylation (40%) in the liver *(60)*. Thus, during critical illness the defects in both receptor abundance and postreceptor signaling responses to growth hormone stimulation may be responsible for the development of growth hormone resistance. The neuroendocrine effects of critical illness on the GH/IGF axis are more thoroughly discussed in Chapter 16, and the effects of IGF proteins on protein balance in Chapter 11.

Cytokines not only reduce the levels of IGF-I but also impair the action of IGF-I. The ability of IGF-I to stimulate protein synthesis is impaired by TNF-α, at serum levels as low as 2 ng/mL and as soon as after 10 min of exposure in human myoblasts *(61)*. In a study with a TNF infusion protocol (20 μg/kg of TNF infusion for 3 h), TNF significantly inhibited the action of IGF-I (200 μg/kg) to lower plasma glucose levels indicated by less glucose required to maintain euglycemia as compared with saline infusion *(62)*. Because this dose of IGF-I did not suppress insulin secretion, it seems the inhibition by TNF on IGF-I-induced glucose utilization is independent of insulin action. Consistent with our findings, Fang et al. reported that cytokines blocked the effects of IGF-I on glucose uptake in incubated muscle *(63)*. However, it also appeared that the inhibition of glucose use by TNF could be readily overcome by the provision of increased amounts of IGF-I (400 μg/kg) even though insulin levels were significantly decreased as compared with low dose of IGF-I (200 μg/kg) *(62)*, suggesting that the resistance to IGF-I might occur at a step distal to IGF-I receptors. In contrast to these findings, Lang *(64)* reported that under euglycemic and hyperinsulinemic conditions the effects of IGF-I on glucose uptake in the gastrocnemius, soleus, and heart muscle were similar between control and septic rats, although the desensitized insulin receptor with association of IRS-1 and IRS-2 may have resulted in cell resistance to both insulin and IGF-I *(65)*.

In the circulation, the levels of free IGF-I are considered to be most relevant to the biologic activity of IGF-I. However, the levels of IGF binding proteins (IGFBPs) also regulate the action of IGF-I. At least six distinct IGFBPs have been characterized (66). IGFBP-3 generally responds in parallel with IGF-I and is most important for the maintenance of IGF-I in the circulation, whereas IGFBP-1 and -2 may inhibit IGF-I activity. TNF, IL-1, and IL-6, produce dose- and time-dependent increases in IGFBP-1 production in HepG2 cells in the liver of C57BL/6 mice *(67,68)*. In a study monitoring IGF-I and IGFBPs levels in intensive care unit patients during a 30-d period, serum levels of IGF-I, IGFBP-3 and acid-labile subunit were low on admission and remained low over 30 d *(69)*. In contrast, IGFBP-I levels were high on admission, correlated with early changes in negative nitrogen balance, and fell rapidly during the first week. Moreover, proteolytic degradation of circulating IGFBP-3 was increased, leading to a reduced ability to form the IGFBP-3 ternary complex *(69,70)*. Taken together, these data suggest that cytokines also inhibit IGF-I action indirectly through alterations in IGFBPs during critical illness.

3. NUTRITIONAL MANAGEMENT IN CRITICAL ILLNESS

3.1. Overview

Critically ill patients are hypermetabolic and have anabolic inefficiencies that lead to increased requirements for certain nutrients. The metabolic changes that characterize the systemic inflammatory response provide a reordering of priorities in relation to metabolic homeostasis. On one level, there are the essential nutrients, some of which like protein and certain vitamins may be required in somewhat greater amounts, whereas others like iron may need to be withheld in the early phase of injury. In addition, the heterogeneity of the patient population, including different degrees of trauma or injury, different types of tumors and different stages of chronic diseases such as hepatic and renal insufficiency, make it more difficult to provide or develop nutritional guidelines applicable to all malnourished patients. Over the past three decades, nutrition support methods by total parenteral nutrition (TPN) or tube feeding (enteral nutrition) have been developed. These invasive feeding techniques provide exciting tools that may allow certain nutrients to perform new and unique roles, such as reducing the intensity of the systemic inflammatory response by their antioxidant (selenium, glutamine, zinc) or anti-inflammatory (omega-3 fatty acids) effects. In general, current nutritional approaches have been designed to respond to special nutritional needs created by the catabolic state. The rationale of nutrition therapy for critically ill patients, therefore, is largely based on clinical judgment. Since nutritional assessment is reviewed in chapter 4, the discussion will be limited to some important aspects of nutritional management, including levels of calories and protein needed, effects of special nutrients on modulation of acute-phase response and the use of anabolic agents in conjunction with adequate nutrition support to critically ill patients.

3.2. Protein Metabolism and Requirements in Critical Illness

The metabolic responses to critical illness differ significantly from those of starvation and food restriction. During starvation and food restriction, the body attempts to adapt to undernutrition by reducing energy expenditure and limiting protein catabolism. With the fall in food intake, glycogen stores are exhausted within the first 24–72 h, suggesting that carbohydrate oxidation rates are altered rapidly to reflect reduced intake. Studies on glucose metabolism have revealed that underweight individuals have higher rates of glucose use per unit of lean body mass accomplished by increasing insulin sensitivity, as compared with normal middle-aged men *(71)*. As an alternate fuel, fat becomes the principal energy source sparing body protein by limiting the need for gluconeogenesis. During longer starvation periods, protein breakdown is further decreased in order to conserve nitrogen and maintain lean body mass. When rates of whole body protein synthesis were measured in the undernourished state (body mass index 16.7 kg/m^2) and a normal state (body mass index 20.8 kg/m^2), total body protein synthesis and breakdown rates per unit of fat free mass were unchanged in the undernourished state *(72)*. This ability, which is essential for conserving nitrogen when intake is reduced, is absent in most critically ill patients. In critical illness, the rate of lean tissue loss can be up to seven times greater than in well-adapted starvation *(73,74)*. Whole-body protein synthesis is diminished in skeletal muscle and connective tissue in animal models of cytokine-produced catabolism *(75)*. Although insulin resistance develops and the percentage contribution of fat to energy expenditure is reduced, total fat oxidation plus protein and carbohydrate oxidation are all increased with the increases in energy expenditure present in critical illness. Interestingly, at the same time, liver fractional rates of protein synthesis are increased in this condition, accounting for the increase in liver size as well as the production of the so-called acute-phase proteins, although there is a concomitant decrease in albumin synthesis. The greatest impact to lower serum albumin concentrations results from the systemic inflammatory response and specifically the IL-6 effects, which reduce albumin synthesis, increase its catabolism, and cause extravascular extravasation. Anorexia limiting protein and energy intake makes only a minor contribution to the development of hypoalbuminemia. Thus, in critical illness conditions, hypoalbuminemia is primarily a marker of the systemic inflammatory response that produces protein-malnutrition, rather than being a direct measure of protein-energy malnutrition per se *(76)*.

In a healthy adult consuming a diet without protein, there is an obligatory loss of 20 to 30 g of protein per day. A level of 55 g of protein intake per day (0.8 g of protein/kg/d) is recommended to prevent a net protein loss in healthy individuals *(77)*. For critically ill patients, substantially more protein is required to account for anabolic inefficiencies. Protein intake ranging from 1.0 to 1.5 g of protein/kg/d is recommended to attenuate protein loss. In the most severe inflammatory states, the delivery of more than 1.75 g of protein/kg/d only increases urea formation *(78–80)* making this the upper effective level of protein intake. Although a positive nitrogen balance is desired, net protein anabolism can usually only be achieved after the systemic inflammatory response subsides. During the acute phase, however, energy intakes that meet energy expenditure and protein intake at 1.5 g/kg will preferentially support the systemic inflammatory response by fostering host immune function and wound healing whereas losses of lean tissue are limited principally to skeletal muscle *(81)*.

3.2.1. Specific Amino Acids

Certain amino acids have unique importance for critically ill patients. The branched-chain amino acids (leucine, isoleucine and valine) are essential amino acids. Studies have shown that these amino acids have additional effects on stimulation of protein synthesis in muscle and on nonbranched chain amino acid uptake in the liver for protein synthesis *(82)*. Glutamine, arginine, and cystine are considered to be conditionally essential amino acids because the levels of these amino acids are often low in plasma and tissues following stress. In studies in rats, a higher protein intake elevates plasma IGF-I levels *(83–84)*, and pharmacological doses of arginine increase serum levels of growth hormone and IGF-I *(85)*. Amino acid limitation, as occurs during dietary protein deficiency, inhibited endogenous IGF-I production *(86)* but induced IGFBP-1 expression in hepatic cells *(87)*. Moreover, a clinical study with glutamine-enriched enteral nutrition in 72 multiple trauma patients demonstrated a significant reduction in infection, although this did not translate into a significant reduction in hospital stay *(88)*. In a second study of trauma patients using a formula, containing not only glutamine but also arginine, omega-3 fatty acid, and nucleotides, there was a significant reduction in infection rate and hospital length of stay *(89)*. Although diets that have enriched concentrations of specific amino acids have not always shown consistent benefits, growing evidence suggests that supplementation with several of these amino acids improves nitrogen balance *(90,91)*, can decrease infectious complications and enhance immune system function *(92–94)*, which is of great potential clinical interest.

3.3. Energy Requirements

Provision of carbohydrate and lipids are also required as sources of energy to minimize protein degradation and lipolysis. Although increasing energy intake above energy requirements may improve protein use in unstressed individuals, there is little evidence for such an effect in critically ill patients. In fact, excess administration of either fat or carbohydrate in this setting can have adverse effects including increasing the risk for infection. Thus, the present recommendation for energy intake is that total energy provision should not exceed energy expenditure in critically ill, malnourished patients. For most medical or surgical patients with mild-to-moderate stress, energy goals are to achieve energy balance, which approximates 25–30 kcal/kg/d. Although patients with severe trauma may have energy expenditures substantially higher, at 35–40 kcal/kg/d, increasingly an upper limit of 30–35 kcal/kg/d is being used in the acute phase of injury to avoid metabolic complications *(95,96)*. In the acute stage of critical illness, metabolic adaptive responses are characterized by hyperglycemia due to central and peripheral insulin resistance, accompanied by a hyperdynamic cardiovascular response including high cardiac output, increased oxygen consumption, high temperature and decreased peripheral vascular resistance. Hyperglycemia is particularly common when patients are fed greater than 35 kcal/kg/d, which can markedly increase the risk for infection *(97)*. For instance, it has been demonstrated that provision of dextrose at rates of 4 mg/kg/min (5.7 g/kg/d) intravenously often is associated with hyperglycemia even in the nondiabetic host *(98)* because of the insulin resistance, which is universal in stressed, hospitalized patients *(96)*. A study from our hospital showed that the presence of a blood glucose >220 mg/dL (12.2 mmol/L) on the first postoperative day was associated with a greater than fivefold increased risk of serious infection in diabetic patients *(99)*. Recent evidence also suggests that hyperglycemia can exacerbate inflammation through either induction of oxidative stress *(100,101)* or acquired immunodepression *(102)*. None of these effects is desirable in the critically ill. Although energy balance may not be achieved in some cases by caloric intakes at 25–30 kcal/kg/d, the lower risk for hyperglycemia may lead to an improved clinical outcome. However, hyperglycemia is usually easily treatable by insulin with substantial clinical benefits in randomized trials in humans *(103–105)* and in endotoxin-induced stress in rats *(106)* and is preventable by limiting caloric intake *(97,107)*. Insulin is a potent anabolic hormone and stimulates muscle protein synthesis. Thus, provision of adequate nutrients with exogenous insulin in prevention of hyperglycemia should enhance muscle anabolism. In general, the goal of nutritional support in the critically ill is to provide support for the systemic inflammatory response including enhancing immune function, repairing injured tissues and healing wounds. Restoration of lost lean tissue is generally not possible until the systemic inflammatory response abates, although the initial losses of lean tissue in the acute phase generally abates and is ultimately reversed by a combination of developing malnutrition and a less intense inflammatory response in those with prolonged illness.

A lower caloric intake approximating resting rather than total energy expenditure while including all other essential nutrients and at least 1 g/kg/d of protein may often be more in accordance with the inflammatory and hormonal mediator climate during the first few days and for up to 10 d of systemic inflammation. Although the effects of hyperglycemia are not often considered in planning nutritional support, it is important to maintain glycemia <220 mg/dL (11.1 mmol/L) in diabetic patients and 180–200 mg/dL (9.1–10.0 mmol/L) in nondiabetic patients to minimize complications in patients receiving enteral and particularly parenteral nutrition support. Even tighter control blood glucose level at 80–110 mg/dL may be justified in the critically ill *(95)*. The nutritional goal for these patients still remains the achievement of net anabolism by advancing caloric intakes to estimated total requirements as tolerated and metabolic homeostasis allows. In general, when a patient's nutritional requirements cannot be met via the oral route for period of 5–7 d (or less if the patients is initially malnourished), parenteral or enteral nutrition is indicated. In chronically malnourished patients, it is well recognized that wound healing and normal immune responses are dependent upon adequate nutrient intake. Therefore, it seems reasonable to start feeding as soon as possible after malnutrition is diagnosed. Early feeding may decrease complication rates and improve quality of life in these patients. For patients with severe stress (multiple trauma, closed head injury, major burns and severe sepsis) who are often well nourished at the onset of their illness, early nutrition support within the first few days should also improve outcome as a result of the intensity and the likelihood for a prolonged duration of the inflammatory response. In patients requiring home TPN, who generally have minimal levels of metabolic stress, a total caloric intake at 35 kcal/kg/d is recommended at the initiation of nutrition support to rapidly replete the cumulative calorie deficit so as to achieve weight gain, and then intake adjusted to a lower level to maintain desired body weight.

3.4. Lipid Metabolism and Recommendations

Lipid is an energy source with high caloric density (9 kcal/g). Compared with diets exclusively of carbohydrate and protein, an adequate intake of fat can result in better nutrient utilization, less CO_2 production and decreased lipogenesis and insulin requirements *(108)*. Provision of fat intake in TPN formulations is also essential to prevent essential fatty acid deficiency *(109–111)*. The ideal ratio of fat and carbohydrate is unknown, but high-fat feeding can enhance stress-stimulated corticosterone levels in the rat *(112)*. In our hospital, 20–40 g fat/d for 40–80 kg body weight is recommended. For intravenous delivery, it is important to control the rate at an upper limit of 0.11 g/kg/h in critically ill patients to avoid the potential for adverse outcomes *(113)*. Malnourished patients with intact gastrointestinal function should be given adequate dietary fat, which can range from 3% to 30% of calories in commercial enteral formulas and usually 30–35% in calories based on food, although surgery or disease may reduce intestinal absorptive capacity. The minimal fat requirements for the prevention of essential fatty acid deficiency are at least 3.2% total calories given as intravenous fat *(114,115)*. The minimal daily requirement for dietary linolenic acid (18:3ω-3) is unknown, because dietary deficiency of 18:3ω-3 in a normal adult consuming food orally has not been described but is assumed to be about 0.5% of total calories.

3.4.1. Omega-3 Fatty Acids (ω-3 Fatty Acids)

As described abovc, thc accelerated catabolism, rapid onset of malnutrition, and immune system failure is related to the excessive production of cytokines underlying the systemic inflammatory response. Substantial evidence has accumulated that fish oil, which is rich in ω-3 fatty acids, can significantly suppress cytokine release from monocytes *(116)* and attenuate the metabolic response to inflammation or infection. Effects noted in experimental studies in animals have included dampening of the febrile response *(117)*, decreasing serum lactate concentration and improving lung morphology *(118)*, decreasing insulin resistance *(116,117)*, and improving survival *(119)*, all after endotoxin challenge. Clinical studies in humans have shown improved outcome in critical illness *(120)*, rheumatoid arthritis *(121,122)*, inflammatory bowel disease *(123,124)*, and renal transplantation *(125)* to name but a few conditions. The intravenous fat currently available for use in United States is soybean oil, which has high content of polyunsaturated fatty acids (mainly ω-6 fatty acids). In rats, it has been demonstrated that dietary ω-6 polyunsaturated fatty acids significantly increase the levels of hepatic IGFBP-1 transcripts and protein, which is independent of any caloric effects of the diets and the levels of insulin *(126)*. Thus, these findings suggest that certain fats can be viewed as potential therapeutic agents during critical illness rather than purely as an energy source.

Although many potential mechanisms have been proposed for the clinical benefits of fish oil feeding, the anti-inflammatory effects of fish oil are thought to principally occur through a reduction in arachidonic acid (AA) content of phospholipids within cell membranes. Eicosapentaenoic acid (EPA, 20:5ω3) and docosahexaenoic acid (22:6ω3), which are enriched in fish oil, are preferentially and rapidly incorporated into membrane phospholipid to displace AA. Moreover, EPA is structurally similar to AA and competes with AA in the cyclo-oxygenase pathway, which leads to the synthesis of a different series of prostaglandins, thromboxanes, and prostacyclins that have substantially less immune suppression, proinflammatory, and hypotensive effects *(127–130)*. These properties of ω-3 fatty acids may have application in the treatment of chronic inflammatory disease, as well as in the more acute situation such as acute respiratory distress syndrome or patients undergoing chemo/radiation therapy *(131–134)*. It is speculated that lipid emulsions with a ω-3/ω-6 fatty acid ratio of 1:2 would induce the highest leukotriene C_5/leukotriene C_4 (LTC_5/LTC_4) ratio and exert the most favorable modulation of lipid mediator synthesis *(135,136)*. Recently, a study in laboratory animals demonstrated that during sepsis a fish oil-supplemented diet with 1:1 fish oil and soybean oil emulsion significantly improved the survival rate and prevented the sepsis-induced suppression of lymphocyte proliferation and IL-2 release *(137)*.

The definition of cancer patients who might benefit from dietary ω-3 fatty acids has only just begun. Clinical studies with EPA-containing fish oil have shown it to be effective in attenuating the development of weight loss in patients with pancreatic cancer. In a trial of 18 patients with unresectable pancreatic cancer orally receiving fish oil capsules (1 g) containing eicosapentaenoic acid 18% and docosahexaenoic acid 12%, 11 patients showed weight gain, three became weight stable, and four continued to lose weight but at a reduced rate *(138)*. Weight gain was seen in other studies where EPA (2.1 g/d) was administered together with adequate calorie and protein supplement *(139,140)*. Moreover, the percentage body water was maintained, suggesting that the weight gain was not the result of the accumulation of water. Body composition analysis further suggested that there was no change in fat mass, opposite to what would be expected from nutritional supplementation alone *(141)*. It appears that provision of a fish oil-enriched nutritional supplement in patients with pancreatic cancer results in some normalization of the metabolic response, in association with an improvement in nutritional status. Such effects might improve the quality of life and increase survival time in these patients. However, further studies are needed to test whether EPA is effective in patients with other types of tumors.

3.5. Anabolic Hormones

The administration of anabolic hormones, such as insulin, growth hormone, IGF-I, and anabolic steroids, in pharmacological amounts represents an approach to overcome the resistance to their actions and reverse the protein energy malnutrition response to acute illness or chronic disease. The availability of recombinant hormones has made some of these agents clinically available for study and use in catabolic states.

Currently, insulin is extensively used only to overcome TPN-induced hyperglycemia as a standard procedure. It has been demonstrated that administration of growth hormone to critically ill patients can enhance the levels of IGF-I and promote tissue anabolism under certain circumstances *(142–147)*. One study even showed that such effects of growth hormone in protein synthesis were achieved in patients receiving only intravenous dextrose or parenteral nutrition with a small amount of nitrogen *(148)*. Schambelan et al *(149)* examined the effect of 12 wk of growth hormone therapy on the body composition and work capacity of HIV-infected individuals who had lost weight. They found that growth hormone increased lean body mass, reduced body fat, and increased treadmill work capacity. However, growth hormone has not consistently demonstrated net anabolic effects on nitrogen economy, because the improvement in nitrogen balance was not always statistically significant. Recent studies *(150)* investigated the effects of high dose growth hormone (range from 0.07 to 8.0 mg/kg/d) on clinical outcome in critically ill adults receiving prolonged intensive care. The results showed that growth hormone administration was associated with an increase in morbidity and mortality. Two potential side effects with growth hormone administration, hyperglycemia and fluid retention, are particularly likely to be a problem for the critically ill. Several other studies also suggest that if patients are severely infected, or have cancer, the response of growth hormone treatment may be impaired *(151,152)*. These results suggest that growth hormone is more likely to be effective when the systemic inflammatory response is mild to moderate. Therefore, despite the fact that growth hormone has proven to be clinically useful in a variety of conditions, it should still be considered as an experimental tool, because its advantages and disadvantages in various conditions need to be defined along with dosage requirements. Its value in reversing catabolic states in cachectic diseases, such as cancer, trauma, infection, and in postoperative care, have not been fully established yet.

IGF-I is an important mediator of the growth promoting effects of growth hormone. Although the effects of IGF-I have also been evaluated, large parenteral doses are required to promote specific anabolic activity. In addition, the action of IGF-I diminishes with time because of enhanced binding activity. Since the negative feedback of IGF-I alters GH and IGF BP elaboration and interacts with insulin effects, it has been suggested that the use of combination therapy of GH + IGF-I or the IGF-I + IGFBP3 molecule might be more beneficial. However, there is no condition of malnutrition where this therapy has been established clinically.

Other anabolic hormones, such as anabolic steroids, have been investigated in a variety of malnourished states, particularly AIDS wasting. The rationale for the use of androgenic steroids in chronic illnesses is based on the fact that there is a high frequency of low testosterone levels in HIV-infected men and that low testosterone levels in these patients are associated with poor disease outcomes and impaired muscle function. Studies in renal failure *(153)* and AIDs *(154,155)* have demonstrated improved restoration of lean tissue structure and function. However, the overall benefits of these drugs are undefined in patients with critical illness.

3.6. Micronutrients and Antioxidants

Micronutrients play a key role in many of the metabolic processes for promotion of survival from critical illness. However, a deficiency state can develop in the critically ill because of decreased nutrient intakes and increased requirements. For instance, sepsis or adult respiratory distress syndrome can dramatically increase the production of reactive oxygen species and lead to oxidative stress and activation of the transcription factor NF-κB). In the rat, burn injury produced cardiac NF-κB nuclear migration 4 h after burn and cardiomyocyte secretion of TNF, IL-1, and IL-6 by 24 h after the burn *(156)*. It has also been demonstrated that vitamin A deficiency results in the decrease of serum IGF-I levels, which is accompanied by lower levels of IGF-I mRNA in rat liver *(157)*. Zinc deficiency produced lower serum IGF-I and liver IGF-I mRNA, lower serum IGFBP3, lower liver growth hormone receptor and its mRNA, and lower serum growth hormone binding protein and its mRNA *(158)*. In these rats, exogenous growth hormone did not enhance the levels of serum IGF-I and its liver mRNA, although the restoration of growth hormone receptor and growth hormone binding protein to normal was achieved by continuously infused bovine growth hormone in these rats. Thus, IGF-I synthesis may require the presence of zinc in addition to growth hormone (discussed in Chapter 5).

In general, serum antioxidant vitamin and trace element concentrations, such as vitamin C, vitamin E, selenium, and zinc, are seen to decrease with systemic inflammation. The logical answer to enhancing micronutrient concentrations is to provide dietary supplementation. There are only a limited number of studies that test the efficacy of antioxidant compounds in critical ill patients. Physiologic selenium replacement in critically ill patients receiving parenteral nutrition restored serum selenium and glutathione peroxidase levels to normal, and reduced the need for hemodialysis as well as mortality although the latter effect was not significant *(159)*. In a prospective, randomized, double-blind, placebo-controlled study *(160)*, 20 patients were randomized to receive a formula supplemented with vitamin A (67 μg/dL), C (13.3 mg/dL), and E (4.94 mg/dL), and 17 patients received an isocaloric and isonitrogenous control solution. Administration of the supplemented solution significantly increased the concentration of plasma β-carotene, plasma and low-density lipoprotein-bound α-tocopherol and improved low-density lipoprotein resistance to oxidative stress compared with controls, as assessed by ex vivo testing. However, there was no clinical benefit identified despite the fact that glutathione status was compromised and correlated with glutathione concentrations in critically ill patients. Parenteral glutamine administration with total parenteral nutrition, which might be expected to enhance glutathione levels, significantly reduced infections and hospital stay in patients undergoing bone marrow transplant *(161)* and major surgery *(162,163)*. Enteral glutamine in trauma patients led to a significant reduction in infection rate in one study *(164)* and in infection rate and length of hospital stay in another *(165)*. However, glutamine has a multitude of other effects that may in some part played a role as well as the unknown contribution of other bioactive compounds contained in the various formulas. All these findings suggest that consideration of dietary components that alter antioxidant/oxidant status may influence the course of inflammatory and/or autoimmune diseases. On one hand, antioxidant levels are diminished but oxidative stress quite clearly increased by severe illness; therefore, reactive oxygen species can be both beneficial and harmful in the critically ill depending on such factors as the nutritional status of the host, the severity of the illness, and the relative balance between the systemic inflammatory response syndrome and compensatory anti-inflammatory response syndrome. Further studies are required to define optimal levels for provision of antioxidants in different diseases as well as the identification of which antioxidants or combinations are effective.

4. SUMMARY AND CONCLUSIONS

Malnutrition is a major contributor to the increased morbidity and mortality seen in critical illness. Percentage weight loss is a sensitive and specific tool that can be used at initial presentation to screen for and identify malnutrition effectively. Nutritional depletion developing subsequently is multifactorial and depends on the interactions among numerous mediators including the proinflammatory cytokines, the stress hormones of intermediary metabolism, along with the decrease in antioxidant defenses and the decreased levels and effectiveness of anabolic hormones. Proinflammatory cytokines, although essential for immune defense, can exert pathologic and even lethal effects when produced in excessive amounts. The catabolic response in certain tissues like muscle, which occurs as a normal part of the inflammatory response in part to support anabolism in other tissues like the liver and hemotopoietic tissue, also bears the risk for the ultimate development of malnutrition. Moreover, the resistance to the effects of anabolic hormones during critical illness impairs the utilization of exogenous nutrients. The precise way in which individual factors interact with each other to determine the outcome of inflammation is largely unknown. It is now widely appreciated however that optimizing the supply of energy, protein, special fatty acids, and the major anabolic hormones and micronutrients so as to support the metabolic responses to injury can significantly affect the outcome in these patients. However, adequate nutrition support and effective therapeutic interventions require an understanding of the pathological processes taking place and the establishment of a balance between the benefits of nutritional/metabolic support and the risks involved with overaggressive feeding. Recent studies also demonstrate that genetic factors can play important roles in the intensity of inflammation and the quality of the response to nutritional therapy in individual patients. Clearly, further studies will be necessary to identify such factors and their interactions so as to achieve the desired efficacy of nutritional therapy in the management of disease-related malnutrition characteristic of critical illness.

5. RECOMMENDATIONS AND FUTURE CHALLENGES

For the future anabolic adjuvant therapy may be directed into other ways to reduce the intensity of the systemic inflammatory response. One way would be the use of anticytokine therapy, such as with IL-1 receptor antagonist (IL-1ra) or anti-TNF therapy, including anti-TNF antibodies, soluble TNF receptors, pentoxifyline, a xanthine-derived agent known to inhibit the production of TNF *(166,167)*, and thalidomide *(168–170)*. Certain pharmacological agents like β-blockers *(171)* and angiotensin-converting enzyme inhibitors *(172)* have been shown to reduce cytokine production in chronic congestive heart failure. Recently, angiotensin-converting enzyme inhibitors have also been shown to improve antioxidant status, nutritional status, and clinical outcome in chronic renal failure, another proinflammatory state *(173)*. Similarly statins, which are widely used to improve cardiovascular outcome by reducing serum cholesterol, have been shown to work as well through their antioxidant action *(174)*. Another potentially promising way is through the use of nutrients that can influence antioxidant status such as selenium, zinc, glutamine, cysteine or vitamin E, since it has now been convincingly shown that reactive oxygen species can exacerbate the systemic inflammatory response *(175)*. The improved clinical outcome in critically ill patients *(176)* using immune-enhancing diets, which contain both immune- and antioxidant-enhancing nutrients and omega 3 fatty acids, which are anti-inflammatory, suggest that combination therapies may be particularly effective. Vitamin E, an important antioxidant nutrient, also has been shown to reduce cardiovascular disease and the cardiovascular end points in chronic renal failure *(177)*. Dietary omega-3 fatty acid pus vitamin E has a significant immunomodulating effect and has been shown to prolong the survival of malnourished patients with generalized malignancy *(178)*. In this regard the combination of anabolic hormones such as growth hormone, and/or IGF-I in conjunction with antioxidant or anti-inflammatory therapies might be worthy of study, particularly since the side effects of the former might be through the promotion of inflammation. Thus, the future looks bright for the development of new methods to improve anabolic nutritional therapies.

REFERENCES

1. Bistrian BR, Blackburn GL, Hallowell E, Heddle R. Protein status of general surgical patients. JAMA 1974;230:858–860.

2. Bistrian BR, Blackburn GL, Vitale J, Cochran D, Naylor J. Prevalence of malnutrition in general medical patients. JAMA 1976;235:1567–1570.
3. Blackburn GL, Bistrian BR, Maini BS, Schlamm HT, Smith MF. Nutritional and metabolic assessment of the hospitalized patient. JPEN J Parenter Enteral Nutr 1977;1:11–22.
4. Blackburn GL, Thornton PA. Nutritional assessment of the hospitalized patient. Med Clin North Am 1979;63:11103–11115.
5. Wilmore DW. Catabolic illness. Strategies for enhancing recovery. N Engl J Med 1991;325:687–702.
6. Shaw JH, Wildbore M, Wolfe RR. Whole body protein kinetics in severely septic patients. The response to glucose infusion and total parenteral nutrition. Ann Surg 1987;205:288 -294.
7. Streat SJ, Beddoe AH, Hill GL. Aggressive nutritional support does not prevent protein loss despite fat gain in septic intensive care patients. J Trauma 1987;27:262–266.
8. Loder PB, Smith RC, Kee AJ, et al. What rate of infusion of intravenous nutrition solution is required to stimulate uptake of amino acids by peripheral tissues in depleted patients? Ann Surg 1990;211:360–368.
9. Lust G. Effect of infection on protein and nucleic acid synthesis in mammalian organs and tissues. Fed Proc 1966;25:1688–1694.
10. Tomkins AM, Garlick PJ, Schofield WN, Waterlow JC. The combined effects of infection and malnutrition on protein metabolism in children. Clin Sci 1983;65:313–324.
11. Wannemacher RW, Jr. Dupont HL, Pekarek RS, et al. An endogenous mediator of depression of amino acids and trace metals in serum during typhoid fever. J Infect Dis 1972;126:77–86.
12. Wannemacher RW Jr, Pekarek RS, Klainer AS, Bartelloni PJ, Dupont HL, Hornick RB, Beisel WR. Detection of a leukocytic endogenous mediator-like mediator of serum amino acid and zinc depression during various infectious illnesses. Infect Immun 1975;11:873–875.
13. Chang HR, Bistrian BR. The role of cytokines in the catabolic consequences of infection and injury. JPEN J Parenter Enteral Nutr 1998;22:156–166.
14. Edwards PD, Moldawer LL. Role of cytokines in the metabolic response to stress. Cur Opin Clin Nutr Metab Care 1998;1:187–190.
15. Blackwell TS, Christman JW. Sepsis and cytokines: current status. Br J Anaesth 1996;77:110–117.
16. Dofferhoff AS, Bom VJ, de Vries-Hospers HG, et al. Patterns of cytokines, plasma endotoxin, plasminogen activator inhibitor and acute phase proteins during the treatment of severe sepsis in humans. Crit Care Med 1992;20:185–192.
17. Yeh FL, Lin WL, Shen HD, Fang RH. Changes in circulating levels of interleukin 6 in burned patients. Burns 1999;25:131–136.
18. Strassmann G, Fong M, Kenney JS, Jacob CO. Evidence for the involvement of interleukin 6 in experimental cancer cachexia. J Clin Invest 1992;89:1681–1684.
19. Gardlund B, Sjolin J, Nilsson A, Roll M, Wickerts CJ, Wretlind B. Plasma levels of cytokines in primary septic shock in humans: correlation with disease severity. J Infect Dis 1995;172:296–301.
20. Damas P, Ledoux D, Nys M, et al. Cytokine serum level during severe sepsis in human IL-6 as a marker of severity. Ann Surg 1992;215:365–362.
21. Pinsky MR, Vincent JL, Deviere J, Alegre M, Kahn RJ, Dupont E. Serum cytokine levels in human septic shock. Relation to multiple-system organ failure and mortality. Chest 1993;103:565–575.
22. Rixen D. Siegel JH, Friedman HP. "Sepsis/SIRS," physiologic classification, severity stratification, relation to cytokine elaboration and outcome prediction in posttrauma critical illness. J Trauma 1996;41:581–598.
23. Stratakis CA, Mastorakos G, Chrousos GP. Interleukin-6 elevation in critically ill infants with sepsis and necrotizing enterocolitis. J Pediatr 1994;125:504.
24. Barton BE. IL-6-like cytokine and cancer cachexia: consequences of chronic inflammation. Immunol Res 2001;23:41–58.
25. Belec L, Meillet D, Gresengnet G, Gherardi RK. Increased tumor necrosis factor-alpha serum levels in patients with HIV wasting syndrome and euthyroid sick syndrome. J Acquir Immune Defic Syndr Hum Retrovirol 1995;8:212–214.
26. Verheul GA, de Jongh-Leuvenink K, Op de Coul AA, van Landeghem AA, van Puyenbroek MJ. Tumor necrosis factor and interleukin-6 in critical illness polyneuromyopathy. Clin Neurol Neurosurg 1994;96:300–304.
27. Aderka D, Englemann H, Hornik V, et al. Increased serum levels of soluble receptors for tumor necrosis factor in cancer patients. Cancer Res 1991;51:5602–5607.

28. Schalkwijk CG, Poland DC, van Dijk W, Kok A, et al. Plasma concentration of C-reactive protein is increased in type I diabetic patients without clinical macroangiopathy and correlates with markers of endothelial dysfunction: evidence for chronic inflammation. Diabetologia 1999;42:351–357.
29. Panichi V, Migliori M, De Pietro S, et al. C-reactive protein as a marker of chronic inflammation in uremic patients. Blood Purif 2000;18:183–190.
30. Flores EA, Bistrian BR, Pomposelli JJ, Dinarello CA, Blackburn GL, Instfan N. Infusion of tumor necrosis factor/cachectin promotes muscle catabolism in the rat. A synergistic effect with interleukin 1. J Clin Invest 1989;83:1614–1622.
31. Ling PR, Schwartz JH, Jeevanandam M, Gauldie J, Bistrian BR. Metabolic changes in rats during a continuous infusion of recombinant interleukin-1. Am J Physiol Endocrinol Metab 1996;270:E305–E312.
32. Waterlow JCP, Garlick PJ, Millward DJ. Protein Turnover in Mammalian Tissues and in the Whole Body. Elsevier/North-Holland, Amsterdan, Netherlands, 1978.
33. Waterlow JC, Stephen JM. The measurement of total lysine turnover in the rat by intravenous infusion of L-[U-14C]lysine. Clin Sci 1967:33:489–506.
34. Pomposelli JJ, Palombo JD, Hamawy KJ, Bistrian BR, Blackburn GL, Moldawer LL. Comparison of different techniques for estimating rates of protein synthesis in vivo in healthy and bacteraemic rats. Biochem J 1985;226:37–42.
35. Ling PR, Bistrian BR, Blackburn GL, Istfan N. Effect of fetal growth on maternal protein metabolism in postabsorptive rat. Am J Physiol Endocrinol Metab 1987;252:E380–E342.
36. Istfan NW, Ling PR, Blackburn GL, Bistrian BR. Enhancement of tumor proteolysis by TNF-alpha: correlation of in vivo isotope estimates with growth. Am J Physiol Endocrinol Metab 1991;261:R106–R116.
37. Ling PR, Schwartz JH, Bistrian BR. Mechanisms of host wasting induced by administration of cytokines in rats. Am J Physiol Endocrinol Metab 1997;272:E333–E339.
38. Lang CH, Fan J, Cooney R, Vary TC. IL-1 receptor antagonist attenuates sepsis-induced alterations in the IGF system and protein synthesis. Am J Physiol Endocrinol Metab 1996;270:E430–E437.
39. Vary TC, Voisin L, Cooney RN. Regulation of peptide-chain initiation in muscle during sepsis by interleukin-1 receptor antagonist. Am J Physiol. 1996;271:E513–E520.
40. Cooney R, Kimball SR, Eckman R, Maish G III, Shumate M, Vary TC. TNF-binding protein ameliorates inhibition of skeletal muscle protein synthesis during sepsis. Am J Physiol 1999;276:E611–E619.
41. Zamir O, Hasselegren PO, James H, Higashiguchi T, Fisher JE. Effect of tumor necrosis factor or interleukin-1 on muscle amino acid uptake and the role of glucocorticoids. Surg Gynecol Obstet 1993;177:27–32.
42. Li YP, Reid MB. NF-kappaB mediates the protein loss induced by TNF-alpha in different skeletal muscle myotubes. Am J Physiol Regul Integr Comp Physiol 2000;279:R1165–R1170.
43. Goodman MN. Interleukin-6 induces skeletal muscle protein breakdown in rats. Proc Soc Exp Biol Med 1994;205:182–185.
44. Ling PR, Istfan NW, Colon E, Bistrian BR. Differential effects of interleukin-1 receptor antagonist in cytokine- and endotoxin-treated rats. Am J Physiol Endocrinol Metab 1995;268:E255–E261.
45. Chai Z, Gatti S, Toniatti C, Poli V, Bartfai T. Interleukin (IL)-6 gene expression in the central nervous system is necessary for fever response to lipopolysaccharide or IL-1β: a study in IL-6-deficient mice. J Exp Med 1996;183:311–316.
46. Tsujinaka T, Fujita J, Ebisui C, et al. Interleukin 6 receptor antibody inhibits muscle atrophy and modulates proteolytic systems in interleukin 6 transgenic mice. J Clin Invest 1996;97:244–249.
47. Ling PR, Bistrian BR, Mendez B, Istfan NW. Effects of systemic infusions of endotoxin, tumor necrosis factor, and interleukin-1 on glucose metabolism in the rat: relationship to endogenous glucose production and peripheral tissue glucose uptake. Metabolism 1994;43:279–284.
48. Mynarcik DC, McNurlan MA, Steigbigel RT, Fuhrer J, Gelato MC. Association of severe insulin resistance with both loss of limb fat and elevated serum tumor necrosis factor receptor levels in HIV lipodystrophy. J Acquir Immune Defic Syndr 2000;25:312–321.
49. Argiles JM, Lopez-Soriano FJ. Insulin and cancer. Int J Oncol 2001;18:683–687.
50. Hotamisligil GS, Peraldi P, Budavari A, Ellis R, White MF, Spiegelman BM. IRS-1-mediated inhibition of insulin receptor tyrosine kinase activity in TNF-alpha- and obesity-induced insulin resistance. Science 1996;271:665–668.
51. Lang CH, Spitzer JA.Glucose kinetics and development of endotoxin tolerance during long-term continuous endotoxin infusion. Metabolism 1987;36:469–474.

52. Fan J, Li YH, Wojnar MM, Lang CH. Endotoxin-induced alteration in insulin-stimulated phosphorylation of insulin receptor, IRS-1, and MAP kinase in skeletal muscle. Shock 1996;6:164–170.
53. Lang CH, Pollard V, Fan J, et al. Acute alterations in growth hormone-insulin-like growth factor axis in humans injected with endotoxin. Am J Physiol Endocrinol Metab 1997;273:R371–R378.
54. McCowen KC, Ling PR, Ciccarone A, et al. Sustained endotoxemia leads to marked down-regulation of early steps in the insulin-signaling cascade. Critical Care Med 2001;29:839–846.
55. Dimitriadis G, Leighton B, Parry-Billings M, et al. Effects of glucocorticoid excess on the sensitivity of glucose transport and metabolism to insulin in rat skeletal muscle. Biochem J 1997;321:707–712.
56. Bessey PQ, Brooks DC, Black PR, Aoki TT, Wilmore DW. Epinephrine acutely mediates skeletal muscle insulin resistance. Surgery. 1983;94:172–179.
57. McGuinness OP, Snowden RT, Moran C, Neal DW, Fujiwara T, Cherrington AD. Impact of acute epinephrine removal on hepatic glucose metabolism during stress hormone infusion. Metabolism. 1999;48:910–914.
58. Defalque D, Brandt N, Ketelslegers JM, Thissen JP. GH insensitivity induced by endotoxin injection is associated with decreased liver GH receptors. Am J Physiol Endocrinol Metab 1999;276:E565–E572.
59. Wolf M, Bohm S, Brand M, Kreymann G. Proinflammatory cytokines interleukin 1 beta and tumor necrosis factor alpha inhibit growth hormone stimulation of insulin-like growth factor I synthesis and growth hormone receptor mRNA levels in cultured rat liver cells. Eur J Endocrinol 1996;135:729–737.
60. Mao Y, Ling RR, Fitzgibbons TP, et al. Endotoxin-induced inhibition of growth hormone receptor signaling in rat liver in vivo. Endocrinology 1999;140:5505–5515.
61. Frost RA, Lang CH, Gelato MC. Transient exposure of human myoblasts to tumor necrosis factor-alpha inhibits serum and insulin-like growth factor-I stimulated protein synthesis. Endocrinology 1997;138:4153–4159.
62. Ling PR, Boyce P, Chow JC, et al. Inhibition of response to a lower but not a higher dose euglycemic infusion of IGF-I in TNF-treated rats. JPEN J Parenter Enteral Nutr 1998;21:S2.
63. Fang CH, Li BG, James JH, Fischer JE, Hasselgren PO. Cytokines block the effects of insulin-like growth factor-I (IGF-I) on glucose uptake and lactate production in skeletal muscle but do not influence IGF-I-induced changes in protein turnover. Shock 1997;8:362–367.
64. Lang CH. IGF-I stimulates muscle glucose uptake during sepsis. Shock. 1996;5:22–27.
65. Auclair M, Vigouroux C, Desbois-Mouthon C, et al. Antiinsulin receptor autoantibodies induce insulin receptors to constitutively associate with insulin receptor substrate-1 and -2 and cause severe cell resistance to both insulin and insulin-like growth factor I. J Clin Endocrinol Metab 1999;84:3197–3206.
66. Shimasaki S, Ling N. Identification and molecular characterization of insulin-like growth factor binding proteins (IGFBP-1, -2, -3, -4, -5, and -6). Prog Growth Factor Res 1991;3:243–266.
67. Samstein B, Hoimes ML, Fan J, Frost RA, Gelato MC, Lang CH. IL-6 stimulation of insulin-like growth factor binding protein (IGFBP)-1 production. Biochem Biophys Res Commun 1996;228:611–615.
68. Benbassat CA, Lazarus DD, Cichy SB, et al. Interleukin-1 alpha (IL-1 alpha) and tumor necrosis factor alpha (TNF alpha) regulate insulin-like growth factor binding protein-1 (IGFBP-1) levels and mRNA abundance in vivo and in vitro. Horm Metab Res 1999;31:209–215.
69. Baxter RC, Hawker FH, To C, Stewart PM, Holman SR. Thirty-day monitoring of insulin-like growth factors and their binding proteins in intensive care unit patients. Growth Horm IGF Res 1998;8:455–463.
70. Firth SM, McDougall F, McLachlan AJ, Baxter RC. Impaired blockade of insulin-like growth factor I (IGF-I)-induced hypoglycemia by IGF binding protein-3 analog with reduced ternary complex-forming ability. Endocrinology 2002;143:1669–1676.
71. Tayek JA, Manglik S, Abemayor E. Insulin secretion, glucose production, and insulin sensitivity in underweight and normal-weight volunteers, and in underweight and normal-weight cancer patients: a Clinical Research Center Study. Metabolism 1997;46:140–145.
72. Soares MJ, Piers LS, Shetty PS, Jackson AA, Waterlow JC. Whole body protein turnover in chronically undernourished individuals. Clin Sci 1994;86:441–446.
73. Duke JH Jr., Jorgensen SB, Broell JR, Long CL, Kinney JM. Contribution of protein to caloric expenditure following injury. Surgery 1970;68:168–174.

74. Kinney M. Metabolic responses of the critically ill patient. Crit Care Clin 1995;11:569–585.
75. Flores EA, Bistrian BR, Pompposelli JJ, Dinarello C, Blackburn GL, Istfan NW. Infusion of tumor necrosis factor/cachectin promotes muscle catabolism in the rat. A synergistic effect with interleukin 1. J Clin Invest 1989;83:1614–1622.
76. Doweiko JP, Nompleggi DL. The role of albumin in human physiology and pathophysiology. Part III: Albumin and disease states. JPEN J Parenter Enteral Nutr. 1991;15:476–483.
77. Dietary Reference. Intakes for energy, carbohydrate, fiber, fat, fatty acids, cholesterol, protein, and amino acid (macronutrient). In: Food and Nutrition Board. Institute of Medicine. The National Academy Press, 2002, p. 465.
78. Wolfe RR, Goodenough RD, Burke JF, Wolfe MH. Response of protein and urea kinetics in burn patients to different levels of protein intake. Ann Surg 1983;197:163–171.
79. Greig P, Elwyn D, Askanazi J, Kinney JM. Parenteral nutrition in septic patients: Effect of increasing nitrogen intake. Am J Clin Nutr 1987;46:1040–1047.
80. Ishibashi N, Plank LD, Sando K, Hill GL. Optimal protein requirements during the first 2 weeks after the onset of critical illness. Crit Care Med 1998;26:1529–1535.
81. Bistrian BR, Babineau T. Optimal protein intake in critical illness? Crit Care Med 1998;26:1476–1477.
82. Montoya A, Gomez-Lechon MJ, Castell JV. Influence of branched-chain amino acid compostion of culture media on the synthesis of plasma proteins by serum-free cultured rat hepatocytes. In Vitro Cell Dev Biol 1989;25:358–364.
83. Kee AJ, Baxter RC, Carlsson AR, Smith RC. Parenteral amino acid intake alters the anabolic actions of insulin-like growth factor I in rats. Am J Physiol Endocrinol Metab 1999;277:E63–E72.
84. Sanchez-Gomez M, Malmlof K, Mejia W, et al. Insulin-like growth factor-I, but not growth hormone, is dependent on a high protein intake to increase nitrogen balance in the rat. Br J Nutr 1999;81:145–152.
85. Isidori A, Lo Monaco A, Cappa M. A study of growth hormone release in man after oral administration of amino acids. Curr Med Res Opin 1981;7:475–481.
86. Yahya ZA, Bates PC, Millward DJ. Responses to protein deficiency of plasma and tissue insulin-like growth factor-I levels and proteoglycan synthesis rates in rat skeletal muscle and bone. J Endocrinol 1990;127:497–530.
87. Jousse C, Bruhat A, Ferrara M, Fafournoux P. Physiological concentration of amino acids regulates insulin-like-growth factor-binding protein 1 expression. Biochem J 1998;334:147–153.
88. Houdijk A, Rijnsburger ER, Jansen J, Wesdorp RI, Weiss JK, McCamish MA, et al. Randomised trial of glutamine-enriched enteral nutrition on infectious morbidity in patients with multiple truama. Lancet 1998;352:772–776.
89. Kudsk KA, Minard G, Croce MA, et al. A randomized trial of isonitrogenous enteral diets after severe trauma. An immune-enhacing diet reduces septic complications. Ann Surg 1996;224:531–540.
90. Wilmore DW. The effect of glutamine supplementation in patients following elective surgery and accidental injury. J Nutr 2001;131:2543S–2549S.
91. Lin MT, Kung SP, Yeh SL, et al. The effect of glutamine-supplemented total parenteral nutrition on nitrogen economy depends on severity of diseases in surgical patients. Clin Nutr 2002;21:213–218.
92. Evoy D, Lieberman MD, Fahey TJ 3rd, Daly JM. Immunonutrition: the role of arginine. Nutrition 1998;14:611–617.
93. Yeh CL, Yeh SL, Lin MT, Chen WJ. Effects of arginine-enriched total parenteral nutrition on inflammatory-related mediator and T-cell population in septic rats. Nutrition 2002;18:631–635.
94. Gil A. Modulation of the immune response mediated by dietary nucleotides. Eur J Clin Nutr 2002;56:S1–S4.
95. van den Berghe G, Wouters P, Weekers F, et al. Intensive insulin therapy in the critically ill patients. N Engl J Med 2001;345:1359–1367.
96. McCowen KC, Malhotra A, Bistrian BR. Stress-induced hyperclycemia. Crit Care Clin 2000;17:107–124.
97. McCowen KC, Friel C, Sternberg J, et al. Hypocaloric total parenteral nutrition: Effectiveness in prevention of hyperglycemia and infectious complications—A randomized clinical trial. Crit Care Med 2000;28:3606–3611.
98. Rosmarin DK, Wardlaw GM, Mirtallo J. Hyperglycemia associated with high, continuous infusion rate of total parenteral nutrition dextrose. Nutr Clin Pract 1996;11:151–156.

99. Pomposelli JJ, Baxter JK III, Babineau TJ, et al. Early postoperative glucose control predicts nosocomial infection rate in diabetic patients. JPEN J Parenter Enteral Nutr 1998;22:77–81.
100. Guha M, Bai W, Nadler JL, Natarajan R. Molecular mechanisms of tumor necrosis factor alpha gene expression in monocytic cells via hyperglycemia-induced oxidant stress-dependent and -independent pathways. J Biol Chem 2000;275:17728–17739.
101. Yerneni KK, Bai W, Khan BV, Medford RM, Natarajan R. Hyperglycemia-induced activation of nuclear transcription factor kappaB in vascular smooth muscle cells. Diabetes 1999;48:855–864.
102. Kwoun MO, Ling PR, Lydon E, et al. Immunologic effects of acute hyperglycemia in nondiabetic rats. J Parenter Enteral Nutr. 1997;21:91–95.
103. Zerr KJ, Furnary AP, Grunkemeier GL, Bookin S, Kanhere V, Starr A. Glucose control lowers the risk of wound infection in diabetics after open heart operations. Ann Thorac Surg. 1997;63:356–361.
104. Furnary AP, Zerr KJ, Grunkemeier GL, Starr A. Continuous intravenous insulin infusion reduces the incidence of deep sternal wound infection in diabetic patients after cardiac surgical procedures. Ann Thorac Surg 1999;67:352–360.
105. Malmberg K. Prospective randomized study of intensive insulin treatment on long term survival after acute myocardial infarction in patients with diabetes mellitus: DIGAMI (Diabetes Mellitus, Insulin Glucose Infusion in Acute Mayocadial Infarction) Study Group. BMJ 1997;314:1512–1515.
106. Ling PR, Lydon E, Qu Zh, Frederich RC, Bistrian BR. Metabolic effects of insulin and insulin-like growth factor-I in endotoxemic rats during total parenteral nutrition feeding. Metabolism 2000;49:611–615.
107. Patino JF, de Pimiento SE, Vergara A, Savino P, Rodriguez M, Escallon J. Hypocaloric support in the critically ill. World J Surg 1999;23:553–559.
108. Macfie J, Smith RC, Hill GL. Glucose or fat as nonprotein energy source ? A controlled clinical trial in gastroenterological patients requiring intravenous nutrition. Gastroenterology 1981;80:103–107.
109. Paulsrud JR, Pensler L, Whitten CF, Stewart S, Holman RT. Essential fatty acid deficiency in infants induced by fat-free intravenous feeding. Am J Clin Nutr 1972;25:897–904.
110. Fleming CR, Smiht LM, Hodges RE. Essential fatty acid deficiency in adults receiving total parenteral nutrition. Am J Clin Nutr 1976;29:976–983.
111. Wene JD, Connor WE, DenBesten L. The development of essential fatty acid deficiency in healthy man fed fat-free diets intravenously and orally. J Clin Invest 1975;56:127–134.
112. Kamara K, Eskay R, Castonguay T. High-fat diets and stress responsivity. Physiol Behav 1998;64:1–6.
113. Klein S, Miles JM. Metabolic effects of long-chain and medium-chain triglyceride emulsions in humans. JPEN J Parenter Enteral Nutr 1994;18:396–397.
114. Barr LH, Dunn GD, Brennan MF. Essential fatty acid deficiency during total parenteral nutrition. Ann Surg 1981;193:304–311.
115. Innis SM. Essential fatty acid requirements in human nutrition. Can J Physiol Pharmacol 1993;71:699–706.
116. Endres S, Ghorbani R, Kelley VE, et al. The effects of dietary supplementation with n-3 polyunsaturated fatty acids on the synthesis of interleukin-1 and tumor necrosis factor by mononuclear cells. N Engl J Med 1989;320:265–271.
117. Pomposelli JJ, Mascioli EA, Bistrian BR, Lopes SM, Blackburn GL. Attenuation of the febrile response in guinea pigs by fish oil enriched diets. J Parenterl Enteral Nutr 1989;13:136–140.
118. Pscheidl EM, Wan JM, Blackburn GL, Bistrian BR, Istfan NM. Influence of omega-3 fatty acids on splanchnic blood flow and lactate metabolism in an endotoxinemic rat model. Metabolism 1992;41:698–705.
119. Ling PR, Istfan N, Colon E, Bistrian BR. Effect of fish oil on glucose metabolism in the interleukin-1 alph-treated rat. Metabolism 1993;42:81–85.
120. Tashiro T, Yamamori H, Takagi K, Hayashi N, Furukawa K, Nakajima N. n-3 versus n-6 polyunsaturated fatty acids in critical illness. Nutrition 1998;14:551–553.
121. Volker D, Fitzgerald P, Major G, Garg M. Efficacy of fish oil concentrate in the treatment of rheumatoid arthritis. J Rheumatol 2000;27:2343–2346.
122. Darlington LG, Stone TW. Antioxidants and fatty acids in the amelioration of rheumatoid arthritis and related disorders. Br J Nutr 2001;85:251–269.
123. Geerling BJ, Badart-Smook A, van Deursen C, van Houwelingen AC, Russel MG, Stockbrugger RW, et al. Nutritional supplementation with N-3 fatty acids and antioxidants in patients with

Crohn's disease in remission: effects on antioxidant status and fatty acid profile. Inflamm Bowel Dis 2000;6:77–84.
124. Ling SC, Griffiths AM. Nutrition in inflammatory bowel disease. Curr Opin Clin Nutr Metab Care 2000;3:339–344.
125. Santos J, Queiros J, Silva F, et al. Effects of fish oil in cyclosporine-treated renal transplant recipients. Transplant Proc. 2000;32:2605–2608.
126. Ghoshal AK, Xu Z, Wood GA, Archer MC. Induction of hepatic insulin-like growth factor binding protein-1 (IGFBP-1) in rats by dietary n-6 polyunsaturated fatty acids. Pro Soc Exp Biol Med. 2000;225:128–135.
127. Curtis-Prior M: Prostaglandins: Biology and Chemistry of Prostaglandins and Related Eicosanoids. Churchill-Livingston, New York,. 1988.
128. Parker CW Lipid mediators produced through the lipoxygenase pathway. Ann Rev Immunol 1987;5:65–84.
129. Kinsella JE, Lokesh B, Broughton S, Whelan J. Dietary polyunsaturated fatty acids and eicosanoids: potential effects on the modulation of inflammatory and immune cells: an overview. Nutrition 1990;6:24–44.
130. Lands WE. Biochemistry and physiology of w3 fatty acids. FASEB J 1992;6:2530–2536.
131. Mayer K, Seeger W, Grimminger F. Clinical use of lipids to control inflammatory disease. Curr Opin Clin Nutr Metab Care 1998;1:179–184.
132. Zadak Z, Cervinkova Z. PUFA n-3 lipid emulsion: a promising agent in ARDS treatment. Nutrition 1997;13:232–233.
133. Baronzio G, Freitas I, Griffini P, et al. Omega-3 fatty acids can improve radioresponse modifying tumor interstitial pressure, blood rheology and membrane peroxidability. Anticancer Res 1994;14:1145–1154.
134. Rose DP, Connolly JM. Omega-3 fatty acids as cancer chemopreventive agents. Pharmacol Ther 1999;83:217–244.
135. Jeffery NM, Newsholme EA, Calder PC. Level of polyunsaturated fatty acids and the n-6 to n-3 polyunsaturated fatty acid ratio in the rat diet alter serum lipid levels and lymphocyte functions. Prostaglandins Leukot Essent Fatty Acids 1997;57:149–160.
136. Wachtler P, Konig W, Senkal M, Kemen M, Koller M. Influence of a total parenteral nutrition enriched omega-3 fatty acids on leukotriene synthesis of peripheral leukocytes and systemic cytokine levels in patients with major surgery. J Trauma 1997;42:191–198.
137. Lanza-Jacoby S, Flynn JT, Miller S. Parenteral supplementation with a fish-oil emulsion prolongs survival and improves rat lymphocyte function during sepsis. Nutrition 2001;17:112–116.
138. Wigmore SJ, Ross JA, Falconer JS, et al. The effect of polyunsaturated fatty acids on the progress of cachexia in patients with pancreatic cancer. Nutrition 1996;12:S27–S30.
139. Barber MD, Ross JA, Voss AC, Tisdale MJ, Fearon KC. The effect of an oral nutrition supplement enriched with fish oil on weight-loss in patients with pancreatic cancer. Br J Cancer 1999;81:80–86.
140. Barber MD, McMillan DC, Preston T, Ross JA, Fearon KC. Metabolic response to feeding in weight-losing pancreatic cancer patients and its modulation by a fish-oil-enriched nutritional supplement. Clin Sci 2000;98:389–399.
141. Wigmore SJ, Barber MD, Ross JA, Tisdale MJ, Fearon KC. Effect of oral eicosapentaenoic acid on weight loss in patients with pancreatic cancer. Nutr Cancer 2000;36:177–184.
142. Ponting GA, Halliday D, Teale JD, Sim AJ. Postoperative positive nitrogen balance with intravenous hyponutrition and growth hormone. Lancet 1988;1:438–440.
143. Manson JM, Smith RJ, Wilmore DW. Growth hormone stimulates protein synthesis during hypocaloric parenteral nutrition: Role of hormonal-substrate environments. Ann Surg 1988;208: 136–142.
144. Gore DC, Honeycutt D, Jahoor F, Wolfe RR, Herndon DN. Effect of exogenous growth hormone on whole-body and isolated-limb protein kinetics in burned patients. Arch Surg 1991;126:38–43.
145. Jeevanandam M, Ali MR, Holaday NJ, Petersen SR. Adjuvant recombinant human growth hormone normalizes plasma amino acids in parenterally fed trauma patients. JPEN J Parenter Enteral Nutr 1995;19:137–144.
146. Voerman BJ, Strack van Schijndel RJ, Groeneveld AB, de Boer H, Nauta JP, Thijs LG. Effects of human growth hormone in critically ill nonseptic patients: results from a prospective, randomized, placebo-controlled trial. Crit Care Med 1995;23:665–673.

147. Carli F, Webster JD, Halliday D. Growth hormone modulates amino acid oxidation in the surgical patient: leucine kinetics during the fasted and fed state using moderate nitrogenous and caloric diet and recombinant human growth hormone. Metabolism. 1997;46:23–28.
148. Carli F, Webster JD, Halliday DA. A nitrogen-free hypocaloric diet and recombinant human growth hormone stimulate postoperative protein synthesis: fasted and fed leucine kinetics in the surgical patients. Metabolism 1997;46:796–800.
149. Schambelan M, Mulligan K, Grunfeld C, et al. Recombinant human growth hormone in patients with HIV-associated wasting. A randomized, placebo-controlled trial. Serostin Study Group. Ann Intern Med. 1996;125:873–882.
150. Takala J, Ruokonen E, Webster NR, et al. Increased mortality associated with growth hormone treatment in critically ill adults. N Eng J Med 1999;341:785–792.
151. Tayek JA, Brasel JA. Failure of anabolism in malnourished cancer patients receiving growth hormone: a clinical research center study. J Clin Endocrino Metab 1995;80:2082–2087.
152. Jenkins RC, Ross RJ. Acquired growth hormone resistance in catabolic states. Baillieres Clin Endocrinol Metab 1996;10:411–419.
153. Handelsman DJ, Liu PY. Androgen therapy in chronic renal failure. Baillieres Clin Endocrinol Metab 1998;12:485–500.
154. Corcoran C, Grinspoon S. The use of testosterone in the AIDS wasting syndrome. AIDS Clin Care 1999;11:25–26, 33–34.
155. Strawford A, Barbieri T, Van Loan M, et al. Resistance exercise and supraphysiologic androgen therapy in eugonadal men with HIV-related weight loss: a randomized controlled trial. JAMA 1999;281:1282–1290.
156. Horton JW, White DJ, Maass DL, Hybki DP, Handek S, Giroir B. Antioxidant vitamin therapy alters burn trauma-mediated cardiac NF-kappaB activation and cardiomyocyte cytokine secretion. J Trauma 2001;50:397–406.
157. Fu Z, Noguchi T, Kato H. Vitamin A deficiency reduces insulin-like growth factor (IGF)-I gene expression and increases IGF-I receptor and insulin receptor gene expression in tissues of Japanese quail (Coturnix coturnix japonica). J Nutr 2001;131:1189–1194.
158. Ninh NX, Maiter D, Lause P, et al. Continuous administration of growth hormone does not prevent the decrease of IGF-I gene expression in zinc-deprived rats despite normalization of liver GH binding. Growth Horm IGF Res 1998;8:465–472.
159. Angstwurm MW, Schottdorf J, Schopohl J, Gaertner R. Selenium replacement in patients with severe systemic inflammatory response syndrome improves clinical outcome. Crit Care Med 1999;27:1807–1813.
160. Preiser JC, Van Gossum A, Berre J, Vincent JL, Carpentier Y. Enteral feeding with a solution enriched with antioxidant vitamins A, C and E enhances the resistance to oxidative stress. Crit Care Med 2000;28:3828–3832.
161. Ziegler TR, Young LS, Benfell K, et al. Clincial and metabolic efficacy of glutamine-supplemented parenteral nutrition after bone marrow transplantation. A randomized, double-blind, controlled study. Ann Intern Med 1992;116:821–828.
162. Schloerb PR, Skikne BS. Oral and parenteral glutamine in bone marrow transplantation: a randomized, double-blind study. JPEN J Parenter Enteral Nutr 1999;23:117–122.
163. Morlion B, Stehle P, Wachtler P, et al. Total parenteral nutrition with glutamine dipeptide after major abdominal surgery: a randomized, double-blind controlled study. Ann Surg 1998;227:302–308.
164. Houdijk AP, Rijnsburger ER, Jansen J, et al. Randomised trial of glutamine-enriched enteral nutrition on infectious morbidity in patients with multiple trauma. Lancet. 1998;352:772–776.
165. Kudsk KA, Minard G, Croce M, et al. A randomized trial of isonitrogenous enteral diets after severe trauma. An immune-enhancing diet reduces septic complications. Ann Surg 1996;224:531–540.
166. Paradowski PT, Zeman K, Pietruszynski R. Pentoxifylline inhibits tumor necrosis factor alpha-induced priming of human neutrophils. Immunol Lett 1996;53:131–134.
167. Porter MH, Hrupka BJ, Altreuther G, Arnold M, Langhans W. Inhibition of TNF-alpha production contributes to the attenuation of LPS-induced hypophagia by pentoxifylline. Am J Physiol Regul Integr Comp Physiol. 2000;279:R2113–2120.
168. Fu CS, Conteas CN, LaRiviere MJ. Successful treatment of idiopathic colitis and proctitis using thalidomide in person infected with human immunodeficiency virus. AIDS Patient Care STDS 1998;12:903–906.

169. Corral LG, Muller GW, Moreira AL, et al. Selection of novel analogs of thalidomide with enhanced tumor necrosis factor alpha inhibitory activity. Mol Med 1996;2:506–515.
170. Keifer JA, Guttridge DC, Ashburner BP, Baldwin AS Jr. Inhibition of NF-kappa B activity by thalidomide through suppression of Ikappa B kinase activity. J Biol Chem 2001;276:22382–22387.
171. Ohtsuka T, Hamada M, Hiasa G, et al. Effect of beta-blockers on circulating levels of inflammatory and anti-inflammatory cytokines in patients with dilated cardiomyopathy. J Am Coll Cardiol 2001;37:412–417.
172. Skudicky D, Bergemann A, Sliwa K, Candy G, Sareli P. Beneficial effects of pentoxifylline in patients with idiopathic dilated cardiomyopaty treated with angiotension-converting enzyme inhibitors and carvedilol: results of a randomized study. Circulation 2001;103:1083–1088.
173. Stenvinkel P, Andersson P, Wang T, et al. Do ACE-inhibitors suppress tumor necrosis factor-alpha production in a advanced chronic renal failure? J Intern Med 1999;246:503–507.
174. Ridker P, Rifai N, Clearfield M, et al. Measurement of C-reactive protein for the targeting of statin therapy in the primary prevention of acute coronary events. N Engl J Med 2001;344:1959–1965.
175. Davies MG, Hagen PO. Systemic inflammatory response syndrome. Br J Surg. 1997;84:920–935.
176. Galban C, Montejo JC, Mesejo A, et al. An immune-enhancing enteral diet reduces mortality rate and episodes of bacteremia in septic intensive care unit patients. Crit Care Med 2000;28:643–648.
177. Mune M, Yukawa S, Kishino M, et al. Effect of vitamin E on lipid metabolism and atherosclerosis in ESRD patients. Kidney Int Suppl 1999;71:S126–S129.
178. Gogos CA, Ginopoulos P, Salsa B, Apostolidou E, Zoumbos NC, Kalfarentzos F. Dietary omega-3 polyunsaturated fatty acids plus vitamin E restore immunodeficiency and prolong survival for severely ill patients with generalized malignancy: a randomized control trial. Cancer 1998;82:395–402.

4 The Insulin-Like Growth Factors and Assessment of Nutritional Status

M. Sue Houston

KEY POINTS

- The regulation of circulating IGF-I and IGFBPs by nutritional intake and the short half-life of these proteins in circulation offer great potential for the IGF proteins to be utilized as exceptionally sensitive acute biochemical markers of nutritional intake, repletion, and metabolic status.
- The value of serum IGF-I as an indicator of short-term response to nutrional intervention has been described in a wide variety of patient populations and experimental conditions.
- The sensitivity and specificity of serum IGF-I as a marker of nutritional status in critical illness is much greater than other visceral markers such as albumin, retinol binding protein, or transthyretin. Continued validation of IGF-I and IGFBPs in critical illness and other acute disorders is anticipated since assessment of appropriate nutritional intervention is both exceedingly important and particularly challenging in these circumstances.
- Because of the acute nature of the response to nutrition, IGFs are much less suited to evaluating chronic nutritional status, body weight, or body composition.
- The dependence of IGF proteins on vitamins, minerals, and other dietary constituents has been less fully investigated; however, deficiencies of specific nutrients clearly influence IGF protein synthesis and concentrations in the serum.
- The IGFBPs, in particular IGFBP-1, IGFBP-2, and perhaps ratios of the IGFBPs and IGF-I, or free IGF-I in relation to nutrition, await further study, but could prove to be valuable markers of nutritional status.

1. INTRODUCTION

The dependency and remarkable sensitivity of the insulin-like growth factor (IGF) proteins and IGF binding proteins (IGFBPs) to nutrient availability has been recognized since the early work on the somatomedins. The fundamental role of IGF proteins in metabolic regulation suggests that the IGF proteins provide a direct functional indicator of sufficient substrates to support anabolism. The regulation of circulating IGF-I and IGFBPs by nutritional intake and the short half-life of these proteins in circulation offers great potential for the IGF proteins to be used as exceptionally sensitive acute

From: *IGF and Nutrition in Health and Disease*
Edited by: M. S. Houston, J. M. P. Holly, and E. L. Feldman © Humana Press Inc., Totowa, NJ

biochemical markers of nutritional and metabolic status. Building upon the fundamental interrelationships between the IGF proteins and nutrition in health and disease, as presented in this volume, the present chapter will review an extensive number of research studies that have examined the IGF proteins as markers of nutritional status. Background about the process of nutritional assessment and the criteria used to evaluate the efficacy of markers is included to provide a context into which research can be examined. The focus of the chapter is the utility of IGF proteins as markers of acute nutritional status and monitors of nutritional repletion. The IGFs are much less suited to evaluating chronic nutritional status, body weight, or body composition. Limitations and the impact of non-nutritional factors on the validity and sensitivity of IGFs are discussed. Although a wide variety of disease states and circumstances have been studied, of particular note is the work demonstrating IGFs as markers of nutritional status in critical illness and other acute disorders in which assessment of appropriate nutritional intervention is both exceedingly important, and particularly challenging.

2. BACKGROUND

The present chapter will focus on the IGF proteins as markers of protein and energy status because much less is known with regard to IGFs as markers of specific vitamin and/or mineral imbalances. An overview of the process and methods available to assess nutritional status is followed by a discussion of the important differences between chronic and acute assessment. The basic concepts of validity, specificity, sensitivity, and precision as they apply to evaluating the appropriateness of nutrition status markers are presented.

2.1. Protein Energy Malnutrition

Protein energy malnutrition (PEM) remains a worldwide problem, particularly in children, but also in institutionalized individuals where the prevalence may reach 40 to 50% of hospitalized patients *(1–5)*. There are two physiological subtypes of protein energy malnutrition, marasmus and kwashiorkor, although combinations of these subtypes are also common *(6)*. Marasmus results from semistarvation and is characterized by inadequate food intake and a balanced lack of both energy and protein. Metabolic adaptation to simple starvation or marasmus is evident with fairly normal serum protein pools, maintenance of immune function, decreased basal metabolic rate, and other metabolic adaptations to preserve body protein. In severe forms, growth failure and a loss of body fat and proteins stores make diagnosis of marasmus PEM fairly obvious. Kwashiorkor, or hypoalbuminemic PEM, in contrast, is a protein deficiency. The metabolic adaptations to fasting and marasmus do not take place with kwashiorkor, and accelerated loss of somatic and visceral proteins results in hypoalbuminemia and edema. Physiological stressors, such as infection or the inflammatory stress response, typically contribute to kwashiorkor by increasing the demand for protein and energy. Immunity is compromised quickly, and both hypermetabolism and hypercatabolism may be present. Kwashiorkor PEM is more difficult to diagnosis because of the rapid onset, lack of obvious clinical signs, masking by normal or excessive body fat stores and/or edema, and presence of other physical stressors. In contrast to marasmus, where chronic and less specific anthropometric markers can be used, detection of kwashiorkor requires the use of sensitive biochemical markers of acute nutritional status *(6–8)*. The ability of IGF proteins to reliably detect PEM in both forms has been demonstrated and is described in more detail in later sections of the chapter.

2.2. Assessment of Nutritional Status: General Considerations

The purpose of nutritional assessment is to accurately detect nutritional disorders as early as possible and to monitor the appropriateness of nutrition intervention *(9)*. Malnutrition generally connotes a deficiency of energy or particular nutrients. However, in its more inclusive meaning, malnutrition indicates "faulty" nutrition, including under, over, and imbalanced nutritional states. The development of malnutrition typically progresses through four stages. The first stage is initiated by such factors as a faulty diet, excessive losses, impaired absorption, or altered energy or nutrient requirements. Although inappropriate food intake may contribute, there are many nondietary factors, and simply testing the "adequacy" of the diet does not reliably predict malnutrition. In the second stage, body stores of the nutrient are altered (increased or decreased). The first and second stages are difficult to discern because tissues indicative of body stores are usually inaccessible (e.g., liver biopsy). In the third stage of malnutrition, function becomes affected. At some threshold of nutrient depletion, excess, or imbalance, biochemical changes become apparent. This is a preclinical stage, symptoms of deficiency are not obvious, but may be detected by acute biochemical markers of nutritional status. In the fourth stage of malnutrition, cellular and tissue deterioration becomes more obvious and can be indicated by clinical signs or chronic markers of nutritional status, such as anthropometrics.

2.2.1. Methods of Nutritional Assessment

The most effective nutritional assessment uses a variety of different types of measurements in combination. Many excellent reviews evaluating nutritional status techniques are available *(9–11)*. The major categories of nutritional assessment methods are outlined in Table 1. Validity, sensitivity, specificity, and reliability are important criteria with which nutrition markers are evaluated (Table 2). Each type of nutrition data provides unique information in the assessment of nutritional status. In many instances a direct correlation between data from two types of method can not be demonstrated. Nutritional assessment indices are not interchangeable, and a single method cannot adequately reflect both long term and acute status. Thus, the validity of a marker is very dependent upon the situation in which it is used. Biochemical indices are generously unreliable in predicting body composition *(9)*. As discussed later in this chapter, serum IGF-I and the IGFBPs in many instances are not valid indicators of body weight or composition.

2.2.2. Methods to Assess Acute Protein and Energy Status: Biochemical Markers

Biochemical (laboratory) assessment is used to detect subclinical deficiency states and can provide the most sensitive information regarding recent status and/or directional changes in both anabolism and catabolism. Concentrations of circulating proteins (indicating visceral protein status) and nitrogen excretion (reflecting changes in metabolism) can provide a picture of current nitrogen balance, but not long-term shifts in somatic protein stores or body composition. With the exception of infants and young children, anthropometric and clinical methods indicate changes in somatic protein and body composition that take a fairly long time to occur. Biochemical tests can be sensi-

Table 1
Types of Data Used in the Assessment of Nutritional Status

Method	*Examples*	*Indicator of acute or chronic malnutrition*
Dietary		
Intake of energy and nutrients	24-h Recall or dietary record	Acute
	Food frequency	Chronic
	Diet history—usual dietary patterns or dietary restrictions	Chronic
Biochemical (laboratory)		
Serum or urinary concentrations of static or functional markers	Serum proteins, such as albumin, transthyretin, transferrin, IGF	Acute
	Serum or urinary vitamins, minerals, electrolytes	Acute
	Urinary nitrogen or metabolites	Acute and chronic
Anthropometric or body composition		
Body dimensions and gross composition (e.g., fat or somatic protein mass)	Body weight, height, body mass index	Chronic
	Triceps skinfold, mid-arm muscle circumference	Chronic
	% Body fat, % fat-free mass,	Chronic
Physical/clinical signs and symptoms		
Overt signs of malnutrition, visual appraisal, reported symptoms	wasting, growth failure, fatigue	Acute and chronic
	chelosis, dermatitis, petechiae, alopecia, anemia and other signs of vitamin/mineral deficiency	Acute and chronic
History		
Factors that influence nutritional risk	Medical diagnoses	Acute and chronic
	Social, psychological, lifestyle, and economic factors	Chronic
	Developmental stage	Chronic
	Medications	Acute and chronic

tive to recent changes and are of two types: static or functional. Static biochemical markers include levels of a nutrient or its metabolite in serum, urine, or other biopsy material. Functional markers indicate the sufficiency of nutrients available to permit cells, tissues, organs, or the whole organism to perform optimally. Functional markers include the activities of enzymes that are dependent upon specific nutrients (e.g., superoxide dismutase), but also include the measure of rapid-turnover visceral proteins in the blood (e.g., transthyretin or IGF-I).

The main site of synthesis for serum proteins used for nutritional assessment is the liver, one of the first organs affected by protein malnutrition. The characteristics of a

Table 2
Criteria to Evaluate the Appropriateness of Nutritional Status Markers

Criteria	*Explanation*	*Example*
Validity	Adequacy with which any measurement truly reflects the parameter of interest	Anthropometric measures are valid markers of chronic but not recent nutritional status Biochemical markers with short half-lives are valid markers to monitor refeeding
Sensitivity	Ability to detect small differences in nutritional status such that there is great ability to identify all persons who are genuinely malnourished (i.e., few false negatives)	Rapid-turnover serum markers with detectable fluctuations that reflect changes in nutritional status. IGF-1 and IGFBP-1 appear to be more sensitive to recent nutrition than IGFBP-3
Specificity	Individuals without malnutrition are correctly identified as normal (i.e. there are few false positives). Reflects the extent to which random errors and non-nutritional factors (e.g., disease, diurnal variations) impact the ability of the index to predict malnutrition.	Serum albumin is nonspecific in critical illness because of extra vascular shifts. Recent weight change related to of edema is not indicative of nutrition
Precision	Reliability or reproducibility. Degree to which repeated measures of a sample give the same value.	Low coefficient of variation for laboratory measurements

marker considered ideal for measuring acute changes in protein status include: a small body pool that can reflect changes quickly; very short biological half-life with a rapid rate of synthesis and a fairly constant catabolic rate; a major pool present within the vascular space with minimal extra vascular shifting; and specificity to protein and energy deprivation with little effect of non-nutritional factors, such as stress and disease *(9,12,13)*. Serum proteins traditionally used as nutrition markers do not necessarily meet these criteria (Table 3). For example, serum albumin has a relatively large body pool, more than 50% of which is present outside of the vascular space. Serum albumin redistributes (unrelated to nutrition) in many circumstances. Albumin has a long half-life, and may be a reasonable prognostic indicator of general health status, morbidity, and hospital stay *(15,16)*, but serum concentrations in adults do not reflect nutrition except in cases of long-term, nonstressed protein and energy deprivation *(17,18)*. In kwashiorkor PEM and metabolic stress, such as severe injury, serum albumin decreases dramatically related to decreased synthesis and increased degradation and trans capillary loss but not nutrition *(15,19–21)*. Other short half-life serum transport proteins, such as transthyretin (thyroxin-binding prealbumin), are widely considered more sensitive markers than serum albumin *(10,22–26)*. However, in the presence of the inflammatory stress response none of the widely used markers of visceral protein

Table 3
Half-Life and Physiochemical Characteristics of Serum Proteins Used to Assess Acute Nutritional Status

	Molecular mass (kDa)	*Normal plasma concentration*	*Approximate normal half-life in serum*	*Approximate body pool*
IGF-I[a]	150–200	100–400 ng/mL	12–15 h	
Albumin	65	3.5–5.2 g/dL	2–3 wk	3–5 g/kg
Transthyretin (prealbumin)	55	19–43 mg/dL	2 d	10 mg/kg
Transferrin	80	200–400 mg/dL	1 wk	<100 mg/kg
Retinol-binding protein	21	2.1–6.4 mg/dL	12–14 h	2 mg/kg

[a]IGF-I as bound in the tertiary complex with IGFBP-3 and ALS. Free IGF-I has an estimated half-life of 10–12 min *(14)*. Serum IGF-I concentrations are age-dependent.

status have sufficient specificity, sensitivity, or validity *(10,15,21,25,27,28)*. In contrast, serum IGF-1 provides a very rapid turnover marker with a small body pool and minimal extra vascular shifting. As discussed later in this chapter under various conditions, serum IGF-1 appears to be less influenced by many disease states than other markers. As suggested in other chapters and research presented in the this chapter, the IGF proteins hold great potential to accurately monitor nutritional interventions in acute stress when avoiding both overfeeding and underfeeding, is particularly critical. Several IGFBPs, free IGF-1, and acute labile subunit (ALS) may also be useful as indices of nutrition but await further study.

2.2.3. Methods to Assess Chronic Nutritional Status: Anthropometric and Body Composition Measures

Anthropometric methods of physical dimension or gross composition of the body are useful in assessing chronic imbalances of protein and/or energy. A reflection of long-term nutritional status, anthropometric methods can detect disturbances in the patterns of physical growth and the relative proportions of body tissues, such as fat, muscle, and body water. Many anthropometric procedures use simple, noninvasive, indirect techniques, such as body weight, height, and triceps skin fold, although more sophisticated techniques of measuring total body potassium, water, or protein are primarily used in research settings. Anthropometric indices are crude markers that indicate advanced malnutrition and are relatively insensitive in detecting subclinical malnutrition or short-term changes in nutrition. For example, acute protein malnutrition with decreased transthyretin can be found in a hospitalized patient with a body mass index (BMI) indicating obesity. Lack of correlation between acute and chronic markers of nutritional status is not uncommon. Mixed disorders commonly occur. In general no single marker can reliably indicate both chronic and acute nutritional status.

3. SENSITIVITY OF IGF PROTEINS TO NUTRITION

This section provides a brief overview of the dependency and sensitivity of circulating IGFs to energy, macronutrient, micronutrient, and other dietary components.

3.1. Protein and Energy

IGF-I and IGF binding proteins are acutely sensitive to nutritional status and recent nutrient intake. The decline in IGF-I as a result of nutritional deprivation is independent of growth hormone (GH) and is a result of decreased gene expression via transcriptional and post-transcriptional mechanisms, reduced hepatic production, increased degradation, and clearance of serum IGF-I (reviewed in Chapter 2). Serum IGF-I falls within 24–48 h of fasting in healthy, normal-weight *(29–31)* adults. A threshold of energy between 11–18 kcal/kg appears to be required in adults to maintain serum IGF-I concentrations irrespective of protein intake *(31,32)*. When energy is adequate (35 kcal/kg), even small increments in protein intake (0.2 g protein/kg) result in post fast increases in serum IGF-I *(31)*. The dependence of serum IGF-I concentrations on both energy and protein intake has been clearly demonstrated in a variety of animal species *(33–41)* as well as adult and pediatric populations *(29–32,42–49)*. Excellent reviews of the sensitivity IGF proteins to protein and energy status are available *(44,50–53)*.

Nutrient deficiency also alters the biological action of IGF-I either directly or indirectly through changes in the IGFBPs. The vast majority of IGF-I (approx 90%) circulates bound to the 150-kDa complex, which consists of IGF-I, IGFBP-3, or IGFBP-5, and an ALS. Likely a storage form of IGF-I, this large complex has an estimated half-life of 12–15 h *(14)* in comparison with free IGF-I with a half-life of 14 min *(54)*. IGFBP-1, IGFBP-2, and IGFBP-4 associate with IGF-I in smaller complexes and may be involved in the delivery of IGF-I to tissues and attachment to cell surface receptors. In addition, IGF-independent actions have been shown for IGFBP-1, -3, and -5. Total serum concentrations of IGF-I correlate positively with ALS and IGFBP-3, but IGFBP-1 and free IGF-I correlate inversely. Nutrient intake is a major regulator of circulating concentrations of the IGFBPs. IGFBP-3 concentration is relatively stable throughout the day, and fasting for 24 h has little observable effect on serum IGFBP-3 and ALS in adults *(55,56)*. With more severe forms of nutritional deprivation (e.g., fasting for 48–72 h, and severe protein and energy restriction), IGFBP-3 and ALS are depressed by the nutrient deprivation *(32,57–62)*, but the magnitude of the change is much less than is reported for other IGF proteins. In contrast, serum IGFBP-1 is elevated in the fasted state *(63)* in energy restriction in adults but not children *(32)* and is markedly and rapidly suppressed by nutrient intake *(64,65)*. Increased insulin, glucose, and perhaps amino acid concentrations mediate the postprandial drop in IGFBP-1, and insulin may stimulate transport of IGFBP-1 to the extravascular space (*see* Chapters 2 and 14). IGFBP-2 concentrations are also elevated by dietary restriction *(32,61)* and are less affected by postprandial changes than IGFBP-1.

3.2. Effects of Specific Nutrients and Dietary Components on the IGF Proteins

Carbohydrate and fat composition of the diet also influence the IGF proteins *(34,66–68)*. The importance of the macronutrients in regulating serum IGF-I and the IGFBPs has been reviewed elsewhere *(44,53,69)*. The dependence of IGF proteins on vitamins, minerals, and other dietary constituents has been less fully investigated; however, deficiencies of specific nutrients clearly influence IGF protein synthesis and concentrations in the serum. The interface between specific nutrient deficiencies, protein synthesis, and growth appears to be mediated via the IGF proteins because alterations in IGF metabolism are observed with deficiencies of zinc *(33,70,71)*, specific amino acids *(72)*, manganese *(73)*, vitamin A *(74–76)*, vitamin D *(77)*, calcium *(77,78)*, iodine *(79,80)*, magnesium *(81,82)*, potassium *(81–83)*, and copper *(84)*. The ability of IGFs to indicate micronutrient deficiencies has not been examined.

Epidemiological evidence suggests that circulating concentrations of IGF proteins may be associated with dietary intake of various electrolytes *(85)*, milk *(86)*, tomato (lycopene) *(87)*, and vegetarian dietary patterns *(88)*. The dietary intake of soy has been related to circulating IGF-I concentrations in some *(89,90)* but not other studies *(91,92)*. The associations suggested by these large population studies are beyond the scope of this chapter and to date do not provide sufficient data to suggest the specificity of IGF proteins in assessing dietary components. Whether the IGF proteins will be useful in assessing specific nutrient deficiencies or the intake of other biologically active components of the diet, such as nutraceuticals, awaits further investigation.

4. IGF PROTEINS AS MARKERS OF ACUTE NUTRITIONAL STATUS

A strong reliable association between serum IGF-I, urinary urea nitrogen, and directional changes in nitrogen balance are observed with fasting and refeeding diets of various quality *(29–31,42)*. Short-term semistarvation, sustained workload, inadequate sleep, thermal strain, and refeeding is reliably reflected in serum IGF concentrations in healthy lean men *(93)*. Short-term restriction of energy or protein in healthy children and adults results in significant changes in serum IGF-I, IGFBP-3, -2, and -1 that are detectable within 1–2 d after the diet is altered and are evident before observable changes in other nutrient-dependent serum proteins *(32)*. Serum IGF-I, IGFBP-3, and IGFBP-2 in premature infants appear to respond to recent dietary intake of energy and protein in a fashion similar to adults *(43)*. The value of serum IGF-I as an indicator of short-term response to nutritional intervention has been described in a wide variety of patient populations *(94–97)*. In malnourished hospitalized patients with diverse diagnoses, serum IGF-I is more attenuated, more sensitive to refeeding, and more strongly correlated to nitrogen balance than serum albumin, transferrin, transthyretin, or retinol binding protein *(46,47,94)*. Serum IGF-I has been shown to be more related to total body water, sodium and potassium, and more sensitive to refeeding than serum albumin and transferrin *(98)* in malnourished patients with biliopancreatic bypass.

4.1. Repletion and Monitoring of Nutritional Interventions

Convincing evidence of the validity, sensitivity, and specificity of a nutritional status marker is the observed changes that are associated with replacement of nutrients after deficiency. The ability to discriminate between deficiency and normality in screening and diagnosis should be distinguished from the utility of a marker in monitoring the response to nutritional intervention. Measurements of body composition and size are generally too crude for monitoring nutrition intervention because they are insensitive to short-term changes in nutrition. Many studies suggest that serum IGF-I is more sensitive to nutrient repletion than albumin, transferrin, or even transthyretin *(46,98,99)*. Relative changes in IGF-I may be even more useful than absolute values as indicators of short-term changes in nutritional status. A large body of evidence demonstrating a prompt, obvious, and reliable response of serum IGF-I to repletion of nutritional deprivation under very diverse circumstances and disease states is now available (Table 4).

Table 4
Studies Demonstrating Increased Serum IGF-I in Response to Nutritional Repletion

Study	*Condition/population*	*Nutritional intervention*
Malnourished children		
Bhutta et al. 1999 *(100)*	Malnourished children with diarrhea	Rice-lentil, yogurt repletion diet
Doherty et al. 2002 *(101)*	Severely malnourished children	Diet, zinc supplement
Hintz et al. 1978 *(102)*	Children with PEM and bacterial infections	Milk-based formula
Kabir et al. 1992 *(103)*	Malnourished children with shigellosis	High or normal protein diet
Lopez-Jaramillo et al. 1992 *(104)*	Schoolboys with low calorie and protein intakes	Animal or vegetable protein supplements
Ninh et al. 1996 *(70)*	Growth-retarded children	Zinc supplementation (10 mg/d)
Palacio et al. 2002 *(105)*	Hospitalized children with PEM	Repletion diet
Pucilowska et al. 1993 *(59)*	Undernourished children with shigellosis	High protein refeeding diet
Smith et al. 1989 *(106)*	Malnourished children with M and K	Vegetable protein repletion diet
Soliman et al. 1986 *(107)*	Malnourished children with M, K, or MK	Nutritional rehabilitation
Zamboni et al. 1996 *(108)*	Malnourished children with M or K	Nutritional rehabilitation
Experimental fasting or semistarvation and repletion		
Clemmons et al. 1985 *(42)*	Healthy normal weight males, fasted 5 d	Diet plus essential amino acids
Clemmons et al. 1981 *(29)*	Healthy obese males fasted for 10 d	Normal diet
Isley et al. 1983 *(30)*	Healthy, normal weight adults fasted 5 d	Normal, protein and/or energy deficient diet
Isley et al. 1984 *(31)*	Healthy, normal weight adults fasted 5 d	Low protein and/or energy refeeding diet
Smith et al. 1995 *(32)*	Healthy adults, protein restriction or energy restriction for 6 d	Normal diet
Smith et al. 1995 *(32)*	Healthy children—protein restriction or energy restriction for 6 d	Normal diet
Friedl et al. 2000 *(93)*	Army Rangers, semistarvation and stress	Normal diet
Critical illness		
Aaberg et al. *(109)*	Intensive care patients with severe injury	TPN and enteral
Baxter et al. 1998 *(110)*	Intensive care patients, diverse diagnoses	TPN and enteral
Burgess 1992 *(97)*	Malnourished surgical patients with sepsis	TPN
Elimam et al. 2001 *(111)*	Normal weight adults, cholecystectomy	TPN
Hawker et al. 1987 *(112)*	Intensive care patients, diverse diagnoses	TPN and enteral
Houston et al. *(62)*	Intensive care patients with severe injury	TPN and enteral
Jeevanandam et al. 1996 *(113)*	Intensive care patients with severe injury	TPN
(Lopez-Hellin et al. 2002 *(114)*	Surgical patients in intensive care	TPN
Marin et al. 1999 *(115)*	Children postsurgery	TPN

(continues)

Table 4
(Continued)

Study	*Condition/population*	*Nutritional intervention*
Mattox et al. 1988) *(116)*	Intensive care patients, diverse diagnoses	Enteral with BCAA
Pittoni et al. 2002 *(117)*	Intensive care patients, trauma and sepsis	TPN and enteral
Eating disorders		
Argente et al. 1997 *(118)*	Anorexia nervosa and bulemia	Refeeding diet
Caregaro et al. 2001 *(95)*	Anorexia nervosa	Refeeding diet
Counts et al. 1992 *(119)*	Anorexia nervosa	Refeeding diet
Fukuda et al. 1999 *(120)*	Anorexia nervosa	Refeeding diet
Golden et al. 1994 *(121)*	Anorexia nervosa	Refeeding diet
Heer et al. 2002 *(122)*	Anorexia nervosa	Refeeding diet
Hill et al. 1993 *(123)*	Anorexia nervosa	Refeeding diet
Hotta et al. 2000 *(124)*	Anorexia nervosa, hospitalized	TPN
Nedvidkova et al. 2000 *(125)*	Anorexia nervosa	Refeeding diet
Pascal et al. 2002 *(126)*	Anorexia nervosa	Refeeding diet
Rappaport et al. 1980 *(127)*	Anorexia nervosa	Refeeding diet
Various chronic diseases		
Beattie et al. 1998 *(128)*	Children and adolescents, Crohn's disease	Enteral nutrition support
Lebl et al. 2001 *(129)*	Children and adults, cystic fibrosis	Oral supplementation
Thomas et al. 1993 *(130)*	Children, Crohn's disease	Elemental diet
Malnourished elderly		
Bachrach-Lindstrom, 2001 *(131)*	Elderly women with hip fractures	Protein–energy supplemented diet
Campillo et al. 2000 *(132)*	Undernourished elderly with hip fractures	Oral diet
Rizzoli et al. 2001 *(49)*	Osteoperotic elderly patients, hip fractures	Oral protein supplement
Schurch et al. 1998 *(133)*	Osteoperotic elderly patients, hip fractures	Oral protein, vitamin, Ca supplement
Salbe et al. 1995 *(134)*	Adult males	Oral, enteral and TPN
Malnourished hospitalized patients		
Donahue and Phillips 1989 *(47)*	Malnourished adult patients	Nutrition support
Raynaud-Simon et al. 2002 *(135)*	Malnourished elderly patients with inflammation	Diet 40 kcal/kg, 15% protein
Clemmons et al. 1985 *(94)*	Malnourished adult patients	Nutrition support
Minuto et al. 1989 *(98)*	Malnourished hospitalized patients with biliopancreatic bypass	Parenteral or enteral nutrition support
Unterman et al. 1985 *(46)*	Malnourished adult patients with M, K, MK	Nutrition support
Newborn infants		
Colonna et al. 1996 *(136)*	Preterm newborn infants	Enteral nutrition
Diaz-Gomez et al. 1997 *(137)*	Preterm newborn infants	Formula supplemented with human milk
Park et al. 2001 *(138)*	Preterm newborn infants	Parenteral nutrition
Price et al. 2001 *(139)*	Premature infants with bronchopulmonary dysplasia	Enteral and parenteral nutrition
Smith et al. 1997 *(43)*	Premature infants	Enteral and parenteral nutrition

PEM, protein energy malnutrition; M, marasmus PEM; K, kwashiorkor PEM; MK, combined marasmus and kwashiorkor PEM; TPN, total parenteral nutrition; enteral, enteral tube feeding; BCAA, branched chain amino acids.

These studies (and there are undoubtedly more) make a compelling case for the use of serum IGF-I to monitor both nutrition intervention and short term variations in nutritional status.

4.2. Relationship Between IGF Proteins and Markers of Chronic Nutritional Status

Cross-sectional data in mixed populations have not demonstrated a consistent association between IGF-I and long-term indicators of nutritional status, body size, and body composition. This is illustrated in an analysis of 790 elderly men and women in the Framingham Heart Study. Serum IGF-I did not correlate with body composition, weight, waist and hip circumferences, past health behaviors, or other long-term indicators but was associated with acute biochemical markers of nutritional status and recent weight loss *(140)*. In many studies, the lack of association between IGF proteins and anthropometric measures may be the presence of mixed chronic and acute nutritional disorders or the inability to predict chronic status with an acute marker.

4.2.1. Healthy Adult Populations

There are discordant data regarding the relationship between serum IGFs and anthropometric and body composition measures in healthy populations. Issues such as adjustment for age, recent dietary intake at the time of sampling, heterogeneity of the sample, and testing only simple linear relationships may explain some of the discrepancies. In studies of small-to-moderately sized populations ($n < 100$), results are conflicting and conclusions difficult. In men, inverse correlations have been noted between IGF-I and BMI, triceps skinfold, and percent body fat *(141–143)*. Similar associations have been found in women in some, but not all studies *(141,143,144)*. Serum IGF-I was weakly correlated with BMI in healthy women, but not with men, after adjustment for age *(145)*. No correlation between IGF-I and BMI was found in healthy elderly persons *(146)*. IGF-I was not predictive of lean body mass in elderly men with varying levels of physical activity *(147)*. However, serum IGF-I was negatively correlated with visceral fat mass, independently of subcutaneous and total fat mass in men with abdominal obesity *(148)*. Positive associations between IGF-I, IGFBP-1, and lean body mass and a negative association between total body fat and IGFBP-1 were observed in normal and growth hormone deficient adults *(149)*.

Data from large mixed healthy cohorts provide an even less convincing argument for the association between serum IGF-I and anthropometrics, other indices of adiposity or lean body mass in healthy populations. In the Baltimore Longitudinal Study of Aging, BMI and waist circumference were not related to serum IGF-I when adjusted for age in healthy, normal weight men or women *(150)*. Serum IGF-I concentrations did not indicate heavier weight, larger waist circumference, body fat, or lean mass in elderly men and women ($n = 790$) from the Framingham Heart Study data *(140)*. After adjustment for age, serum IGF-I was not associated with height, BMI, total or central body fat, or lean body mass in the Rancho Bernardo Study, which included 420 healthy men and 419 women aged 50 years and older *(151)*. In a recent study of a large group of healthy women ($n = 1037$), serum IGFBP-3, but not IGF-I, was positively associated with BMI *(152)*. BMI did not correlate significantly with serum IGF-I in 1030 healthy children, adolescents, and adults *(153)*.

4.2.2. Other Developmental Stages

The relationship between IGF-I and body size or composition may be developmentally dependent. Studies of healthy, growing infants have demonstrated that serum IGF-I and IGFBPs are related to gestational age, birth weight, body weight, and nutritional intake during gestation and early postnatal life *(154–157)*. Serum IGF-I and IGFBP-3 increase with increasing caloric and protein intake; these changes correlate with anthropometric measurements in growing preterm infants *(43,136,137)* and premature infants with bronchopulmonary dysplasia *(139)*. During infancy, research suggests that IGF-I levels are primarily regulated by nutrition *(157)*. Before puberty, serum IGF-I concentrations may reflect overall somatic size, that is, weight, height, BMI, and fat free mass in nonobese healthy girls. However, with sexual maturation, the relationship between circulating IGF-I and body size is diminished *(158)*. Other studies have found that after adjusting for pubertal development, serum IGF-I was not related to BMI, body weight, or other anthropometric measurements in a sample of 325 healthy girls *(159)*.

4.2.3. Obesity

Alterations in the IGF/GH axis, although difficult to characterize, are commonly observed in obesity *(160–162)*. Despite alterations in the IGF system, measurement of serum IGF-I or the IGFBPs have not been shown to be sensitive indicators of body weight, adiposity, or body fatness, and in that manner not able to identify obesity *(163–165)*. In children, before puberty, IGF-I concentrations are greater in obese compared with normal weight children in some *(166,167)* but not other reports *(163)*. IGFBP-3, IGFBP-1, IGFBP-2, and free IGF-I are also significantly different between normal weight and obese prepubertal children *(163,166)*. In obese children, IGF-I and IGFBP-3 concentrations are greater after puberty compared to prepuberty *(166,167)*. However, the ability of serum IGF-I or IGFBP3 to reflect BMI in normal weight or obese children is very inconsistent *(163,166,167)*. Interestingly, with short-term changes in nutrition (caloric restriction and 25% reduction of BMI standard deviation score), IGF-I, free IGF-I, BP-1, and BP-2 were associated with BMI in obese children *(163)*. Weight loss has also been shown to cause at least a temporary increase in IGF-I concentration in adults *(164)*.

4.2.4. Severe Malnutrition

In extreme circumstances of undernutrition, the IGF proteins appear to be more predictive of body composition and size than in healthy populations. There may be a threshold under which IGF-I (and perhaps other IGF proteins) may reflect BMI, body weight, and other indicators of body size and composition. Whether the IGF proteins are responsive to recent nutritional inadequacies or reflect decreased body stores of protein or fat is difficult to discern. In any case, with severe malnutrition, IGF-I is predictive of BMI and/or other markers of body composition in conditions, such as anorexia nervosa *(95,118–120,123,124,168–170)*, end-stage renal disease *(171–174)*, cystic fibrosis *(175,176)*, AIDS *(134)*, malnourished elderly patients with hip fractures *(132,177,178)*, and children with PEM *(100,107,179–182)*.

Thus, in conditions of chronic malnutrition resulting in decreased body weight and diminished fat stores, serum IGF-I does correspond to anthropometric measurements in a fashion that is not evident in normal weight or obese individuals. Even so, serum IGF-

I may not be a reliable indicator of chronic nutritional status in diverse clinical populations that vary in severity of illness and/or levels of adiposity. For example, serum IGF-I does not consistently correspond to BMI or anthropometric markers in cancer patients with diverse clinical status and varying percentages of body fat *(183–185)*, and the relationship between IGF-I and indices of adiposity may be gender specific *(184)*.

5. IGF PROTEINS AS MARKERS OF NUTRITIONAL STATUS IN UNDERNOURISHED CHILDREN

Some of the earliest observations recognizing the relationship between somatomedin activity and nutritional status were of chronically malnourished children with marasmus and/or kwashiorkor PEM *(102,186–188)*. A very consistent finding in populations of children with any of these forms of PEM is initial observations of significantly depressed serum IGF-I that responds to nutritional repletion and is correlated with weight and height gains and general improvement in health status. The responsiveness of serum IGF-I (somatomedin C bioactivity in early studies) to nutritional depletion and repletion has been documented in children in South Africa *(186)*, Thailand *(102)*, India *(187)*, Nigeria *(106,179)*, Morocco *(180)*, Egypt *(107)*, Malaysia *(181)*, Vietnam *(70)*, Equador *(104)*, Pakistan *(100)*, Chile *(105)*, and Bangladesh *(59,103)*. Serum IGF-I is a better marker of nutritional recovery than serum albumin, transthyretin, and retinol-binding protein *(100)* and dramatic increases in serum IGF-I and IGFBP-3 are observed with as little as 10% weight gain. Serum IGFBP-3 has also been associated with body weight and height in recovering malnourished children *(100,181)*. Although difficult to separate in many studies, serum IGF-I tends to be lower in children with kwashiorkor compared to marasmic protein energy malnutrition and supports animal work that demonstrates that not only the lack of protein and/or energy, but the imbalance of protein to energy intake has a negative impact on circulating concentrations of serum IGF-I *(189)*.

6. IGF PROTEINS IN ASSESSING NUTRITIONAL STATUS AND MONITORING THE RESPONSE TO NUTRITION SUPPORT IN CRITICAL ILLNESS

The sensitivity and specificity of serum IGF-I as a nutritional marker in critical illness has been strongly supported by several studies that made comparisons to traditional markers of nutritional status. Correlations between nitrogen balance and serum IGF-I concentrations are preserved during the acute response to critical illness *(97,112,116)* in a manner similar to malnourished patients requiring parenteral or enteral nutrition support *(46,47)*. Serum IGF proteins are significantly associated with accepted markers of nutritional status *(110,190)*. However, serum albumin, transthyretin, transferrin, and retinol binding protein are affected by the stress response during early critical illness. Thus, many investigators have concluded that serum IGF-I is a more useful index of nutritional status, particularly in indicating acute directional changes in the early phases of critical illness and while monitoring the response to nutritional support *(62,97,112,114–116,191)*.

Serum IGF-I responds to the initiation of nutrition support and the protein and energy intake received in early critical illness *(62,112,114,116)*. In a study of severely injured patients, serum IGF-I was significantly less in patients receiving <12 kcal/kg compared with patients receiving >20 kcal/kg by d 4 after trauma despite a similar severity of injury. During the first week, energy intake was a significant predictor of serum IGF-I, even after adjusting for age and BMI by using multiple regression analysis *(62)*.

Less direct evidence of the sensitivity of nutrition on serum IGF-I levels to nutrition in critical illness is suggested by observational studies demonstrating depressed IGF levels that reach a nadir after several days of minimal nutritional intake and increase towards normal in conjunction with increased protein and energy intake over the next week to 10 d *(110,113,115–117,192–198)*.

Response of serum IGF-I to nutritional support in critically ill patients has not been clear in all studies. However, factors such as comparison to anthropometric measures, small or diverse groups of patients, variations in time observed, or several days of fasting or minimal feeding prior to initiation of full nutritional support *(193,198–200)* may explain some of the lack of observed effect. Non-nutritional factors affecting IGF proteins that have been observed in critically ill patients include age, severity of illness, gender, and obesity *(201–203)*. Another important consideration is the distinctive metabolic environment that occurs after 7–10 d or in prolonged critical illness (Chapter 16). When data from several weeks of hospitalization, which encompass several neuroendocrine and metabolic phases are averaged, direct relationships between serum IGF-I concentrations and nutrient intake or nitrogen balance are not observed *(62,110,204–206)*.

Convincing confirmation of the validity of IGF-I as a marker of nutritional status in critical illness was demonstrated in a carefully designed study aimed at determining the efficiency of several short-lived proteins in assessing nutrition intake in surgical patients *(114)*. Patients were randomized to receive four different parenteral nutrition solutions that varied in protein (0 to 1.5 g/kg/d), energy (approx 7, 11, 18, 33 kcal/kg/d), carbohydrate, and fat content after surgery and 48 h of fasting. Serum IGF-I was sensitive to nutritional intake, able to discern between the four different levels of energy and protein intake, and was not influenced by the stress response at adequate levels of nutritional intake. Only IGF-I was able to indicate nutritional intake as clearly as nitrogen balance.

Changes in IGFBPs during critical illness are just beginning to be characterized *(59,110,197,207–211)*. Preliminary observations indicate that several IGFBPs are quite responsive to the metabolic shift that occurs from fasting or hypocaloric feeding to adequate nutritional support in severely injured patients. Marked changes in IGF-I, IGFBP-1, ALS, and free IGF-I occur in severely injured patients over a 24- to 48-h period as nutrition support is initiated following a period of fasting or minimal intravenous dextrose administration during the first few days after trauma *(109)*. Even in the presence of inflammatory stress, IGFBP2 is an independent predictor of protein intake *(139)*. Further investigation of observations indicating alterations of IGFBPs and IGFBP-3 proteolysis and their sensitivity to nutrition appear to be warranted.

7. THE IGFS AS SENSITIVE MARKERS OF STARVATION AND REPLETION IN ANOREXIA NERVOSA

Anorexia nervosa is a circumstance of starvation, a marasmus PEM. Not typically related to other catabolic illnesses, anorexia nervosa is simple starvation resulting in profound alterations in body composition and dimensions. The GH/IGF axis is dramatically altered in anorexia nervosa, with approx 50% lower basal IGF-I levels than found in critically ill, obese, or normal subjects *(127,212)*, elevated IGFBP-1, and lower ALS and IGFBP3 concentrations *(120,168)*. Distinctly different patterns of GH and IGF proteins are found in anorexia nervosa when compared with hypopituitarism or acromegaly, reinforcing the major role of nutrition in affecting the GH/IGF axis. GH/IGF and insulin are altered and related to energy and dietary fat intake even in subclinical eating disorders with amenorrhea *(67,213)*.

The ability of the body to maintain near-normal concentrations of some liver-derived serum proteins (including those used to assess nutritional status) in the presence of marasmus-type protein energy malnutrition has been well documented in both early *(214)* and more recent *(93)* controlled studies of starvation. Indeed, in recently diagnosed patients with severe anorexia nervosa, serum albumin, transthyretin, and retinol-binding protein are remarkably normal, and do not reflect the presence of profound malnutrition *(95,123,215)*. In contrast, IGF-I, IGFBP-1, -2, -3, and ALS are markedly changed and are considered good indicators of nutritional state in individuals with eating disorders *(118–121,170)*.

This extreme degree of malnutrition is a circumstance in which IGF proteins appear to be predictive of BMI and other markers of body size and composition. At the initiation of therapy, both recent nutrient intake and chronic nutritional deprivation are present and strong positive correlations are observed between total IGF-I, free IGF-I, ALS, IGFBP3, and negative correlations between IGFBP2, IGFBP1, IGF-I receptors, and BMI or body weight *(95,118–121,124,168–170)*. With repletion, changes in IGF proteins correspond to increases in body weight *(123,126)* and eventually with BMI *(95,120,121,123)*. IGF-I has been shown to be more sensitive to weight gain with repletion than proteins commonly used to assess nutritional status, such as retinol-binding protein, albumin, and transthyretin, *(95,123)*.

8. THE IGF PROTEINS IN ASSESSING NUTRITION IN CHRONIC DISEASES ASSOCIATED WITH MALNUTRITION

The validity of IGF proteins as sensitive markers of nutritional status has been proposed in individuals with various conditions that contribute to malnutrition and wasting, such as HIV infection or AIDS *(134)*, and hip fractures *(132,177)*. Below are several conditions for which more thorough investigation of the IGF proteins has occurred.

8.1. Renal Disease

The GH/IGF axis is altered in renal failure. Trapping of IGF-I by the kidney, increases in IGFBPs, metabolic acidosis, diabetes, uremia, catabolism, and PEM can all contribute to attenuated serum IGF-I in renal disease (reviewed in Chapter 13). Despite other influences, serum IGF-I has consistently predicted the presence and severity of malnutrition in chronic renal disease *(52,171,172,174,216–218)*. Serum IGF-I has been proposed as a valid, sensitive marker of nutrition, with advantages compared with serum albumin and other visceral protein markers in children and adults with end-stage renal disease, on either predialysis, hemodialysis, or peritoneal dialysis *(171–173,219–222)*. Furthermore, serum IGF-I and the IGF-I/IGFBP-1 ratio are related to protein intake calculated from urea kinetics (protein catabolic rate) *(221)*.

8.2. Liver Disease

Disturbed hepatic synthesis, toxic effects of ethanol, as well as other pathological changes and concomitant malnutrition contribute to the very low circulating concentration of IGF-I in liver disease *(223–226)*. Protein energy malnutrition is a common finding in patients with liver disease *(227,228)*, but few studies have tested the significance of IGF-I as a marker of nutrition in this population. In one study of alcoholic cirrhosis, malnutrition correlated with IGF-I independently of liver dysfunction *(229)*. In a more recent study, serum IGF-I correlated with the degree of liver failure was a useful marker of survival, was more suppressed in patients with the most severe liver disease and malnutrition, was closely correlated with other serum markers of nutritional status, but was not related to anthropometric indicators of chronic energy malnutrition *(99)*. Serum IGF-I remained very low in patients with cirrhosis who had 2–4 wk of refeeding *(230)*. IGF-I and other markers of nutrition increased significantly in malnourished alcohol abusers after hospitalization *(231)*. Although tempting to assume that circulating IGF proteins are not related to nutrition in liver disease, more specific studies are needed.

8.3. Cystic Fibrosis

Malnutrition in cystic fibrosis (CF) is related to increased energy expenditure, decreased energy intakes, pulmonary disease, malabsorption of ingested nutrients, pancreatic insufficiency and chronic inflammation. IGF-I concentrations are diminished and related to the poor growth, catabolic state, altered GH responsiveness, and malnutrition that accompany cystic fibrosis *(232,233)*. A well-designed cross-sectional and longitudinal study of CF patients (3–33 yr) found very depressed IGF-I and IGFBP-3 concentrations that correlated with markers of nutritional status, anthropometrics and serum vitamin E concentrations. With intensive nutrition and antibiotic therapy, IGF-I and IGFBP3 increased significantly *(129)*. The close association between IGF-I and IGFB-3 and nutrition has been demonstrated in other studies of patients with CF *(175,176)*.

9. NORMAL STANDARDS, NON-NUTRITIONAL FACTORS, AND LIMITATIONS OF IGF PROTEINS AS MARKERS OF NUTRITIONAL STATUS

Relative rather than absolute values are very useful in indicating the response of IGFs to nutritional interventions. However, the use of IGFs for nutritional screening, diagnosis, or cross-sectional assessment requires a comparison to a reference distribution, i.e., normal range or pre-determined cutoff points. Reference values are obtained from a healthy sample group. Ideally, comparison of an individual observation to the reference distribution involves matching factors such as age, sex, race, physiological state, fasting, and analysis methods. An extensive reference distribution continues to be developed to enable sophisticated and reliable interpretation of serum IGF values under multiple circumstances *(118,145,153,158,234–240)*. Establishing a normal range in each laboratory has become less of an issue for IGF-I with the advent of commercially available kits and automated systems that provide fairly standardized procedures for extraction of the binding proteins. Important analytical differences are still possible however, particularly in testing free IGF-I and some of the IGFBPs.

The choice of a cut-off point to differentiate between malnourished and well-nourished states for a particular index critically affects both sensitivity and specificity. Lowering the cut-off, that is, enlarging the normal reference range, will increase the specificity (less likely to miss a malnourished individual), but decreases the sensitivity (more classified as malnourished). This remains a challenge for IGF proteins for which normal reference standards continue to evolve, and in the case of IGF-I, a fairly large range (generally 200–400 ng/mL) is considered "normal." Normal ranges and cut-off points for the IGF-BPs and free IGF-I are much less established and await further research.

Many non-nutritional factors affect IGF proteins and their levels in circulation *(241,242)*. Age, gender, growth hormone status, and diabetes have recognized influences on the IGF proteins (Chapters 1, 2, 9, and 14). Consideration of other factors may include estrogen status and parity *(152,243)*, other sex hormone *(244)*, menstrual cycle *(245)*, thyroid status *(246)*, alcohol ingestion *(151,247)*, and exercise *(248–250)*. Whether these factors are actually limitations in interpreting nutritional status will likely need to be determined under each specific circumstance.

Recent work in animal models suggests that local production of the IGF peptides may compensate for changes in circulating levels of the IGF proteins in response to protein or dietary restriction *(251,252)*. The biological and clinical significance of the autocrine and paracrine responses to nutrient availability are unknown.

Interactions of IGFBPs, both independently and in ratio with IGF-I have important, but not fully understood, effects on the bioavailability, biological activity, and circulating concentrations of IGF-I. Further research may demonstrate that concentrations of IGFBPs, particularly IGFBP-1 and/or -2, or the molar ratios of IGF/IGFBP-3 may provide a more reliable nutritional status marker than IGF-I.

10. SUMMARY AND CONCLUSIONS

Serum IGF-I is acutely sensitive to recent protein and energy nutritional status in adults, children, infants, and many animal species. This observation is well documented in healthy individuals under experimental conditions, but also in individuals in a wide variety of disease and stressed conditions. A large body of evidence supports the use of serum IGF-I as a sensitive, reliable marker to monitor repletion and nutritional support. Serum IGF-I appears to be more sensitive and perhaps a more useful marker of acute nutritional status than conventionally used serum proteins such as albumin, transthyretin, transferrin, and retinol binding protein. This is particularly evident in critical illness and extreme starvation such as anorexia nervosa.

As biochemical markers of nutritional status, serum IGF-I and the IGFBPs are less suited to indicating chronic nutritional status and body composition. Before puberty, in extreme malnutrition, or the presence of both chronic and acute deprivation, IGF proteins may correlate with anthropometric measures. However, in mixed populations serum IGF-I is not a reliable indicator of body weight or composition. The IGFBPs hold promise as assessment markers of nutrition as well, and await further study.

11. FUTURE DIRECTIONS

Current evidence supports the use of serum IGF-I as a valid marker of acute nutritional status and monitor of nutritional interventions in several situations including critical illness, and in repletion of severe PEM. The use of IGF-I and the IGFBPs in other populations and clinical situations requires further validation. A better understanding of the strengths and limitations of the nutritional assessment process and appropriate application of specific types of methods will enhance the design of research studies investigating the IGFs as nutritional status markers.

The study of the IGFBPs, in particular IGFBP-1, IGFBP-2, and perhaps ratios of the IGFBPs and IGF-I, or free IGF-I in relation to nutrition is just beginning. As the understanding of the interface between the GH/IGF axis and nutrition continues to expand, additional markers, and perhaps better markers may become evident. The transition from parameters that are used in a research setting to widespread availability and reasonable cost will be necessary to fully use the IGF proteins in nutritional assessment.

REFERENCES

1. Bistrian BR, Blackburn GL, Vitale J, Cochran D, Naylor J. Prevalence of malnutrition in general medical patients. JAMA 1976;235:1567–1570.
2. Bistrian BR, Blackburn GL, Hallowell E, Heddle R. Protein status of general surgical patients. JAMA 1974;230:858–860.
3. Butterworth CE, Jr. Editorial: Malnutrition in the hospital. JAMA 1974;230:879.
4. McWhirter JP, Pennington CR. Incidence and recognition of malnutrition in hospital. Brit Med J 1994;308:945–948.
5. Edington J, Boorman J, Durrant ER, et al. Prevalence of malnutrition on admission to four hospitals in England. The Malnutrition Prevalence Group. Clin Nutr 2000;19:191–195.
6. McClave SA, Mitoraj TE, Thielmeier KA, Greenburg RA. Differentiating subtypes (hypoalbuminemic vs marasmic) of protein-calorie malnutrition: incidence and clinical significance in a university hospital setting. J Parenter Enteral Nutr 1992;16:337–342.
7. Fleck A. Plasma proteins as nutritional indicators in the perioperative period. Br J Clin Pract Suppl 1988;63:20–24.
8. Tayek JA, Blackburn GL. Goals of nutritional support in acute infections. Am J Med 1984;76:81–90.
9. Gibson RS. Principles of Nutritional Assessment. Oxford University Press, New York, 1990.
10. Shenkin A. Impact of disease on markers of macronutrient status. Proc Nutr Soc 1997;56:433–441.
11. Shenkin A, Cederblad G, Elia M, Isaksson B. Laboratory assessment of protein energy status. J Int Fed Clin Chem 1996;9:58–61.
12. Laboratory Utilization for Nutrition Support: Current Practice, Requirements, Expectations. Ross Laboratories, Columbus, OH, 1994.
13. Fischer J. Plasma proteins as indicators of nutritional status. In: Nutritional Assessment—Present Status, Future Directions and Prospects. Levenson S (ed.). Ross Laboratories, Columbus, OH, 1981, p. 25–26.
14. Guler HP, Zapf J, Schmid C, Froesch ER. Insulin-like growth factors I and II in healthy man. Estimations of half-lives and production rates. Acta Endocrinol (Copenh) 1989;121:753–758.
15. Boosalis MG, Ott L, Levine AS, et al. Relationship of visceral proteins to nutritional status in chronic and acute stress. Crit Care Med 1989;17:741–747.
16. Buzby GP, Mullen JL, Matthews DC, Hobbs CL, Rosato EF. Prognostic nutritional index in gastrointestinal surgery. Am J Surg 1980;139:160–167.
17. Shetty PS, Watrasiewicz KE, Jung RT, James WP. Rapid-turnover transport proteins: an index of subclinical protein-energy malnutrition. Lancet 1979;2:230–232.
18. Bistrian BR. Acute phase proteins and the systemic inflammatory response. Crit Care Med 1999;27:452–453.
19. Klein S. The myth of serum albumin as a measure of nutritional status. Gastroenterology 1990;99:1845–1846.
20. Doweiko JP, Nompleggi DJ. Role of albumin in human physiology and pathophysiology. J Parenter Enteral Nutr 1991;15:207–211.

21. Fleck A. Clinical and nutritional aspects of changes in acute-phase proteins during inflammation. Proc Nutr Soc 1989;48:347–354.
22. Ingenbleek Y, Barclay D, Dirren H. Nutritional significance of alterations in serum amino acid patterns in goitrous patients. Am J Clin Nutr 1986;43:310–319.
23. Ingenbleek Y, Young V. Transthyretin (prealbumin) in health and disease: nutritional implications. Annu Rev Nutr 1994;14:495–533.
24. Cavarocchi NC, Au FC, Dalal FR, Friel K, Mildenberg B. Rapid turnover proteins as nutritional indicators. World J Surg 1986;10:468–473.
25. Carpentier YA, Barthel J, Bruyns J. Plasma protein concentration in nutritional assessment. Proc Nutr Soc 1982;41:405–417.
26. Fletcher JP, Little JM, Guest PK. A comparison of serum transferrin and serum prealbumin as nutritional parameters. J Parenter Enteral Nutr 1987;11:144–147.
27. Raguso CA, Dupertuis YM, Pichard C. The role of visceral proteins in the nutritional assessment of intensive care unit patients. Curr Opin Clin Nutr Metab Care 2003;6:211–216.
28. Ingenbleek Y, Bernstein L. The stressful condition as a nutritionally dependent adaptive dichotomy. Nutrition 1999;15:305–320.
29. Clemmons DR, Klibanski A, Underwood LE, et al. Reduction of plasma immunoreactive somatomedin C during fasting in humans. J Clin Endocrinol Metab 1981;53:1247–1250.
30. Isley WL, Underwood LE, Clemmons DR. Dietary components that regulate serum somatomedin-C concentrations in humans. J Clin Invest 1983;71:175–182.
31. Isley WL, Underwood LE, Clemmons DR. Changes in plasma somatomedin-C in response to ingestion of diets with variable protein and energy content. J Parenter Enteral Nutr 1984;8:407–411.
32. Smith WJ, Underwood LE, Clemmons DR. Effects of caloric or protein restriction on insulin-like growth factor- I (IGF-I) and IGF-binding proteins in children and adults. J Clin Endocrinol Metab 1995;80:443–449.
33. Bolze MS, Reeves RD, Lindbeck FE, Elders MJ. Influence of selected amino acid deficiencies on somatomedin, growth and glycosaminoglycan metabolism in weanling rats. J Nutr 1985;115:782–787.
34. Reeves RD, Dickinson L, Lee J, Kilgore B, Branham B, Elders MJ. Effects of dietary composition on somatomedin activity in growing rats. J Nutr 1979;109:613–620.
35. Phillips LS, Orawski AT, Belosky DC. Somatomedin and nutrition. IV. Regulation of somatomedin activity and growth cartilage activity by quantity and composition of diet in rats. Endocrinology 1978;103:121–127.
36. Price DA, Wit JM, van Buul-Offers S, et al. Serum somatomedin activity and cartilage metabolism in acutely fasted, chronically malnourished, and refed rats. Endocrinology 1979;105:851–861.
37. Prewitt TE, D'Ercole AJ. Modest dietary restriction and serum somatomedin-C/insulin like growth factor-I in young, mature and old rats. Prog Clin Biol Res 1989;287:157–162.
38. Simmen FA, Badinga L, Green ML, Kwak I, Song S, Simmen RC. The porcine insulin-like growth factor system: at the interface of nutrition, growth and reproduction. J Nutr 1998;128:315S–320S.
39. Beccavin C, Chevalier B, Simon J, Duclos MJ. Circulating insulin-like growth factors (IGF-I and -II) and IGF binding proteins in divergently selected fat or lean chickens: effect of prolonged fasting. Growth Horm IGF Res 1999;9:187–194.
40. Maxwell A, Butterwick R, Yateman M, Batt RM, Cotterill A, Camacho-Hubner C. Nutritional modulation of canine insulin-like growth factors and their binding proteins. J Endocrinol 1998;158:77–85.
41. Oldham JM, Martyn JA, Hua KM, MacDonald NA, Hodgkinson SC, Bass JJ. Nutritional regulation of IGF-II, but not IGF-I, is age dependent in sheep. J Endocrinol 1999;163:395–402.
42. Clemmons DR, Seek MM, Underwood LE. Supplemental essential amino acids augment the somatomedin-C/insulin- like growth factor I response to refeeding after fasting. Metabolism 1985;34:391–395.
43. Smith WJ, Underwood LE, Keyes L, Clemmons DR. Use of insulin-like growth factor I (IGF-I) and IGF-binding protein measurements to monitor feeding of premature infants. J Clin Endocrinol Metab 1997;82:3982–3988.
44. Thissen JP, Ketelslegers JM, Underwood LE. Nutritional regulation of the insulin-like growth factors. Endocr Rev 1994;15:80–101.

45. Savendahl L, Underwood LE. Fasting increases serum total cholesterol, LDL cholesterol and apolipoprotein B in healthy, nonobese humans. J Nutr 1999;129:2005–2008.
46. Unterman TG, Vazquez RM, Slas AJ, Martyn PA, Phillips LS. Nutrition and somatomedin. XIII. Usefulness of somatomedin-C in nutritional assessment. Am J Med 1985;78:228–234.
47. Donahue SP, Phillips LS. Response of IGF-I to nutritional support in malnourished hospital patients: a possible indicator of short-term changes in nutritional status. Am J Clin Nutr 1989;50:962–969.
48. Bonofiglio D, Maggiolini M, Catalano S, Marsico S, Aquila S, Ando S. Bone mineral density is inversely related to parathyroid hormone in adolescent girls. Horm Metab Res 2001;33:170–174.
49. Rizzoli R, Ammann P, Chevalley T, Bonjour JP. Protein intake and bone disorders in the elderly. Joint Bone Spine 2001;68:383–392.
50. Underwood LE, Clemmons DR, Maes M, D'Ercole AJ, Ketelslegers JM. Regulation of somatomedin-C/insulin-like growth factor I by nutrients. Horm Res 1986;24:166–176.
51. Underwood LE, Thissen JP, Lemozy S, Ketelslegers JM, Clemmons DR. Hormonal and nutritional regulation of IGF-I and its binding proteins. Horm Res 1994;42:145–151.
52. Rabkin R. Nutrient regulation of insulin-like growth factor-I. Miner Electrolyte Metab 1997;23:157–160.
53. Estivariz CF, Ziegler TR. Nutrition and the insulin-like growth factor system. Endocrine 1997;7:65–71.
54. Frystyk J, Hussain M, Skjaerbaek C, Porksen N, Froesch ER, Orskov H. The pharmacokinetics of free insulin-like growth factor-I in healthy subjects. Growth Horm IGF Res 1999;9:150–156.
55. Frystyk J, Delhanty PJ, Skjaerbaek C, Baxter RC. Changes in the circulating IGF system during short-term fasting and refeeding in rats. Am J Physiol 1999;277:E245–E252.
56. Baxter RC, Martin JL, Tyler MI, Howden ME. Growth hormone-dependent insulin-like growth factor (IGF) binding protein from human plasma differs from other human IGF binding proteins. Biochem Biophys Res Commun 1986;139:1256–1261.
57. Baxter RC. The binding protein's binding protein—clinical applications of acid- labile subunit (ALS) measurement. J Clin Endocrinol Metab 1997;82:3941–3943.
58. Delhanty PJ, Baxter RC. The regulation of acid-labile subunit gene expression and secretion by cyclic adenosine 3',5'-monophosphate. Endocrinology 1998;139:260–265.
59. Pucilowska JB, Davenport ML, Kabir I, et al. The effect of dietary protein supplementation on insulin-like growth factors (IGFs) and IGF-binding proteins in children with shigellosis. J Clin Endocrinol Metab 1993;77:1516–1521.
60. Blum WF, Ranke MB (ed.) Modern Concepts of Insulin-Like Growth Factors: Elsevier Science Publishing Co., Inc., New York, 1991.
61. Savendahl L, Underwood LE. Decreased interleukin-2 production from cultured peripheral blood mononuclear cells in human acute starvation. J Clin Endocrinol Metab 1997;82:1177–11780.
62. Houston MS, Levis N, Knotts FB. Initial response of serum IGF-I to severe injury is related to adequacy of nutrition support, FASEB J 1998;12:A249.
63. Cotterill AM, Holly JM, Wass JA. The regulation of insulin-like growth factor binding protein (IGFBP)-1 during prolonged fasting. Clin Endocrinol (Oxf) 1993;39:357–362.
64. Baxter RC, Cowell CT. Diurnal rhythm of growth hormone-independent binding protein for insulin-like growth factors in human plasma. J Clin Endocrinol Metab 1987;65:432–440.
65. Busby WH, Snyder DK, Clemmons DR. Radioimmunoassay of a 26,000-dalton plasma insulin-like growth factor- binding protein: control by nutritional variables. J Clin Endocrinol Metab 1988;67:1225–1230.
66. Musey VC, Goldstein S, Farmer PK, Moore PB, Phillips LS. Differential regulation of IGF-I and IGF-binding protein-1 by dietary composition in humans. Am J Med Sci 1993;305:131–138.
67. Laughlin GA, Yen SS. Nutritional and endocrine-metabolic aberrations in amenorrheic athletes. J Clin Endocrinol Metab 1996;81:4301–4309.
68. Snyder DK, Clemmons DR, Underwood LE. Dietary carbohydrate content determines responsiveness to growth hormone in energy-restricted humans. J Clin Endocrinol Metab 1989;69:745–752.
69. Clemmons DR. Use of growth hormone and insulin-like growth factor I in catabolism that is induced by negative energy balance. Horm Res 1993;40:62–67.
70. Ninh NX, Thissen JP, Collette L, Gerard G, Khoi HH, Ketelslegers JM. Zinc supplementation increases growth and circulating insulin-like growth factor I (IGF-I) in growth-retarded Vietnamese children. Am J Clin Nutr 1996;63:514–519.

71. Devine A, Rosen C, Mohan S, Baylink D, Prince RL. Effects of zinc and other nutritional factors on insulin-like growth factor I and insulin-like growth factor binding proteins in postmenopausal women. Am J Clin Nutr 1998;68:200–206.
72. Bolze MS, Reeves RD, Lindbeck FE, Elders MJ. Influence of zinc on growth, somatomedin, and glycosaminoglycan metabolism in rats. Am J Physiol 1987;252:E21–E26.
73. Bolze MS, Reeves RD, Lindbeck FE, Kemp SF, Elders MJ. Influence of manganese on growth, somatomedin and glycosaminoglycan metabolism. J Nutr 1985;115:352–358.
74. Bolze MS, Reeves RD, Lindbeck FE, Elders MJ. Influence of vitamin A on somatomedin and glycosaminoglycan metabolism. Nutr Res 1986;6:395–405.
75. Gabbitas B, Canalis E. Retinoic acid regulates the expression of insulin-like growth factors I and II in osteoblasts. J Cell Physiol 1997;172:253–264.
76. Fu Z, Yoneyama M, Noguchi T, Kato H. Response of the insulin-like growth factor system to vitamin A depletion and repletion in rats. J Nutr Sci Vitaminol (Tokyo) 2002;48:453–460.
77. Fatayerji D, Mawer EB, Eastell R. The role of insulin-like growth factor I in age-related changes in calcium homeostasis in men. J Clin Endocrinol Metab 2000;85:4657–4662.
78. Yoo A, Tanimoto H, Akesson K, Baylink DJ, Lau KH. Effects of calcium depletion and repletion on serum insulin-like growth factor I and binding protein levels in weanling rats. Bone 1998;22:225–232.
79. Alikasifoglu A, Ozon A, Yordam N. Serum insulin-like growth factor-I (IGF-I) and IGF-binding protein-3 levels in severe iodine deficiency. Turk J Pediatr 2002;44:215–218.
80. Aydin K, Bideci A, Kendirci M, Cinaz P, Kurtoglu S. Insulin-like growth factor-I and insulin-like growth factor binding protein-3 levels of children living in an iodine- and selenium-deficient endemic goiter area. Biol Trace Elem Res 2002;90:25–30.
81. Dorup I, Flyvbjerg A, Everts ME, Clausen T. Role of insulin-like growth factor-1 and growth hormone in growth inhibition induced by magnesium and zinc deficiencies. Br J Nutr 1991;66:505–521.
82. Dorup I. Magnesium and potassium deficiency. Its diagnosis, occurrence and treatment in diuretic therapy and its consequences for growth, protein synthesis and growth factors. Acta Physiol Scand Suppl 1994;618:1–55.
83. Flyvbjerg A, Dorup I, Everts ME, Orskov H. Evidence that potassium deficiency induces growth retardation through reduced circulating levels of growth hormone and insulin-like growth factor I. Metabolism 1991;40:769–775.
84. Roughead ZK, Lukaski HC. Inadequate copper intake reduces serum insulin-like growth factor-I and bone strength in growing rats fed graded amounts of copper and zinc. J Nutr 2003;133:442–448.
85. Giovannucci E, Pollak M, Liu Y, et al. Nutritional predictors of insulin-like growth factor I and their relationships to cancer in men. Cancer Epidemiol Biomarkers Prev 2003;12:84–89.
86. Holmes MD, Pollak MN, Willett WC, Hankinson SE. Dietary correlates of plasma insulin-like growth factor I and insulin-like growth factor binding protein 3 concentrations. Cancer Epidemiol Biomarkers Prev 2002;11:852–861.
87. Mucci LA, Tamimi R, Lagiou P, et al. Are dietary influences on the risk of prostate cancer mediated through the insulin-like growth factor system? BJU Int 2001;87:814–820.
88. Allen NE, Appleby PN, Davey GK, Kaaks R, Rinaldi S, Key TJ. The associations of diet with serum insulin-like growth factor I and its main binding proteins in 292 women meat-eaters, vegetarians, and vegans. Cancer Epidemiol Biomarkers Prev 2002;11:1441–1448.
89. Khalil DA, Lucas EA, Juma S, Smith BJ, Payton ME, Arjmandi BH. Soy protein supplementation increases serum insulin-like growth factor- I in young and old men but does not affect markers of bone metabolism. J Nutr 2002;132:2605–2608.
90. Probst-Hensch NM, Wang H, Goh VH, Seow A, Lee HP, Yu MC. Determinants of circulating insulin-like growth factor I and insulin-like growth factor binding protein 3 concentrations in a Cohort of Singapore men and women. Cancer Epidemiol Biomarkers Prev 2003;12:739–746.
91. Nagata C, Shimizu H, Takami R, Hayashi M, Takeda N, Yasuda K. Dietary soy and fats in relation to serum insulin-like growth factor-1 and insulin-like growth factor-binding protein-3 levels in premenopausal Japanese women. Nutr Cancer 2003;45:185–189.
92. Adams KF, Newton KM, Chen C, et al. Soy isoflavones do not modulate circulating insulin-like growth factor concentrations in an older population in an intervention trial. J Nutr 2003;133:1316–1319.
93. Friedl KE, Moore RJ, Hoyt RW, Marchitelli LJ, Martinez-Lopez LE, Askew EW. Endocrine markers of semistarvation in healthy lean men in a multistressor environment. J Appl Physiol 2000;88:1820–1830.

94. Clemmons DR, Underwood LE, Dickerson RN, et al. Use of plasma somatomedin-C/insulin-like growth factor I measurements to monitor the response to nutritional repletion in malnourished patients. Am J Clin Nutr 1985;41:191–198.
95. Caregaro L, Favaro A, Santonastaso P, et al. Insulin-like growth factor 1 (IGF-I), a nutritional marker in patients with eating disorders. Clin Nutr 2001;20:251–257.
96. Spiekerman AM. Proteins used in nutritional assessment. Clin Lab Med 1993;13:353–369.
97. Burgess EJ. Insulin-like growth factor 1: a valid nutritional indicator during parenteral feeding of patients suffering an acute phase response. Ann Clin Biochem 1992;29:137–144.
98. Minuto F, Barreca A, Adami GF, et al. Insulin-like growth factor-I in human malnutrition: relationship with some body composition and nutritional parameters. J Parenter Enteral Nutr 1989;13:392–396.
99. Caregaro L, Alberino F, Amodio P, et al. Nutritional and prognostic significance of insulin-like growth factor 1 in patients with liver cirrhosis. Nutrition 1997;13:185–190.
100. Bhutta ZA, Bang P, Karlsson E, Hagenas L, Nizami SQ, Soder O. Insulin-like growth factor I response during nutritional rehabilitation of persistent diarrhoea. Arch Dis Child 1999;80:438–442.
101. Doherty CP, Crofton PM, Sarkar MA, et al. Malnutrition, zinc supplementation and catch-up growth: changes in insulin-like growth factor I, its binding proteins, bone formation and collagen turnover. Clin Endocrinol (Oxf) 2002;57:391–399.
102. Hintz RL, Suskind R, Amatayakul K, Thanangkul O, Olson R. Plasma somatomedin and growth hormone values in children with protein- calorie malnutrition. J Pediatr 1978;92:153–156.
103. Kabir I, Butler T, Underwood LE, Rahman MM. Effects of a protein-rich diet during convalescence from shigellosis on catch-up growth, serum proteins, and insulin-like growth factor-I. Pediatr Res 1992;32:689–692.
104. Lopez-Jaramillo P, Lopez de Garcia A, Prevot C, et al. Effect of social class and nutrient intake on height and plasma insulin- like growth factor in Andean Equadorian children. Eur J Clin Nutr 1992;46:137–142.
105. Palacio AC, Perez-Bravo F, Santos JL, Schlesinger L, Monckeberg F. Leptin levels and IgF-binding proteins in malnourished children: effect of weight gain. Nutrition 2002;18:17–19.
106. Smith IF, Taiwo O, Payne-Robinson HM. Plasma somatomedin-C in Nigerian malnourished children fed a vegetable protein rehabilitation diet. Eur J Clin Nutr 1989;43:705–713.
107. Soliman AT, Hassan AE, Aref MK, Hintz RL, Rosenfeld RG, Rogol AD. Serum insulin-like growth factors I and II concentrations and growth hormone and insulin responses to arginine infusion in children with protein-energy malnutrition before and after nutritional rehabilitation. Pediatr Res 1986;20:1122–1130.
108. Zamboni G, Dufillot D, Antoniazzi F, Valentini R, Gendrel D, Tato L. Growth hormone-binding proteins and insulin-like growth factor-binding proteins in protein-energy malnutrition, before and after nutritional rehabilitation. Pediatr Res 1996;39:410–414.
109. Aaberg ML, Houston MS, Meserve LA, Williford JH, Knotts FB. Alterations in serum IGF-1, IGFBP-1, IGFBP-3, and ALS in response to nutrition support in severe injury, Endocrine Society Annual Meeting, Denver, CO, June, 2002, p3–553.
110. Baxter RC, Hawker FH, To C, Stewart PM, Holman SR. Thirty-day monitoring of insulin-like growth factors and their binding proteins in intensive care unit patients. Growth Horm IGF Res 1998;8:455–463.
111. Elimam A, Tjader I, Norgren S, et al. Total parenteral nutrition after surgery rapidly increases serum leptin levels. Eur J Endocrinol 2001;144:123–128.
112. Hawker FH, Stewart PM, Baxter RC, et al. Relationship of somatomedin-C/insulin-like growth factor I levels to conventional nutritional indices in critically ill patients. Crit Care Med 1987;15:732–736.
113. Jeevanandam M, Holaday NJ, Petersen SR. Integrated nutritional, hormonal, and metabolic effects of recombinant human growth hormone (rhGH) supplementation in trauma patients. Nutrition 1996;12:777–787.
114. Lopez-Hellin J, Baena-Fustegueras JA, Schwartz-Riera S, Garcia-Arumi E. Usefulness of short-lived proteins as nutritional indicators surgical patients. Clin Nutr 2002;21:119–125.
115. Marin VB, Rebollo MG, Castillo-Duran CD, et al. Controlled study of early postoperative parenteral nutrition in children. J Pediatr Surg 1999;34:1330–1335.
116. Mattox TW, Brown RO, Boucher BA, Buonpane EA, Fabian TC, Luther RW. Use of fibronectin and somatomedin-C as markers of enteral nutrition support in traumatized patients using a modified amino acid formula. J Parenter Enteral Nutr 1988;12:592–596.

117. Pittoni G, Gallioi G, Zanello M, et al. Activity of GH/IGF-I axis in trauma and septic patients during artificial nutrition: different behavior patterns? J Endocrinol Invest 2002;25:214–223.
118. Argente J, Caballo N, Barrios V, et al. Disturbances in the growth hormone-insulin-like growth factor axis in children and adolescents with different eating disorders. Horm Res 1997;48:16–18.
119. Counts DR, Gwirtsman H, Carlsson LM, Lesem M, Cutler GB, Jr. The effect of anorexia nervosa and refeeding on growth hormone-binding protein, the insulin-like growth factors (IGFs), and the IGF-binding proteins. J Clin Endocrinol Metab 1992;75:762–767.
120. Fukuda I, Hotta M, Hizuka N, et al. Decreased serum levels of acid-labile subunit in patients with anorexia nervosa. J Clin Endocrinol Metab 1999;84:2034–2036.
121. Golden NH, Kreitzer P, Jacobson MS, et al. Disturbances in growth hormone secretion and action in adolescents with anorexia nervosa. J Pediatr 1994;125:655–660.
122. Heer M, Mika C, Grzella I, Drummer C, Herpertz-Dahlmann B. Changes in bone turnover in patients with anorexia nervosa during eleven weeks of inpatient dietary treatment. Clin Chem 2002;48:754–760.
123. Hill KK, Hill DB, McClain MP, Humphries LL, McClain CJ. Serum insulin-like growth factor-I concentrations in the recovery of patients with anorexia nervosa. J Am Coll Nutr 1993;12:475–478.
124. Hotta M, Fukuda I, Sato K, Hizuka N, Shibasaki T, Takano K. The relationship between bone turnover and body weight, serum insulin- like growth factor (IGF) I, and serum IGF-binding protein levels in patients with anorexia nervosa. J Clin Endocrinol Metab 2000;85:200–206.
125. Nedvidkova J, Papezova H, Haluzik M, Schreiber V. Interaction between serum leptin levels and hypothalamo-hypophyseal-thyroid axis in patients with anorexia nervosa. Endocr Res 2000;26:219–230.
126. Pascal N, Amouzou EK, Sanni A, et al. Serum concentrations of sex hormone binding globulin are elevated in kwashiorkor and anorexia nervosa but not in marasmus. Am J Clin Nutr 2002;76:239–244.
127. Rappaport R, Prevot C, Czernichow P. Somatomedin activity and growth hormone secretion. I. Changes related to body weight in anorexia nervosa. Acta Paediatr Scand 1980;69:37–41.
128. Beattie RM, Camacho-Hubner C, Wacharasindhu S, Cotterill AM, Walker-Smith JA, Savage MO. Responsiveness of IGF-I and IGFBP-3 to therapeutic intervention in children and adolescents with Crohn's disease. Clin Endocrinol (Oxf) 1998;49:483–489.
129. Lebl J, Zahradnikova M, Bartosova J, Zemkova D, Pechova M, Vavrova V. Insulin-like growth factor-I and insulin-like growth factor-binding protein-3 in cystic fibrosis: a positive effect of antibiotic therapy and hyperalimentation. Acta Paediatr 2001;90:868–872.
130. Thomas AG, Holly JM, Taylor F, Miller V. Insulin like growth factor I, insulin like growth factor binding protein-1, and insulin in childhood Crohn's disease. Gut 1993;34:944–947.
131. Bachrach-Lindstrom M, Unosson M, Ek AC, Arnqvist HJ. Assessment of nutritional status using biochemical and anthropometric variables in a nutritional intervention study of women with hip fracture. Clin Nutr 2001;20:217–223.
132. Campillo B, Paillaud E, Bories PN, Noel M, Porquet D, Le Parco JC. Serum levels of insulin-like growth factor-1 in the three months following surgery for a hip fracture in elderly: relationship with nutritional status and inflammatory reaction [In Process Citation]. Clin Nutr 2000;19:349–354.
133. Schurch MA, Rizzoli R, Slosman D, Vadas L, Vergnaud P, Bonjour JP. Protein supplements increase serum insulin-like growth factor-I levels and attenuate proximal femur bone loss in patients with recent hip fracture. A randomized, double-blind, placebo-controlled trial. Ann Intern Med 1998;128:801–809.
134. Salbe AD, Kotler P, Tierney AR, Wang J, Pierson R, Campbell RG. Correlation between serum insulin-like growth factor 1 (IGF1) concentrations and nutritional status in HIV-infected individuals. Nutr Res 1995;15:1437–1443.
135. Raynaud-Simon A, Perin L, Meaume S, et al. IGF-I, IGF-I-binding proteins and GH-binding protein in malnourished elderly patients with inflammation receiving refeeding therapy. Eur J Endocrinol 2002;146:657–665.
136. Colonna F, Pahor T, de Vonderweid U, Tonini G, Radillo L. Serum Insulin-like growth factor-I (IGF-I) and IGF binding protein-3 (IGFBP-3) in growing preterm infants on enteral nutrition. J Pediatr Endocrinol Metab 1996;9:483–489.
137. Diaz-Gomez NM, Domenech E, Barroso F. Breast-feeding and growth factors in preterm newborn infants. J Pediatr Gastroenterol Nutr 1997;24:322–327.
138. Park MJ, Namgung R, Kim JN, Kim DH. Serum leptin, IGF-I and insulin levels in preterm infants receiving parenteral nutrition during the first week of life. J Pediatr Endocrinol Metab 2001;14:429–433.

139. Price WA, Lee E, Maynor A, Stiles AD, Clemmons DR. Relation between serum insulinlike growth factor-1, insulinlike growth factor binding protein-2, and insulinlike growth factor binding protein- 3 and nutritional intake in premature infants with bronchopulmonary dysplasia. J Pediatr Gastroenterol Nutr 2001;32:542–549.
140. Harris TB, Kiel D, Roubenoff R, et al. Association of insulin-like growth factor-I with body composition, weight history, and past health behaviors in the very old: the Framingham Heart Study. J Am Geriatr Soc 1997;45:133–139.
141. Copeland KC, Colletti RB, Devlin JT, McAuliffe TL. The relationship between insulin-like growth factor-I, adiposity, and aging. Metabolism 1990;39:584–587.
142. Veldhuis JD, Liem AY, South S, et al. Differential impact of age, sex steroid hormones, and obesity on basal versus pulsatile growth hormone secretion in men as assessed in an ultrasensitive chemiluminescence assay. J Clin Endocrinol Metab 1995;80:3209–3222.
143. Landin-Wilhelmsen K, Wilhelmsen L, Lappas G, et al. Serum insulin-like growth factor I in a random population sample of men and women: relation to age, sex, smoking habits, coffee consumption and physical activity, blood pressure and concentrations of plasma lipids, fibrinogen, parathyroid hormone and osteocalcin. Clin Endocrinol (Oxf) 1994;41:351–357.
144. Kelly PJ, Eisman JA, Stuart MC, Pocock NA, Sambrook PN, Gwinn TH. Somatomedin-C, physical fitness, and bone density. J Clin Endocrinol Metab 1990;70:718–723.
145. Nystrom FH, Ohman PK, Ekman BA, Osterlund MK, Karlberg BE, Arnqvist HJ. Population-based reference values for IGF-I and IGF-binding protein-1: relations with metabolic and anthropometric variables. Eur J Endocrinol 1997;136:165–172.
146. Darling-Raedeke M, Thornton WH, Jr., MacDonald RS. Growth hormone and IGF-I plasma concentrations and macronutrient intake measured in a free-living elderly population during a one-year period. J Am Coll Nutr 1998;17:392–397.
147. Rudman D, Drinka PJ, Wilson CR, et al. Relations of endogenous anabolic hormones and physical activity to bone mineral density and lean body mass in elderly men. Clin Endocrinol (Oxf) 1994;40:653–661.
148. Marin P, Kvist H, Lindstedt G, Sjostrom L, Bjorntorp P. Low concentrations of insulin-like growth factor-I in abdominal obesity. Int J Obes Relat Metab Disord 1993;17:83–89.
149. Jorgensen JO, Vahl N, Hansen TB, et al. Determinants of serum insulin-like growth factor I in growth hormone deficient adults as compared to healthy subjects. Clin Endocrinol (Oxf) 1998;48:479–486.
150. O'Connor KG, Tobin JD, Harman SM, et al. Serum levels of insulin-like growth factor-I are related to age and not to body composition in healthy women and men. J Gerontol A Biol Sci Med Sci 1998;53:M176–M182.
151. Goodman-Gruen D, Barrett-Connor E. Epidemiology of insulin-like growth factor-I in elderly men and women. The Rancho Bernardo Study. Am J Epidemiol 1997;145:970–976.
152. Holmes MD, Pollak MN, Hankinson SE. Lifestyle correlates of plasma insulin-like growth factor I and insulin-like growth factor binding protein 3 concentrations. Cancer Epidemiol Biomarkers Prev 2002;11:862–867.
153. Juul A, Bang P, Hertel NT, et al. Serum insulin-like growth factor-I in 1030 healthy children, adolescents, and adults: relation to age, sex, stage of puberty, testicular size, and body mass index. J Clin Endocrinol Metab 1994;78:744–752.
154. Ogilvy-Stuart AL, Hands SJ, Adcock CJ, et al. Insulin, insulin-like growth factor I (IGF-I), IGF-binding protein-1, growth hormone, and feeding in the newborn. J Clin Endocrinol Metab 1998;83:3550–3557.
155. Fall CH, Pandit AN, Law CM, et al. Size at birth and plasma insulin-like growth factor-1 concentrations. Arch Dis Child 1995;73:287–293.
156. Yang SW, Yu JS. Relationship of insulin-like growth factor-I, insulin-like growth factor binding protein-3, insulin, growth hormone in cord blood and maternal factors with birth height and birthweight. Pediatr Int 2000;42:31–36.
157. Ong K, Kratzsch J, Kiess W, Dunger D. Circulating IGF-I levels in childhood are related to both current body composition and early postnatal growth rate. J Clin Endocrinol Metab 2002;87:1041–1044.
158. Beckett PR, Wong WW, Copeland KC. Developmental changes in the relationship between IGF-I and body composition during puberty. Growth Horm IGF Res 1998;8:283–288.
159. Wilson DM, Killen JD, Hammer LD, et al. Insulin-like growth factor-I as a reflection of body composition, nutrition, and puberty in sixth and seventh grade girls. J Clin Endocrinol Metab 1991;73:907–912.

160. Jorgensen JO, Pedersen SB, Borglum J, et al. Serum concentrations of insulin-like growth factors (IGFs), IGF binding proteins 1 and 3 and growth hormone binding protein in obese women and the effects of growth hormone administration: a double-blind, placebo- controlled study. Eur J Endocrinol 1995;133:65–70.
161. Nam SY, Lee EJ, Kim KR, et al. Effect of obesity on total and free insulin-like growth factor (IGF)-1, and their relationship to IGF-binding protein (BP)-1, IGFBP-2, IGFBP-3, insulin, and growth hormone. Int J Obes Relat Metab Disord 1997;21:355–359.
162. Attia N, Tamborlane WV, Heptulla R, et al. The metabolic syndrome and insulin-like growth factor I regulation in adolescent obesity. J Clin Endocrinol Metab 1998;83:1467–1471.
163. Argente J, Caballo N, Barrios V, et al. Multiple endocrine abnormalities of the growth hormone and insulin-like growth factor axis in prepubertal children with exogenous obesity: effect of short- and long-term weight reduction. J Clin Endocrinol Metab 1997;82:2076–2083.
164. Rasmussen MH, Frystyk J, Andersen T, Breum L, Christiansen JS, Hilsted J. The impact of obesity, fat distribution, and energy restriction on insulin-like growth factor-1 (IGF-I), IGF-binding protein-3, insulin, and growth hormone. Metabolism 1994;43:315–319.
165. Saitoh H, Kamoda T, Nakahara S, Hirano T, Nakamura N. Serum concentrations of insulin, insulin-like growth factor(IGF)-I, IGF binding protein (IGFBP)-1 and -3 and growth hormone binding protein in obese children: fasting IGFBP-1 is suppressed in normoinsulinaemic obese children. Clin Endocrinol (Oxf) 1998;48:487–492.
166. Falorni A, Bini V, Cabiati G, et al. Serum levels of type I procollagen C-terminal propeptide, insulin-like growth factor-I (IGF-I), and IGF binding protein-3 in obese children and adolescents: relationship to gender, pubertal development, growth, insulin, and nutritional status. Metabolism 1997;46:862–871.
167. Bideci A, Cinaz P, Hasanoglu A, Elbeg S. Serum levels of insulin-like growth factor-I and insulin-like growth factor binding protein-3 in obese children. J Pediatr Endocrinol Metab 1997;10:295–299.
168. Hall K, Lundin G, Povoa G. Serum levels of the low molecular weight form of insulin-like growth factor binding protein in healthy subjects and patients with growth hormone deficiency, acromegaly and anorexia nervosa. Acta Endocrinol (Copenh) 1988;118:321–326.
169. Hochberg Z, Hertz P, Colin V, et al. The distal axis of growth hormone (GH) in nutritional disorders: GH- binding protein, insulin-like growth factor I (IGF-I), and IGF-I receptors in obesity and anorexia nervosa. Metabolism 1992;41:106–112.
170. Argente J, Caballo N, Barrios V, et al. Multiple endocrine abnormalities of the growth hormone and insulin-like growth factor axis in patients with anorexia nervosa: effect of short- and long-term weight recuperation. J Clin Endocrinol Metab 1997;82:2084–2092.
171. Besbas N, Ozdemir S, Saatci U, et al. Nutritional assessment of children on haemodialysis: value of IGF-I, TNF-alpha and IL-1beta. Nephrol Dial Transplant 1998;13:1484–1488.
172. Qureshi AR, Alvestrand A, Danielsson A, et al. Factors predicting malnutrition in hemodialysis patients: a cross- sectional study. Kidney Int 1998;53:773–782.
173. Sanaka T, Shinobe M, Ando M, Hizuka N, Kawaguchi H, Nihei H. IGF-I as an early indicator of malnutrition in patients with end-stage renal disease. Nephron 1994;67:73–81.
174. Abdullah MS, Wild G, Jacob V, et al. Cytokines and the malnutrition of chronic renal failure. Miner Electrolyte Metab 1997;23:237–242.
175. Taylor AM, Bush A, Thomson A, et al. Relation between insulin-like growth factor-I, body mass index, and clinical status in cystic fibrosis. Arch Dis Child 1997;76:304–309.
176. Taylor AM, Thomson A, Bruce-Morgan C, et al. The relationship between insulin, IGF-I and weight gain in cystic fibrosis. Clin Endocrinol (Oxf) 1999;51:659–665.
177. Ponzer S, Tidermark J, Brismar K, Soderqvist A, Cederholm T. Nutritional status, insulin-like growth factor-1 and quality of life in elderly women with hip fractures. Clin Nutr 1999;18:241–246.
178. Sullivan DH, Carter WJ. Insulin-like growth factor I as an indicator of protein-energy undernutrition among metabolically stable hospitalized elderly. J Am Coll Nutr 1994;13:184–191.
179. Smith IF, Latham MC, Azubuike JA, et al. Blood plasma levels of cortisol, insulin, growth hormone and somatomedin in children with marasmus, kwashiorkor, and intermediate forms of protein-energy malnutrition. Proc Soc Exp Biol Med 1981;167:607–611.
180. Bouhaddioui L, Brun JF, Jacquemin JL, et al. Immunoreactive somatomedin C in children from Morocco: a biological marker of nutritional growth retardation? Biomed Pharmacother 1989;43:59–63.

181. Wan Nazaimoon WM, Osman A, Wu LL, Khalid BA. Effects of iodine deficiency on insulin-like growth factor-I, insulin- like growth factor-binding protein-3 levels and height attainment in malnourished children. Clin Endocrinol (Oxf) 1996;45:79–83.
182. Thibault H, Souberbielle JC, Taieb C, Brauner R. Idiopathic prepubertal short stature is associated with low body mass index. Horm Res 1993;40:136–140.
183. Attard-Montalto SP, Hadley J, Kingston JE, Eden OB, Saha V. Ongoing assessment of nutritional status in children with malignant disease. Pediatr Hematol Oncol 1998;15:393–403.
184. Colletti RB, Copeland KC, Devlin JT, Roberts JD, McAuliffe TL. Effect of obesity on plasma insulin-like growth factor-I in cancer patients. Int J Obes 1991;15:523–527.
185. Brennan BM, Gill M, Pennells L, Eden OB, Thomas AG, Clayton PE. Insulin-like growth factor I, IGF binding protein 3, and IGFBP protease activity: relation to anthropometric indices in solid tumours or leukaemia. Arch Dis Child 1999;80:226–30.
186. Grant DB, Hambley J, Becker D, Pimstone BL. Reduced sulphation factor in undernourished children. Arch Dis Child 1973;48:596–600.
187. Mohan PS, Jaya Rao KS. Plasma somatomedin activity in protein calorie malnutrition. Arch Dis Child 1979;54:62–64.
188. Dai ZK, Huang MY, Huang TY. [Somatomedin-C in infantile nutritional assessment with comparison with prealbumin, insulin and growth hormone]. Gaoxiong Yi Xue Ke Xue Za Zhi 1995;11:110–116.
189. Bolze MS, Osborne JM, Vecbastiks KA, White ME. Insulin-like growth factor binding proteins in rats respond to fasting and the protein and energy content of the re-feeding diet. J Nutr Biochem 1991;2:623–628.
190. Clark MA, Hentzen BT, Plank LD, Hill GI. Sequential changes in insulin-like growth factor 1, plasma proteins, and total body protein in severe sepsis and multiple injury. JPEN J Parenter Enteral Nutr 1996;20:363–370.
191. Jeevanandam M, Holaday NJ, Petersen SR. Posttraumatic hormonal environment during total parenteral nutrition. Nutrition 1993;9:333–338.
192. Della Corte F, Mancini A, Valle D, et al. Provocative hypothalamopituitary axis tests in severe head injury: correlations with severity and prognosis. Crit Care Med 1998;26:1419–1426.
193. Cotterill AM, Mendel P, Holly JM, et al. The differential regulation of the circulating levels of the insulin- like growth factors and their binding proteins (IGFBP) 1, 2 and 3 after elective abdominal surgery. Clin Endocrinol (Oxf) 1996;44:91–101.
194. Jeevanandam M, Shamos RF, Petersen SR. Substrate efficacy in early nutrition support of critically ill multiple trauma victims. J Parenter Enteral Nutr 1992;16:511–520.
195. Petersen SR, Holaday NJ, Jeevanandam M. Enhancement of protein synthesis efficiency in parenterally fed trauma victims by adjuvant recombinant human growth hormone. J Trauma 1994;36:726–733.
196. Petersen SR, Jeevanandam M, Holaday NJ. Adjuvant recombinant human growth hormone stimulates insulin-like growth factor binding protein-3 secretion in critically ill trauma patients. J Trauma 1995;39:295–300; discussion 300–302.
197. Nygren J, Sammann M, Malm M, et al. Distributed anabolic hormonal patterns in burned patients: the relation to glucagon. Clin Endocrinol (Oxf) 1995;43:491–500.
198. Timmins AC, Cotterill AM, Hughes SC, et al. Critical illness is associated with low circulating concentrations of insulin-like growth factors-I and -II, alterations in insulin-like growth factor binding proteins, and induction of an insulin-like growth factor binding protein 3 protease. Crit Care Med 1996;24:1460–1466.
199. Wojnar MM, Fan J, Frost RA, Gelato MC, Lang CH. Alterations in the insulin-like growth factor system in trauma patients. Am J Physiol 1995;268:R970–R977.
200. Ross RJ, Miell JP, Holly JM, et al. Levels of GH binding activity, IGFBP-1, insulin, blood glucose and cortisol in intensive care patients. Clin Endocrinol (Oxf) 1991;35:361–367.
201. Houston-Bolze MS, Downing MT, Sayed AM, Williford JH. Serum insulin-like growth factor binding protein-3 responds differently to trauma in men and women. Crit Care Med 1996;24:1988–1992.
202. Houston-Bolze MS, Downing MT, Sayed AM, Meserve LA. Gender differences in the responses of serum insulin-like growth factor-1 and transthyretin (prealbumin) to trauma. Crit Care Med 1996;24:1982–1987.
203. Jeevanandam M, Holaday NJ, Shamos RF, Petersen SR. Acute IGF-I deficiency in multiple trauma victims. Clin Nutr 1992;11:352–357.

204. Abribat T, Nedelec B, Jobin N, Garrel DR. Decreased serum insulin-like growth factor-I in burn patients: relationship with serum insulin-like growth factor binding protein-3 proteolysis and the influence of lipid composition in nutritional support. Crit Care Med 2000;28:2366–2372.
205. Abribat T, Brazeau P, Davignon I, Garrel DR. Insulin-like growth factor-I blood levels in severely burned patients: effects of time post injury, age of patient and severity of burn. Clin Endocrinol (Oxf) 1993;39:583–589.
206. Buonpane EA, Brown RO, Boucher BA, Fabian TC, Luther RW. Use of fibronectin and somatomedin-C as nutritional markers in the enteral nutrition support of traumatized patients [see comments]. Crit Care Med 1989;17:126–132.
207. Davies SC, Wass JA, Ross RJ, et al. The induction of a specific protease for insulin-like growth factor binding protein-3 in the circulation during severe illness. J Endocrinol 1991;130:469–473.
208. Bang P, Nygren J, Carlsson-Skwirut C, Thorell A, Ljungqvist O. Postoperative induction of insulin-like growth factor binding protein-3 proteolytic activity: relation to insulin and insulin sensitivity. J Clin Endocrinol Metab 1998;83:2509–2515.
209. Davenport ML, Isley WL, Pucilowska JB, et al. Insulin-like growth factor-binding protein-3 proteolysis is induced after elective surgery. J Clin Endocrinol Metab 1992;75:590–595.
210. Skjaerbaek C, Frystyk J, Orskov H, et al. Differential changes in free and total insulin-like growth factor I after major, elective abdominal surgery: the possible role of insulin- like growth factor-binding protein-3 proteolysis. J Clin Endocrinol Metab 1998;83:2445–2449.
211. Maile LA, Holly JM. Insulin-like growth factor binding protein (IGFBP) proteolysis: occurrence, identification, role and regulation. Growth Horm IGF Res 1999;9:85–95.
212. Gianotti L, Broglio F, Ramunni J, et al. The activity of GH/IGF-I axis in anorexia nervosa and in obesity: a comparison with normal subjects and patients with hypopituitarism or critical illness. Eat Weight Disord 1998;3:64–70.
213. Laughlin GA, Dominguez CE, Yen SS. Nutritional and endocrine-metabolic aberrations in women with functional hypothalamic amenorrhea. J Clin Endocrinol Metab 1998;83:25–32.
214. Keys A, Brozek J, Henschel A, Mickelsen O, Taylor H. The Biology of Human Starvation. University of Minnesota Press, Minneapolis, 1950.
215. Smith G, Robinson PH, Fleck A. Serum albumin distribution in early treated anorexia nervosa. Nutrition 1996;12:677–684.
216. Suliman ME, Qureshi AR, Barany P, et al. Hyperhomocysteinemia, nutritional status, and cardiovascular disease in hemodialysis patients. Kidney Int 2000;57:1727–1735.
217. Lu F, Li P, Zheng F, Zhang Z, Tomino Y. Serum insulin-like growth factor 1 level and nutritional assessment in nondialytic patients with chronic renal failure. Kidney Blood Press Res 2002;25:116–119.
218. Nanba K, Nagake Y, Miyatake N, et al. Relationships of serum levels of insulinlike growth factors with indices of bone metabolism and nutritional conditions in hemodialysis patients. Nephron 2001;89:145–152.
219. Jacob V, Marchant PR, Wild G, Brown CB, Moorhead PJ, el Nahas AM. Nutritional profile of continuous ambulatory peritoneal dialysis patients. Nephron 1995;71:16–22.
220. Jacob V, Le Carpentier JE, Salzano S, et al. IGF-I, a marker of undernutrition in hemodialysis patients. Am J Clin Nutr 1990;52:39–44.
221. Lindgren BF, Friis K, Ericsson F. Insulin-like growth factor I correlates with protein intake estimated from the normalized protein catabolic rate in hemodialysis patients. Am J Nephrol 2000;20:255–262.
222. Parker TF, 3rd, Wingard RL, Husni L, Ikizler TA, Parker RA, Hakim RM. Effect of the membrane biocompatibility on nutritional parameters in chronic hemodialysis patients. Kidney Int 1996;49:551–556.
223. Hong-Brown LQ, Frost RA, Lang CH. Alcohol impairs protein synthesis and degradation in cultured skeletal muscle cells. Alcohol Clin Exp Res 2001;25:1373–1382.
224. Eriksson S. Insulin-like growth factor in chronic liver disease. J Intern Med 1994;235:93–94.
225. Inaba T, Saito H, Inoue T, et al. Growth hormone/insulin-like growth factor 1 axis alterations contribute to disturbed protein metabolism in cirrhosis patients after hepatectomy. J Hepatol 1999;31:271–276.
226. Santolaria F, Gonzalez-Gonzalez G, Gonzalez-Reimers E, et al. Effects of alcohol and liver cirrhosis on the GH-IGF-I axis. Alcohol Alcohol 1995;30:703–708.

227. Mendenhall CL, Anderson S, Weesner RE, Goldberg SJ, Crolic KA. Protein-calorie malnutrition associated with alcoholic hepatitis. Veterans Administration Cooperative Study Group on Alcoholic Hepatitis. Am J Med 1984;76:211–222.
228. Caregaro L, Alberino F, Amodio P, et al. Malnutrition in alcoholic and virus-related cirrhosis. Am J Clin Nutr 1996;63:602–609.
229. Mendenhall CL, Chernausek SD, Ray MB, et al. The interactions of insulin-like growth factor I(IGF-I) with protein- calorie malnutrition in patients with alcoholic liver disease: V.A. Cooperative Study on Alcoholic Hepatitis VI. Alcohol Alcohol 1989;24:319–329.
230. Kondrup J, Nielsen K, Juul A. Effect of long-term refeeding on protein metabolism in patients with cirrhosis of the liver. Br J Nutr 1997;77:197–212.
231. Santolaria F, Perez-Cejas A, Aleman MR, et al. Low serum leptin levels and malnutrition in chronic alcohol misusers hospitalized by somatic complications. Alcohol Alcohol 2003;38:60–66.
232. Laursen EM, Lanng S, Rasmussen MH, Koch C, Skakkebaek NE, Muller J. Normal spontaneous and stimulated GH levels despite decreased IGF-I concentrations in cystic fibrosis patients. Eur J Endocrinol 1999;140:315–321.
233. Laursen EM, Juul A, Lanng S, et al. Diminished concentrations of insulin-like growth factor I in cystic fibrosis. Arch Dis Child 1995;72:494–497.
234. Barrios V, Pozo J, Munoz MT, Buno M, Argente J. Normative data for total and free acid-LabileSubunit of the human insulin-like growth factor-binding protein complex in pre- and full- term newborns and healthy boys and girls throughout postnatal development [In Process Citation]. Horm Res 2000;53:148–153.
235. Juul A, Flyvbjerg A, Frystyk J, Muller J, Skakkebaek NE. Serum concentrations of free and total insulin-like growth factor-I, IGF binding proteins -1 and -3 and IGFBP-3 protease activity in boys with normal or precocious puberty. Clin Endocrinol (Oxf) 1996;44:515–523.
236. Juul A, Holm K, Kastrup KW, et al. Free insulin-like growth factor I serum levels in 1430 healthy children and adults, and its diagnostic value in patients suspected of growth hormone deficiency. J Clin Endocrinol Metab 1997;82:2497–2502.
237. Argente J, Barrios V, Pozo J, et al. Normative data for insulin-like growth factors (IGFs), IGF-binding proteins, and growth hormone-binding protein in a healthy Spanish pediatric population: age- and sex-related changes. J Clin Endocrinol Metab 1993;77:1522–1528.
238. Juul A, Moller S, Mosfeldt-Laursen E, et al. The acid-labile subunit of human ternary insulin-like growth factor binding protein complex in serum: hepatosplanchnic release, diurnal variation, circulating concentrations in healthy subjects, and diagnostic use in patients with growth hormone deficiency. J Clin Endocrinol Metab 1998;83:4408–4415.
239. Janssen JA, Stolk RP, Pols HA, Grobbee DE, de Jong FH, Lamberts SW. Serum free IGF-I, total IGF-I, IGFBP-1 and IGFBP-3 levels in an elderly population: relation to age and sex steroid levels. Clin Endocrinol (Oxf) 1998;48:471–478.
240. Janssen JA, Jacobs ML, Derkx FH, Weber RF, van der Lely AJ, Lamberts SW. Free and total insulin-like growth factor I (IGF-I), IGF-binding protein-1 (IGFBP-1), and IGFBP-3 and their relationships to the presence of diabetic retinopathy and glomerular hyperfiltration in insulin-dependent diabetes mellitus [see comments]. J Clin Endocrinol Metab 1997;82:2809–2815.
241. Hall K, Hilding A, Thoren M. Determinants of circulating insulin-like growth factor-I. J Endocrinol Invest 1999;22:48–57.
242. Hong Y, Pedersen NL, Brismar K, Hall K, de Faire U. Quantitative genetic analyses of insulin-like growth factor I (IGF-I), IGF-binding protein-1, and insulin levels in middle-aged and elderly twins. J Clin Endocrinol Metab 1996;81:1791–1797.
243. Cardim HJ, Lopes CM, Giannella-Neto D, da Fonseca AM, Pinotti JA. The insulin-like growth factor-I system and hormone replacement therapy. Fertil Steril 2001;75:282–287.
244. Leifke E, Gorenoi V, Wichers C, Von Zur Muhlen A, Von Buren E, Brabant G. Age-related changes of serum sex hormones, insulin-like growth factor-1 and sex-hormone binding globulin levels in men: cross-sectional data from a healthy male cohort. Clin Endocrinol (Oxf) 2000;53:689–695.
245. Juul A, Scheike T, Pedersen AT, et al. Changes in serum concentrations of growth hormone, insulin, insulin- like growth factor and insulin-like growth factor-binding proteins 1 and 3 and urinary growth hormone excretion during the menstrual cycle. Hum Reprod 1997;12:2123–2128.

246. Seck T, Scheidt-Nave C, Ziegler R, Pfeilschifter J. Positive association between circulating free thyroxine and insulin- like growth factor 1 concentrations in euthyroid elderly individuals. Clin Endocrinol (Oxf) 1998;48:361–366.
247. Rojdmark S, Rydvald Y, Aquilonius A, Brismar K. Insulin-like growth factor (IGF)-1 and IGF-binding protein-1 concentrations in serum of normal subjects after alcohol ingestion: evidence for decreased IGF-1 bioavailability. Clin Endocrinol (Oxf) 2000;52:313–318.
248. Nindl BC, Kraemer WJ, Marx JO, et al. Overnight responses of the circulating IGF-I system after acute, heavy- resistance exercise. J Appl Physiol 2001;90:1319–1326.
249. Koziris LP, Hickson RC, Chatterton RT, Jr., et al. Serum levels of total and free IGF-I and IGFBP-3 are increased and maintained in long-term training. J Appl Physiol 1999;86:1436–1442.
250. Anthony TG, Anthony JC, Lewitt MS, Donovan SM, Layman DK. Time course changes in IGFBP-1 after treadmill exercise and postexercise food intake in rats. Am J Physiol Endocrinol Metab 2001;280:E650–E656.
251. Tomita M, Shimokawa I, Higami Y, et al. Modulation by dietary restriction in gene expression related to insulin- like growth factor-1 in rat muscle. Aging (Milano) 2001;13:273–281.
252. Naranjo WM, Yakar S, Sanchez-Gomez M, Perez AU, Setser J, D LE. Protein calorie restriction affects nonhepatic IGF-I production and the lymphoid system: studies using the liver-specific IGF-I gene-deleted mouse model. Endocrinology 2002;143:2233–2241.

III GROWTH AND DEVELOPMENT

5 Regulation of Growth and the Insulin Growth Factor System by Zinc

Ruth S. MacDonald

KEY POINTS

- Zinc deficiency results in impaired growth of animals.
- Zinc deprivation is rapidly sensed before tissue stores are depleted.
- Changes in zinc-dependent enzymes do not correlate with the rapid growth suppression.
- The IGF axis, including GH, IGF-I, and the IGF binding proteins, are affected directly and indirectly by zinc depletion.
- Restoration of depressed IGF-I fails to restore growth of zinc-deficient animals.
- Defects in calcium uptake and protein kinase C signaling occur in zinc deficiency.
- Zinc depletion may alter intracellular signaling pathways that regulate growth.
- Zinc binding domains on regulatory proteins that affect gene expression may provide the brake for mitogenic activity in response to zinc depletion.

1. INTRODUCTION

The regulation of growth is a complex integration of endocrinology, nutrition, and physiology. Delayed or suboptimal growth is characteristic of many endocrine disorders as well as nutritional deficiencies. Because the insulin growth factor system is intimately associated with growth regulation, many studies have investigated the interrelationships among nutrient intake, the IGF system, and growth. It has been well documented that decreased protein or energy intake results in decreased circulating IGF-I *(1)*. Whereas a prolonged deficiency of most essential nutrients will ultimately affect growth rate, inadequate zinc intake has rapid and severe effects on growth. Because the growth inhibition occurs before tissue depletion of zinc, a more rapid, perhaps circulating sensor of zinc status is implied. Zinc is an essential component of many enzymes, provides a functional role in gene transcription factors, and may affect growth hormone (GH) and IGF-I production. Hence, the IGF axis would be a likely mechanism to explain the rapid growth inhibition associated with zinc deprivation.

2. OVERVIEW OF ZINC AND GROWTH

Zinc deficiency was associated with growth retardation and delay of sexual maturation in boys in the 1960s *(2)*. In animals, feeding a zinc-deficient diet induces decreased

From: *IGF and Nutrition in Health and Disease*
Edited by: M. S. Houston, J. M. P. Holly, and E. L. Feldman © Humana Press Inc., Totowa, NJ

food intake within 4 d and delayed growth rate *(3)*. Restoration of zinc to the diet rapidly restores growth rate and food intake. Although zinc is essential for growth, the specific zinc-dependent cellular mechanisms that affect growth have not been identified. Because zinc forms stable complexes with amino acids and is resistant to oxidation and reduction it has catalytic, structural, and regulatory roles in more than 300 metalloenzymes. The wide range of distribution of zinc metalloenzymes covers all aspects of metabolism; however, the growth inhibition associated with zinc depletion has not been found to correlate with enzyme activity *(4)*. Furthermore, amino acid sequences that bind zinc to form functional domains (zinc fingers) have been found in DNA binding segments of many eukaryotic regulatory proteins. Bunce *(5)* has proposed that many of the clinical symptoms of zinc deficiency can be associated with defects in activation of the nuclear steroid receptor superfamily, which may be regulated via zinc-finger DNA-binding domains. Hence, altered gene activation caused by inadequate zinc nutriture may provide the signal that results in growth inhibition. However, to date no specific genetic pathway has been shown to correlate with the immediate growth inhibition observed in animals in response to feeding a zinc-depleted diet.

3. RESPONSE OF IGF-I AND GH TO ZINC DEPLETION

Serum growth hormone (GH) *(6)* was found to be reduced by zinc deficiency in rats fed zinc-deficient diets compared with zinc-adequate diets. Serum somatomedin C correlated with tibia zinc levels, a good marker of zinc status, in rats *(7)*. And decreased IGF activity, measured using $^{35}SO_4$ incorporation, was significantly depressed in cartilage of zinc-deficient rats *(8)*. These early findings suggested impaired GH/IGF activity could explain the growth inhibition of zinc deficiency. Because rats fed zinc-deficient diets voluntarily reduce food intake, and decreased energy intake reduces IGF-I levels *(1)*, it is difficult to distinguish effects of zinc depletion from caloric restriction on the IGF system. The typical experiment controls for this variable by including a pair-fed group: each animal fed the zinc-depleted diet is paired with an animal that receives the identical quantity of food (containing zinc) consumed by the zinc-depleted animal. Although this model controls for energy consumption, it is not entirely adequate for separating the effect of decreased energy intake from decreased zinc intake, as both groups are energy deprived. A force-feeding model, in which animals are gavaged with a zinc-depleted diet to ensure adequate energy intake, does correct energy intake while inducing a zinc deficiency. We have also found administration of megestrol acetate stimulates food intake of zinc-deficient male rats *(3,9)*. In both of these models, however, maintaining adequate food intake does not correct the growth suppression of zinc depletion, which suggests zinc depletion is the primary mediator of growth inhibition. Zinc deficiency does appear to have direct effects on the GH/IGF axis, although the mechanisms for this are not well defined. Decreased serum IGF-I in rats fed a low-zinc diet compared with a zinc-adequate diet is consistently observed. Some studies have found serum IGF-I to be lower in zinc-deficient rats compared with zinc-adequate and pair-fed controls *(8,10–12)*, whereas others found serum IGF-I was decreased similarly in zinc-deficient and pair-fed controls *(13,14)*. Droke et al. *(15)* observed lower serum IGF-I in lambs that were fed a zinc-deficient diet compared to marginal or adequate zinc diets, with similar food intake in each group. It is difficult to reconcile these results, although differences in diet composition or age of animals used may be factors.

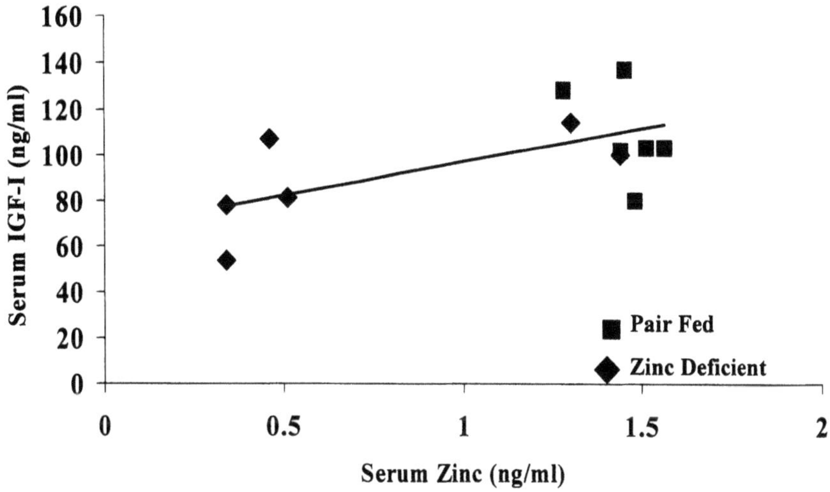

Fig. 1. Zinc deficiency directly induces decreased serum IGF-I concentration. Rats fed a zinc-deficient diet or pair fed a zinc-adequate diet at a reduced level to match the intake of the zinc-deficient rats (pair fed) were followed for 32 d. Serum zinc and IGF-I concentrations were measured on d 0, 2, 7, 12, 22, and 32.

Cossack *(7)* found that somatomedin C levels in rats fed a low protein diet were increased by adding zinc to the diet, although adding protein to a low-zinc diet did not affect somatomedin C levels. Furthermore, restoration of serum somatomedin C after a 72-h fast was dependent on adequate zinc nutriture in rats *(16)*. In contrast with these findings, Clegg et al. *(14)* found serum IGF-I concentration in rats was similarly decreased by food restriction and zinc depletion and that IGF-I levels did not correlate with serum zinc at one time point (17 d). The time course of changes in serum IGF-I in ad libitum-fed, pair-fed, and zinc-deficient rats was determined by Roth and Kirchgessner *(12)*. Serum IGF-I was similar among the three groups until d 7, when the level began to increase in the ad libitum-fed animals. In zinc-deficient rats, serum IGF-I levels begin to decrease at this time point, whereas it remained constant or slightly increased in the pair-fed animals. A negative correlation between serum IGF-I and zinc concentration was observed in the zinc-deficient animals but not the pair-fed, as shown in Fig. 1. These data support the hypothesis that zinc deficiency affects serum IGF-I concentration independently of energy intake.

Changes in IGFBP levels in zinc-deficient rats compared with zinc-adequate rats have also been observed, but the same effects were found in the food-restricted animals *(14)*. In contrast, Ninh et al. *(17)* found that zinc-deficient rats had significantly lower serum IGFBP-3 levels compared with control or pair-fed rats, and although administration of IGF-I increased IGFBP-3 levels in all rats, the levels remained lower in the zinc-deficient animals compared to controls. Hence, serum IGFBP may also be directly affected by zinc deficiency but adequate study of this relationship has not been done.The pattern of changes in serum GH in response to zinc depletion was further examined by Roth and Kirchgessner *(12)*. Two days after feeding a zinc-depleted diet to rats, serum GH was significantly lower compared with zinc-adequate rats. Serum

GH remained lower in zinc-depleted animals through d 32, whereas serum IGF-I was not different among the three groups at d 7, then decreased in both pair-fed and zinc-depleted rats thereafter. In the zinc-depleted rats, pituitary GH concentrations were slightly greater compared with controls after 3 wk, whereas liver IGF-I concentration was not affected until d 12, when it began to decrease.

Using the force-feeding model, Roth and Kirchgessner *(18)* attempted to separate the effects of zinc deficiency from impaired food intake. Despite a similar macronutrient intake, rats fed the zinc-deficient diet gained less body weight and had lower serum IGF-I concentrations than the zinc-adequate animals. A similar response was reported in humans. Serum IGF-I (measured as somatomedin C) was decreased by 50% in healthy adult volunteers who consumed a low-zinc diet for 12 wk *(19)*. The subjects maintained constant caloric intake during the study but all experienced weight loss. Similarly, in postmenopausal women, serum IGF-I concentration was positively correlated with zinc intake *(20)*. Overall, the majority of the data suggest that dietary zinc depletion results in a more severe decrease in serum IGF-I than does food restriction alone. Clearly, zinc deficiency in the presence of adequate energy intake results in decreased serum IGF-I concentration, and restoring energy intake without correcting zinc deficiency fails to reverse decreased serum IGF-I concentrations.

4. RESPONSE TO GH OR IGF-I DURING ZINC DEPLETION

Evidence suggests that zinc deficiency impairs GH and/or IGF-I responsiveness in animals. Administration of GH to rats fed a zinc-depleted diet failed to restore body weight or tibia epiphysis width *(10)*. Similarly, hGH treatment of rats fed a zinc-deficient diet did not correct growth rate *(13)*, and rats fed a zinc-deficient diet for 5 wk failed to increase body weight in response to 2 wk of GH administration compared with rats fed a zinc-replete diet *(21)*. Zinc deficiency was found to reduce bone growth in response to GH infusion in rats *(22)*. Rats were fed a zinc-deficient or adequate diet or pair-fed the adequate diet and GH was infused into the artery of one hindlimb by an implanted osmotic pump. In zinc-adequate and pair-fed rats, GH infusion resulted in increased epiphyseal plate width compared with the noninfused limb. Rats fed the zinc-deficient diet had no change in plate width in response to GH infusion, suggesting that zinc deficiency induces GH resistance in bone. Using hypophysectomized and normal rats, Prasad et al. *(21)* concluded that zinc and GH had independent but additive effects on growth.

The defect in GH response in zinc deficiency is not simply the result of impaired IGF-I activation, as zinc deficiency also prevents the mitogenic response to IGF-I. Infusion of IGF-I for 1 wk to rats fed a zinc-depleted diet for 4 wk failed to stimulate growth, despite normalization of serum IGF-I concentration *(17)*. We also found that maintaining serum IGF-I levels delivered by implanted mini-osmotic pumps during zinc depletion of rats failed to correct the growth inhibition or depression of food intake *(3)*. These findings suggest that decreased IGF-I and/or GH levels that occur during zinc depletion are not the primary factors associated with growth inhibition. It is clear that zinc acts independently of GH and IGF-I to regulate growth and that maintaining normal serum IGF-I and/or GH fails to prevent the growth inhibition induced by zinc deficiency.

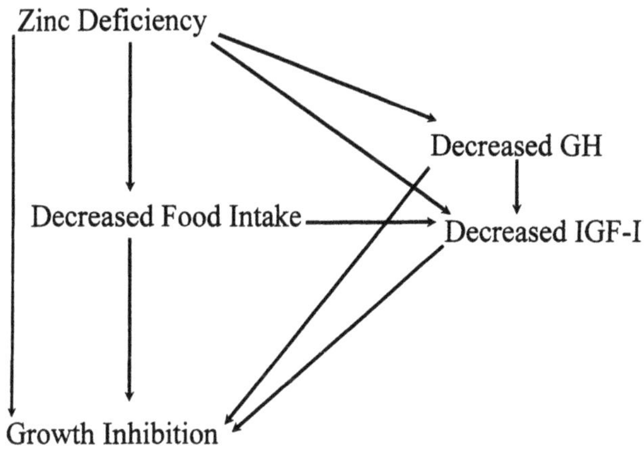

Fig. 2. Inadequate zinc intake results in decreased food intake and growth inhibition by direct effects on these processes and through altered GH and IGF-I activity.

5. ZINC SUPPLEMENTATION WITH GH OR IGF THERAPY

Based on the hypothesis that zinc, IGF-I, and GH are independent mediators of growth but perhaps may have synergistic relationships, several studies have examined the IGF axis during zinc administration to growth-impaired children. Figure 2 depicts the complex interrelationships between zinc, IGF, and growth. Zinc administration (10 mg/d) to Vietnamese children increased growth and serum IGF-I concentrations *(23)*. Treatment resulted in reduced infectious disease and improved appetite, both of which may have contributed to the elevation in IGF-I. Evidence from clinical studies suggests that some children with impaired growth and exhibiting below normal serum IGF-I and/or GH levels, respond to zinc supplementation by increasing growth and restoration of serum IGF-I and GH levels. Collipp et al. *(24)* reported that zinc supplementation (220 mg daily) to two children with clinically determined growth hormone deficiency resulted in improved growth rate and increased growth hormone levels. Similarly, Nishi et al. *(25)* observed zinc supplementation to improve appetite, GH levels, and growth in a 13-yr-old boy with delayed growth. Ghavami-Maibodi et al. *(26)* also observed improved growth and increased serum IGF-I and GH in short but healthy children given zinc supplementation (100 mg/d). When Japanese children with short stature were treated with zinc (5 mg/kg/d) for 6 mo, their growth rate was improved and serum IGF-I levels were increased *(27)*. Measurements of zinc status of these children demonstrated normal levels of serum zinc but elevated clearance of an intravenously administered dose of zinc. Therefore, zinc depletion or increased zinc requirement may occur in children without overt zinc deficiency, and the administration of zinc may correct growth without hormone treatment. In contrast with these positive reports, no difference in response to GH treatment was observed in children given a zinc supplement (220 mg/d) compared with children who were not *(28)*. Also, zinc supplementation (2 mg/kg/d) in infants with nonorganic failure to thrive increased serum IGF-I levels but did not improve growth *(29)*.

6. GH AND IGF EFFECTS ON ZINC HOMEOSTASIS

GH appears to influence zinc homeostasis in humans. Administration of GH to GH-deficient children resulted in reduced excretion of zinc in the urine and increased hair zinc concentration but did not affect serum zinc concentration *(30)*. Children with GH deficiency had normal plasma zinc but elevated erythrocyte and urinary zinc levels compared with age-matched controls *(31)*. After GH treatment, urinary zinc excretion was reduced but remained higher than controls, whereas erythrocyte zinc fell into the normal range. Aihara et al. *(31)* also found elevated plasma and urinary copper in patients before GH treatment but, unlike zinc, plasma copper remained elevated and urinary copper increased after GH therapy. Erythrocyte manganese was below normal and plasma selenium was above normal before treatment but both were corrected by GH treatment. Patients with acromegaly were found to have lower plasma zinc and higher urinary zinc excretion compared with controls *(31)*. After adenectomy, plasma zinc increased and urinary zinc decreased; however, both were higher than in controls. In these patients, copper, selenium, and manganese levels were within the normal range both before and after surgery. These studies suggest that GH treatment or excessive endogenous GH induces a negative zinc balance. It has been suggested that the increased zinc turnover reflects the accelerated use of zinc in catch-up or accelerated growth.

7. ZINC EFFECTS ON GH AND IGF HOMEOSTASIS

Rat anterior pituitary was found to contain high amounts of zinc and regions of the pituitary responsible for hormone storage and release contained measurable amounts of unbound zinc *(32)*. Zinc and other divalent cations inhibited the release of GH and prolactin from bovine adenohypophysial secretory granules in an in vitro assay *(33)*. Somatotropin (GH) release in response to growth hormone releasing-factor analog administration was greater in zinc-deficient lambs compared with either marginal or adequate zinc lambs, although basal levels were not affected by zinc status *(15)*. The response of the pituitary to zinc deprivation was compared in sexually mature and immature male rats *(6)*. In both mature and immature rats, zinc deprivation resulted in decreased circulating GH and increased LH concentrations. In the immature rats zinc depletion also resulted in impaired gonadal growth, and increased levels of pituitary gonadotropins (luteinizing hormone and follicle-stimulating hormone).

Using an in vitro assay of bovine pituitary gland extracts, LaBella et al. *(34)* found the release of pituitary hormones (thyroid-stimulating hormone, luteinizing hormone, adrenocorticotropic hormone and GH) was increased by addition of zinc, whereas the release of prolactin was inhibited. These responses were also observed with copper and nickel. Similarly, prolactin release from rat pituitary glands was also inhibited by zinc in an in vitro assay *(35)*. Cunningham et al. *(36)* found zinc induced dimerization of human growth hormone and proposed that this was a mechanism to increase stability of GH during storage and reduce interaction of GH with receptors in the pituitary. Furthermore, Cunningham et al. *(37)* found that the binding of hGH to the prolactin receptor, a mechanism that is thought to explain the ability of GH to affect lactation, involves the formation of a hormone-zinc-receptor "sandwich." The zinc interaction is likely to occur via zinc ligands identified as three residues on GH (His18, His21, and Glu174) and His188 on the prolactin receptor. Notably, this ligand domain is conserved in all prolactin receptors across species. Based on experiments using hGH variants, produced by site-directed mutagenesis, it was found that zinc plays a role in mediating GH-mediated priming of neutrophils for an enhancement of superoxide radical secretion *(38)*. Because the GH and prolactin receptors are members of the cytokine receptor gene superfamily, this finding implies that zinc may also be involved as a mediator of other cytokines perhaps by providing receptor binding recognition domains.

Incubation of isolated rat hepatocytes with a zinc chelator, diethylenetrinitrilopentaacetate (DTPA), did not alter basal or GH stimulated IGF-I mRNA expression *(39)*. However, hepatocytes isolated from zinc-depleted rats had significantly lower IGF-I, growth hormone receptor (GHR) and growth hormone binding protein (GHBP) mRNA than hepatocytes from zinc-adequate rats, despite no difference in total zinc concentration in the hepatocytes. McNall et al. *(40)* also observed reduced IGF-I, GHR, and GHBP mRNA in liver obtained from rats fed a zinc-deficient diet compared with pair-fed or ad libitum fed controls. The addition of zinc to the culture media of hepatocytes from the zinc-deficient rats did not reverse IGF-I, GHR, or GHBP mRNA levels, whereas metallothionein expression was recovered *(39)*. In contrast, supplementation of the culture media with 50 μ*M* zinc resulted in reduced basal and GH stimulated IGF-I mRNA expression. The authors conclude from these studies that the IGF-I gene is not responsive to decreased zinc concentration, although high zinc concentrations specifically inhibited this gene. In animals fed a zinc-deficient diet, depressed hepatic expression of IGF-I, GHR, and GHBP was an indirect consequence and not owing directly to reduced zinc availability. It was speculated that the stability of the IGF-I mRNA transcript is reduced by zinc deficiency *(40)*. Using cultured GH3 rat pituitary cells, Sciaudone et al. *(41)* observed that chelation of zinc resulted in increased expression of GH mRNA in response to thyroid or retinoic acid activation. The authors suggest that reduced availability of zinc may increase the response of nuclear receptors that regulate GH gene expression.

8. ZINC AND INTRACELLULAR SIGNALING PATHWAYS

There is evidence to suggest that zinc influences aspects of the intracellular signaling pathway associated with the regulation of cell proliferation. Chesters et al. *(42)* used the Swiss 3T3 epithelial cell culture model to examine cell cycle progression in cells deprived of zinc by addition of the chelator, DTPA. When DTPA was present, fetal bovine serum, as a source of growth factors, failed to stimulate thymidine incorporation into DNA. The addition of zinc specifically restored the rate of proliferation. Furthermore, Chesters and Boyne *(43)* observed decreased RNA and protein synthesis in zinc-deprived cells. They postulated that the defective DNA synthesis resulted from failure to produce and maintain a specific protein required for progression of the cells from the G_1 to the S phase of the cell cycle. In a review, Chesters *(44)* suggested that lack of zinc restricts gene expression of proteins directly involved with the initiation of DNA synthesis, such as thymidine kinase. Although this is a valid conclusion, the same results would occur if mitotic signal transduction were impaired by lack of zinc. To explore this possibility, MacDonald et al. *(45)* extended the Chesters model and showed that thymidine incorporation was stimulated by sequential treatment of 3T3 cells with platelet-derived growth factor (PDGF), epidermal growth factor (EGF), and IGF-I to a level equal that achieved by fetal bovine serum supplementation. Cells stimulated with PDGF and EGF are considered to be primed and competent for IGF-I stimulation of cell proliferation. In this model, depletion of extracellular zinc by DTPA had no affect on the PDGF or EGF response but completely eliminated IGF-I stimulation of cell proliferation. Impairment of the IGF-I response could result from failure of receptor expression or of signal transduction. Thornton et al. *(46)* found that IGF-I receptor expression in 3T3 cells was not significantly affected by zinc deprivation but that the proliferative fraction, that is, the proportion of cells in the S and G_2/M phases of the cycle, was greatly decreased. To further define the defect in IGF-I signaling associated with zinc depletion, MacDonald et al. *(47)* found decreased extracellular calcium uptake in response to IGF-I when zinc was depleted by DTPA. This observation agrees with the fact that calcium uptake is impaired in other zinc-deficient systems, including platelets *(48,49)* and brain synaptic vesicles *(50,51)* prepared from zinc-deficient animals. In some cells, IGF-I signaling of mitogenic events requires activation of extracellular calcium uptake *(52)*. Hence, impaired IGF-I activation of extracellular calcium uptake because of zinc depletion may be a mechanism through which the mitogenic effect of IGF-I is impaired by zinc deficiency.

Using MC3T3-E1 cells as a model of osteoblasts, Matsui and Yamaguchi *(53)* observed zinc (10 μ*M*) and IGF-I (10 n*M*) to increase cell proliferation individually and in combination to have a synergistic effect on these cells. Staurosporin, an inhibitor of protein kinase C (PKC), inhibited the ability of zinc but not IGF-I to increase cell protein concentration. The authors conclude that zinc may activate PKC in these cells. PKC is a family of serine-threonine kinases that are involved in signal transduction pathways in numerous cell types. Quest et al. *(54)* found that PKC is a zinc metalloenzyme that incorporates four zinc atoms per molecule. The zinc is bound within the lipid binding regulatory domain of the enzyme that is thought to be the site for phorbol ester (a PKC-activating compound) binding. However, when zinc was chelated with 1,10-phenanthroline the ability of phorbol 12-myristate 13-acetate to induce phospholipase D-mediated hydrolysis of phosphatidylcholine was enhanced rather than inhibited *(55)*. The addition of zinc to the reaction reversed the stimulatory response. Hence, the role of the zinc containing domain of PKC remains unclear.

In cultured rat osteoblasts, chelation of zinc with NNN-tetrakis (2-pyridylmethyl) ethylenediamine induced apoptosis *(56)*. The zinc-depleted cells also demonstrated reduced formation of the PKC metabolite, inositol-1,4,5-triphosphate (IP_3), leading the authors to conclude that apoptosis induced by zinc deficiency in these cells was the result of decreased PKC activity. Using the force-fed zinc-deficient rat model, Kirchgessner et al. *(57)* observed that whereas the specific activity of PKC/mg of protein in skeletal muscle was not reduced, a significant reduction of PKC in the particulate fraction occurred. A reduced PKC activity was suggested in these rats as platelets from the zinc-deficient rats had significantly less IP_3 compared with zinc-adequate animals *(58)*. Platelet aggregation requires PKC and zinc-deficient rats demonstrate reduced platelet aggregation *(49)*. However, no change in subcellular distribution of PKC, as determined by phorbol ester binding, occurred in platelets from zinc-deficient rats *(59)*. The authors found significantly impaired calcium uptake by platelets from the zinc-deficient rats and therefore concluded that the defect in platelet aggregation with zinc deficiency was caused primarily by impaired calcium uptake, which subsequently resulted in defective PKC activation.

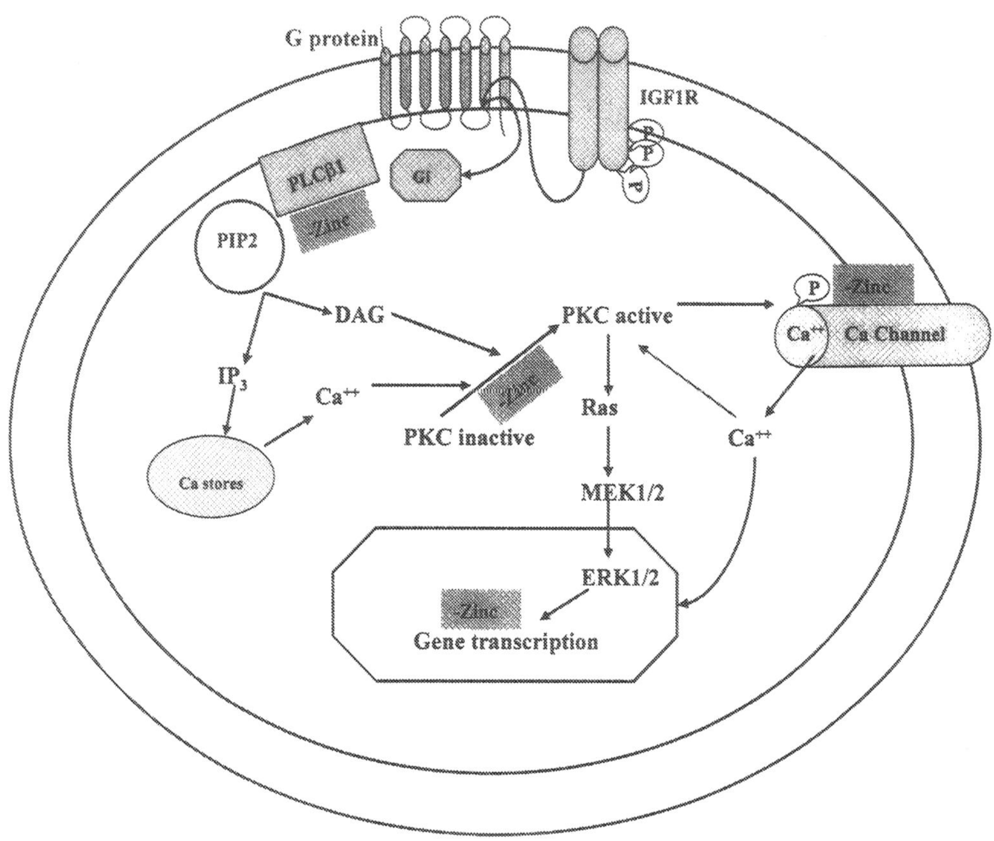

Fig. 3. Proposed mechanisms through which zinc deficiency affects intracellular signaling pathways associated with mitogenic responses to IGF-I. Symbols indicate IGF-I receptor (IGF-IR), phosphorylation sites (P), G protein subunit (Gi), phospholipase C β1 (PLCβ1), phosphoinositol (PIP_2), diacylglycerol (DAG), inositol-1,4,5 triphosphate (IP_3), calcium (Ca^{2+}), protein kinase C (PKC), and intracellular signaling proteins (RAS, MEK1/2, ERK1/2). The rectangles indicated by zinc are potential sites where zinc may be involved as a regulator either directly or indirectly.

Overall, these studies suggest that zinc status affects intracellular signaling cascades associated with IGF-I and PKC. A model that depicts hypothetical roles for calcium and PKC in IGF-I-stimulated proliferation of 3T3 cells is shown in Fig. 3. Binding of IGF-I results in autophosphorylation of the receptor protein and activation of its intrinsic tyrosine kinase activity *(60)*. Receptor tyrosine kinases, including the IGF-I receptor, activate G_i-coupled receptors *(61)*. Subsequent release of $G_{\beta\gamma}$ causes activation of $PLC\beta_1$, a zinc-dependent enzyme *(62)*, which catalyzes the production of diacylglycerol and IP_3 from phosphoinositol. IP_3 stimulates release of intracellular calcium stores, which, together with diacylglycerol and phosphatidylserine, mediate the activation of PKC_a. Activated PKC_a phosphorylates the calcium channel, leading to calcium uptake *(63)*. Furthermore, activated PKC couples with Ras to activate mitogenic proteins such as Mek-1/2 and Erk1/2, which activate transcription factors in the nucleus. Evidence from our work and others suggests in the absence of zinc, the calcium channel is impaired. The inhibition of calcium uptake observed in zinc depletion may occur at several points in this pathway, including steps involved with activation of PKC or the calcium channel directly. Recently, a zinc-sensing receptor has been proposed in colonocytes, which induces intracellular calcium release in response to increased extracellular zinc concentration *(64)*. It was proposed that this zinc receptor was coupled to a G-protein because inhibition of phospholipase C blocked calcium release. These studies suggest that zinc may be involved at several points in the highly complex network of intracellular signaling cascades that regulate cell proliferation and metabolism.

It is likely that additional zinc-responsive enzymes and signaling proteins will be identified to further extend this scenario. For example, recently Kim et al. *(65)* found zinc-activated p70S6k, a kinase that regulates phosphorylation of the ribosomal protein S6, in Swiss 3T3 cells. Activation of p70S6k is thought to mediate cell growth at the G1 to S transition. Furthermore, zinc was found to activate the phosphoinositide 3-kinase (PI3K) pathway in these cells via a tyrosine kinase-dependent mechanism. In this model, zinc activation of p70S6k was independent of calcium. Another recent report also suggests that zinc mediates the PI3K pathway. Addition of zinc to primary mouse cortical cultures was found to induce stimulation of c-Jun N-terminal kinase and this effect was blocked by inhibitors of PI3K *(66)*. The large number of transcription factors that possess zinc finger motifs, such as the SP1 family of the Kruppel type zinc finger proteins *(67)*, the zinc RING (really interesting new gene) finger proteins *(68)*, and tumor suppressor genes such as p53 *(69)*. which mediate cell cycle progression and apoptosis, suggest that changes in zinc availability may alter the function of these proteins.

9. OTHER TRACE METALS AND THE IGF SYSTEM

The metabolism of other trace minerals may also be affected by GH and IGF, although there has been little research in this area. Manganese is an essential nutrient associated with glucose and lipid metabolism, as well as growth. A dietary induced manganese deficiency was associated with reduced serum IGF-I concentrations in rats *(70)*. No changes in IGF binding proteins were observed in the manganese-deficient animals. Iron is a critical component of heme containing proteins, which are involved in many metabolic reactions. Iron deficiency results in impaired growth, however iron depletion of veal calves did not affect plasma IGF-I, nor GH secretion *(71)*.

10. SUMMARY AND CONCLUSIONS

Zinc is an essential nutrient for mammals and a deficiency of zinc results in impaired growth. The IGF axis, including GH, IGF-I, and the IGF binding proteins, are affected both directly and indirectly by zinc depletion. Decreased circulating IGF-I is characteristic of zinc deficient animals and humans. However, impaired growth because of zinc deficiency cannot be restored by the addition of GH or IGF-I, which suggests zinc alters the ability of these mitogens to affect growth. Current evidence suggests that zinc depletion is rapidly sensed, even before tissue stores are affected, and mitogenic signaling pathways are inhibited. Specific intracellular signaling pathways that are zinc responsive have not been fully characterized, although calcium uptake and PKC are likely candidates. Changes in zinc-dependent enzymes have not been found to correlate with the rapid growth inhibition observed in animals. Zinc associates with amino acid residues on proteins and provides linkages that create functional domains. Such zinc-binding domains have been found in many regulatory proteins that affect gene expression. It is currently not known if the zinc ions associated with such regulatory proteins are responsive to subtle changes in intracellular zinc availability. However, these zinc-dependent proteins may provide the brake for mitogenic activity in response to zinc depletion.

11. RECOMMENDATIONS AND CHALLENGES FOR THE FUTURE

The limiting cellular role for zinc in growth remains poorly defined. Many zinc-dependent enzymes have been identified and characterized; yet, alteration of enzyme activity cannot explain the rapid onset of growth inhibition observed when animals are fed zinc-depleted diets. Exciting recent evidence suggests zinc may be involved in many intracellular signaling pathways that provide rapid response to changes in zinc concentrations. The IGF system is influenced by zinc availability, but future studies are needed to identify how these systems interact. It is known that within cells, free zinc concentrations are very low; however the transport, storage, and distribution of zinc are not fully understood. As advances in understanding zinc transport progress, potential relationships to the IGF and other mitogenic systems can be made. Understanding the role of zinc in regulatory proteins will also provide keys to identify genetic targets for zinc.

ACKNOWLEDGMENTS

The research cited by the author was funded by the USDA-NRI. The author thanks Dr. Boyd O'Dell and Mr. Jimmy Browning for their contribution to this work.

REFERENCES

1. Underwood LE. Nutritional regulation of IGF-I and IGFBPs. J Pediatr Endocr Metab 1996;9(Suppl 3):303–312.
2. Prasad AS. Importance of zinc in human nutrition. Am J Clin Nutr 1967;20:648–652.
3. Browning JD, MacDonald RS, Thornton WH, O'Dell BL. Reduced food intake in zinc deficient rats is normalized by megestrol acetate but not by insulin-like growth factor-I. J Nutr 1998;128:136–142.
4. Chesters JK, Will M. Effect of age, weight and adequacy of zinc intake on the balance between alkaline ribonuclease and ribonuclease inhibitor in various tissues of the rat. Br J Nutr 1978;39:375–382.
5. Bunce GE. Interactions between zinc, vitamins A and D and hormones in the regulation of growth. Adv Exp Med Biol 1994;352:257–264.
6. Root AW, Duckett G, Sweetland M, Reiter EO. Effects of zinc deficiency upon pituitary function in sexually mature and immature male rats. J Nutr 1979;109:958–964.
7. Cossack ZT. Somatomedin-C and zinc status in rats as affected by Zn, protein and food intake. Br J Nutr 1986;56:163–169.
8. Bolze MS, Reeves RD, Lindbeck FE, Elders MJ. Influence of zinc on growth, somatomedin, and glycosaminoglycan metabolism in rats. Am J Physiol 1987;252:E21–E26.
9. Williamson PS, Browning JD, MacDonald RS. Megestrol acetate increases short-term food intake in zinc-deficient rats. Physiol Behav 2002;75:323–330.
10. Oner G, Bhaumick B, Bala RM. Effect of zinc deficiency on serum somatomedin levels and skeletal growth in young rats. Endocrinology 1984;114:1860–1863.
11. Cossack ZT. Somatomedin-C in zinc deficiency. Experientia 1984;40:498–500.

12. Roth HP, Kirchgessner M. Course of concentration changes of growth hormone, IGF-1, insulin and C-peptide in serum, pituitary and liver of zinc-deficient rats. J Anim Physiol Anim Nutr 1997;77:91–101.
13. Dicks D, Rojhani A, Cossack ZT. The effect of growth hormone treatment on growth in zinc deficient rats. Nutr Res 1993;13:701–713.
14. Clegg MS, Keen CL, Donovan SM. Zinc deficiency-induced anorexia influences the distribution of serum insulin-like growth factor-binding proteins in the rat. Metab Clin Exp 1995;44:1495–1501.
15. Droke EA, Spears JW, Armstrong JD, Kegley EB, Simpson RB. Dietary zinc affects serum concentrations of insulin and insulin-like growth factor I in growing lambs. J Nutr 1993;123:13–19.
16. Cossack ZT. Effect of zinc level in the refeeding diet in previously starved rats on plasma somatomedin C levels. J Pediatr Gastroenterol Nutr 1988;7:441–445.
17. Ninh NX, Maiter D, Verniers J, Lause P, Ketelslegers JM, Thissen JP. Failure of exogenous IGF-I to restore normal growth in rats submitted to dietary zinc deprivation. J Endocrinol 1998;159:211–217.
18. Roth HP, Kirchgessner M. Influence of alimentary zinc deficiency on the concentration of growth hormone (GH), insulin-like growth factor I (IGF-I) and insulin in the serum of force-fed rats. Hormone Metab Res 1994;26:404–408.
19. Cossack ZT. Decline in somatomedin-C, insulin-like growth factor-1, with experimentally induced zinc deficiency in human subjects. Clin Nutr (Edinburgh) 1991;10:284–291.
20. Devine A, Rosen C, Mohan S, Baylink D, Prince RL. Effects of zinc and other nutritional factors on insulin-like growth factor I and insulin-like growth factor binding proteins in postmenopausal women. Am J Clin Nutr 1998;68:200–206.
21. Prasad AS, Oberleas D, Wolf P, Horwitz JP. Effect of growth hormone on nonhypophysectomized zinc-deficient rats and zinc on hypophysectomized rats. J Lab Clin Med 1969;73:486–494.
22. Cha MC, Rojhani A. Zinc deficiency inhibits the direct growth effect of growth hormone on the tibia of hypophysectomized rats. Biol Trace Elem Res 1997;59:99–111.
23. Ninh NX, Thissen JP, Collette L, Gerard G, Khoi HH, Ketelslegers JM. Zinc supplementation increases growth and circulating insulin-like growth factor I (IGF-I) in growth-retarded Vietnamese children. Am J Clin Nutr 1996;63:514–519.
24. Collipp PJ, Castro-Magana M, Petrovic M, Thomas J, Cheruvanky T, Chen SY, Sussman H. Zinc deficiency: improvement in growth and growth hormone levels with oral zinc therapy. Ann Nutr Metab 1982;26:287–290.
25. Nishi Y, Hatano S, Aihara K, Fujie A, Kihara M. Transient partial growth hormone deficiency due to zinc deficiency. J Am Coll Nutr 1989;8:93–97.
26. Ghavami-Maibodi SZ, Collipp PJ, Castro-Magana M, Stewart C, Chen SY. Effect of oral zinc supplements on growth, hormonal levels, and zinc in healthy short children. Ann Nutr Metab 1983;27:214–219.
27. Nakamura T, Nishiyama S, Futagoishi-Suginohara Y, Matsuda I, Higashi A. Mild to moderate zinc deficiency in short children: effect of zinc supplementation on linear growth velocity. J Pediatr 1993;123:65–69.
28. Richards GE, Marshall RN. The effect of growth hormone treatment alone or growth hormone with supplemental zinc on growth rate, serum, and urine zinc and copper concentrations and hair zinc concentration in patients with growth hormone deficiency. J Am Coll Nutr 1983;2:133–140.
29. Hershkovitz E, Printzman L, Segev Y, Levy J, Phillip M. Zinc supplementation increases the level of serum insulin-like growth factor-I but does not promote growth in infants with nonorganic failure to thrive. Hormone Res 1999;4:200–204.
30. Cheruvanky T, Castro-Magana M, Chen SY, Collipp PJ, Ghavami-Maibodi Z. Effect of growth hormone on hair, serum, and urine zinc in growth hormone-deficient children. Am J Clin Nutr 1982;35:668–670.
31. Aihara K, Nishi Y, Hatano S, Kihara M, Ohta M, Sakoda K, Uozumi T, Usui T. Zinc, copper, manganese, and selenium metabolism in patients with human growth hormone deficiency or acromegaly. J Pediatr Gastroenterol Nutr 1985;4:610–615.
32. Thorlacius-Ussing O, Flyvbjerg A, Esmann J. Evidence that selenium induces growth retardation through reduced growth hormone and somatomedin C production. Endocrinology 1987;120:659–663.
33. Lorenson MY, Robson DL, Jacobs LS. Divalent cation inhibition of hormone release from isolated adenohypophysial secretory granules. J Biol Chem 1983;258:8618–8622.
34. LaBella F, Dular R, Vivian S, Queen G. Pituitary hormone releasing or inhibiting activity of metal ions present in hypothalamic extracts. Biochem Biophys Res Commun 1973;52:786–791.

35. Judd AM, MacLeod RM, Login IS. Zinc acutely, selectively and reversibly inhibits pituitary prolactin secretion. Brain Res 1984;294:190–192.
36. Cunningham BC, Mulkerrin MG, Wells JA. Dimerization of human growth hormone by zinc. Science 1991;253:545–548.
37. Cunningham BC, Bass S, Fuh G, Wells JA. Zinc mediation of the binding of human growth hormone to the human prolactin receptor. Science 1990;250:1709–1712.
38. Fu YK, Arkins S, Fuh G, Cunningham BC, Wells JA, Fong S, Cronin MJ, Dantzer R, Kelley KW. Growth hormone augments superoxide anion secretion of human neutrophils by binding to the prolactin receptor. J Clin Invest 1992;89:451–457.
39. Lefebvre D, Beckers F, Ketelslegers JM, Thissen JP. Zinc regulation of insulin-like growth factor-I (IGF-I), growth hormone receptor (GHR) and binding protein (GHBP) gene expression in rat cultured hepatocytes. Mol Cell Endocrinol 1998;138:127–136.
40. McNall AD, Etherton TD, Fosmire GJ. The impaired growth induced by zinc deficiency in rats is associated with decreased expression of the hepatic insulin-like growth factor I and growth hormone receptor genes. J Nutr 1995;125:874–879.
41. Sciaudone MP, Chattopadhyay S, Freake HC. Chelation of zinc amplifies induction of growth hormone mRNA levels in cultured rat pituitary tumor cells. J Nutr 2000;130:158–163.
42. Chesters JK, Petrie L, Vint H. Specificity and timing of the Zn2+ requirement for DNA synthesis by 3T3 cells. Exp Cell Res 1989;184:499–508.
43. Chesters JK, Boyne R. Nature of the Zn2+ requirement for DNA synthesis by 3T3 cells. Exp Cell Res 1991;192:631–634.
44. Chesters JK. Trace element-gene interactions. Nutr Rev 1992;59:217–223.
45. MacDonald RS, Wollard-Biddle LC, Browning JD, Thornton WH Jr, O'Dell BL Zinc deprivation of murine 3T3 cells by use of diethylenetrinitrilopentaacetate impairs DNA synthesis upon stimulation with insulin-like growth factor-1 (IGF-1). J Nutr 1998;128:1600–1605.
46. Thornton WH Jr, MacDonald RS, Wollard-Biddle LC, Browning JD, O'Dell BL. Chelation of extracellular zinc inhibits proliferation in 3T3 cells independent of insulin-like growth factor-I receptor expression. Proc Soc Exp Biol Med 1998;219:64–68.
47. MacDonald RS, Browning JD, Wollard-Biddle L, O'Dell BL. Calcium uptake and proliferation of IGF-I stimulated 3T3 cells are impaired by DTPA-induced zinc deprivation. FASEB J. 1999;13:A570.
48. Emery MP, O'Dell BL. Low zinc status in rats impairs calcium uptake and aggregation of platelets stimulated by fluoride. Proc Soc Exp Biol Med 1993;203:480–484.
49. Xia J, O'Dell BL. Zinc deficiency in rats decreased thrombin-stimulated platelet aggregation by lowering protein kinase C activity secondary to impaired calcium uptake. J Nutr Biochem 1995;6:661–666.
50. Browning JD, O'Dell BL. Low zinc status in guinea pigs impairs calcium uptake by brain synaptosomes. J Nutr 1994;124:436–443.
51. Browning JD, O'Dell BL. Low zinc status impairs calcium uptake by hippocampal synaptosomes stimulated by potassium but not by N-methyl-D-aspartate. J Nutr Biochem 1995;6:588–594.
52. Kojima I, Matsunaga H, Kurokawa K, Ogata E, Nishimoto I. Calcium influx: an intracellular message of the mitogenic action of insulin-like growth factor-I. J Biol Chem 1988;263:16561–16567.
53. Matsui T, Yamaguchi M. Zinc modulation of insulin-like growth factor's effect in osteoblastic MC3T3-E1 cells. Peptides 1995;6:1063–1068.
54. Quest AF, Bloomenthal J, Bardes ES, Bell RM. The regulatory domain of protein kinase C coordinates four atoms of zinc. J Biol Chem 1992;267:10193–10197.
55. Kiss Z. The zinc chelator 1,10-phenanthroline enhances the stimulatory effects of protein kinase C activators and staurosporine, but not sphingosine and H2O2, on phospholipase D activity in NIH 3T3 fibroblasts. Biochem J 1994;298:93–98.
56. Cen XB, Wang RS, Wang H. Apoptosis induced by zinc deficiency in rat osteoblast: possible involvement of protein kinase C. Biomed Environ Sci 1999;12:161–169.
57. Kirchgessner M, Moser C, Roth HP. Activity and subcellular distribution of protein kinase C (PKC) in muscle and brain of force-fed zinc-deficient rats. Biol Trace Element Res 1996;52:273–280.
58. Roth HP, Moser C, Kirchgessner M. Subcellular distribution of protein kinase C (pKC) in erythrocytes and concentration of D-myo-inositol-1,4,5-trisphosphate (IP3) in platelets and monocytes of force-fed zinc-deficient rats. Biol Trace Element Res 1996;53:225–234.

59. Xia J, Emery M, O'Dell BL. Zinc status and distribution of protein kinase C in rat platelets. J Nutr Biochem 1994;5:536–541.
60. LeRoith D, Werner H, Neuenschwander S, Kalebic T, Helman LJ. The role of the insulin-like growth factor-I receptor in cancer. Ann NY Acad Sci 1995;766:402–408.
61. Kuemmerle JF, Murthy KS. Coupling of the insulin-like growth factor-I receptor tyrosine kinase to Gi2 in human intestinal smooth muscle: Gbetagamma-dependent mitogen-activated protein kinase activation and growth. J Biol Chem 2001;276:7187–7194.
62. Martin SF, Follows BC, Hergenrother PJ, Franklin CL. A novel class of zinc-binding inhibitors for the phosphatidylcholine-preferring phospholipase C from Bacillus cereus. J Org Chem 2000;65:4509–4514.
63. Cooper CB, Arnot MI, Feng ZP, Jarvis SE, Hamid J, Zamponi GW. Cross-talk between G-protein and protein kinase C modulation of N-type calcium channels is dependent on the G-protein beta subunit isoform. J Biol Chem 2000;275:40777–40781.
64. Hershfinkel M, Moran A, Grossman N, Sekler I. A zinc-sensing receptor triggers the release of intracellular Ca2+ and regulates ion transport. Proc Natl Acad Sci USA 2001;98:11749–11754.
65. Kim S, Jung Y, Kim D, Koh H, Chung J. Extracellular zinc activates p70 S6 kinase through the phosphatidylinositol 3-kinase signaling pathway. J Biol Chem 2000;275:25979–25984.
66. Eom SJ, Kim EY, Lee JE, Kang HJ, Shim J, Kim SU, Gwag BJ, Choi EJ. Zn(2+) induces stimulation of the c-Jun N-terminal kinase signaling pathway through phosphoinositide 3-Kinase. Mol Pharm 2001;59:981–986.
67. Shields JM, Christy RJ, Yang VW. Identification and characterization of a gene encoding a gut-enriched Kruppel-like factor expressed during growth arrest. J Biol Chem 1996;271:20009–20017.
68. Sun Y, Tan M, Duan H, Swaroop M. SAG/ROC/Rbx/Hrt, a zinc RING finger gene family: molecular cloning, biochemical properties, and biological functions. Antioxidants Redox Signal 2001;3:635–650.
69. Hainaut P, Mann K. Zinc binding and redox control of p53 structure and function. Antioxidants Redox Signal 2001;3:611–623.
70. Clegg MS, Donovan SM, Monaco MH, Baly DL, Ensunsa JL, Keen CL. The influence of manganese deficiency on serum IGF-1 and IGF binding proteins in the male rat. Proc Soc Exp Biol Med 1998;219:41–47.
71. Ceppi A, Mullis PE, Eggenberger E, Blum JW Growth hormone concentration and disappearance rate, insulin-like growth factors I and II and insulin levels in iron-deficient veal calves. Ann Nutr Metab 1994;38:281–286.

6 The Role of the Insulin-Like Growth Factor System in Pre- and Postnatal Growth, Development, and Tumorigenesis

Charles T. Roberts, Jr.

KEY POINTS

- IGF action is an important regulator of pre- and postnatal growth in both experimental animals and in humans.
- The complexity of the IGF signaling system of ligands, receptors, and binding proteins and their developmental and tissue-specific patterns of expression affords a powerful and finely orchestrated control mechanism throughout the life of the organism.
- As a result of its ability to control growth and cell survival, the IGF system has the ability to affect, and has been implicated in, tumorigenesis in many types of cancer.
- The IGF system has many components and aspects that make it an attractive therapeutic target for treatment of a number of disorders, including those affecting growth, cancer, and diabetes.

1. INTRODUCTION

The insulin-like growth factor (IGF) signaling system plays a critical role in the growth and development of many tissues and is an important mediator of overall growth, particularly prenatal growth. The IGF system is also implicated in pathophysiology and plays an important role in tumorigenesis. As described in Chapter 1, the IGF system is composed of the IGF ligands (IGF-I and IGF-II), cell-surface receptors that mediate the biological effects of the IGFs, and a family of IGF binding proteins (IGFBPs) that affect the half-lives and bioavailability of the IGFs in the circulation and in extracellular fluids. This review will focus on the contribution of the IGF axis to growth and development and its role in tumorigenesis, with an emphasis on human data. The original somatomedin hypothesis that posited that IGF-I is the principal mediator of the growth-promoting actions of growth hormone is still considered to be valid overall *(1)*. Thus, it is not entirely accurate to discuss the actions of the IGF system without considering them in the greater context of the hypothalamic-pituitary axis. With this caveat, this chapter focuses more narrowly on the IGF system *per se* and its

From: *IGF and Nutrition in Health and Disease*
Edited by: M. S. Houston, J. M. P. Holly, and E. L. Feldman © Humana Press Inc., Totowa, NJ

physiological and pathophysiological effects. The following section reviews some basic aspects of the IGF system that are of particular relevance to the topic of this chapter.

2. BACKGROUND

2.1. IGF-I and IGF-II Expression

The expression of the IGF-II gene in rodents is widespread prenatally, but diminishes drastically after birth, with the choroid plexus and the leptomeninges being the persistent sites of synthesis in adult animals. Murine expression of IGF-I, however, is low prenatally and significantly increases during puberty, with hepatic production being a major contributor to overall IGF-I levels in the circulation. IGF-I is produced by numerous other adult organs, however, including kidney, lung, and bone, and exerts endocrine, paracrine, and autocrine effects. This inverse pattern of IGF-I and IGF-II expression in rats and mice initially led to the concept of IGF-II as a fetal growth factor and IGF-I as an adult growth factor. This is not the situation in humans, however, because both IGF-I and IGF-II are produced throughout life by multiple tissues. In fact, the circulating levels of IGF-II are consistently several-fold higher than those of IGF-I, which supports that concept that there are potentially divergent roles for the two IGFs in human physiology.

2.2. The IGF Receptors

Most, if not all, of the effects of IGF-I result from its activation of the IGF-I receptor (IGF-IR) *(2)*. IGF-I is not thought to crossreact with the insulin receptor (IR), except at pharmacological doses, because the relative affinity of IGF-I for the IGF-IR vs the IR differs by an order of magnitude. It was initially thought that IGF-II, like IGF-I, only bound appreciably to the IGF-IR as compared with the IR. Studies in knockout mice lacking various combinations of the IGF system and the IR suggested that IGF-II acted through the IR in early development, prior to detectable IGF-IR gene expression *(3)*. The molecular basis for this phenomenon was revealed when it was discovered that a splice variant of the IR displayed high affinity for IGF-II. The IR transcript is subject to alternative splicing of exon 11, which encodes a 12-amino acid segment at the C-terminus of the extracellular α subunit. Previous studies had shown that the IR isoform encoded by the mRNA lacking the exon-11 sequence (IR-A) displayed a twofold higher affinity for insulin than the IR-B isoform specified by the exon 11-containing mRNA. More recently, it has been reported that the IR-A isoform, in fact, functions as a high-affinity receptor for IGF-II and produces predominantly proliferative effects as compared to the principally metabolic effects elicited by insulin stimulation of IR-B *(4)*. Thus, IGF-I functions primarily by activating the IGF-IR, while IGF-II can act through either the IGF-IR or through the A form of the IR.

2.3. Hybrid Receptors

IGF signaling is made considerably more complex by the existence of hybrid receptors that result from the dimerization of IGF-IR and IR hemireceptors, each consisting of a single α- and β-subunit linked by disulfide bonds. These hybrid receptors are formed by the formation of intra-α subunit disulfide bonds in the Golgi apparatus of cells expressing both the IGF-IR and IR genes. Although originally considered to represent a small proportion of the total number of IGF-IR and IR in a given cell, recent evidence suggests that the formation of hybrids may be preferred over the formation of classical IGF-IR and IR heterotetramers. This could be the result of the preferential formation of disulfide bonds between cysteine residues in IGF-IR and IR α subunits themselves. Thus, in some circumstances, hybrid receptors may outnumber "pure" IGF-IR or IR molecules at the cell surface.

IGF-IR/IR hybrid receptors retain high affinity for IGF-I, but exhibit severely reduced affinity for insulin. This is thought to reflect the ability of IGF-I to efficiently bind to either IGF-IR α subunit, while tight insulin binding requires its interaction with both of the α subunits found in the IR. As a consequence, the existence of significant number of hybrid receptors may preferentially diminish cellular responsiveness to insulin, but not IGF-I. This has, in fact, been proposed as a mechanism through which upregulation of IGF-IR expression could result in insulin resistance in cells expressing the IR. The situation with hybrid receptors is further complicated by the existence and the IGF-II-binding characteristics of IR-A and IR-B. Both IR-A/IGF-IR and IR-B/IGF-IR hybrids probably occur because most cell express both splice variants. It has been recently demonstrated that IGF-IR/IR-A hybrids bind IGF-I, IGF-II and insulin, whereas IGF-IR/IR-B hybrids bind IGF-I with high affinity, IGF-II with low affinity, and do not bind insulin *(5)*. Therefore, the relative expression of the IGF-IR and IR genes and the degree of alternative splicing of exon 11 of the IR gene governs the ability of a given cell to respond to IGF-I, IGF-II, and insulin.

2.4. *IGFBPs*

The biological activities of the IGF ligands are modulated by a family of high-affinity IGFBPs (IGFBP-1 through -6) that are found in the circulation and in extracellular fluids *(6)*. IGFBP-3 is the predominant IGFBP in serum, and most circulating IGF-I and IGF-II is not found in a free form, but in a ternary complex with IGFBP-3 and a third component, acid-labile subunit, in a 1:1:1 molar ratio. IGFBP-5 also forms ternary complexes with IGFs and acid-labile subunit. Although IGFBPs-1 through 4 exhibit generally similar affinities for IGF-I and IGF-II, IGFBP-5 and 6 bind IGF-II with 10- and 100-fold greater affinities, respectively, than IGF-I. The IGFBPs do not bind insulin. The IGFBPs control IGF action by increasing the half-lives of circulating IGFs by controlling their availability for receptor binding and, in the case of cell surface-associated IGFBPs, by potentially influencing their direct interaction with receptors. Each of the IGFBPs is subject to limited and potentially regulated proteolysis by various proteases. Thus, ligand-receptor interactions in the IGF system are subject to complex regulation as a result of IGFBP levels, expression profile, degree of cell-surface association, and extent of proteolysis.

3. THE ROLE OF THE IGF SYSTEM IN GROWTH AND DEVELOPMENT

The contributions of IGF action to growth and development have been discerned from studies in transgenic mice in which various components of the IGF signaling system have been ablated or overexpressed and from human studies of populations, such as pygmies and rare individuals with mutations affecting the IGF-IR and IGF-I genes. These findings are discussed below.

3.1. Evidence from Transgenic Animals

3.1.1. Prenatal Growth

The role of IGF action in prenatal growth has been deduced from the phenotypes of transgenic and knockout mice in which the expression of the IGF-I, IGF-II, IGF-IR, and IGF-II/M6P receptor genes has been manipulated *(7–10)*. IGF-I and IGF-II deficiency each results in a 40% decrease in birthweight, with IGF-II knockout mice also exhibiting placental growth retardation. Double knockouts exhibit an additive growth deficiency of 80%. IGF-I knockouts can exhibit general perinatal lethality, depending on the genetic background. IGF-IR knockout mice exhibit a 55% decrease in growth rate, which is less than that seen in the IGF-I/IGF-II knockouts, and invariably die of suffocation at birth because of inadequate development of the musculature of the diaphragm. Additional loss of IGF-I in IGF-IR knockout animals does not further decrease birth weight, suggesting that IGF-I functions exclusively through the IGF-IR. In contrast, IGF-II and IGF-IR double knockouts are more growth-retarded than single IGF-IR knockouts, suggesting that IGF-II effects can be mediated by another receptor during embryogenesis. Analysis of IGF-IR/IR knockouts *(3)* suggested that the IR was responsible for IGF-II signaling not mediated by the IGF-IR. As mentioned above, it was subsequently found that alternative splicing of exon 11 produces an IR isoform that exhibits high affinity for IGF-II. An indirect role for the IGF-II/M6P receptor in prenatal growth *(11–13)* was inferred from the phenotype of IGF-II/M6P receptor knockout mice, which exhibit modest fetal and placental overgrowth (25–40%). This phenotype has been interpreted as resulting from the excess IGF-II that is seen in the serum and tissues of these animals from lack of the clearance function of the IGF-II/M6P receptor.

3.1.2. Postnatal Growth

IGF-I-deficient mice that do not die perinatally exhibit severely reduced postnatal growth, whereas IGF-II-deficient mice, although smaller than normal at birth, have normal growth velocities postnatally. These findings support the concept that IGF-I is the principal mediator of postnatal growth. The lack of a postnatal phenotype in IGF-II-deficient mice is not surprising in light of the normal shutoff of IGF-II expression in almost all mouse tissues postnatally.

Global overexpression of IGF-I in transgenic mice produces generalized hyperplasia and organomegaly, resulting in adult animals that are 30% larger than normal *(14)*. Conversely, postnatal overexpression of IGF-II does not result in increased somatic growth *(15,16)*. Again, the lack of a growth phenotype in IGF-II transgenics may reflect the lack of postnatal IGF-II expression in postnatal rodents.

To date, no convincing phenotype has been observed in knockouts of any of the six IGFBPs, including several double knockouts. This puzzling lack of an effect may reflect the redundancy of function among the six IGFBPs.

3.2. IGF System Effects in Humans

The role of IGF action in human growth and development has come from several lines of evidence, including analysis of African Pygmies, a patient with mutational loss of the IGF-I gene, and a series of patients with hemizygosity of the IGF-IR gene resulting from loss of the distal arm of chromosome 15.

3.2.1. Efe Pygmies

Initial cross-sectional studies of Mbuti and Babinga Pygmies concluded that the short stature of these populations was caused by the lack of the pubertal growth spurt *(17)*. Subsequent longitudinal studies of Efe Pygmies demonstrated growth retardation at birth that increased in the first 5 yr of life *(18,19)*. More recently, it has been shown that immortalized T- and B-cell lines from Efe Pygmies are IGF-I-resistant *(20–22)*. The molecular basis for this IGF-I resistance and, potentially, the growth phenotype of the Efe population, appears to be a defect in IGF-IR gene expression *(23)*. Thus, decreased IGF action from decreased IGF-IR levels causes pre- and postnatal growth retardation in humans.

3.2.2. Human Mutations Affecting the IGF-I and IGF-IR Genes

One patient has been described who was homozygous for a partial deletion of the IGF-I gene *(24)*. This patient made no active IGF-I, exhibited severe pre- and postnatal growth retardation and also presented with deafness, mental retardation, and microcephaly, characteristics not found in patients with growth hormone deficiency or resistance. This patient's parents were heterozygous for the IGF-I gene mutation, had extremely low circulating IGF-I levels, and also exhibited short stature. These findings provide additional support for a role of IGF-I in both pre- and postnatal growth and development.

A number of patients have been described that are hemizygous for the IGF-IR gene as the result of deletion of the distal arm of chromosome 15 *(25,26)* or ring chromosome 15 syndrome *(27,28)*. All of these patients exhibited intrauterine growth retardation and postnatal growth failure, as well as other developmental abnormalities. Although the growth-deficiency phenotype consistently manifested by these patients is consistent with decreased IGF-IR levels, the fact that no direct demonstration of IGF resistance in cells derived from these patients has been reported makes this data supportive, but not definitive, evidence for a role of IGF-IR action in human pre- and postnatal growth and development.

4. THE ROLE OF THE IGF SYSTEM IN TUMORIGENESIS

An important aspect of the IGF system in postnatal human physiology is its involvement in tumorigenesis. This is hardly unexpected, based upon the demonstrated role of IGF-I, in particular, as a potent growth regulator. Reports over the last several years of a strong association of circulating IGF-I levels with the risk of developing a number of important human cancers, as well as the ongoing studies of the molecular mechanisms of IGF action in cancer cells, has renewed interest in the therapeutic and diagnostic possibilities of the IGF system in cancer therapy. The sections below summarize these molecular and epidemiological data. The topic is discussed further, and with reference to nutrition, in Chapter 18.

4.1. Molecular Studies

4.1.1. IGF-II and the IGF-IR in Tumorigenesis

Numerous studies performed over the last 20 yr have suggested that transformed cells express higher levels of the IGF-IR. The molecular mechanisms responsible for the increased expression of the IGF-IR gene in tumors, however, remain largely unidentified. Amplification of the IGF-IR locus at band 15q26 has been reported in a small number of breast and melanoma cases *(29)*. Most primary tumors and transformed cell lines express easily detectable levels of IGF-II mRNA and protein, whereas some tumors overexpress the IGF-I gene. The IGF-II gene is imprinted in mouse and human, which restricts expression to the paternal allele *(7)*. A number of human cancers exhibit relaxation of IGF-II gene imprinting, including Beckwith-Wiedemann syndrome, Wilms tumor, rhabdomyosarcoma, and lung cancer *(30–32)*. Altered imprinting may lead to overexpression of IGF-II, which could contribute to the development of the tumors as a consequence of increased proliferative signaling. The presumed role of the IGF-IR in tumorigenesis involves increased IGF-IR expression and concomitant increased responsiveness to IGF in terms of proliferation and inhibition of apoptosis. Although this picture is probably accurate with respect to the pediatric tumors that are often associated with chromosomal translocations, such as Wilms tumor and rhabdomyosarcoma, the situation in the epithelial tumors that are more prevalent in adults is more complex *(33)*. The original suggestion that the IGF-IR itself functions as an oncogene was based upon the behavior of fibroblasts in which the IGF-IR had been overexpressed *(34)*, a system with limited relevance to human cancer. Other studies suggesting that increased IGF-IR expression modulates radiosensitivity have also used IGF-IR overexpression in fibroblasts *(35)*. It should be noted, however, that a recent report has demonstrated that inhibition of IGF-IR activity by a selective kinase inhibitor in MCF-7 breast cancer cells resulted in increased radiosensitivity *(36)*.

The multitude of studies describing overexpression of the IGF-IR in breast, prostate, and other tumor types have been, for the most part, based on analyses of tissue homogenates or established cancer cell lines for which appropriate normal controls do not exist. The apparent IGF-IR content of homogenates, in particular, can be affected by contamination with stroma, which would dilute IGF-IR content in normal epithelium or small tumors. More focused studies of IGF-IR expression in breast and prostate that employed immunohistochemistry, or matched cell lines corresponding to normal and tumor tissue, revealed that normal epithelium and early-stage tumors both express abundant IGF-IR, and that IGF-IR expression is significantly reduced in advanced, metastatic cancer *(37–41)*. This view has been challenged by a recent report by Hellawell et al. *(42)*, who observed that IGF-IR expression was decreased in some metastatic prostate cancer samples as compared with benign or carcinoma tissue but was increased in a majority of samples studied (8 of 12). In this study, however, the immunostaining for IGF-IR using a single β-subunit antibody was diffusely cytoplasmic in most samples, in contrast to the expected membrane localization reported by Chott et al. *(39)* using two different α-subunit antibodies. Thus, the issue of the extent of IGF-IR over- or underexpression in prostate cancer progression is not completely settled.

The activation of the IGF-IR present in normal epithelium by elevated circulating levels of IGF-I may underlie the epidemiological data cited below, whereas the subsequent decrease in IGF-IR (if substantiated by additional studies) may represent an attempt by established cancer cells to avoid the potential differentiating effects of IGF-I at sites of metastasis. Alternatively, decreased expression of the IGF-IR may protect tumor cells from a novel, nonapoptotic form of programmed cell death that has been recently described as being triggered by the unliganded IGF-IR *(43)*. It is clear, however, that the prevailing notion that the IGF-IR is routinely overexpressed in transformed cells is somewhat of an overgeneralization.

4.2. Epidemiological Studies

4.2.1. Prostate Cancer

4.2.1.1. IGF-I and Prostate Cancer. The potent mitogenic activity of IGF-I in cell culture made it an obvious candidate risk factor in cancer development, but it was not until 1998 that several prospective studies suggested that high circulating levels of IGF-I were associated with an increased risk of developing prostate cancer *(44–47)*.

A significant amount of data had been accumulated that suggested that the IGF system plays an important role in the prostate. Prostatic stromal cells and epithelial cells in primary culture secrete IGFBPs and stromal cells produce IGF-II, and both stromal and epithelial cells express the IGF-I receptor and are responsive to IGF-I with respect to proliferation *(48–51)*. In vivo, it is likely that the prostate epithelial cells that are the precursors to prostatic intraepithelial neoplasia and prostatic adenocarcinoma respond to both locally produced IGF-II and circulating IGF-I through paracrine and endocrine mechanisms, respectively. Further support for the role of IGF action in prostate growth has come from recent reports that systemic administration of IGF-I increases rat prostate growth *(52)*, that modulation of rat ventral prostate weight by finasteride is associated with altered levels of IGF-I receptors and IGFBP-3 gene expression *(53)*, and that IGF-I-deficient mice exhibit decreased prostate size and complexity of prostate structure *(54)*.

The strength of the association between IGF-I levels and prostate cancer risk was questioned in subsequent cross-sectional studies *(55,56)*, whereas Djavan et al. *(57)*, in a prospective study, found that the IGF-I/PSA ratio was superior to IGF-I or PSA measurements alone for predicting prostate cancer risk. A meta-analysis of the data available to date in 2000 *(58)* concluded that high-circulating IGF-I levels posed a risk equivalent to that associated with high testosterone.

In a screening trial, Finne et al. *(59)* did not find an association between serum IGF-I levels and prostate cancer risk, whereas Baffa et al. *(60)* actually found that circulating IGF-I levels were lower in a group of patients undergoing radical prostatectomy as compared to age-matched controls. In additional prospective studies, however, Harman et al. *(61)* and Stattin et al. *(62)* found that IGF-I levels were associated with prostate cancer risk, and that this association was especially evident in younger men. A second meta-analysis of 14 case-controlled studies *(63)* concluded that high circulating IGF-I levels are indeed associated with prostate cancer risk.

In a subsequent cross-sectional study, Latif et al. *(64)* did not find a correlation between levels of IGF-I or IGFBP-3 and prostate cancer stage, whereas in the latest prospective study *(65)*, circulating IGF-I levels appeared to be most predictive of advanced prostate cancer.

Although the conclusions of this extensive series of studies appear contradictory, there is, in fact, some consistency. Prospective studies have consistently demonstrated an association between high circulating IGF-I levels and prostate cancer risk, whereas cross-sectional studies have generated variable results. These data are consistent with the hypothesis that high serum IGF-I levels in younger men predict the occurrence of advanced prostate cancer years later, whereas IGF-I levels at the time of diagnosis may not be informative. This hypothesis suggests that long-term exposure of prostate epithelial cells to high levels of serum-derived IGF-I increases the probability of initiating hyperplasia in the cellular precursors of prostatic intraepithelial neoplasia and subsequent prostate adenocarcinoma.

Corroboration of the relationship between IGF-I levels and prostate carcinogenesis at the molecular level has now come from analysis of transgenic mice with targeted expression of IGF-I in the basal prostatic epithelium. This dysregulated IGF-I biosynthesis resulted in the appearance of hyperplastic lesions resembling prostatic intraepithelial neoplasia by 6 mo of age *(66)*, and prostatic adenocarcinomas or small cell carcinomas were eventually seen in 50% of the transgenics. Specifically, deregulated expression of IGF-I and constitutive activation of IGF-I receptors in basal epithelial cells resulted in tumor progression similar to that seen in human disease. These studies also provide additional evidence for the prostate basal epithelial cell as a precursor to prostate cancer.

4.2.1.2. IGF-II and Prostate Cancer. A potential contribution of IGF-II levels to prostate cancer risk is of potential interest, given that levels of circulating IGF-II in humans are consistently several-fold higher than those of IGF-I throughout life. The only study to date to directly address the relationship of IGF-II levels to prostate cancer risk *(61)* found that serum levels of IGF-II were inversely related to risk. These authors suggest that IGF-II may actually inhibit prostate cancer development. It is intriguing that Gnanapragasam et al. *(67)* report that IGF-II increases androgen receptor expression in prostate stromal cells and LNCaP prostate carcinoma cells, because loss of wild-type androgen receptor function and androgen insensitivity is a hallmark of advanced disease.

4.2.2. Breast and Other Cancers

In 1998, Hankinson et al. *(68)* and Bohlke et al. *(69)* reported that premenopausal but not postmenopausal women in the highest tertile of serum IGF-I levels had a significantly increased risk of developing breast cancer. These findings have been generally supported by most *(70–72)* but not all *(73)*, subsequent studies. Racial factors may play a role in the IGF-I-breast cancer association, in that Agurs-Collins et al. *(74)* found that high serum IGF-I levels were strongly associated with breast cancer risk in postmenopausal African-American women.

With respect to colorectal cancer, Ma et al. *(75)*, Manousos et al. *(76)*, Kaaks et al. *(77)*, and Palmqvist et al. *(78)* have reported positive associations between serum IGF-I and colorectal cancer risk in the US, Greek, and Swedish cohorts, whereas Probst-Hensch et al. *(79)* found an association between IGF-I or IGFBP-3 levels and colorectal cancer risk in a Chinese cohort. The role of IGF-II is unclear, being positively associated in the Greek and Chinese studies, but not in the US cohort.

Yu et al. *(80)* reported a positive association between high IGF-I and low IGFBP-3 levels (but not IGF-II) and lung cancer risk. Lukanova et al. *(81)*, however, found no correlation between serum IGF-I or IGFBPs in a large female cohort.

Collectively, these studies continue to suggest a role for IGF-I as a risk factor for breast, colorectal, and lung cancer, but its utility as a pragmatic marker is potentially limited by ethnic and (for colorectal and lung cancer) gender factors.

5. RECOMMENDATIONS AND CHALLENGES FOR THE FUTURE

Despite decades of intensive investigation, there remain basic aspects of the IGF system that are poorly understood. Principal among these is the role of IGF-II in human physiology. Additionally, the effects of IGF-I and IGF-II in combination at a cellular level are entirely unknown, although most human tissues are routinely exposed to a combination of endocrine, paracrine, and, often, autocrine IGF-I and IGF-II. Finally, the strength of the association between circulating IGF-I and cancer risk requires additional careful analysis in order to ascertain its usefulness in predicting disease.

REFERENCES

1. Le Roith D, Bondy C, Yakar S, Liu JL, Butler A. The somatomedin hypothesis: 2001. Endocr Rev 2001;22:53–74.
2. LeRoith D, Werner H, Beitner-Johnson D, Roberts CT. Molecular and cellular aspects of the insulin-like growth factor I receptor. Endocr Rev 1995;16:143–163.
3. Louvi A, Accili D, Efstratiadis A. Growth-promoting interaction of IGF-II with the insulin receptor during mouse embryonic development. Dev Biol 1997;189:33–48.
4. Frasca F, Pandini G, Scalia P, et al. Insulin receptor isoform A, a newly recognized, high-affinity insulin-like growth factor II receptor in fetal and cancer cells. Mol Cell Biol 1999;19:3278–3288.
5. Pandini G, Frasca F, Mineo R, Sciacca L, Vigneri R, Belfiore A. Insulin/insulin-like growth factor I hybrid receptors have different biological characteristics depending on the insulin receptor isoform involved. J Biol Chem 2002;277:39684–39695.
6. Jones JI, Clemmons DR. Insulin-like growth factors and their binding proteins: biological actions. Endocr Rev 1995;16:3–34.
7. DeChiara TM, Robertson EJ, Efstratiadis A. Parental imprinting of the mouse insulin-like growth factor II gene. Cell 1991;64:849–859.
8. Liu J, Baker J, Perkins AS, Robertson EJ, Efstratiadis A. Mice carrying null mutations of the genes encoding insulin-like growth factor I (Igf-1) and type 1 IGF receptor (Igf1r). Cell 1993;75:59–72.
9. Baker J, Liu JP, Robertson EJ, Efstratiadis A. Role of insulin-like growth factors in embryonic and postnatal growth. Cell 1993;75:73–82.
10. Powell-Braxton L, Hollingshead P, Warburtin C, et al. IGF-I is required for normal embryonic growth in mice. Genes Dev 1993;7:2609–2617.
11. Lau MMH, Stewart CEH, Liu Z, Bhatt H, Rotwein P, Stewart CL. Loss of the imprinted IGF2 cation-independent mannnose 6-phosphate receptor results in fetal overgrowth and perinatal lethality. Genes Dev 1994;8:2953–2963.
12. Wang Z-Q, Fung MR, Barlow DP, Wagner EF. Regulation of embryonic growth and lysosomal targeting by the imprinted Igf2/Mpr gene. Nature 1994;372:464–467.
13. Ludwig T, Eggenschwiler J, Fisher P, D'Ercole AJ, Davenport ML, Efstratiadis A. Mouse mutant embryos overexpressing IGF-II exhibit phenotypic features of the Beckwith-Wiedemann and Simpson-Gloabi-Behmel syndromes. Genes Dev 1997;11:3128–3142.
14. Mathews LS, Hammer RE, Behringer RR, D'Ercole AJ, Bell GI, Brinster RL. Growth enhancement of transgenic mice expressing human insulin-like growth factor I. Endocrinology 1988;123:2827–2833.
15. Rogler CE, Yang D, Rosetti L, et al. Altered body composition and increased frequency of diverse malignancies in insulin-like growth factor transgenic mice. J Biol Chem 1994;269:13779–13784.
16. Wolf E, Rapp K, Blum WF, Kolb H, Brem G. Skeletal growth of transgenic mice with elevated levels of circulating insulin-like growth factor-II. Growth Regul 1995;5:177–183.
17. Mann GV. The riddle of Pygmy stature. N Engl J Med 1987;317:709–710.
18. Bailey RC. The comparative growth of Efe Pygmies and African farmers from birth to age 5 years. Ann Hum Biol 1991;18:113–120.
19. Bailey RC. Growth of African Pygmies in early childhood. N Engl J Med 1990;323:1146.
20. Geffner ME, Bailey RC, Bersch N, Vera J, Golde DW. Insulin-like growth factor-I unresponsiveness in an Efe Pygmy. Biochem Biophys Res Commun 1993;193:1216–1223.
21. Geffner ME, Bersch N, Bailey RC, Golde DW. Insulin-like growth factor-I resistance in immortalized T-cell lines from African Efe Pygmies. J Clin Endocrinol Metab 1995;80:3732–3738.
22. Cortez AB, Van Dop C, Bailey RC, et al. IGF-I resistance in virus-transformed B-lymphocytes from African Efe Pygmies. Biochem Mol Med 1996;58:31–36.

23. Hattori Y, Vera JC, Rivas CI, et al. Decreased insulin-like growth factor-I (IGF-I) receptor expression and function in immortalized African pygmy T-cells. J Clin Endocrinol Metab 1996;81:2257–2263.
24. Woods KA, Camacho-Huebner C, Savage MO, Clark AJ. Intrauterine growth retardation and postnatal growth failure associated with the insulin-like growth factor I gene. N Engl J Med 1996;335:1363–1367.
25. Roback EW, Baraket AJ, Dev VG, Mbikay M, Chretien M, Butler MG. An infant with deletion of the distal long arm of chromosome 15 (q26.1→qter) and loss of insulin-like growth factor I receptor gene. Am J Med Genet 1991;38:74–79.
26. Siebler T, Wlodzimierz L, Terry CL, et al. Insulin-like growth factor I receptor expression and function in fibroblasts from two patients with deletion of the distal long arm of chromosome 15. J Clin Endocrinol Metab 1995;80:3447–3457.
27. Tamura T, Tohma T, Ohta T, et al. Ring chromosome 15 involving deletion of the insulin-like growth factor 1 receptor gene in a patient with features of Russell-Silver syndrome. Clin Dysmorphol 1993;2:106–113.
28. Peoples R, Milatorich A, Francke U. Hemizygosity at the insulin-like growth factor I receptor (IGF1R) locus and growth failure in the ring chromosome 15 syndrome. Cytogenet Cell Genet 1995;70:228–234.
29. Almeida A, Muleris M, Dutrillaux B, Malfoy B. The insulin-like growth factor I receptor gene is the target for the 15q26 amplicon in breast cancer. Genes Chrom Cancer 1994;11:63–65.
30. Ogawa O, Becroft DM, Morison IM, et al. Constitutional relaxation of insulin-like growth factor II gene imprinting associated with Wilms' tumor and gigantism. Nat Genet 1993;5:40812.
31. Suzuki H, Veda R, Takahashi T. Altered imprinting in lung cancer. Nat Genet 1994;6:332–333.
32. Zhan S, Shapiro DN, Helman LJ. Activation of an imprinted allele of the insulin-like growth factor II gene implicated in rhabbdomyosarcoma. J Clin Invest 1994;94:445–448.
33. DePhino RA. The age of cancer. Nature 2000;408:248–254.
34. Kaleko M, Rutter WJ, Miller AD. Overexpression of the human insulin-like growth factor I receptor promotes ligand-dependent neoplastic transformation. Mol Cell Biol 1990;10:464–473.
35. Turner BC, Haffty BG, Narayanan L, et al. Insulin-like growth factor-I receptor overexpression mediates cellular radioresistance and local breast cancer recurrence after lumpectomy and radiation. Cancer Res 1997;57:3079–3083.
36. Wen B, Deutsch E, Marangoni E, et al. Tyrphostin AG1024 modulates radiosensitivity in human breast cancer cells. Br J Cancer 2001;85:2017–2021.
37. Tennant MK, Thrasher JB, Twomey PA, Drivdahl RH, Birnbaum RS, Plymate S. Protein and mRNA for the type 1 insulin-like growth factor (IGF) receptor is decreased and IGF-II mRNA is increased in human prostate carcinoma compared to benign prostate epithelium. J Clin Endocrinol Metab 1996;81:3774–3782.
38. Happerfield LC, Miles DW, Barnes DM, Thomsen LL, Smith P, Hhanby AM. The localization of the insulin-like growth factor receptor 1 (IGFR-1) in benign and malignant breast tissue. J Pathol 1997;183:412–417.
39. Chott A, Sun Z, Morganstern D, et al. Tyrosine kinases expressed in vivo by human prostate cancer bone marrow metastases and loss of type 1 insulin-like growth factor receptor. Am J Pathol 1999;155:1271–1279.
40. Schnarr B, Strunnz K, Ohsam J, Benner A, Wacker J, Mayer D. Down-regulation of insulin-like growth factor-I receptor and insulin receptor substrate-1 expression in advanced human breast cancer. Int J Cancer 2000;89:506–513.
41. Damon SE, Plymate SR, Carroll JM, et al. Transcriptional regulation of insulin-like growth factor-I receptor gene expression in prostate cancer cells. Endocrinology 2001;142:21–27.
42. Hellawell GO, Turner GD, Davies DR, Poulsom R, Brewster SF, Macaulay VM. Expression of the type 1 insulin-like growth factor receptor is up-regulated in primary prostate cancer and commonly persists in metastatic disease. Cancer Res 2002;62:2942–2950.
43. Sperandio S, de Belle I, Bredesen DE. An alternative, nonapoptotic form of programmed cell death. Proc Natl Acad Sci USA 2000;97:14376–14381.
44. Mantzoros CS, Tzonou A, Signorello LB, Stampfer M, Trichopoulos D, Adami HO. Insulin-like growth factor 1 in relation to prostate cancer and benign prostatic hyperplasia. Br J Cancer 1997;76:1115–1118.

45. Chan JM, Stampfer MJ, Giovannucci E, et al. Plasma insulin-like growth factor-I and prostate cancer risk: A prospective study. Science 1998;279:563–566.
46. Wolk A, Mantzoros CS, Andersson SO, et al. Insulin-like growth factor 1 and prostate cancer risk: A population-based, case-control study. J Natl Cancer Inst 1998;90:911–915.
47. Cohen P. Serum insulin-like growth factor I levels and prostate cancer risk—interpreting the evidence. J Natl Cancer Inst 1998;90:876–879.
48. Cohen P, Peehl DM, Lamson G, Rosenfeld RG. Insulin-like growth factors (IGFs), IGF receptors, and IGF-binding proteins in primary cultures of prostate epithelial cells. J Clin Endocrinol Metab 1991;73:401–407.
49. Peehl DM, Cohen P, Rosenfeld RG. The insulin-like growth factor system in the prostate. World J Urol 1994;13:306–311.
50. Cohen P, Peehl DM, Rosenfeld RG. The IGF axis in the prostate. Horm Metab Res 1994;26:81–84.
51. Boudon C, Rodier G, Lechevallier E, Mottet N, Barenton B, Sultan C. Secretion of insulin-like growth factors and their binding proteins by human normal and hyperplastic prostatic cells in primary culture. J Clin Endocrinol Metab 1996;81:612–617.
52. Torring N, Vinter-Jensen L, Pederson SB, Sorensen FB, Flyvbjerg A, Nexo E. Sytemic Administration of insulin-like growth factor I (IGF-I) causes growth of the rat prostate. J Urol 1997;158:222–227.
53. Huynh H, Seyam RM, Brock GB. Reduction of ventral prostate weight by finasteride is associated with suppression of insulin-like growth factor I (IGF-I) and IGF-I receptor genes and with an increase in IGF binding protein 3. Cancer Res 1998;58:215–218.
54. Ruan W, Powell-Braxton L, Kopchick JJ, Kleinberg DL. Evidence that insulin-like growth factor I and growth hormone are required for prostate gland development. Endocrinology 1999;140:1984–1989.
55. Cutting CW, Hunt C, Nisbet JA, Bland JM, Dalgleish AG, Kirby RS. Serum insulin-like growth factor-1 is not a useful marker of prostate cancer. BJU Int 1999;83:996–999.
56. Kurek R, Tunn UW, Eckart O, Aumuller G, Wong J, Renneberg H. The significance of serum levels of insulin-like growth factor-1 in patients with prostate cancer. BJU Int 2000;85:125–129.
57. Djavan G, Bursa B, Seitz C, et al. Insulin-like growth factor 1 (IGF-1), IGF-1 density, and IGF-1/PSA ratio for prostate cancer detection. Urology 1999;54:603–606.
58. Shaneyfelt T, Husein R, Bubley G, Mantzoros CS. Hormonal predictors of prostate cancer: A meta-analysis. J Clin Oncol 2000;18:847–853.
59. Finne P, Auvinen A, Koistinen H, et al. Insulin-like growth factor I is not a useful marker of prostate cancer in men with elevated levels of prostate-specific antigen. J Clin Endocrinol Metab 2000;85:2744–2747.
60. Baffa R, Reiss K, El-Gabry EA, et al. Low serum insulin-like growth factor 1 (IGF-1): A significant association with prostate cancer. Tech Urol 2000;6:236–239.
61. Harman SM, Metter EJ, Blackman MR, Landis PK, Carter HB. Serum levels of insulin-like growth factor I (IGF-I), IGF-II, IGF-binding protein-3, and prostate-specific antigen as predictor of clinical prostate cancer. J Clin Endocrinol Metab 2000;85:4258–4265.
62. Stattin P, Bylund A, Rinaldi S, et al. Plasma insulin-like growth factor-I, insulin-like growth factor-binding proteins, and prostate cancer risk; a prospective study. J Natl Cancer Inst 2000;92:1910–1917.
63. Shi R, Berkel HJ, Yu H. Insulin-like growth factor-I and prostate cancer: a meta-analysis. Br J Cancer 2001;85:991–996.
64. Latif Z, McMillan DC, Wallace AM, et al. The relationship of circulating insulin-like growth factor 1, its binding protein-3, prostate-specific antigen and C-reactive protein with disease stage in prostate cancer. BJU Int 2002;89:396–399.
65. Chan JM, Stampfer MJ, Ma J, et al. Insulin-like growth factor-I (IGF-I) and IGF binding protein-3 as predictors of advanced-stage prostate cancer. J Natl Cancer Inst 2002;94:1099–1106.
66. DiGiovanni J, Kiguchi K, Frijhoff A, et al. Deregulated expression of insulin-like growth factor 1 in prostate epithelium leads to neoplasia in transgenic mice. Proc Natl Acad Sci USA 2000;97:3455–60.
67. Gnanapragasam VJ, McCahy PJ, Neal DE, Robson CN. Insulin-like growth factor II and androgen receptor expression in the prostate. BJU Int 2000;86:731–735.
68. Hankinson SE, Willett WC, Colditz GA, et al. Circulating concentrations of insulin-like growth factor-I and risk of breast cancer. Lancet. 1998;351:1393–1396.
69. Bohlke K, Cramer DW, Trichopoulos D, Mantzoros, CS. Insulin-like growth factor-I in relation to pre-menopausal ductal carcinoma in situ of the breast. Epidemiology 1998;9:570–573.

70. Vadgama JV, Wu Y, Datta G, Khan H, Chillar R. Plasma insulin-like growth factor-I and serum IGF-binding protein 3 can be associated with the progression of breast cancer, and predict the risk of recurrence and the probability of survival in African-American and Hispanic women. Oncology 1999;57:330–340.
71. Byrne C, Colditz GA, Willett WC, Speizer FE, Pollak M, Hankinson SE. Plasma insulin-like growth factor (IGF) I, IGF-binding protein 3, and mammographic density. Cancer Res 2000;60:3744–3748.
72. Li BD, Khosravi MJ, Berkel HJ, et al. Free insulin-like growth factor-I and breast cancer risk. Int J Cancer 2001;91:736–739.
73. Jernstrom H, Barrett-Connor E. Obesity, weight change, fasting insulin, proinsulin, C-peptide, and insulin-like growth factor-1 levels in women with and without breast cancer: the Rancho Bernardo Study. J Womens Health Gend Based Med 1999;8:1265–1272.
74. Agurs-Collins T, Adams-Campbell LL, Kim KS, Cullin KJ. Insulin-like growth factor-1 and breast cancer risk in postmenopausal African-American women. Cancer Detect Prev 2000;24:199–206.
75. Ma J, Pollak MN, Giovannucci E, et al. Prospective study of colorectal cancer risk in men and plasma levels of insulin-like growth factor (IGF)-I and IGF-binding protein-3. J Natl Cancer Inst 1999;91:579–581.
76. Manousos O, Souglakos J, Bosetti C, et al. IGF-I and IGF-II in relation to colorectal cancer. Int J Cancer 1999;83:15–17.
77. Kaaks R, Toniolo P, Akhmedkhanov A, et al. Serum C-peptide, insulin-like growth factor (IGF)-I, IGF-binding proteins, and colorectal cancer risk in women. J Natl Cancer Inst 2000;92:1592–1600.
78. Palmqvist R, Hallmans G, Rinaldi S, et al. Plasma insulin-like growth factor 1, insulin-like growth factor binding protein 3, and risk of colorectal cancer: A prospective study in north Sweden. Gut 2002;50:642–646.
79. Probst-Hensch NM, Yuan JM, Stanczyk FZ, Gao YT, Ross RK, Yu MC. IGF-1, IGF-2 and IGFBP-3 in prediagnostic serum: association with colorectal cancer in a cohort of Chinese men in Shanghai. Br J Cancer 2001;85:1695–1699.
80. Yu H, Spitz MR, Mistry J, Gu J, Hong WK, Wu X. Plasma levels of insulin-like growth factor-I and lung cancer risk: a case-control analysis. J Natl Cancer Inst 1999;91:151–156.
81. Lukanova A, Toniolo P, Akhmedkhanov A, et al. A prospective study of insulin-like growth factor-I, IGF-binding proteins-1, -2 and -3 and lung cancer risk in women. Int J Cancer 2001;92:888–892.

7 The Insulin-Like Growth Factor Axis in the Fetus and Neonate

Cynthia L. Blanco and Robert J. Ferry, Jr.

KEY POINTS

- The IGF system plays a central role in somatic growth *in utero* and after birth. Plasma IGF-I concentrations correlate with birth weight, birth length, and gestational age.
- Maternal nutrition, growth hormone, IGF-binding proteins, and genetic factors comprise the primary modulators of IGF action in the fetus.
- Congenital IGF-I deficiency (owing to gene depletion) presents with severe IUGR, glucose intolerance, and impaired postnatal growth.
- Serum IGF-I, IGFBP-2, and IGFBP-3 levels indicate nutritional status in premature and term infants.
- IGF-I plays a major role on retinal vessel growth in retinopathy of prematurity.
- IGF-I exerts a trophic effect on the gastrointestinal tract and may contribute to the pathophysiology of bronchopulmonary dysplasia.
- Animal studies of variations to IGF-I gene expression suggest an association between low birth weight, diabetes, and cardiovascular disease.
- Most sick neonates display normal serum IGF-I and IGFBP levels, despite cachexia and serious illness.

1. INTRODUCTION

Insulin-like growth factors (IGF-I and IGF-II) and their high-affinity binding proteins (IGFBPs) comprise the major regulators of somatic growth during both intrauterine and extrauterine life. IGFs exert their mitogenic actions via paracrine and endocrine mechanisms at IGF receptors on the cell surface. IGFBPs regulate the bioavailability of IGFs for the IGF receptors. Current and mounting evidence support the novel concept that IGFBPs exert IGF receptor-independent actions related to programmed cell death (apoptosis) and glucose metabolism. Fetal origins lay the foundation for health and disease in infancy and childhood. Thus, this chapter integrates current concepts of IGF biology and pathophysiology during early life.

2. IGF CELLULAR BIOLOGY

IGFs and the high-affinity IGF binding proteins (IGFBPs) display tight regulation across gestational age and tissue type. Animal models suggest that IGFs exert their

From: *IGF and Nutrition in Health and Disease*
Edited by: M. S. Houston, J. M. P. Holly, and E. L. Feldman © Humana Press Inc., Totowa, NJ

Table 1
Functions of the Insulin-Like Growth Factor-Binding Proteins

Limit bioavailability of free IGFs to bind type 1 IGF receptors
Prevent IGF-induced hypoglycemia
Regulate transport of IGFs between intra-and extra vascular spaces
Prolong the half-life of IGFs in circulation
Enhance actions of IGFs by forming a slow-releasing pool of IGFs
Modulate cellular proliferation/death via putative IGFBP receptors

Table 2
Modulators of Fetal IGF-I Action

Maternal nutrition
Growth hormone-mediated induction of IGF-I
Indirect, rapid regulation of free IGFs via insulin's suppression of IGFBP-1
Chronic regulation of free IGFs via other IGFBPs
Genetic factors (*IGF1* gene deletion)

actions during postnatal life primarily via the type 1 IGF receptors. Type 1 IGF receptors are cell surface tetramers composed of two α subunits (identical to the α subunits of the insulin receptor) and two β subunits. IGF binding to these protein tyrosine kinase receptors activates several key intracellular phosphorelays, primarily the mitogen-activated protein kinase relays.

To date, six high-affinity IGFBPs and four low-affinity IGFBP-related proteins (IGFBP-rPs) have been reported *(1)*. IGFBPs are postulated to inhibit or enhance the actions of IGFs (Table 1), respectively, by transporting IGFs to target tissues and by sequestration of IGFs. Sequestration inhibits IGF binding to IGF receptors and also, by reducing exposure of the IGFs to proteolysis, prolongs the half-life of IGFs in circulation *(1)*.

In addition to regulation of IGF and IGFBP release in patterns specific to tissue and developmental stage, specific enzymes have been identified that proteolyze the IGF-BPs, including prostate-specific antigen and members of the matrix metalloproteinase family *(2)*. Additional levels of regulation within the complex GH–IGF–IGF-BP axis include the induction of IGF release by growth hormone (somatotropin) and variable IGF binding affinity with the IGFBPs and the IGF receptors under local conditions affected by pH and IGFBP proteolysis (Table 2). More extensive review of the molecular aspects of the IGF axis is provided in chapter 1.

3. FETAL IGF AXIS

Recent mouse models that manipulate components of the IGF system and clinical reports have provided key support for the central role of IGFs in somatic growth *in utero* and after birth (also discussed in chapters 6). The null IGF-I mouse displays severe intrauterine growth retardation, resulting in birth weights that are just 60% that of their wild-type counterparts *(4,15)*. A boy with congenital IGF-I gene deletion at 12*q* was born at 37 wk gestation with length z-score –5.4, head circumference z-score

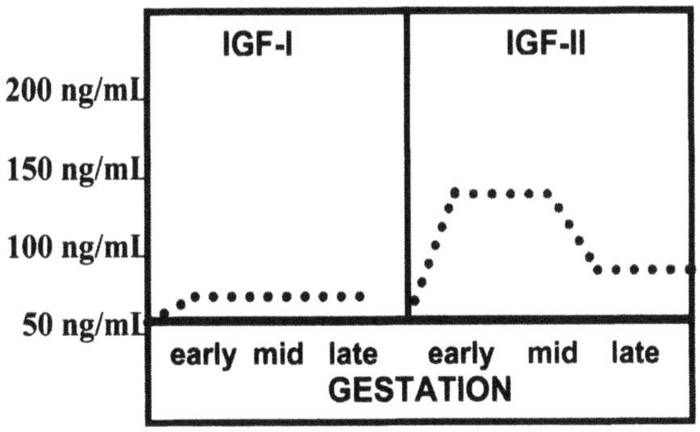

Fig. 1. IGF axis profiles in human amniotic fluid. Early gestation = 15–20 wk; midgestation = 26–33 wk; late gestation = 37–40 wk (adapted from ref. *19* with permission).

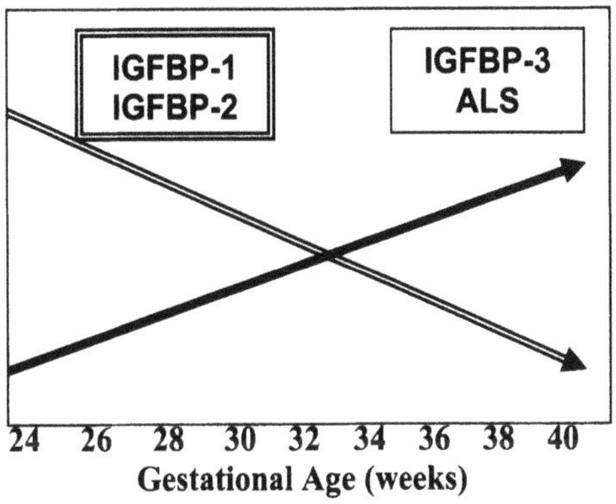

Fig. 2. Fetal serum IGF axis profile.

–4.9, and weight z-score –3.9 *(24)*. Although IGF-II is clearly essential for prenatal growth in mice, its role in the human fetus remains uncertain. No clinical report of IGF-II gene deletion exists, although one would predict, based on the mouse models, that the clinical phenotype of congenital IGF-II deficiency will include severe intrauterine growth retardation and possibly insulin resistance *(3,10)*.

Low plasma concentrations of IGF-I and IGF-II in the preterm fetus rise by term and correlate closely with birth weight, length, and gestational age (Fig. 1) *(9)*. Glucose and insulin significantly regulate the prenatal IGF axis. Insulin has been shown to increase fetal uptake of glucose and amino acids from the placenta (in sheep), and fetal IGF-I increases glucose transport from the placenta *(10)*. Pancreatectomy of the ovine fetus decreases the serum IGF-I level, suggesting that insulin exerts an important role on fetal IGF-I release or turnover. Maternal malnutrition results in decreased concentrations of IGF-I in maternal serum and cord blood. Clearly, fetal IGF-I and maternal nutrition are key regulators of intrauterine growth.

Human fetal serum contains significant amounts of IGFBP-1 and IGFBP-2, whereas IGFBP-3 is the predominant IGFBP species in postnatal serum (Fig. 2). With advancing gestational age, serum levels of IGFBP-1 fall, whereas IGFBP-3 and ALS rise, par-

Table 5
Serum IGFBP Profiles in the Pediatric Population

	IGFBP-1		*IGFBP-2*		*IGFBP-3*	
Age	*Range ng/mL*	*Mean ng/mL*	*Range ng/mL*	*Mean ng/mL*	*Range ng/mL*	*Mean ng/mL*
0–4 wk	na	na	321–1000	587	0.2–0.5	0.37
0–1 yr	348–922	567	271–814	470	0.7–2.5	1.3
1–2 yr	280–750	460	260–778	449	na	na
2–6 yr	275–700	435	250–727	426	1.4–3.0	2.1
6–10 yr	255–540	370	226–568	358	1.5–4.2	2.7
10–15 yr	200–470	305	200–490	315	2–5.8	4.2
15–25 yr	215–518	325	180–490	300	2.5–4.8	3.8

Normative data courtesy of Mark Skene, PhD, Esoterix Endocrinology, Calabasas Hills, CA. Na, not available.

able to IGF-I and IGF-II action *(3,4)*. Congenital IGF-I deficiency in a human appears to be comparable with the mouse models. The absence of IGF-I in serum and other tissues was observed in a boy with IGF-I gene deletion. The primary consequence of congenital IGF-I deficiency was severe intrauterine growth retardation, which continued throughout postnatal development *(5)*. In addition, IGF-I deficiency resulted in glucose intolerance, which was ameliorated by recombinant human (rh) IGF-I replacement therapy in a dose-dependent manner. Chronic (over 15 yr), untreated, congenital IGF-I deficiency was also associated with sensorineural hearing loss; however, the absence of supporting data from animal models limit the association that can be made between hearing loss and IGF deficiency.

Current in vivo evidence and clinical studies of term and preterm infants associate the IGF–IGFBP axis with specific disorders that are associated with intrauterine growth restriction, such as pre-eclampsia. Based on extensive epidemiologic data gathered by Barker since he proposed the fetal origins hypothesis of adult-onset insulin resistance in 1963, small size at birth is associated with increased risk of cardiovascular disease in adulthood *(6)*. Small size appears to be one marker for the fetal origins of life-long programming within the IGF axis *(1,7)*.

7. REGULATION OF THE IGF AXIS DURING INFANCY

Immaturity of the growth hormone–IGF–IGFBP axis in the premature infant contributes to morbidity and mortality *(9)*. Euthyroid infants with congenital panhypopituitarism display birth weight and length within the normal range *(10)*. Newborns with anencephaly also display normal serum IGF-I levels and normal birth weights adjusted for gestational age. These clinical observations imply that intrauterine IGF action can be independent of growth hormone (somatotropin) in humans. Follow-up of somatic growth and serum IGF levels in euthyroid infants with growth hormone deficiency suggest that beyond the sixth month of postnatal life, IGF production becomes dependent on somatotropin. This may explain why caloric hyperalimentation can enhance linear growth only during the first few months of life. Gender does not appear to affect serum levels of IGFs or IGFBPs in the human fetus or infant *(9)*.

8. PERINATAL NUTRITION AND IGF ACTION

Birth marks the transition from continuous placental glucose delivery to the extrauterine pattern of fasting interrupted by feedings. Insulin is a potent regulator of hepatic IGFBP-1 release, and fasting-induced hypoglycemia is a potent stimulus for adrenal cortisol release *(25)*. Acute suppression of serum IGFBP-1 release upon feeding may integrate an increase in free IGF level with the increased caloric availability. Total serum IGF-I level has been shown to decrease in normal adults during a fast, and both in adults and children by short-term decrements in dietary protein or calories (*see* Chapter 2). The latter, diet-related changes are detectable within 1–2 d after the diet alters *(11)*.

Both protein intake and total caloric intake determine circulating IGF concentrations in premature infants. IGF-I values are reduced more than 50% when calorie intake is low, an effect that can be independent of protein intake. As dietary protein increases, serum IGF-I levels increase fourfold, with the most pronounced effect observed when 12–15% of dietary calories are derived from protein *(11)* Serum IGF-I may be a useful nutritional assessment marker to monitor feeding in the early postnatal period (reviewed in Chapter 4). Serum concentrations of IGFBP-3 are reduced by protein-caloric malnutrition and rise with refeeding. The associations between dietary protein with gestational age and postnatal age are significantly stronger with IGF-I than for IGFBP-3 *(11)*.

Serum levels of IGFBP-2 are highest in infancy and decline with age. Serum IGFBP-2 concentrations appear to be the highest at 24-wk gestation in live infants, with a linear decrement to the nadir values at 34 wk of gestation. Protein is a major regulator of prenatal serum IGFBP-2 concentrations. Serum IGFBP-2 levels increase with protein-calorie malnutrition in young children and declines markedly upon refeeding with a protein-enriched diet. Premature infants display over 50% decrease in serum IGFBP-2 levels as the dietary protein intake increases from 6% to 15%. This effect is observed regardless of gestation age. Thus, serum IGF-I and IGFBP-2 levels appear to be useful indicators of nutritional status during premature and postnatal life *(11)*.

9. BRONCHOPULMONARY DYSPLASIA

Bronchopulmonary dysplasia (BPD) is a chronic illness associated commonly with prematurity. Appropriate nutrient intake in these infants promotes lung growth and development. Current methods for assessing the adequacy of protein and calorie intake for these infants have numerous limitations. Weight gain is not a sensitive indicator of short-term changes in lean body mass, particularly when edema or dehydration is present *(12)* Serum IGFBP-2 concentration is a suitable marker of protein intake in infants with BPD, but the determinants of weight gain are more complex in other premature infants. IGF-I appears to exert a key role to facilitate the actions of vascular endothelial growth factor with respect to vascular endothelial growth in vitro. Further work is needed to determine the role of IGFs in vascularization of the premature or prenatal lung to determine its contributions to the etiopathophysiology of BPD *(12,22)*.

10. RETINOPATHY OF PREMATURITY

Retinopathy of prematurity (ROP) is a blinding disease initiated by lack of retinal vascular growth associated with premature birth. Lack of IGF-I in knockout mice prevents normal retinal vascular growth despite the presence of vascular endothelial growth factor *(13,22)*. Patients with IGF-I deficiency (despite normal somatotropin receptors) display less retinal vascularization with lower number of vascular branching points *(22)*.

Clinical and animal studies suggest that when tissue IGF-I levels fall for an extended time in premature infants, the vessels cease to grow, and this maturing avascular retina becomes hypoxic. Vascular endothelial growth factor (VEGF) accumulates in the hypoxic vitreous. As serum IGF-I levels rise above threshold in the presence of high concentrations of VEGF, a rapid growth of new blood vessels is triggered. IGF-I and VEGF complement endothelial cell function through the aforementioned mitogen-activated protein kinase and AKT signal-transduction pathways. Patients who do not develop ROP have higher levels of IGF-I from birth and reach higher levels of IGF-I faster than patients with ROP, which has led to some controversy in the etiopathophysiologic role of IGF-I in retinopathy *(13,22)*.

It is reasonable to conclude that the timing of the increased IGF-I level is a critical determinant of IGF action. Normalization of the IGF-I level during the first few weeks of postnatal life might prevent ROP, while bearing in mind the therapeutic complications of hyperoxygenation *(13)*.

11. IGF ACTION ON THE GASTROINTESTINAL TRACT

Mammals are the only mothers who control development of the intestine through breast milk. The effect of growth factors and polyamines on intestinal development has been studied most intensively in terms of intestinal repair, or restitution from short bowel syndrome. Amniotic fluid exerts growth-promoting activity in cultured human fetal small intestinal cells, but human milk possesses a greater trophic effect than amniotic fluid *(14,23)*.

The mitogenic activity attributed to human milk is related to the presence of several growth factors, including epidermal growth factor, IGF-I, fibroblast growth factor, human growth factor, and transforming growth factor-β *(14)*. Intestinal cell growth-promoting activity equal to that of amniotic fluid or human milk has not yet been duplicated artificially, even with recombinant growth factors. Many of these growth factors also alter the proliferation of epithelial cells and their expression of brush border enzymes. Numerous growth factors have been identified in human milk, but additional growth factors are likely to be identified and linked to intestinal cell growth *(14,23)*.

12. IGF AND DEXAMETHASONE

In adults, dexamethasone increases serum IGFBP-3 levels, induces protein catabolism, and induces growth hormone release. Dexamethasone decreases the activity of circulating IGF-I concentrations, which may explain the negative correlation of serum IGF-I level with weight gain observed in infants treated with dexamethasone. Dexamethasone disrupts the relations between nutritional intake and serum IGF-I and IGFBP-3 concentrations *(12)*.

13. GENE VARIATIONS

Severe IGF deficiency results in severe intrauterine growth retardation; perinatal lethality; postnatal growth retardation; delayed development in brain, muscle, bone, and lung; and infertility in mice. Overexpression of IGF-I in transgenic mice is coupled with widespread tissue hypertrophy in the brain, heart, muscle, and intestine. The conventional gene knockout mice demonstrate the crucial role of IGF-I in intrauterine development and perinatal survival. This model is unsuitable for postnatal studies on animal growth because most of the mice die after birth *(15)*.

It has been postulated that fetal genetic factors could underline the relationship between low birth weight and predisposition of an infant to diabetes and cardiovascular disease. Vaessen et al. reported that absence of the wild-type IGF-I (192-bp allele of a polymorphism in the promoter region of the IGF-I gene) associates significantly with low circulating IGF-I concentrations, reduced height in adulthood, diminished insulin-secreting capacity, and a high risk of type 2 diabetes mellitus and myocardial infarction *(16)*. Individuals without the wild-type allele showed a strong postnatal gain in weight up to that of wild-type carriers. Although genetically established expression of IGF-I and insulin are important determinants of growth during the fetal period, other genetic factors and environmental factors (like nutrition) exert greater regulatory effects on weight. These observations do suggest that association between low birth weight, diabetes, and cardiovascular disease could be a result of genetic variation of IGF expression *(16)*.

14. THE SICK NEONATE

Numerous studies have demonstrated a positive correlation between serum IGF concentrations and nutritional variables. Illness has shown to increase IGFBP-3 proteolytic activity. This mechanism potentially maintains IGF bioavailability to critical tissues during periods of caloric stress, thus ensuring survival, even growth. A recent study comparing 24 hospitalized sick neonates to 8 newborn infants with congenital growth hormone deficiency revealed normal serum IGF-I and IGFBP-3 levels in sick hospitalized neonates even in the face of cachexia and serious illness. These results suggest that patients with congenital growth hormone deficiency could be diagnosed by assessment of serum IGFBP-3 levels despite severe illness *(17)*.

15. SUMMARY AND CONCLUSIONS

William Salmon and William Daughaday *(21)* first reported in June 1957 "a hormonally controlled serum factor which stimulates sulfate incorporation by cartilage in vitro." The molecular revolution of the 1970s revealed the genetic basis of these factors as protein molecules sharing high levels of structural homology with insulin: the insulin-like growth factors. IGFBPs and their own partners have been rapidly identified throughout the 1980s and 1990s. With the 21st century well underway, the IGF-IGFBP axis still remains provocative nearly 50 yr after its discovery.

ACKNOWLEDGMENTS

This work was supported in part by NIH grant K08 DK 02876 (to R. J. F.) and the Genentech Clinical Scholar Award of the Lawson Wilkins Pediatric Endocrine Society (to R. J. F.). The authors gratefully thank Mark Stene, PhD of Esoterix Endocrinology (Calabasas Hills, CA) for sharing current normative IGF and IGFBP data in the pediatric population (http://www.esoterix.com).

REFERENCES

1. Kajantie E, Dunkel L, Rutanen E, Seppala M. IGF-I, IGF binding protein-3, phosphoisoforms of igfbp-1, and postnatal growth in very low birth weight infants. J Clin Endocrinol Metab 2002;87:2171–2179.
2. Ferry RJ Jr, Cohen P. The insulin-like growth factor axis in pediatrics. Clin Pediatr Endocrinol 1999;8:1–10.
3. Liu JP, Baker J, Perkins AS, Robertson EJ, Efstratiadis A. Mice carrying null mutations of the genes encoding insulin-like growth factor I (IGF-1) and type 1 IGF receptor (IGF1r). Cell 1993;75:59–72.
4. Liu J, Gringerg A, Westphal H. Insulin-like growth factor-I affects perinatal lethality and postnatal development n a gene dosage-dependent manner: manipulation using the Cre/IoxP system in transgenic mice. Mol Endocrinol 1998;12:1452–1462.
5. Woods KA, Camacho-Hübner C, Savage MO, Clark AJ. Intrauterine growth retardation and postnatal growth failure associated with deletion of the insulin-like growth factor 1 gene. N Engl J Med 1996;335:1363–1367.
6. DeChiara TM, Efstratiadis A, Robertson EJ. A growth-deficiency phenotype in heterozygous mice carrying an insulin-like growth factor II gene disrupted by targeting. Nature 1990;345:78–80.
7. Hibi I, Tanaka T. Hormonal regulation of growth and maturation: the effect of hormones on fetal growth. Clin Pediatr Endocrinol 1997;6:57–71.
8. Lo H, Tsao L. Relation of cord serum levels of growth hormone, insulin-like growth factors, insulin-like growth factor binding proteins, leptin, and interleukin-6 with birth weight, birth length and head circumference in term and preterm neonates. Nutrition 2002;18:604–608.
9. Prosser CG. Insulin-like growth factors in milk and mammary gland. J Mammary Gland Biol Neoplasia 1996;1:298–306.
10. Nagashima K, Itoh K, Kuroume T. Levels of insulin-like growth factor I in full- and preterm human milk in comparison to levels in cow's milk and in milk formulas. Biol Neonate 1990;58:343–346.
11. Donovan SM, Hintz RL, Rosenfeld RG. Insulin-like growth factors I and II and their binding proteins in human milk: effect of heat treatment on IGF and IGF binding protein stability. J Pediatr Gastroenterol Nutr 1991;13:242–253.
12. Merimee TJ, Grant M. Insulin-like growth factors in amniotic fluid. J Clin Endocrinol Metab 1984;59:752–755.
13. Bennett A, Wilson DM, Liu F, Nagashima R, Rosenfeld RG, Hintz RL. Levels of insulin-like growth factors I and II in human cord blood. J Clin Endocrinol Metab 1983;57:609.
14. Camacho-Hübner C, Woods KA, Miraki-Moud F, Clark A, Savage MO. Effects of recombinant human insulin-like growth factor I (IGF-I) therapy on the growth hormone-IGF system of a patient with a partial IGF-I gene deletion. J Clin Endocrinol Metab 1999 May;84:1611–1616.
15. Barker DJ, Hales CN, Fall CH, Osmond C, Phipps K, Clark PM. Type 2 (non-insulin-dependent) diabetes mellitus, hypertension and hyperlipidemia (syndrome X): relation to reduced fetal growth. Diabetologia 1993;36:62–67.
16. Fall CH, Pandit AN, Law CM, Yajnik CS, Clark PM, Breier B, et al. Size at birth and plasma insulin-like growth factor-1 concentrations. Arch Dis Child 1995;73:287–293.
17. Katz LE, Satin-Smith MS, Collett-Solberg P, Baker L, Stanley CA, Cohen P. Dual regulation of insulin-like growth factor binding protein-1 levels by insulin and cortisol during fasting. J Clin Endocrinol Metab 1998;83:4426–4430.
18. Smith WJ, Underwood LE, Keyes L, Clemmons DR. Use of insulin-like growth factor I (IGF-I) and IGF binding protein measurements to monitor feeding of premature infants. J Clin Endocrinol Metab 1997;82:3982–3988.
19. Price WA, Lee E, Maynor A, Stiles A, Clemmons DR. Relation between serum insulin like growth factor-1, insulin like growth factor binding protein-2, and insulin like growth factor binding protein-3 and

nutritional intake in premature infants with bronchopulmonary dysplasia. J Pediatr Gastroenterol Nutr 2001;32:542–549.

20. Hellstrom A, Carlsson B, Niklasson A, Segnestam K, Boguszewski M, de Lacerda L, et al. IGF-I is critical for normal vascularization of the human retina. J Clin Endocrinol Metab 2002;87:3413–3416.
21. Hellstrom A, Peruzzi C, Ju M, Engstrom E. Low IGF-I suppresses VEGF survival signaling in retinal endothelial cells: direct correlation with clinical retinopathy of prematurity. Proc Natl Acad Sci USA 2001;98:5804–5808.
22. Hirai C, Ichiba H, Saito M. Trophic effect of multiple growth factors in amniotic fluid or human milk on cultured human fetal small intestinal cells. J Pediatr Gastroenterol Nutr 2002;34:524–528.
23. Sanderson IR. Vascular endothelial growth factor in human milk. NeoReviews 2003;4:e125–126.
24. Vaessen N, Janssen J. Association between genetic variation in the gene for insulin-like growth factor-I and low birthweight. Lancet 2002;359:1036–1037.
25. Bhala A, Harris MD, Zirin S, Corcoran L, Cohen P. Insulin-like growth factor axis parameters in sick hospitalized neonates. J Pediatr Endocrinol Metab 1998;11:451–459.
26. Salmon WD, Daughaday WH. A hormonally controlled serum factor which stimulates sulfate incorporation by cartilage in vitro. J Lab Clin Med 1990;116:408–419.

8 Nutrition and the IGF System in Reproduction

Frank A. Simmen, Inseok Kwak, Jason L. Blum, and Rosalia C. M. Simmen

KEY POINTS

- Nutrition interacts with the IGF system to modify reproductive processes.
- The relative roles of the circulating vs tissue IGF systems in nutritional control of reproduction remains to be elucidated.
- There are profound species differences in IGF system expression and actions in reproduction.
- Use of multiple models and approaches is required to elucidate fundamental aspects of IGFs in nutrition and reproduction of humans and domestic animals.

1. INTRODUCTION

Evidence has been steadily emerging to indicate that the "IGF system," which consists of two secreted growth factor ligands (insulin growth factor [IGF]-I and -II), six secreted and/or membrane-localized IGF binding proteins (IGFBP-1, -2, -3, -4, -5, and -6), the IGFBP-3 acid-labile subunit (ALS), two cell-surface receptors (type I and type II IGF receptors), and potentially numerous ancillary participatory IGF and IGFBP proteases, is a critical regulatory component for the orchestration of successful reproduction in mammals and other vertebrates *(1)*. The IGF system can be functionally divided into two parallel entities, by virtue of whether its components are present in the circulation ("endocrine IGF") or are synthesized and act locally ("autocrine/paracrine" or "tissue IGF"). In many instances, the two IGF systems are not functionally equivalent or at most are partially overlapping. Many of the IGF system components present in the circulation, microvasculature, and extravascular spaces are under nutritional control with respect to their concentrations, and in some cases this involves noncoordinate or even opposing effects on different family members in the face of changing nutritional inputs or overall energy balance. The physiological effects and endpoints of such changes are only now being elucidated; similarly, questions of how nutritional status affects the expression and functions of individual tissue IGF Systems have just recently emerged as an area of intense investigation. Here, we review the present state of research that has implicated

From: *IGF and Nutrition in Health and Disease*
Edited by: M. S. Houston, J. M. P. Holly, and E. L. Feldman © Humana Press Inc., Totowa, NJ

IGF Systems (IGFs, IGFBPs and IGF Receptors) in Reproduction	Demonstrated Direct or Indirect Linkage with Nutritional State
Endocrine	√√
Liver (Maternal, Fetal)	√√
Mammary Glands & Secretions	√
Uterus: Endometrium, Myometrium	?
Ovary, Follicles, Oocytes	√√
Testes, Prostate, Seminal Fluid	?
Preimplantation Embryo/Fetus/Placenta	√

Fig. 1. Linkages: the IGF system, nutrition, and reproductive tissue functions.

the IGF system in reproduction and how nutrition interacts with and/or modifies such reproductive actions where known (Fig. 1). Lastly, we attempt to formulate possible directions for future research that may have the potential to impact human reproductive medicine as well as animal growth and reproduction via nutritional means.

2. OVARY

The functions of the ovary, among the reproductive organs/tissues of many species, be it a human, mouse, or fruit fly, are affected in particular by the relative nutritional state of the organism *(2)*. The ovary is known to have a self-contained and fully operational IGF system, which is integral to the dynamic processes of folliculogenesis (proliferation and differentiation), corpora lutea (CL) development and function (transdifferentiation), and CL regression (apoptosis) during the estrous cycle and pregnancy (Fig. 2). In this tissue, local and/or systemic IGF-I and IGF-II are synergistic with the gonadotropins luteinizing hormone (LH) and follicle-stimulating hormone to stimulate growth and differentiation of ovarian follicles and the subsequent synthesis and secretion of estradiol, via induction and action of the P450 aromatase enzyme in the granulosa cells. Local IGF-I appears to have as one of its key actions the stimulation of expression of follicle-stimulating hormone receptors in ovarian follicles, thereby making the developing follicles more responsive to gonadotropin *(3)*. It seems obvious based on studies using multiple animal models that the intraovarian IGF system relies heavily on temporally regulated production as well as regulated proteolysis of IGFBPs (the latter via serine proteases and metalloproteases) to affect the relative IGF bioactivity, which likely underlies proliferation and differentiation in the developing follicle *(4,5)*. In the rat ovary, the tissue-specific expression and functions of the individual IGFBPs are suggested by the distinct expression of IGFBP-2, -3, and -4 in specific cell types, which include the IGFBP-2 transcript mainly in thecal interstitial

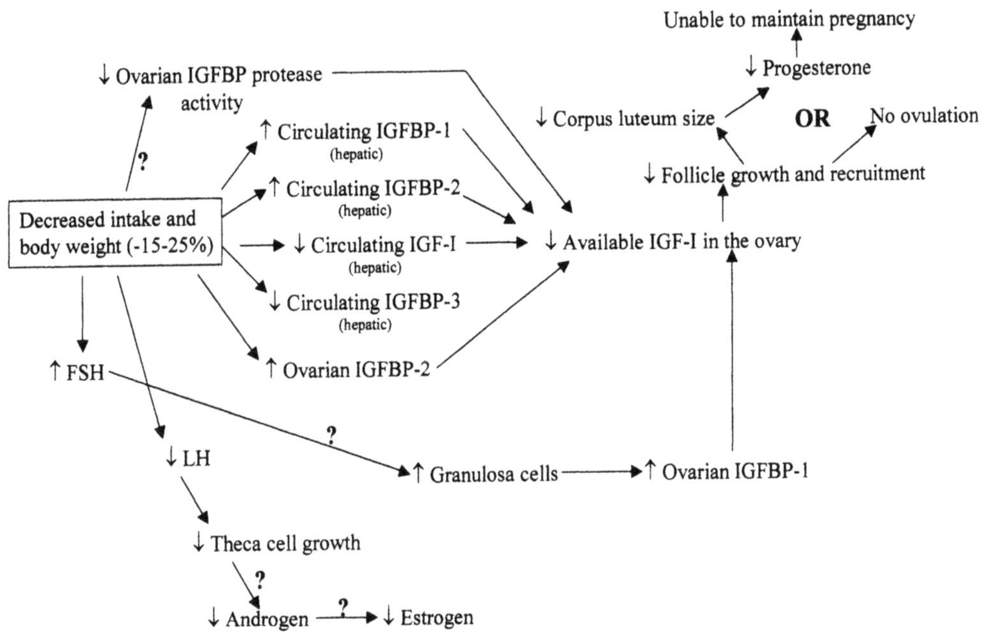

Fig. 2. Mechanistic aspects of how the "intra-ovarian" and "systemic" IGF systems respond to altered nutritional states to affect folliculogenesis.

cells of Graafian follicles, the IGFBP-3 transcript in corpora lutea, and the IGFBP-4 transcript in granulosa cells of atretic follicles *(6)*.

Lactating sows that are feed-restricted have reduced frequency of LH pulses, smaller ovaries, and smaller and fewer number of follicles than do normally fed counterparts *(7)*. In addition, aspirated follicular fluids from the former group have lower IGF-I concentrations than do those from the latter group *(7)*. Similarly, nutritionally induced anovulation in cows is characterized by decreased growth rate of the ovulatory follicle and lowered serum concentrations of LH, estradiol, and IGF-I *(8)*. Cows underfed to induce weight loss have smaller CLs than those fed to gain weight; interestingly, the difference in growth of ovarian tissues between these two systems is not accompanied by any changes in luteal IGF-I mRNA abundance *(9)*. In a study using sheep, it was found that under- as well as overfeeding affects the follicular fluid concentrations of both IGF-I and IGF-II *(10)*. This collective group of studies suggests that the systemic as well as intraovarian IGF systems are under nutritional control and that such controls may mediate, at least in part, the effects of altered nutrition on ovulation rate, ovarian function, early embryo development, circulating reproductive hormone concentrations, and overall pregnancy success.

3. OVIDUCT

The oviduct provides the site for fertilization and an optimal microenvironment for the early cleavage stages of embryo development. Oviducts from human, pig, sheep, and rat have documented expression of IGFs, IGFBPs, and IGF receptors, suggesting a functional locally acting IGF system in this tissue *(11–13)*. Rat oviduct expresses genes for many of the IGFBPs, with IGFBP-2, -4, -5, and -6 exhibiting stage of estrous cycle and/or cell-type (epithelial, fibroblast, smooth muscle)-specific mRNA expression patterns *(14)*. Interestingly, these same IGFBPs can be identified in oocyte–cumulus complexes collected from oviducts, suggesting their possible uptake from oviduct luminal fluid and targeted actions in early developing embryos because the corresponding mRNAs cannot be detected in the complexes *(14)*. Similarly, oviductal fluid contains both IGF-I and IGF-II *(15)*, a finding that has significance for the various developmental processes (i.e., cell division, metabolism, or apoptosis) occurring in the early preimplantation embryo. Sheep oviduct at periestrus exhibits expression of IGFs, IGFBPs-3 and -4, and type I IGF receptors *(16)*. In this model, IGF-I gene expression was localized primarily to the subepithelial stroma and the muscle layer and was maximal just before ovulation, coincident with high circulating estrogens. IGF-I receptor mRNAs, in contrast, are maximally expressed in the mucosal epithelium, consistent with the occurrence of a paracrine-type, stromal-epithelial communication mediated by IGF-I *(16)*. Human oviduct primarily expresses IGFBPs-2, -3, and -4 *(12)*. With regard to the possible effects of nutrition on the expression and/or actions of the IGF system components in the oviduct, there is a virtual absence of published studies that have examined such questions. In the same vein, although it is clear that serum steroid hormones (estrogens [E2], progesterone) can exert a major effect on oviductal IGF levels and bioactivity, the ramifications of such effects on overall reproductive efficiency remain unexplored.

4. UTERUS

The complete IGF system is operative in the uterus of humans, rodents, and domestic farm animals, which strongly suggests autocrine and/or paracrine physiology but with demonstrable species differences *(1,11,17–24)*. The two IGF ligands are differentially expressed in the uterine endometrium during pregnancy and the estrous cycle *(11,20)*, indicative of their unique as well as overlapping activities in the corresponding uterine tissue(s). In the pig, endometrial IGF-I mRNA abundance is correlated with circulating progesterone (mid-luteal stage of the cycle), whereas IGFBP-2 mRNA abundance is best correlated with circulating estrogens (periestrus) *(11)*. In this animal model, abundance of endometrial IGF-I mRNA declines after implantation whereas that for endometrial IGF-II increases *(11)*. Correspondingly, parallel induction of endometrial IGFBP-2 and placental IGF-II transcripts occur. In the sheep, cow, and rat, however, uterine IGF-I transcript abundance is greatest at estrus and is correlated with circulating estrogen *(19,24,25)*; by contrast, the expression of endometrial IGF-II and IGFBP-2 transcripts is positively correlated with presence of the embryo/fetus and progesterone, respectively *(17)*. In those species examined, the majority of the endometrial IGF-I transcripts originate from the subepithelial stroma *(19,20,24)*. The corresponding receptor (type I IGF receptor) mRNAs, in contrast, are more enriched in the endometrial epithelium *(19)*, illustrating the prominent role of IGF-I as a stromal-derived epithelial mitogen under distinct hormonal and perhaps nutritional control (Fig. 3). The mitogenic actions of IGF-I in the uterus appear to involve its own receptor (type I IGF receptor) as well as that for estrogen *(26)*. Interestingly, IGFBP-2 also acts as a uterine endometrial epithelial cell mitogen *(27)*.

The stage of estrous cycle- or pregnancy-dependent uterine expression of a number of the IGFBPs has also been described. In the rat, the temporal and cell type-specific

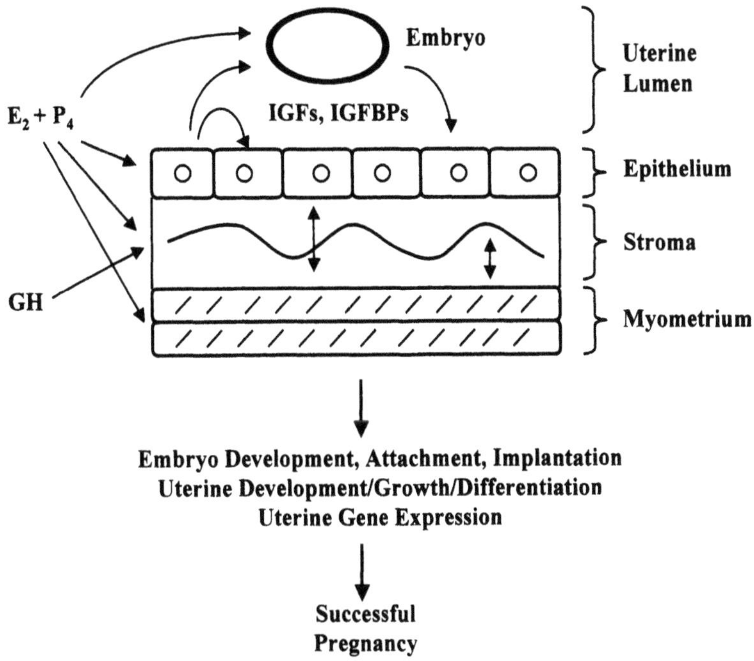

Fig. 3. The IGF system: a paracrine mediator of embryo–maternal communication essential to early development and implantation. The extent of nutritional impact on the expression and/or actions of this local system during pregnancy remains unknown.

expression of IGFBPs-2 through -6 during the estrous cycle are distinct *(18)*. The IGFBP-2 and IGFBP-4 genes, for example, are mainly expressed in this tissue's epithelial cells. In the pig, endometrial IGFBP-2 mRNAs are induced soon after embryo attachment to the uterine endometrial epithelium *(11)*, whereas, a transient expression of IGFBP-1 mRNA is observed in uterine endometrium at or near the time of embryo implantation/attachment in the human and ruminant species (sheep, cow) *(21,24)*. IGFBP-1 is considered to be a placental trophoblast integrin ligand *(28)* and is expressed in endometrial epithelium at pregnancy d 14 and 15 in the sheep *(21)* and cow *(22,24)*, and in the human endometrium at the secretory phase of the estrous cycle *(20)*. These periods of expression represent the early stages of embryo–maternal interaction during which time the trophoblast attaches to the uterine epithelium. Species differences in the type(s) of endometrial IGFBPs expressed at early pregnancy may well be tied to differences in the type of placentation exhibited. In this regard, the pig, which exhibits a very noninvasive type of placentation, does not have detectable endometrial expression of the IGFBP-1 gene at any time during pregnancy (F. A. Simmen, unpublished observations).

A myriad of studies now indicate that there is a dynamic aspect to the regulated expression of the IGF and IGFBP genes during early pregnancy, a time characterized by significant embryo mortality in humans and animals. This effect is particularly evident within the oviduct and uterus. Moreover, the embryo–maternal interface appears to be an important site of action for IGF ligands and IGFBPs *(11,28–30)*. The tissue targeting, as well as the timing, of the actions of uterine-elicited IGFs and IGFBPs relative to the embryo/trophoblast and endometrial epithelium, appears to also involve the actions of IGFBP-specific proteases. Human, porcine, ovine, and bovine uterine luminal fluids have IGFs, IGFBPs (mainly IGFBPs-1, -2 and -3), and IGFBP proteases as part of their components *(22,30–33)*. The physiological regulation of proteolysis of IGF:IGFBP complexes in the uterine lumen involves the actions of IGFBP-specific proteases under the control of maternal progesterone *(30,31)* and may also be dependent on the overall phosphorylation state of the target IGFBP *(33)*.

As noted for the oviduct, it is similarly unclear whether the nutritional status of the organism has a major impact, if any, on the uterine IGF system. However, given the plasticity of this system it is likely that its regulation by nutrition results in key effects on multiple processes involving implantation, fetal development and pregnancy outcome.

5. TESTES

Male reproductive tissues, with the notable exception of prostatic tumor cells, have not been as extensively examined with respect to a functioning IGF system as female reproductive tissues. However, there are some provocative indications that the IGF system is important to male reproductive success and that nutritional status may constitute a primary interacting factor. In rams, testis size, plasma testosterone, plasma IGF-I, peak pubertal reproductive activity, and body weight are positively correlated with feed intake *(34)*. There is a significant amount of IGFBP-3 immunoreactivity in human seminal fluids, which appears to be the result of IGFBP-3 secretion from the prostate and subsequent partial proteolysis via prostate-specific antigen *(35)*. Physiological concentrations of IGF-I are also found in bovine seminal plasma *(36)*. Moreover, bovine sperm displays receptors for IGF-I localized to the acrosomal region. Perhaps most interestingly, recombinant IGF-I or IGF-II can increase bovine sperm motility in vitro, presumably by acting through sperm IGF receptors *(36,37)*.

6. THE CIRCULATING IGF SYSTEM

GH, besides being a somatogenic hormone, is an important endocrine factor for reproduction *(38)*. This hormone affects male and female sexual development, gonadal steroidogenesis, gametogenesis, ovulation, fetal and placental growth, mammogenesis, and lactation, all of which undoubtedly involve IGF system-dependent and -independent pathways. Exogenous GH stimulates the circulating levels of IGF-I, IGFBP-3, and ALS while suppressing that for IGFBP-2 *(38)*. Conversely, feeding restriction leads to an induction in circulating IGFBP-2 and a concomitant decrease in circulating IGF-I/IGFBP-3 *(9)*. Under these two physiological conditions, IGF-I and IGFBP-2 may constitute counter-regulatory principles. IGF-I, IGFBP-2, and IGFBP-3 concentrations in the circulation are relatively constant during a normal estrous cycle *(39)* and would therefore appear to be independent of or uninvolved with cyclical changes in ovarian and uterine physiology. However, it is very likely that nutritional deficits that affect circulating IGF and/or IGFBP levels may contribute to changes in reproductive physiology. Treatment of pregnant pigs with recombinant GH can, in some cases, augment fetal growth *(29)*, but this effect does not appear to involve any changes in endometrial production of IGF-I, IGF-II, or IGFBP-2 *(29)*.

The studies described previously point to an association between nutritional status and reproductive physiology with the circulating IGF system serving as the link between the two. In postpartum cattle subject to nutrient restriction, circulating concentrations of IGF-I and IGFBP-3 are depressed, whereas that of IGFBP-2 is increased *(40)*. Moreover, nutrient restriction leads to decreased resumption of estrous cycles in this same model. Long-term food restriction of guinea pigs has no effect on the relative size of the uterus, and although circulating IGF-I, IGF-II, IGFBP-1, IGFBP-3, and IGFBP-4 levels are severely depressed, IGFBP-2 levels are increased and many tissues are either increased or decreased in relative size under these conditions *(41)*. In fetal and neonatal sheep, the relative state of nutrition can markedly affect the hepatic expression of many IGF system components. In these animals, undernutrition leads to increased expression of the IGFBP-2 gene and decreased expression of the IGF-I and ALS genes in the liver *(42)*.

7. TRANSGENIC AND KNOCKOUT MOUSE MODELS: "REPRODUCTIVE PHENOTYPES"

Growth hormone receptor-null mutant ("knockout") mice exhibit a reduced or complete lack of circulating IGF-I and have markedly reduced fertility *(43,44)*. In males, this partial defect in fertility resides at the levels of the hypothalamus, pituitary gland, and testes and involves reduced basal as well as LH-stimulated testosterone release from the testes *(44)*. Female GH receptor knockouts have delayed sexual maturation, which can be corrected with exogenous IGF-I treatment *(43)*. Litter size and newborn body weights are reduced for progeny of GH receptor-null females *(43)*. Interestingly, the administration of IGF-I leads to an increase in uterine weights *(43)*. These data clearly indicate that in mice, GH and/or IGF-I are determinants of fertility for both genders.

That IGF-I is indeed critical for reproductive tissue development is demonstrated by the phenotypes of IGF-I knockout mice. Male and female mice that have null mutations of the IGF-I locus are infertile and exhibit severe reductions in the size of reproductive organs *(45,46)*. IGF-I-deficient males have reduced testes size, produce markedly less testosterone, and fail to manifest mating behavior *(46)*. Females do not ovulate, even after the administration of gonadotropins, and have an infantile uterus caused mostly by hypoplasia of the myometrium *(46)*. More recently, Cre-induced, liver-specific IGF-I gene targeting has been used to examine effects of hepatic IGF-I gene knockouts on postnatal growth and development. These mice typically have massive decreases in liver IGF-I gene expression postnatally and manifest a decline in, or the complete absence of, circulating IGF-I. Interestingly, these mice are normal with respect to growth and development and are fertile, leading to the conclusion that although liver is the main source of circulating IGF-I, it is not important for fertility in mice *(47,48)*. Consistent with this, mice lacking the acid-labile subunit gene had no fertility defect despite a major deficit in postnatal circulating IGF-I levels *(49)*.

Female mice genetically engineered for global overexpression of IGFBP-1 have reduced reproductive performance characterized by decreased ovulation rate and increased embryo mortality (reviewed in ref. *50*). However, mice homozygous for the null IGFBP-2 allele and thus completely lacking IGFBP-2 mRNA and protein are fully viable and fertile *(51)*. Moreover, global overexpression of IGFBP-2 in tissues and in the circulation leads to postnatal growth inhibition but without reported effects on fertility *(50,52)*. Despite the lack of experimental confirmation, one might hypothesize from these experiments that circulating IGFBP-1 and IGFBP-2 are not functionally equivalent and that nutritional deficits, which are known to lead to an induction in circulating IGFBP-1 (as well as IGFBP-2), might be deleterious to female reproductive function.

8. SUMMARY AND CONCLUSIONS

Although it is apparent that the IGF system is used in the endocrine and paracrine regulation of male and female reproductive processes, much less is known about how nutrition specifically interacts with these processes. Results from multiple animal models have suggested that ovarian and testicular functions in particular may be compromised under conditions of chronic under- or overnutrition. Attempts to link IGF system gene products to these tissue phenotypes have, as in the cases of large animal models, pointed to circulating IGF-I as being an important component in this regard. However, the recent elegant gene targeting experiments in mice suggest that the locally expressed IGFs might have more crucial roles in reproductive processes. This is an interesting dichotomy that awaits further resolution. Consequently, it is not possible to conclusively state whether ovarian and testicular IGF system components exhibit any profound degrees of nutritional regulation either at the levels of synthesis, secretion, processing, and/or signal reception.

9. RECOMMENDATIONS AND CHALLENGES FOR THE FUTURE

It is obvious that nutrition is an important determinant of reproductive success. It is equally apparent that conditions of low nutrient availability are not advantageous to reproduction. One checkpoint for molecular control of reproduction might reside at the level of gametogenesis. Perhaps the IGF system functions in this biological process by serving as a stimulus under conditions of adequate nutrients and by restricting such effects under low nutrient conditions. Once fertilization and early development have been initiated, the IGF system may serve in numerous other important regulatory capacities such as ensuring for adequate fetal nutrition by the stimulation of placental growth, among other effects. The temporal linkage of the "early" and "late" components of these IGF effects is suggested by the intriguing observation that exposure to undernutrition at precisely the time of conception has profound effects on the circulating levels of IGF-I and IGFBP-3 in the fetus near term *(53)*. Likewise, undernutrition, specifically during later stages of fetal development, may delay the onset of the circulating IGF System postnatally *(42)*. Together, these observations may point to the existence of "nutritional imprinting" of the fetus as a consequence of maternal nutrition and involving this fascinating growth factor-associated system *(54–56)*. By necessity, much of the published work to date is descriptive in nature. Clearly, future work is needed to clarify more of the mechanistic aspects of how nutrients, energy, and the IGF system interact during reproduction and pre- and postnatal development. Such studies may eventually provide for novel nutritional means to augment reproduction of animals and alleviate infertility in women.

10. ACKNOWLEDGMENTS

We regret that many important contributions to this area of research could not be cited because of space limitations. Research in the authors' laboratories has been supported by grants from the NIH (HD-21961), the USDA NRICGP, and by USDA-CRIS-6251-5100-002-06S to the Arkansas Children's Nutrition Center.

REFERENCES

1. Wang H-S, Chard T. IGFs and IGF-binding proteins in the regulation of human ovarian and endometrial function. J Endocrinol 1999;161:1–13.
2. Drummond-Barbosa D, Spradling AC. Stem cells and their progeny respond to nutritional changes during Drosophila oogenesis. Dev Biol 2001;231:265–278.
3. Zhou J, Kumar TR, Matzuk MM, Bondy C. Insulin-like growth factor I regulates gonadotropin responsiveness in the murine ovary. Mol Endocrinol 1997;11:1924–1933.
4. Besnard N, Pisselet C, Zapf J, Hornebeck W, Monniaux D, Monget P. Proteolytic activity is involved in changes in intrafollicular insulin-like growth factor-binding protein levels during growth and atresia of ovine ovarian follicles. Endocrinology 1996;137:1599–1607.
5. Besnard N, Pisselet C, Monniaux D, Monget P. Proteolytic activity degrading insulin-like growth factor-binding protein-2, -3, -4, and -5 in healthy growing and atretic follicles in the pig ovary. Biol Reprod 1997;56:1050–1058.
6. Nakatani A, Shimasaki S, Erickson GF, Ling N. Tissue-specific expression of four insulin-like growth factor-binding proteins (1, 2, 3, and 4) in the rat ovary. Endocrinology 1991;129:1521–1529.
7. Quesnel H, Pasquier A, Mounier AM, Prunier A. Influence of feed restriction during lactation on gonadotropic hormones and ovarian development in primiparous sows. J Anim Sci 1998;76:856–863.
8. Bossis I, Wettemann RP, Welty SD, Vizcarra JA, Spicer LJ, Diskin MG. Nutritionally induced anovulation in beef heifers: ovarian and endocrine function preceding cessation of ovulation. J Anim Sci 1999;77:1536–1546.
9. Vandehaar MJ, Sharma BK, Fogwell RL. Effect of dietary energy restriction on the expression of insulin-like growth factor-I in liver and corpus luteum of heifers. J Dairy Sci 1995;78:832–841.
10. O'Callaghan D, Yaakub H, Hyttel P, Spicer LJ, Boland MP. Effect of nutrition and superovulation on oocyte morphology, follicular fluid composition and systemic hormone concentrations in ewes. J Reprod Fertil 2000;118:303–313.
11. Simmen FA, Simmen RCM, Geisert RD, Martinat-Botte F, Bazer FW, Terqui M. Differential expression, during the estrous cycle and pre- and postimplantation conceptus development, of messenger ribonucleic acids encoding components of the pig uterine insulin-like growth factor system. Endocrinology 1992;130:1547–1556.
12. Giudice LC, Dsupin BA, Irwin JC, Eckert RL. Identification of insulin-like growth factor binding proteins in human oviduct. Fertil Steril 1992;57:294–301.
13. Carlsson B, Hillsjö T, Nilsson A, Törnell J, Billig H. Expression of insulin-like growth factor-I (IGF-I) in the rat Fallopian tube: possible autocrine and paracrine action of Fallopian tube-derived IGF-I on the Fallopian tube and on the preimplantation embryo. Endocrinology 1993;133:2031–2039.
14. Erickson GF, Girvigian MR, Sadighian AR, Nakatani A, Ling N, Shimasaki S. Tissue specific and cyclic expression of insulin-like growth factor binding proteins -1, -2, -3, -4, -5, -6 in the rat oviduct. Endocrine 1995;3:667–676.
15. Wiseman DL, Henricks DM, Eberhardt DM, Bridges WC. Identification and content of insulin-like growth factors in porcine oviductal fluid. Biol Reprod 1992;47:126–132.
16. Stevenson KR, Wathes DC. Insulin-like growth factors and their binding proteins in the ovine oviduct during the oestrous cycle. J Reprod Fertil 1996;108:31–40.
17. Geisert RD, Lee C-Y, Simmen FA, Zavy MT, Fliss AE, Bazer FW, Simmen RCM. Expression of messenger RNAs encoding insulin-like growth factor-I, -II, and insulin-like growth factor binding protein-2 in bovine endometrium during the estrous cycle and early pregnancy. Biol Reprod 1991;45:975–983.
18. Girvigian MR, Nakatani A, Ling N, Shimasaki S, Erickson GF. Insulin-like growth factor-binding proteins show distinct patterns of expression in the rat uterus. Biol Reprod 1994;51:296–302.
19. Stevenson KR, Gilmour RS, Wathes DC. Localization of insulin-like growth factor-I (IGF-I) and -II messenger ribonucleic acids and type 1 IGF receptors in the ovine uterus during the estrous cycle and early pregnancy. Endocrinology 1994;134:1655–1664.
20. Zhou J, Dsupin BA, Giudice LC, Bondy CA. Insulin-like growth factor system gene expression in human endometrium during the menstrual cycle. J Clin Endocrinol Metab 1994;79:1723–1734.
21. Cann CH, Fairclough RJ, Sutton R, Gow CB. Endometrial expression of mRNA encoding insulin-like growth factors I and II and IGF-binding proteins 1 and 2 in early pregnant ewes. J Reprod Fertil 1997;111:7–13.

22. Keller ML, Roberts AJ, Seidel GE Jr. Characterization of insulin-like growth factor-binding proteins in the uterus and conceptus during early conceptus elongation in cattle. Biol Reprod 1998;59:632–642.
23. Rutanen EM. Insulin-like growth factors in endometrial function. Gynecol Endocrinol 1998;12:399–406.
24. Robinson RS, Mann GE, Gadd TS, Lamming GE, Wathes DC. The expression of the IGF system in the bovine uterus throughout the oestrous cycle and early pregnancy. J Endocrinol 2000;165:231–243.
25. Murphy LJ, Ghahary A. Uterine IGF-I: regulation of expression and its role in estrogen-induced uterine proliferation. Endocr Rev 1990;11:443–453.
26. Klotz DM, Curtis-Hewitt SC, Ciana P, Raviscioni M, Lindzey JK, Foley J, et al. Requirement of estrogen receptor-alpha in insulin-like growth factor-1(IGF-1)-induced uterine responses and in vivo evidence for IGF-1/estrogen receptor cross-talk. J Biol Chem 2002;277:8531–8537.
27. Badinga L, Song S, Simmen RCM, Clarke JB, Clemmons DR, Simmen FA. Complex mediation of uterine endometrial epithelial cell growth by insulin-like growth factor-II (IGF-II) and IGF-binding protein-2. J Mol Endocrinol 1999;23:277–285.
28. Giudice LC. Multifaceted roles for IGFBP-1 in human endometrium during implantation and pregnancy. Ann N Y Acad Sci 1997;828:146–156.
29. Sterle JA, Boyd C, Peacock JT, Koenigsfeld AT, Lamberson WR, Gerrard DE, Lucy MC. Insulin-like growth factor (IGF)-I, IGF-II, IGF-binding protein-2 and pregnancy-associated glycoprotein mRNA in pigs with somatotropin-enhanced fetal growth. J Endocrinol 1998;159:441–450.
30. Lee CY, Green ML, Simmen RCM, Simmen FA. Proteolysis of insulin-like growth factor-binding proteins (IGFBPs) within the pig uterine lumen associated with peri-implantation conceptus development. J Reprod Fertil 1998;112:369–377.
31. Peterson AJ, Ledgard AM, Hodgkinson SC. The proteolysis of insulin-like growth factor binding proteins in ovine uterine fluid. Reprod Fertil Dev 1998;10:309–314.
32. Cann CH, Fairclough RJ, Browne CA, Gow CB. Uterine luminal content of insulin-like growth factor (IGF)-I and endometrial expression of mRNA encoding IGF-binding proteins 1 and 2 during the oestrus cycle and early pregnancy in the ewe. Reprod Fertil Dev 1998;10:155–163.
33. Gibson JM, Aplin JD, White A, Westwood M. Regulation of IGF bioavailability in pregnancy. Mol Hum Reprod 2001;7:79–87.
34. Adam CL, Findlay PA. Effect of nutrition on testicular growth and plasma concentrations of gonadotrophins, testosterone and insulin-like growth factor I (IGF-I) in pubertal male Soay sheep. J Reprod Fertil 1997;111:121–125.
35. Plymate SR, Rosen CJ, Paulsen CA, Ware JL, Chen J, Vessella RE, Birnbaum RS. 1996. Proteolysis of insulin-like growth factor-binding protein-3 in the male reproductive tract. J Clin Endocrinol Metab 1996;81:618–624.
36. Henricks DM, Kouba AJ, Lackey BR, Boone WR, Gray SL. Identification of insulin-like growth factor I in bovine seminal plasma and its receptor on spermatozoa: influence on sperm motility. Biol Reprod 1998;59:330–337.
37. Lackey BR, Boone WR, Gray SL, Henricks DM. Computer-assisted sperm motion analysis of bovine sperm treated with insulin-like growth factor I and II: implications as motility regulators and chemokinetic factors. Arch Androl 1998;41:115–125.
38. Hull KL, Harvey S. Growth hormone: a reproductive endocrine-paracrine regulator? Rev Reprod 2000;5:175–182.
39. Funston RN, Moss GE, Roberts AJ. Insulin-like growth factor-I (IGF-I) and IGF-binding proteins in bovine sera and pituitaries at different stages of the estrous cycle. Endocrinology 1995;136:62–68.
40. Roberts AJ, Nugent RA III, Klindt J, Jenkins TG. Circulating insulin-like growth factor I, insulin-like growth factor binding proteins, growth hormone, and resumption of estrus in postpartum cows subjected to dietary energy restriction. J Anim Sci 1997;75:1909–1917.
41. Sohlstrom A, Katsman A, Kind KL, Grant PA, Owens PC, Robinson JS, Owens JA. Effects of acute and chronic food restriction on the insulin-like growth factor axis in the guinea pig. J Endocrinol 1998;157:107–114.
42. Rhoads RP, Greenwood PL, Bell AW, Boisclair YR. Nutritional regulation of the genes encoding the acid-labile subunit and other components of the circulating insulin-like growth factor system in the sheep. J Anim Sci 2000;78:2681–2689.
43. Danilovich N, Wernsing D, Coschigano KT, Kopchick JJ, Bartke A. Deficits in female reproductive function in GH-R-KO mice: role of IGF-I. Endocrinology 1999;140:2637–2640.

44. Chandrashekar V, Bartke A, Awoniyi CA, Tsai-Morris CH, Dufau ML, Russell LD, Kopchick JJ. Testicular endocrine function in GH receptor gene disrupted mice. Endocrinology 2001;142:3443–3450.
45. Baker J, Liu J-P, Robertson EJ, Efstratiadis A. Role of insulin-like growth factors in embryonic and postnatal growth. Cell 1993;75:73–82.
46. Baker J, Hardy MP, Zhou J, Bondy C, Lupu F, Bellvé AR, Efstratiadis A. Effects of an IGF1 gene null mutation on mouse reproduction. Mol Endocrinol 1996;10:903–918.
47. Yakar S, Liu J-L, Stannard B, Butler A, Accili D, Sauer B, LeRoith D. 1999. Normal growth and development in the absence of hepatic insulin-like growth factor I. Proc Natl Acad Sci USA 1999;96:7324–7329.
48. Liu J-L, Yakar S, LeRoith D. Conditional knockout of mouse insulin-like growth factor-1 gene using the Cre/loxP system. Proc Soc Exp Biol Med 2000;223:344–351.
49. Ueki I, Ooi GT, Tremblay ML, Hurst KR, Bach LA, Boisclair YR. Inactivation of the acid labile subunit gene in mice results in mild retardation of postnatal growth despite profound disruptions in the circulating insulin-like growth factor system. Proc Natl Acad Sci USA 2000;97:6868–6873.
50. Schneider MR, Lahm H, Wu M, Hoeflich A, Wolf E. Transgenic mouse models for studying the functions of insulin-like growth factor-binding proteins. FASEB J 2000;14:629–640.
51. Wood TL, Rogler LE, Czick ME, Schuller AGP, Pintar JE. Selective alterations in organ sizes with a targeted disruption of the insulin-like growth factor binding protein-2 gene. Mol Endocrinol 2000;14:1472–1482.
52. Hoeflich A, Wu M, Mohan S, Föll J, Wanke R, Froehlich T, Arnold GJ, Lahm H, Kolb HJ, Wolf E. Overexpression of insulin-like growth factor-binding protein-2 in transgenic mice reduces postnatal body weight gain. Endocrinology 1999;140:5488–5496.
53. Gallaher BW, Breier BH, Keven CL, Harding JE, Gluckman PD. Fetal programming of insulin-like growth factor (IGF)-I and IGF-binding protein-3: evidence for an altered response to undernutrition in late gestation following exposure to periconceptual undernutrition in the sheep. J Endocrinol 1998;159:501–508.
54. Brameld JM, Mostyn A, Dandrea J, Stephenson TJ, Dawson JM, Buttery PJ, Symonds ME. Maternal nutrition alters the expression of insulin-like growth factors in fetal sheep liver and skeletal muscle. J Endocrinol 2000;167:429–437.
55. Vickers MH, Ikenasio BA, Breier BH. IGF-I treatment reduces hyperphagia, obesity, and hypertension in metabolic disorders induced by fetal programming. Endocrinology 2001;142:3964–3973.
56. Osgerby JC, Wathes DC, Howard D, Gadd TS. The effect of maternal undernutrition on ovine fetal growth. J Endocrinol 2002;173:131–141.

9 The Insulin Growth Factor System and Nutrition in Adulthood and Aging

Moira S. Lewitt and Kerstin Hall

KEY POINTS

- After puberty there is a continuous decline in IGF-I concentrations with age.
- Alterations in the IGF axis during aging contribute to age-related decreases in muscle and bone mass.
- The fall in IGF-I may relate to reduced nutritional intake, as well as a decline in GH levels.
- The relative excess of circulating IGFBPs during aging may contribute to a further decline in IGF availability to tissues.
- Survival to very old age (> 80 yr) is associated with higher IGF-I levels than predicted.
- The nutritional requirements for an appropriate IGF-I concentration at each stage of life should be the focus of future research.

1. INTRODUCTION

Changes in the insulin growth factor (IGF) system are thought to have a major impact on the altered body composition and cellular function that occurs with age. Alterations in the growth hormone (GH)–IGF axis are believed to be responsible for many age-related disabilities. Factors other than GH may contribute to the change in IGF activity with age. Other components of the GH–IGF axis that may be altered by the aging process include IGF sensitivity at the receptor and postreceptor level and the profile of the IGF-binding proteins in the circulation and target tissues. Nutritional factors have an important influence at each of these levels.

2. SCOPE AND AIM

In this chapter, we outline what is known about the changes in the IGF system with aging in adulthood and the effect of nutrition. The physiology of the IGF system is covered in detail in chapter 1 and other chapters. Here, we will highlight aspects that are relevant to aging. We emphasize the importance of this system in age-related disabilities. Finally, we discuss the somewhat controversial area of the role of the IGF system in longevity. In our concluding remarks, we will attempt to identify some key

From: *IGF and Nutrition in Health and Disease*
Edited by: M. S. Houston, J. M. P. Holly, and E. L. Feldman © Humana Press Inc., Totowa, NJ

areas for future study. In this review we have used the terms "young adulthood" for the ages 20 to 40 yr, "middle age" for 40 to 60 yr, "old age" for 60 to 80 yr and "very old age" for over 80 yr.

3. PHYSIOLOGY

IGF-I and -II, acting through the IGF-I receptor and insulin receptors, have a wide spectrum of activity, which is regulated to a large extent by a family of six specific IGF-binding proteins. The IGFs have both endocrine and paracrine roles *(1)*. GH stimulates IGF-I expression, and IGF-I contributes to the regulation of GH by feedback inhibition. Rodent studies suggest the pattern of gene expression during aging is similar to that of GH deficiency and can be partly restored with GH treatment *(2)*. Factors other than GH are important in the regulation of the IGF system with aging. Insulin may be of particular importance in the positive regulation of IGF-I. The relative impact of insulin in the maintenance of IGF-I concentrations in aging is yet to be clarified.

The clinical studies that we review in this chapter focus on the changes in the endocrine IGF system with aging. Most of the circulating IGFs are in a ternary complex, in association with IGFBP-3 and the acid labile subunit (ALS), which are also both GH-dependent proteins. ALS circulates in excess of the other components of the ternary complex, whereas IGF-I and IGFBP-3 can directly and positively influence each other's circulating concentrations by promoting ternary complex formation *(3)*. Thus the endocrine IGF level is dependent on ALS production. All six IGFBPs participate in binary complex formation that influences the delivery of IGFs to their target cells. Alterations in the endocrine profile of the IGFBPs with age could significantly influence IGF tissue activity. The availability of IGF at the target tissue is also dependent on IGF release from IGFBPs, which may be influenced by the action of proteases. IGFBP-1, because of its dynamic nutritional regulation, may be of specific importance in the relationship between nutrition, aging, and IGF availability. Paracrine IGFs and IGFBPs and the sensitivity of the tissues to IGF signaling through receptors are also important considerations in the impact of age and nutrition. The tissue levels and activity of the components of the IGF system are unknown in most circumstances. However, it is generally assumed that the fraction of unbound IGFs in the circulation represents the biologically active pool available to the periphery.

In interpreting the results of clinical studies, one should be familiar with the assay method, not only for the "free" IGF assays, but also for all the IGF system components. For example, it is often important to consider what posttranslationally modified form of IGFBP is being measured, the time of day, the relationship to a meal, and so on.

4. THE IGF SYSTEM THROUGHOUT ADULTHOOD

4.1. Overview

Normal IGF and IGFBP levels in healthy aging human populations have been determined from cross-sectional data. This introduces bias related to survival selection as well as decreasing ability of even relatively healthy elderly individuals to participate in a routine study assessment. At all postnatal ages most of the IGFs circulate in the

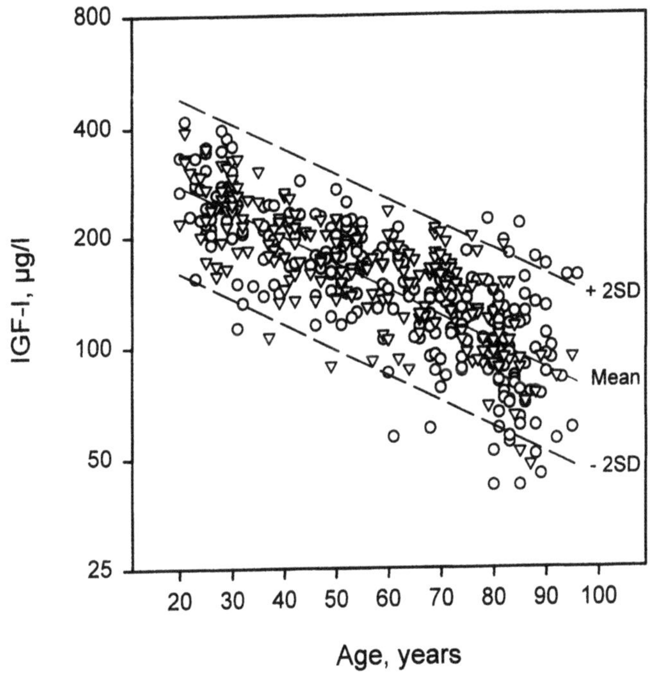

Fig. 1. Progressive decline in total serum IGF-I concentrations in 448 healthy subjects from young adulthood to old age. The correlation coefficient between IGF-I and age was r = –0.774, $p < 0.001$. The regression lines for the mean and 2 SD are shown. Women are represented by the circles and men by the triangles.

ternary complex with IGFBP-3 and ALS. Total IGF-I concentrations fall with increasing age. The net fall in IGFBPs is less pronounced, so that there is a relative increase in IGF-binding. Although clinical studies give us an idea of changes in the endocrine IGF system with age, the profile of paracrine IGFs, IGFBPs and receptors are important in determining the available IGF activity. In rodents IGF-I receptor expression declines with aging *(4)*. In humans it is not yet known whether the paracrine IGF-I expression in different tissues follows the age-dependent pattern of endocrine IGF-I. It is known that IGFBP-3 secretion by fibroblasts increases with the age of the donor *(5)*. This contrasts with the changes in endocrine IGFBP-3 described below. Overall, the patterns that we describe suggest that with age there is a fall in endocrine IGF bioavailability. The contribution of nutritional changes to this fall has not yet been defined.

4.2. Total IGFs and the Ternary Complex

The progressive decline of total serum IGF-I concentrations from young adulthood to old age is well established in several studies using different immunoassays *(6–14)*. In our own reference material of 448 healthy adults *(13)*, we have found an inverse linear correlation between logarithmic transformed IGF-I levels and age (Fig. 1). From 20 yr of age, the geometrical mean of total IGF-I decreased by 50% for each 30 yr of aging. Thus the mean IGF-I value at 80 yr of age is only 25% of the mean level at 20 yr. In the very elderly, this age dependency may be lost. In healthy centenarians, the IGF-I levels in fact were higher than in elderly aged 80 yr *(15)*. In each decade of life the variation of IGF-I levels around the mean is wide. In our healthy reference material the –2 SD value is 57% of the mean. Because of the lack of longitudinal studies, it is unknown whether each individual follows a fixed IGF-I SD score throughout life as a result of a genetically determined set point in IGF-I expression. Studies in twins, however, suggest that at least 40% of the variability in IGF-I is genetic *(16,17)*.

Circulating IGF-II concentrations are less dependent on GH. Some studies document a progressive fall in circulating IGF-II with age in middle to old age *(10,12)*; however, others show no variation *(9,18)*.

Any fall in IGF-I and/or IGF-II could be secondary to changes in IGFBPs in the circulation. IGFBP-3, which accounts for most of the IGF-binding in the circulation, declines progressively during middle and old age *(9–12,19)*, as does IGFBP-5, which can also associate with ALS *(20)*. Notably, the changes in IGFBP-3 and -5 are less pronounced than the fall in IGF-I. Thus, there is a relative excess of IGFBP-3 and the IGF-I/IGFBP-3 ratio decreases *(9)*, although this pattern is not observed in centenarians *(15)*. An excess of IGFBP-3 in relation to IGF-I is also seen in GH deficiency *(21)*. Most of the IGF-I bound to IGFBP-3 circulates in a complex with ALS. There is a body of evidence supporting the role of GH as the primary transcriptional regulator of ALS *(22)*. It is surprising therefore that ALS concentrations decline only slightly with age in adult men and remain constant in females *(23)*. This observation supports the concept that factors other than declining GH are important in determining the changes in ALS and IGF-I with age.

4.3. Binary Complexes and Free IGFs

IGFBP-1, which displays a slight increase throughout adulthood *(9,19)*, is an important determinant of the dynamic availability of endocrine and tissue IGF activity *(24,25)*. Insulin is the most important regulator of hepatic IGFBP-1 secretion. An inverse relationship with insulin is maintained throughout life *(9,26)* but with an upward shift in the regression line *(9,19)*. This has been attributed to hepatic insulin resistance *(27)* and this is further discussed in Chapter 14.

IGFBP-4 concentrations increase with age *(20)*. Thus, there is excess of each of IGFBP-1 to -5 in relation to the changes in IGF-I in studies of aging *(20,28)*. IGF-I that is not bound to IGFBPs or can be easily displaced from IGFBPs is considered to be more biologically active. Overall, a relative excess of IGFBPs would be expected to contribute to a decline in IGF bioavailability. When "free" IGF-I is measured by ultrafiltration, it is found to fall progressively from young adulthood to old age, in parallel with the total IGF-I concentration, so that there is no change in the percentage of total IGF-I *(29)*. In this study, total and free IGF-II concentrations were found to be independent of age. Within an older study population (55–80 yr), using a different assay that measures both free IGF-I and the fraction that is readily dissociated from IGFBPs, the concentrations did not decrease with age and in fact increased in individuals above 70 yr *(26)*. Thus it is not yet clear whether the amount of IGF available from the circulation changes with aging.

4.4. Hormonal Regulation of the IGF System During Aging

The mean IGF-I value in a 90-yr-old individual corresponds to <4 SD of healthy young adults. This is as low as that found in GH-deficient patients of younger age *(13)*, who share many phenotypic features with those of old age *(30)*. Because the amplitude and duration of GH pulses decline with advancing age *(31)*, it has been postulated that the age-dependent decline in circulating IGF-I levels during adulthood is caused by a decrease in GH secretion. However, in a recent study, a positive association between IGF-I and integrated 24-h GH concentrations was observed in young and not old subjects *(32)*. In this study abdominal visceral fat and fasting insulin concentrations were consistently the most important predictors of GH secretion.

Alteration of the set point in the hypothalamus or pituitary to the IGF feedback of the GH axis is an attractive hypothesis to explain an age-dependent decline in IGF-I. We do not believe it has been definitively excluded that in old age the pituitary is more sensitive to the suppressive effect of IGF-I on GH release. One study has shown that the GH levels achieved after IGF-I infusion did not differ between fasting old and young subjects despite higher basal GH levels in the young individuals *(33)*. However, it was not possible to clearly determine sensitivity to suppression in this study. We speculate that increasing free fatty acid (FFA) concentrations with age may have potentiating effects on IGF-I-induced suppression of GH release. A nicotinic acid derivative, which suppresses FFAs, is a strong stimulator of GH release in adults *(34)*, restores the GH response to GH-releasing hormone in elderly subjects *(35)*, and partially prevents GH-induced insulin resistance in GH-deficient subjects *(36,37)*. Hyperinsulinemia induces a similar fall in FFAs but impairs the GH response to GH releasing hormone *(38)*. The role of FFAs and insulin in determining the set point between GH and IGF-I will need to be elucidated in the future.

A decline in the peripheral IGF-I response to GH with age has been considered to contribute to the fall in IGF-I levels with age. One study has documented a reduced IGF-I response in older men to a single dose of GH *(39)*. Against this concept GH replacement doses do not change with age in GH-deficient patients *(40)*.

Age-related changes of other hormones could inhibit IGF-I expression or attenuate the GH-induced IGF-I response in the liver. A small attenuation of hepatic insulin sensitivity or insulin production *(41)* could decrease both basal and GH-induced hepatic IGF-I release in response to GH. Total IGF-I is inversely correlated to sex hormone binding globulin *(26,42,43)*, which is an insulin-regulated protein and which can change the availability of gonadal steroids. However, estrogens, despite their stimulatory effect on GH, are generally considered to attenuate IGF-I levels *(39,44)*, and a higher GH replacement dose is required in women than men *(45)*. Administration of testosterone in high concentrations has been reported to increase serum IGF-I levels when used in young healthy men *(46)*. Some researchers suggest that adrenal androgens have age-related effects via the IGF system *(47–49)*. The role of thyroid hormones *(50)* and leptin *(12)*, both of which correlate positively with IGF-I in older subjects, is yet to be defined. Also worthy of consideration is the hypothalamus–pituitary–adrenal system, the activity of which declines with age in humans *(51,52)*. In rats glucocorticoids have been shown to suppress hepatic IGF-I expression when adequate nutrition is provided *(53)*.

5. NUTRITION AND THE IGF SYSTEM IN AGING

5.1. Overview

In the switch in metabolism from the use of exogenous nutrients to endogenous sources, insulin, GH, IGFs, and IGFBPs are important signaling factors. During fasting

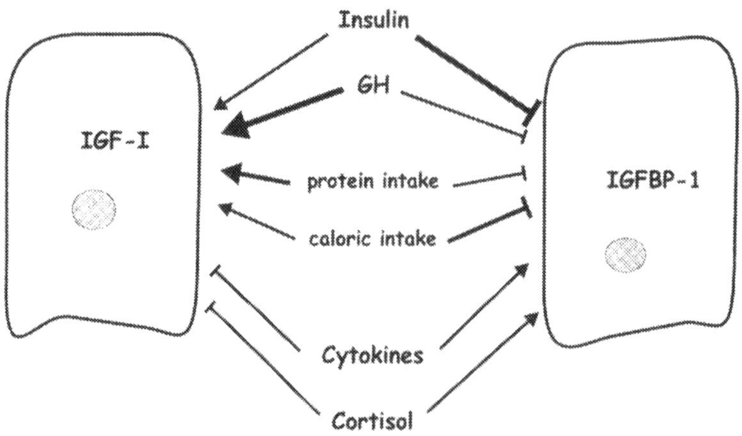

Fig. 2. Hepatic IGF-I and IGFBP-1 are inversely controlled by common regulators.

declining insulin levels lead to a decrease in glucose uptake in muscle and adipose tissue. There is also a contribution from decreased IGF-I expression and bioavailability caused by increased IGFBP-1. Reduced bioavailability of IGFs also leads to feedback inhibition in the pituitary and GH increases with fasting in humans. GH mobilizes FFA from the adipose stores and causes insulin resistance. Concomitantly, there is induction of GH resistance further reducing IGF-I expression. Humans and rats have different patterns of GH regulation during fasting *(54)* and therefore extrapolation from rodent studies to the human should be made with caution. There are additional differences in the GH–IGF axis between species. For example in the rat, IGF-II is highest in the fetus, declines rapidly and has disappeared from the circulation at the time of weaning *(55)*.

An inverse relationship between IGF-I and IGFBP-1 is seen throughout the lifespan, in health and in disease. Common nutritional regulators may have opposite effects on the expression of IGF-I and IGFBP-1 (Fig. 2).

5.2. Effect of Nutrition on the IGF System

The IGF-I assays, first developed to evaluate GH status, have proven to be valuable tools in the evaluation of undernutrition. The effect of prolonged fasting on IGF-I in adults, and its correlation with the change in urinary urea nitrogen excretion, were noted 20 yr ago *(56,57)*. This occurs despite increased GH levels, leading to the concept of acquired GH resistance leading to IGF-I deficiency (*see* Chapter 2). The rate of decline in IGF-I level during fasting in patients with acromegaly (K. Brismar et al, personal communication) is similar to that previously reported in healthy nonobese adults *(58)*. The increase in IGF-I levels during refeeding after fasting requires both calories and proteins containing essential amino acids *(54)*. The balance between protein and caloric intake and energy expenditure to optimize IGF levels has been studied in healthy young adults and newborns but similar studies in older individuals are notably lacking. There is a lesser effect of prolonged fasting on IGF-II *(54)*, although this has not been studied specifically in the elderly.

With age, there may be different IGFBP responses to caloric and protein restriction. For example, during protein restriction, IGFBP-3 decreases in young adults but not in children, while the opposite occurs during caloric restriction *(59)*. In both age groups IGFBP-2 increased during protein restriction, but a rapid response to refeeding was observed only in children. An increase in IGFBP-2 has also been observed in patients with anorexia nervosa *(60)*, suggesting that it might a useful marker of protein restriction. In the latter study ALS concentrations were found to be decreased throughout life. The effect of short term nutrition changes on ALS requires additional studies.

Reduced nutrition may make an important contribution to the wide variation of IGF-I levels in elderly and to the fall in IGF-I with aging. It is well known that food intake and its quality declines in later life. Aging is also associated with decreased nutrient absorption, although this appears to relate to the diseases associated with aging, rather than aging *per se (61)*. In the Framingham study, in subjects 72 yr of age and older, IGF-I was not related to body composition but strongly related to nutritional status *(62)*. In an ongoing longitudinal study of elderly above 80 yr, we have observed a significant correlation between changes in IGF-I levels over a 3-yr period and changes in the consumption of dairy products and fish, but not with changes in body weight *(63)*. Low insulin levels associated with low caloric content in the diet may contribute to an IGF-I decrease. The role of insulin in the regulation of IGF-I may change with age, as insulin resistance increases to peak at around 80 yr and is markedly decreased in survivors above 90 yr *(41)*.

Specific nutritional components may have a marked effect on the IGF system. Impaired IGF-I responses to protein malnutrition are due to a postreceptor defects in GH action *(64–66)*. During malnutrition, the concentrations of several essential amino acids are decreased both in plasma and red blood cells in a pattern similar to hemodialysis patients *(67)*. Rat studies have shown that a low protein diet decreases IGF-I and increases the hepatic expression of IGFBP-1 and -2 *(68)*. In primary cultured hepatocytes withdrawal of single amino acids stimulates the expression of IGFBP-1 *(69)* and a response element to amino acid withdrawal has been observed in the IGFBP-1 promoter *(70)*. Specific nutrient effects on the IGF system are reviewed more extensively in Chapters 2 and 5.

5.3. The IGF System as a Marker of Nutrition

Serum IGF-I concentrations have been used in the assessments of nutritional status of elderly. Some researchers who have used reliable assays without interference of IGFBPs report that IGF-I is a better marker of nutritional status than commonly used markers, while others have not found any advantage of using IGF-I determination. The role of IGF-I as a marker of nutritional status is covered in more detail in Chapter 4.

Amongst the IGFBPs in the circulation only IGFBP-1 displays rapid variation, reflecting the insulin levels and insulin sensitivity of the liver (Chapter 14). In short-term studies of fasting and refeeding IGFBP-1 reflects prevailing insulin concentrations. Although IGFBP-1 levels display this diurnal variation, the fasting IGFBP-1 level in the morning can be used as a marker of mean insulin levels throughout the day *(71)*. Elevated IGFBP-1 levels in relation to insulin levels are seen in many catabolic conditions, such as GH deficiency and renal failure *(67,71)*. Other regulators of IGFBP-1, such as cytokines, glucagon, and catecholamines, may contribute to the stimulation in these conditions *(25)*. IGFBP-1 is a predictor of survival in severe catabolic stress *(72)*. The cause of the increase in IGFBP-1 with age in not known. One possibility is relative protein malnutrition, because amino acids activate a pathway that inhibits IGFBP-1 *(73,74)*.

6. AGING-RELATED DISORDERS

A change in the IGF system has been observed in a variety of disorders associated with aging. Whether these changes are a cause or an effect of the disease is not established. Many diseases are covered in detail in other chapters. Therefore, we will discuss briefly only a few conditions with a specific impact in the elderly.

6.1. Dementia

The role of the IGF system in brain function, as proposed by Sara et al. *(75)*, is now well documented in animal studies. It is postulated that many of the effects of brain aging, including behavior and memory, are an outcome of IGF-I deficiency and decreased IGF-I receptor expression *(76,77)*. In a study in humans, lower IGF-I levels are associated with a higher prevalence of dementia *(78)*. Nutritional status may also be important in cognitive function, although this is less clear in aging *(79)*, and its interaction with the IGF system needs to be defined. IGFBPs may have specific roles in the aging nervous system. IGFBPs are measurable in cerebral spinal fluid, where there are clear age-related changes, including decreasing IGFBP-2 and -4 and increasing IGFBP-3 and -5 *(80)*.

6.2. Osteoporosis

Apart from gonadal steroids, the IGFs and their binding proteins have been proposed to play a role in the development of osteoporosis. There is conflicting evidence in the literature of a relationship between bone composition and IGF-I with age with some studies showing an association *(81)*, and others none *(78,82)*. Only longitudinal studies can clarify whether IGF-I is a predictor of bone loss. Local IGF-I in iliac crest cancellous bone predicts the bone volume better than circulating IGF-I *(83)*. Study of femoral cortical bone from men and women aged 20–64 yr shows linear declines in IGF-I, transforming growth factor-β, and IGFBP-5 *(84)*. The relationships among IGF proteins, nutrition and osteoporosis are reviewed more extensively in Chapter 10.

6.3. Muscle Wasting

Clinical studies suggest that in old women IGF-I concentrations are associated with poor muscle strength and reduced mobility *(85)*. Studies in aging rodents have documented increasing skeletal muscle resistance to IGF-I, particularly to the stimulation of protein synthesis *(86)*, as the result of a decrease in IGF-I receptor number *(87)*. In old rats, continued exercise training can restore the lack of response in IGF-I and IGF-I receptor mRNA to a mechanical load *(88)*. Localized IGF-I transgene expression also preserves muscle architecture and regenerative capacity during aging *(89)*.

6.4. Insulin Resistance, Diabetes, and Cardiovascular Disease

Although the IGF system is a useful marker for insulin resistance in older age *(90)*, its role as a predictor of cardiovascular risk is less clear. Low serum IGFBP-1 has been associated with an unfavorable cardiovascular marker risk profile in old subjects *(11,19)*. In contrast to studies that use cardiovascular markers as end points, we have observed that low IGFBP-1 levels, high levels of IGF-I, and high concentrations of total cholesterol are significant predictors of 3-yr survival in 82- to 97-yr-olds. When the IGFBP-1 level was used as continuous variable in logistic analyses, each doubling of IGFBP-1 levels increased 3-year mortality threefold *(91)*. This also suggests that the relevance of cardiovascular markers, such as plasma lipid profiles, should be reevaluated in very old age. A more detailed discussion of insulin resistance, diabetes mellitus, and cardiac failure is presented in Chapters 14 and 17.

6.5. Reduced Immune Function

One study in old compared with young adults has suggested that reduction in circulating IGF-I concentrations may contribute to a decrease in immunocompetence because concentrations correlate with a number of immune parameters *(92)*. The connection between the neuroendocrine and immune systems is well described. The effect of GH or IGF-I on thymus architecture and cell function has been reviewed elsewhere *(93)*. The administration of IGF-I appears to improve immune function in aged female monkeys *(94)*.

7. LONGEVITY AND THE IGF SYSTEM

The observation that caloric restriction can extend the life span in many species provides evidence of another possible link to IGF-regulated pathways in aging. It should be noted that the "caloric restriction" in animal studies is defined as the controlled provision of a balanced caloric intake, which is 60 to 70% of ad libitum feeding, and does not infer acute starvation or malnutrition, which decreases life expectancy. The fall in IGF-I with age may contribute to the aging phenotype, but it may play an important role in reducing the risk of pathologies, including malignancy (*see* Chapter 18). It is important that these interrelationships are clarified before recommendations can be made regarding manipulation of this system in human aging.

The IGF system is clearly involved in highly conserved pathways regulating longevity in many organisms. However, whether IGFs are central to the aging process in mammals is far from proven. Not all mutations in the insulin-IGF-I pathway extend lifespan, and some decrease it *(95)*. IGF-I has been shown to enhance telomerase activity in mononuclear cells and may play an essential role in the regulation of telomere length, thus participating in the cell's capacity for replication *(96)*. Some patients with progeria, which is a disease characterized by several features of premature aging, have reduced telomere length *(97)*. It has been reported that these patients also have low IGF-I levels *(98)*.

7.1. Animal Models of Decelerated Aging

The insulin/IGF-I signaling system has been implicated in the control of longevity. Single gene mutations in yeast, nematodes, and insects increase life span independently of growth and body size *(95)*. For example, in *Caenorhabditis elegans*, mutation of *daf-2*, which encodes an insulin/IGF receptor, increases lifespan by 200% *(99)*. In the fruit fly, mutation of the insulin-like receptor *(100)* and loss of insulin receptor substrate protein *(101)* significantly extends longevity.

Some IGF activity is essential for life. Many IGF-I and IGF-I receptor null mice die in the early neonatal period *(102)*. A number of mouse models of decelerated aging have been described. Most notably, those with decreased GH secretion or absent GH receptor have increased life expectancy. The Ames dwarf mouse, which has the homozygous mutation *Prop-1df (103)*, and the Snell dwarf mice, which is homozygous for the *Pit1dw* mutation show similar extensions of lifespan *(104)*. These mouse models have a propensity to obesity and, in the Snell dwarf mice, the increased longevity is most pronounced when combined with caloric restriction *(105)*. Animals with targeted disruption of the GH receptor have longevity associated with decreased IGF-I and IGFBP-3 concentrations and small size *(106)*. The phenotype of each of these animal model shares many of the characteristics described in animal models of caloric restriction.

7.2. Caloric Restriction in Rodents

Reductions in caloric intake have been shown to reduce age-related pathologies and increase lifespan *(77,107)*. In rodents it has been shown that caloric restriction prevents the age-related decline in GH pulses. Although plasma IGF-I concentrations decrease by about 40% early in life in relation to reduced food intake, there is no further age-related decline *(108)*. There are clear decreases in insulin concentrations and increases in insulin sensitivity. Sonntag and coworkers propose that there is an increase in IGF activity through increased paracrine IGF production and IGF receptor expression *(4)*. These effects of caloric restriction and aging on the GH/IGF axis in rodents are illustrated in Fig. 3. Because evidence points to an obligatory role for the IGF-I receptor in carcinogenesis, it is also proposed that a decrease in IGF-I signaling mediates the anti-carcinogenic effects of caloric restriction *(109)*.

7.3. Longevity in Primates

At first glance, conclusions about survival from studies in rodents seem to be contradictory to what we know in humans. Although there is anecdotal evidence that, similar to the Ames mice *(103)*, *Prop-1* mutations in humans may be associated with delayed aging *(110)*, GH-deficient humans have increased mortality from cardiovascular disease *(111)*.

Individuals who survive above 100 yr have higher-than-predicted IGF levels *(15)*. In the age group above 80 yr, the 3-yr survival is positively associated with IGF-I levels and inversely related to IGFBP-1 levels *(91)*. We should therefore be cautious about extrapolating from the studies of caloric restriction in animals to humans. Studies of dietary restriction in primates are underway *(112)*.

8. SUMMARY AND CONCLUSIONS

Total IGF-I concentrations in adults decrease with age. IGFBP-3 and ALS, important determinants of the ternary complex, decline to a lesser extent than IGF-I with aging. It is not clear whether tissue IGF activity changes with age. The fall in circulating IGF-I has been attributed to a decline in GH activity but other factors are likely to be involved. There is no definite evidence of a decrease in GH sensitivity with increasing age. In caloric and protein malnutrition IGF-I also decreases and there is a clear decline in GH-stimulated hepatic IGF-I production. Insulin could play a role in the response to caloric undernutrition, whereas in protein deficiency post-receptor GH resistance may predominate. IGFBP-1 is nutritionally regulated throughout life, with a pattern that is opposite to IGF-I. In addition to IGF-I, IGFBP-1 has been used as a marker of nutritional status as well as survival.

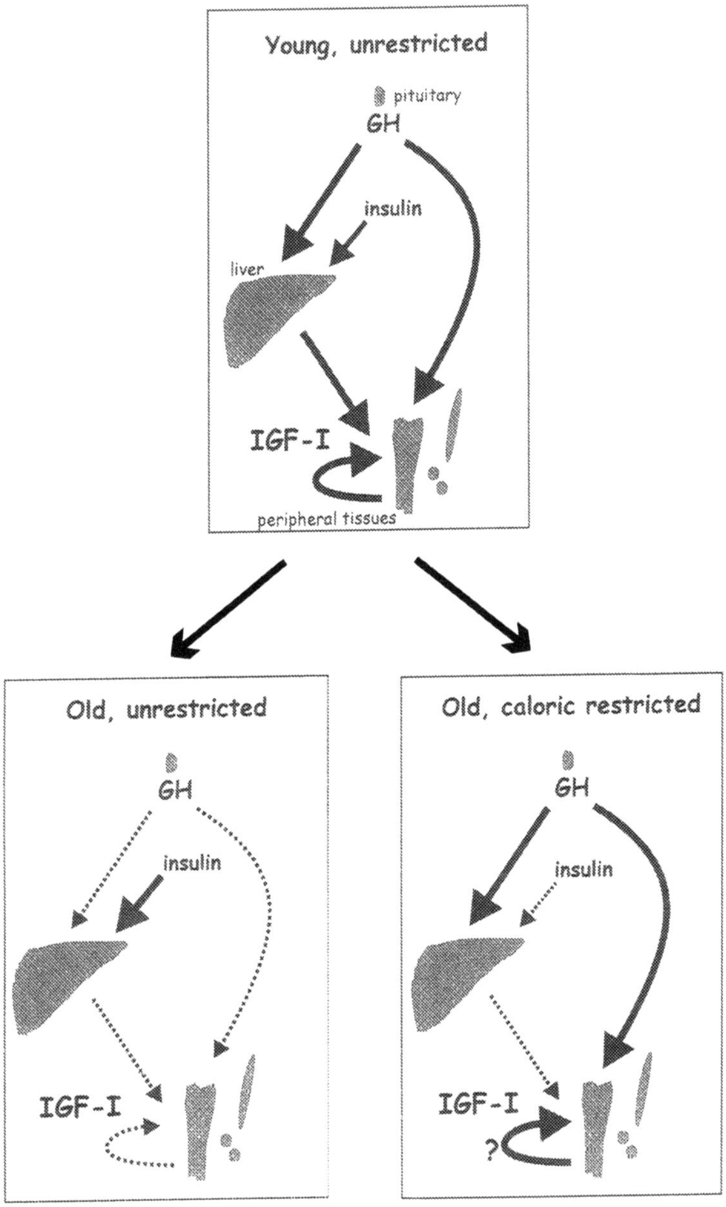

Fig. 3. Effect of caloric restriction on the IGF system in old mice and rats. The figures are based on the work by Sonntag and coworkers *(4)*, with addition of the changes in insulin.

9. CHALLENGES AND RECOMMENDATIONS FOR THE FUTURE

It is clear that we are a long way from understanding the relationship between various nutritional factors and the IGF system during the aging process. Specific nutritional recommendations that might optimally modify the IGF system or IGF-specific therapies that might ameliorate aging-related problems are therefore impossible at this stage. Nevertheless, age-related disabilities are a growing social and economic burden that may ultimately be addressed by such interventions.

9.1. Are the IGF/IGFBPs Better Indicators of Malnutrition in Adults Than Other Assessments?

A simple method of evaluating anabolism is needed for adults in the same way that growth rate is used in children. The recently developed reliable IGF and IGFBP assays are candidates and the levels need to be carefully validated in relation to lean body mass and compared with currently used methods.

9.2. What Are the Nutritional Requirements Throughout Adulthood?

It is likely that nutritional requirements change with age, so that the optimum caloric, protein, and micronutrient intake need to be defined for each decade of life. This will only be achieved by well controlled longitudinal studies, such as those performed in children.

9.3. Why Do IGF-I Levels Decline With Age?

Is a fall in GH production really the main cause of age-dependent decline in IGF-I? How does increasing age change the effect of insulin and its sensitivity on the GH-induced hepatic IGF-I release? More studies are required to determine the factors that induce endocrine or paracrine IGF-I expression and secretion.

9.4. What Role Has IGF-I Sensitivity for the Wide Variation of IGF-I Levels?

Only longitudinal studies can clarify whether each healthy individual maintains their IGF-I SD score throughout life. The presence and determinants of IGF resistance have not received much attention compared to the study of insulin resistance. Further research should focus on the changes in IGF sensitivity with age.

9.5. Is High IGF-I Appropriate and of Benefit in Older Age?

The finding of relatively high IGF-I levels in healthy centenarians may indicate a beneficial effect of IGF-I for longevity, but we are lacking information about the IGF-I SD score of these individuals earlier in life. Possible deleterious effects of more bioavailable IGF with age should not be overlooked, such as the risk of malignancy or cardiovascular disease.

9.6. If High IGF-I Is Good, Then How Do We Effectively Increase It?

At present, trials of exogenous treatment with GH alone or IGF-I alone in the elderly should not be undertaken. The former has been linked to increased mortality in catabolic patients and the latter would suppress endogenous GH with unknown effects on paracrine IGF-I. We believe that the best approach would be one that promotes endogenous IGF-I secretion and this may be achieved by providing optimal nutrition.

9.7. Is IGFBP-1 a Marker of Longevity?

The predictive value of IGFBP-1, as well as IGF-I, on survival and longevity needs to be evaluated in prospective population-based studies.

9.8. What Is the Role of Changes in the Profile and Function of IGFBPs Throughout Life?

Study of the modulation and activity of IGFBP at the tissue level is a developing field of research from which new therapeutic approaches might arise.

ACKNOWLEDGMENTS

We acknowledge the support from the Swedish Medical Foundation (04224) and the Torsten and Ragnar Söderberg Foundation. We are grateful to Agneta Hilding for data analysis.

REFERENCES

1. Le Roith D, Bondy C, Yakar S, Liu JL, Butler A. The somatomedin hypothesis: 2001. Endocr Rev 2001;22:53–74.
2. Tollet-Egnell P, Flores-Morales A, Odeberg J, Lundeberg J, Norstedt G. Differential cloning of growth hormone-regulated hepatic transcripts in the aged rat. Endocrinology 2000;141:910–921.
3. Zapf J, Hauri C, Waldvogel M, Futo E, Häsler H, Binz K, Guler HP, Schmid C, Froesch ER. Recombinant human insulin-like growth factor I induces its own specific carrier protein in hypophysectomized and diabetic rats. Proc Natl Acad Sci USA 1989;86:3813–3817.
4. Sonntag WE, Lynch CD, Cefalu WT, Ingram RL, Bennett SA, Thornton PL. Pleiotropic effects of growth hormone and insulin-like growth factor (IGF)-1 on biological aging: inferences from moderate caloric restricted animals. J Gerontol 1999;54:B521–B538.
5. Goldstein S, Moerman EJ, Baxter RC. Accumulation of insulin-like growth factor binding protein-3 in conditioned medium of human fibroblasts increases with chronologic age of donor and senescence in vitro. J Cell Physiol 1993;156:294–302.
6. Yamamoto H, Sohmiya M, Oka N, Kato Y. Effects of aging and sex on plasma insulin-like growth factor I (IGF-I) levels in normal adults. Acta Endocrinol (Copenh) 1991;124:497–500.
7. Juul A, Bang P, Hertel NT, Main K, Dalgaard P, Jorgensen K, Muller J, Hall K, Skakkebaek NE. Serum insulin-like growth factor-I in 1030 healthy children, adolescents, and adults: Relation to age, sex, stage of puberty, testicular size, and body mass index. J Clin Endocrinol Metab 1994;78:744–752.
8. Kitano M, Shimizu T, Yamazaki Y, Umezu Y, Arakawa Y, Daimon Y. Serum insulin-like growth factor-I (IGF-I) in normal Japanese adults. Endocr J 1995;42:767–770.
9. Benbassat CA, Maki KC, Unterman TC. Circulating levels of insulin-like growth factor (IGF) binding protein-1 and -3 in aging men: relationships to insulin, glucose, IGF, and 18 dehydroepiandrosterone sulfate levels and andropometric measures. J Clin Endocrinol Metab 1997;82:1484–1491.
10. Ceda GP, Dallaglio E, Magnacavallo A, Vargas N, Fontana V, Maggio M, Valenti G, Lee PDK, Hintz RL, Hoffman AR. The insulin-like growth factor axis and plasma lipid levels in the elderly. J Clin Endocrinol Metab 1998;83:499–502.
11. Janssen JAMJL, Stolk RP, Pols H, Grobbee DE, Lamberts SWJ. Serum total IGF-I, free IGFI, and IGFBP-1 levels in an elderly population—relation to cardiovascular risk factors and disease. Arterioscler Thromb Vasc Biol 1998;18:277–282.
12. Seck T, Englaro P, Blum WF, Scheidtnave C, Rascher W, Ziegler R, Pfeilschifter J. Leptin concentrations in serum from a randomly recruited sample of 50- to 80-year-old men and women—positive association with plasma insulin-like growth factors (IGFs) and IGF-binding protein-3 in lean, but not in obese, individuals. Eur J Endocrinol 1998;138:70–75.
13. Hilding A, Hall K, Wivall-Helleryd IL, Saaf M, Melin AL, Thorén M. Serum levels of insulinlike growth factor I in 152 patients with growth hormone deficiency, aged 19–82 years, in relation to those in healthy subjects. J Clin Endocrinol Metab 1999;84:2013–2019.
14. Clemmons DR. Commercial assays available for insulin-like growth factor I and their use in diagnosing growth hormone deficiency. Horm Res 2001;55:73–79.
15. Paolisso G, Ammendola S, Delbuono A, Gambardella A, Riondino M, Tagliamonte MR, Rizzo MR, Carella C, Varricchio M. Serum levels of insulin-like growth factor-I (IGF-I) and IGF-binding pro-

tein-3 in healthy centenarians—relationship with plasma leptin and lipid concentrations, insulin action, and cognitive function. J Clin Endocrinol Metab 1997;82:2204–2209.
16. Harrela M, Koistinen H, Kaprio J, Lehtovirta M, Tuomilehto J, Eriksson J, Tolvanen L, Koskenvuo M, Leinonen P, Koistinen R, Seppälä M. Genetic and environmental components of interindividual variation in circulating levels of IGF-I, IGF-II, IGFBP-1, and IGFBP-3. J Clin Invest 1996;98:2612–2615.
17. Hong Y, Pedersen NL, Brismar K, Hall K, de Faire U. Quantitative genetic analyses of insulin-like growth factor I (IGF-I), IGF-binding protein-1, and insulin levels in middle –aged and elderly twins. J Clin Endocrinol Metab 1996;81:1791–1797.
18. Zapf J, Walter H, Froesch ER. Radioimmunological determination of insulinlike growth factors I and II in normal subjects and in patients with growth disorders and extrapancreatic tumor hypoglycemia. J Clin Invest 1981;68:1321–1330.
19. Harrela M, Koistinen R, Tuomilehto J, Nissinen A, Seppälä M. Low serum insulin-like growth factor-binding protein-1 is associated with an unfavourable cardiovascular risk profile in elderly men. Ann Med 2000;32:424–428.
20. Mohan S, Farley JR, Baylink DJ. Age-related changes in IGFBP-4 and IGFBP-5 levels in human serum and bone: implications for bone loss with aging. Prog Growth Factor Res 1995;6:465–473.
21. Baum HB, Biller BM, Katznelson L, Oppenheim DS, Clemmons DR, Cannistraro KB, Schoenfeld DA, Best SA, Klibanski A. Assessment of growth hormone (GH) secretion in men with adult-onset GH deficiency compared with that in normal men—a clinical research center study. J Clin Endocrinol Metab 1996;81:84–92.
22. Boisclair YR, Rhoads RP, Ueki I, Wang J, Ooi GT. The acid-labile subunit (ALS) of the 150 kDa IGF-binding protein complex: an important but forgotten component of the circulating IGF system. J Endocrinol 2001;170:63–70.
23. Juul A, Moller S, Mosfeldt-Laursen E, Rasmussen MH, Scheike T, Pedersen SA, Kastrup KW, Yu H, Mistry J, Rasmussen S, Muller J, Henriksen J, Skakkebaek NE. The acid-labile subunit of human ternary insulin-like growth factor binding protein complex in serum: hepatosplanchnic release, diurnal variation, circulating concentrations in healthy subjects, and diagnostic use in patients with growth hormone deficiency. J Clin Endocrinol Metab 1998;83:4408–4415.
24. Lewitt MS. Role of the insulin-like growth factors in the endocrine control of glucose homeostasis. Diab Res Clin Pract 1994;23:3–15.
25. Lee PDK, Giudice LC, Conover CA, Powell DR. Insulin-like growth factor binding protein-1: recent findings and new directions. Proc Soc Exp Biol Med 1997;216:319–357.
26. Janssen JA, Stolk RP, Pols HA, Grobbee DE, de Jong FH, Lamberts SW. Serum free IGF-I, total IGF-I, IGFBP-1 and IGFBP-3 levels in an elderly population: relation to age and sex steroid levels. Clin Endocrinol 1998;48:471–8.
27. Rutanen EM, Kärkkäinen T, Stenman UH, Yki-Järvinen H. Aging is associated with decreased suppression of insulin-like growth factor binding protein-1 by insulin. J Clin Endocrinol Metab 1993;77:1152–1155.
28. Juul A, Main K, Blum WF, Lindholm J, Ranke MB, Skakkebaek NE. The ratio between serum levels of insulin-like growth factor (IGF)-I and the IGF binding proteins (IGFBP-1, 2 and 3) decreases with age in healthy adults and is increased in acromegalic patients. Clin Endocrinol 1994;41:85–93.
29. Frystyk J, Skjaerbaek C, Dinesen B, Ørskov H. Free insulin-like growth factors (IGF-I and IGF-II) in human serum. FEBS Lett 1994;348:185–191.
30. Hoffman AR, Pyka G, Lieberman SA, Ceda GP, Marcus R. The somatopause. In: Growth Hormone and Somatomedins During Lifespan. Muller EE, Cocchi D, Locatelli V (eds.). Springer-Verlag, New York, 1992, pp. 265–274.
31. Corpas E, Harman SM, Blackman MR. Human growth hormone and human ageing. Endocr Rev 1993;14:20–39.
32. Clasey JL, Weltman A, Patrie J, Weltman JY, Pezzoli S, Bouchard C, Thorner MO, Hartman ML. Abdominal visceral fat and fasting insulin are important predictors of 24-hour GH release independent of age, gender, and other physiological factors. J Clin Endocrinol Metab 2001;86:3845–3852.
33. Chapman IM, Hartman ML, Pezzoli SS, Harrell FE, Hintz RL, Alberti KGMM, Thorner MO. Effect of aging on the sensitivity of growth hormone secretion to insulin-like growth factor-I negative feedback. J Clin Endocrinol Metab 1997;82:2996–3004.

34. Peino R, Cordido F, Penalva A, Alvarez CV, Dieguez C, Casanueva FF. Acipimox-mediated plasma free fatty acid depression per se stimulates growth hormone (GH) secretion in normal subjects and potentiates the response to other GH-releasing stimuli. J Clin Endocrinol Metab 1996;81:909–913.
35. Pontiroli AE, Manzoni MF, Malighetti ME, Lanzi R. Restoration of growth hormone (GH) response to GH-releasing hormone in elderly and obese subjects by acute pharmacological reduction of plasma free fatty acids. J Clin Endocrinol Metab 1996;81:3998–4001.
36. Nielsen S, Møller N, Christiansen JS, Jorgensen JO. Pharmacological antilipolysis restores insulin sensitivity during growth hormone exposure. Diabetes 2001;50:2301–8.
37. Segerlantz M, Bramnert M, Manhem P, Laurila E, Groop LC. Inhibition of the rise in FFA by Acipimox partially prevents GH-induced insulin resistance in GH-deficient adults. J Clin Endocrinol Metab 2001;86:5813–5818.
38. Lanzi R, Manzoni MF, Andreotti AC, Malighetti ME, Bianchi E, Sereni LP, Caumo A, Luzi L, Pontiroli AE. Evidence for an inhibitory effect of physiological levels of insulin on the growth hormone (GH) response to GH-releasing hormone in healthy subjects. J Clin Endocrinol Metab 1997;82:2239–2243.
39. Lieberman SA, Mitchell AM, Marcus R, Hintz RL, Hoffman AR. The insulin-like growth factor I generation test: resistance to growth hormone with aging and estrogen replacement therapy. Horm Metab Res 1994;26:229–233.
40. Fernholm R, Bramnert M, Hagg E, Hilding A, Baylink DJ, Mohan S, Thorén M. Growth hormone replacement therapy improves body composition and increases bone metabolism in elderly patients with pituitary disease. J Clin Endocrinol Metab 2000;85:4104–4112.
41. Barbieri M, Rosaria Rizzo M, Manze lla D, Paolisso G. Age-related insulin resistance: is it an obligatory finding? The lesson from healthy centenarians. Diabetes Metab Res Rev 2001;17:19–26.
42. Pfeilschifter J, Scheidtnave C, Leidigbruckner G, Woitge HW, Blum WF, Wuster C, Haack D, Ziegler R. Relationship between circulating insulin-like growth factor components and sex hormones in a population-based sample of 50- to 80-year-old men and women. J Clin Endocrinol Metab 1996;81:2534–2540.
43. Lecomte P, Lecureuil N, Lecureuil M, Lemonnier Y, Mariotte N, Valat C, Garrigue MA. Sex differences in the control of sex-hormone-binding globulin in the elderly: role of insulin-like growth factor-I and insulin. Eur J Endocrinol 1998;139:178–183.
44. Duursma SA, Bijlsma JWJ, Van Paassen HC, van Buul-Offers S, Skottner-Lundin A. Changes in serum somatomedin and growth hormone concentrations after 3 weeks oestrogen substitution in post-menopausal women. Acta Endocrinol (Copenh) 1984;106:527–531.
45. Johansson AG, Engstrom BE, Ljunghall S, Karlsson FA, Burman P. Gender differences in the effects of long term growth hormone (GH) treatment on bone in adults with GH deficiency. J Clin Endocrinol Metab 1999;84:2002–2007.
46. Bhasin S, Woodhouse L, Casaburi R, Singh AB, Bhasin D, Berman N, Chen X, Yarasheski KE, Magliano L, Dzekov C, Dzekov J, Bross R, Phillips J, Sinha-Hikim I, Shen R, Storer TW. Testosterone dose-response relationships in healthy young men. Am J Physiol Endocrinol Metab 2001;281:E1172-E1181.
47. Orentreich N, Brind JL, Rizer RL, Vogelman JH. Age changes and sex differences in serum dehydroepiandrosterone sulfate concentrations throughout adulthood. J Clin Endocrinol Metab 1984;59:551–555.
48. Nestler JE, Barlascini CL, Clore JN, Blackard WG. Dehydroepiadnrosterone reduces serum low density lipoprotein levels and body fat but does not alter insulin sensitivity in normal men. J Clin Endocrinol Metab 1988;66:57–61.
49. Morales AJ, Nolan JJ, Nelson JC, Yen SSC. Effects of replacement dose of dehydroepiandrosterone in men and women of advancing age. J Clin Endocrinol Metab1994;78:1360–1367.
50. Seck T, Scheidtnave C, Ziegler R, Pfeilschifter J. Positive association between circulating free thyroxine and insulin-like growth factor I concentrations in euthyroid elderly individuals. Clin Endocrinol 1998;48:361–366.
51. Van Cauter E, Leproult R, Kupfer DJ. Effects of gender and age on the levels and circadian rhythmicity of plasma cortisol. J Clin Endocrinol Metab 1996;81:2468–2473.
52. Deuschle M, Gotthardt U, Schweiger U, Weber B, Korner A, Schmider J, Standhardt H, Lammers CH, Heuser I. With aging in humans the activity of the hypothalamus-pituitary adrenal system increases and its diurnal amplitude flattens. Life Sci 1997;61:2239–2246.

53. Kritsch KR, Murali S, Adamo ML, Ney DM. Dexamethasone decreases serum and liver IGF-I and maintains liver IGF-I mRNA in parenterally fed rats. Am J Physiol Regul Integr Comp Physiol 2002;282:R528-R536.
54. Thissen JP, Ketelslegers JM, Underwood LE. Nutritional regulation of the insulin-like growth factors. Endocr Rev 1994;15:80–101.
55. Moses AC, Nissley SP, Short PA, Rechler MM, White RM, Knight AB, Higa OZ. Increased levels of multiplication-stimulating activity, an insulin-like growth factor, in fetal rat serum. Proc Natl Acad Sci USA 1980;77:3649–3653.
56. Clemmons DR, Klibanski A, Underwood LE, McArthur JW, Ridgway EC, Beitins IZ, Van Wyk JJ. Reduction of plasma immunoreactive somatomedin C during fasting in humans. J Clin Endocrinol Metab 1981;53:1247–1250.
57. Merimee TJ, Zapf J, Froesch ER. Insulin-like growth factors in the fed and fasted states. J Clin Endocrinol Metab 1982;55:999–1002.
58. Bang P, Brismar K, Rosenfeld RG, Hall K. Fasting affects serum insulin-like growth factors (IGFs) and IGF-binding proteins differently in patients with noninsulin-dependent diabetes mellitus versus healthy nonobese and obese subjects. J Clin Endocrinol Metab 1994;78:960–967.
59. Smith WJ, Underwood LE, Clemmons DR. Effects of caloric or protein restriction on insulinlike growth factor-I (IGF-I) and IGF-binding proteins in children and adults. J Clin Endocrinol Metab 1995;80:443–449.
60. Fukuda I, Hotta M, Hizuka N, Takano K, Ishikawa Y, Asakawa-Yasumoto K, Tagami E, Demura H. Decreased serum levels of acid-labile subunit in patients with anorexia nervosa. J Clin Endocrinol Metab 1999;84:2034–2036.
61. Russell RM. Factors in aging that effect the bioavailability of nutrients. J Nutr 2001;131:1359S–1361S.
62. Harris TB, Kiel D, Roubenoff R, Langlois J, Hannan M, Havlik R, Wilson P. Association of insulin-like growth factor-I with body composition, weight history, and past health behaviors in the very old: The Framingham Heart Study. J Am Geriatr Soc 1997;45:133–139.
63. Sääf M, Melin AL, Hansson L-O, Hilding A, Jacobsson H, Hall K. Bone density of femoral neck is associated to IGF-I, IGFBP-1 and cystatin C in elderly above 80 years of age. J Clin Endocrinol Metab (manuscript in preparation)
64. Smith SR, Edgar PJ, Pozefsky T, Chhetri MK, Prout TE. Growth hormone in adults with protein calorie malnutrition. Endocrinology 1974;39:53–62.
65. Maes M, Amand Y, Underwood LE, Maiter D, Ketelslegers J-M. Decreased serum insulinlike growth factor I response to growth hormone in hypophysectomized rats fed a low protein diet: evidence for a postreceptor defect. Acta Endocrinol (Copenh) 1988;117:320–326.
66. Maiter D, Fliesen T, Underwood LE, Maes M, Gerard G, Davenport ML, Ketelslegers JM. Dietary protein restriction decreases insulin-like growth factor I independent of insulin and liver growth hormone binding. Endocrinology 1989;124:2604–2611.
67. Divino Filho JC, Hazel SJ, Furst P, Bergstrom J, Hall K. Glutamate concentration in plasma, erythrocyte and muscle in relation to plasma levels of insulin-like growth factor (IGF)-I, IGF binding protein-1 and insulin in patients on haemodialysis. J Endocrinol 1998;156:519–527.
68. Hazel SJ, Nordqvist A-CS, Hall K, Nilsson M, Schalling M. Differential expression of IGF-I and IGF-binding protein-1 and -2 in periportal and perivenous zones of rat liver. J Endocrinol 1998;1–10.
69. Jousse C, Bruhat A, Ferrara M, Fafournoux P. Physiological concentration of amino acids regulates insulin-like-growth-factor-binding protein 1 expression. Biochem J 1998;334:147–53.
70. Takenaka A, Komori K, Morishita T, Takahashi SI, Hidaka T, Noguchi T. Amino acid regulation of gene transcription of rat insulin-like growth factor-binding protein-1. J Endocrinol 2000;164:R11–R16.
71. Hilding A, Brismar K, Degerblad M, Thorén M, Hall K. Altered relation between circulating levels of insulin-like growth factor-binding protein-1 and insulin in growth hormone-deficient patients and insulin-dependent diabetic patients compared to that in healthy subjects. J Clin Endocrinol Metab 1995;80:2646–2652.
72. Van den Berghe G. IGFBPs in critical illness. Growth Horm IGF Res 2000;10:A34 (Abstract).
73. Pao CI, Farmer PK, Begovic S, Villafuerte BC, Wu GJ, Robertson DG, Phillips LS. Regulation of insulin-like growth factor-I (IGF-I) and IGF-binding protein 1 gene transcription by hormones and provision of amino acids in rat hepatocytes. Mol Endocrinol 1993;7:1561–1568.

74. Straus DS, Burke EJ, Marten NW. Induction of insulin-like growth factor binding protein-1gene expression in liver of protein-restricted rats and in rat hepatoma cells limited for a single amino acid. Endocrinology 1993;132:1090–1100.
75. Sara VR, Hall K, Von Holtz H, Humbel R, Sjogren B, Wetterberg L. Evidence for the presence of specific receptors for insulin-like growth factors 1 (IGF-1) and 2 (IGF-2) and insulin throughout the adult human brain. Neurosci Lett 1982;34:39–44.
76. Aleman A, Verhaar HJ, De Haan EH, De Vries WR, Samson MM, Drent ML, Van der Veen EA, Koppeschaar HP. Insulin-like growth factor I and cognitive function in healthy older men. J Clin Endocrinol Metab 1999;84:471–475.
77. Sonntag WE, Lynch C, Thornton P, Khan A, Bennett S, Ingram R. The effects of growth hormone and IGF-1 deficiency on cerebrovascular and brain ageing. J Anat 2000;197:575–585.
78. Arai Y, Hirose N, Yamamura K, Shimizu K, Takayama M, Ebihara Y, Osono Y. Serum insulin-like growth factor-1 in centenarians: implications of IGF-1 as a rapid turnover protein. J Gerontol A Biol Sci Med Sci 2001;M79-M82.
79. Gonzalez-Gross M, Marcos A, Pietrzik K. Nutrition and cognitive impairment in the elderly. Br J Nutr 2001;86:313–321.
80. Arnold PM, Ma JY, Citron BA, Festoff BW. Insulin-like growth factor binding proteins in cerebrospinal fluid during human development and aging. Biochem Biophys Res Commun 1999;264:652–656.
81. Langlois JA, Rosen CJ, Visser M, Hannan MT, Harris T, Wilson PW, Kiel DP. Association between insulin-like growth factor-I and bone mineral density in older women and men: The Framingham Heart Study. J Clin Endocrinol Metab 1998;83:4257–4262.
82. Ravalia G, Forti P, Maioli F, Nesi B, Pratelli L, Cucinotta D, Bastagli L, Cavalli G. Body composition, sex steroid, IGF-I, and bone mineral status in aging men. J Gerontol A Biol Sci Med Sci 2000;55:M516-M521.
83. Seck T, Scheppach B, Scharla S, Diel I, Blum WF, Bismar H, Schmid G, Krempien B, Ziegler R, Pfeilschifter J. Concentration of insulin-like growth factor (IGF)-I and -II in iliac crest bone matrix from pre- and postmenopausal women: relationship to age, menopause, bone turnover, bone volume, and circulating IGFs. J Clin Endocrinol Metab 1998;83:2331–2337.
84. Nicolas V, Mohan S, Honda Y, Prewett A, Finkelman RD, Baylink DJ, Farley JR. An agerelated decrease in the concentration of insulin-like growth factor binding protein-5 in human cortical bone. Calcified Tissue International 1995;57:206–212.
85. Cappola AR, Bandeen-Roche K, Wand GS, Volpato S, Fried LP. Association of IGF-I levels with muscle strength and mobility in older women. J Clin Endocrinol Metab 2001;86:4139–4146.
86. Dardevet D, Sornet C, Attaix D, Baracos VE, Grizard J. Insulin-like growth factor-1 and insulin resistance in skeletal muscles of adult and old rats. Endocrinology 1994;134:1475–1484.
87. Dardevet D, Manin M, Balage M, Sornet C, Grizard J. Influence of low- and high-protein diets on insulin and insulin-like growth factor-I binding to skeletal muscle and liver in the growing rat. Br J Nutr 1991;65:47–60.
88. Owino V, Yang SY, Goldspink G. Age-related loss of skeletal muscle function and the inability to express the autocrine form of insulin-like growth factor-I (MGF) in response to mechanical overload. FEBS Lett 2001;505:259–263.
89. Musaro A, McCullagh K, Paul A, Houghton L, Dobrowolny G, Molinaro M, Barton ER, Sweeney HL, Rosenthal N. Localized IGF-1 transgene expression sustains hypertrophy and regeneration in senescent skeletal muscle. Nat Genet 2001;27:195–200.
90. Paolisso G, Tagliamonte MR, Rizzo MR, Carella C, Gambardella A, Barbieri M, Varricchio M. Low plasma insulin-like growth factor-1 concentrations predict worsening of insulinmediated glucose uptake in older people. J Am Geriat Soc 1999;47:1312–1318.
91. Hall K, Hilding A, Melin A, Sääf M. IGFBP-1 as survival marker in the elderly (abstract). Growth Horm IGF Res 2000;19:A34.
92. Krishnaraj R, Zaks A, Unterman T. Relationship between plasma IGF-I levels, in vitro correlates of immunity, and human senescence. Clin Immunol Immunopathol 1998;88:264–270.
93. Burgess W, Liu Q, Zhou J, Tang Q, Ozawa A, VanHoy R, Arkins S, Dantzer R, Kelley KW. The immune-endocrine loop during aging: role of growth hormone and insulin-like growth factor-I. Neuroimmunomodulation 1999;6:56–68.

94. Le Roith D, Yanowski J, Kaldjian EP, Jaffe ES, Leroith T, Purdue K, Cooper BD, Pyle R, Adler W. The effects of growth hormone and insulin-like growth factor I on the immune system of aged female monkeys. Endocrinology 1996;137:1071–1079.
95. Kenyon C. A conserved regulatory system for aging. Cell 2001;105:165–168.
96. Tu W, Zhang DK, Cheung PT, Tsao SW, Lau YL. Effect of insulin-like growth factor 1 on PHA-stimulated cord blood mononuclear cell telomerase activity. Br J Haematol 1999;104:785–794.
97. Allsopp RC, Vaziri H, Patterson C, Goldstein S, Younglai EV, Futcher AB, Greider CW, Harley CB. Telomere length predicts replicative capacity of human fibroblasts. Proc Natl Acad Sci USA 1992;89:10114–10118.
98. Abdenur JE, Brown WT, Fabre JMea. Endogenous growth hormone resistance and malnutrition in children with Hutchinson-Guildford progeria syndrome (HGP) (abstract). Pediatr Res 1991;29:73A.
99. Guarente L, Kenyon C. Genetic pathways that regulating ageing in model organisms. Nature 2000;408:255–262.
100. Tatar M, Kopelman A, Epstein D, Tu M-P, Yin C-M, Garofalo RS. A mutant Drosophila insulin receptor homolog that extends life-span and impairs neuroendocrine function. Science 2001;292:107–110.
101. Clancy DJ, Gems D, Harshman LG, Oldham S, Stocker H, Hafen E, Leevers SJ, Partridge L. Extension of life-span by loss of CHICO, a *Drosophila* insulin receptor substrate protein. Science 2001;292:104–106.
102. Liu J-P, Baker J, Perkins AS, Robertson EJ, Efstratiadis A. Mice carrying null mutations of the genes encoding insulin-like growth factor I (*Igf-1*) and the type 1 IGF receptor (*Igf1r*). Cell 1993;75:59–72.
103. Dozmorov I, Bartke A, Miller RA. Array-based expression analysis of mouse liver genes: effect of age and of the longevity mutant Prop1df. J Gerontol A Biol Sci Med Sci 2001;56:B72–B80.
104. Miller RA. Kleemier Award lecture: are there genes for aging? J Gerontol Biol Sci 1999;54A:B297–B307.
105. Flurkey K, Papaconstantinou J, Miller RA, Harrison DE. Lifespan extension and delayed immune and collagen aging in mutant mice with defects in growth hormone production. Proc Natl Acad Sci USA 2001;98:6736–6741.
106. Coschigano KT, Clemmons DR, Bellush LL, Kopchick JJ. Assessment of growth parameters and life span of GHR/BP gene-disrupted mice. Endocrinology 2000;14:2608–2613.
107. Weindruch R. The retardation of aging by caloric restriction: studies in rodents and primates. Toxicol Pathol 1996;24:742–745.
108. Breese CR, Ingram RL, Sonntag WE. Influence of age and long-term dietary restriction on plasma insulin-like growth factor-I (IGF-I), IGF-I gene expression, and IGF-I binding proteins. J Gerontol Biol Sci 1991;46:B180–B187.
109. Kari FW, Dunn SE, French JE, Barrett JC. Roles fror insulin-like growth factor-1 in mediating the anti/carcinogenic effects of caloric restriction. J Nutr Health Aging 1999;3:92–101.
110. Krzisnik C, Kolacio Z, Battelino T, Brown M, Parks J, Laron Z. The 'little people' of the Island of Krk—revisited. Etiology of hypopituitarism revealed. J Endocr Genet 1999;1:9–19.
111. Rosen T. Premature mortality due to cardiovascular disease in hypopituitarism. Lancet 1990;336:285–288.
112. Ramsey JJ, Colman RJ, Binkley NC, Christiansen JD, Gresl TA, Kemnitz JW, Weindruch R. Dietary restriction and aging in rhesus monkeys: the University of Wisconsin study. Exp Gerontol 2000;35:1131–1149.

IV IGF AND ORGAN SYSTEMS

10 Nutrition and Insulin Growth Factor-I in Relation to Bone Health and Disease

Jean-Philippe Bonjour, Patrick Ammann, Thierry Chevalley, and René Rizzoli

KEY POINTS

- At the skeletal level, IGF-I exerts a positive effect on bone mineral mass by a direct action on osteogenic cells.
- At the kidney level, IGF-I enhances both the renal reabsorption of inorganic phosphate (Pi) and the production of calcitriol, the hormonal form of vitamin D that stimulates the intestinal absorption of calcium and Pi, the two main bone mineral elements.
- Protein undernutrition reduces IGF-I production, decreases skeletal acquisition during growth, and accelerates bone loss during adulthood.
- The stimulation of bone formation in response to IGF-I is impaired in presence of an inadequately low intake of proteins.
- Protein undernutrition, probably by influencing negatively IGF-I production and action, contributes to the pathogenesis of osteoporotic fractures in elderly.

1. INTRODUCTION

The impact of nutrition on the insulin growth factor (IGF) system in relation to bone mineral mass gain and loss has been the subject of increasing attention over the last decade. Accumulating evidence strongly suggests that IGF-I plays an important role in bone metabolism. Both the production and action of this growth factor are selectively influenced by the dietary supply of proteins. Deficiency in protein intake is associated with low plasma IGF-I, decreased bone mineral mass, and increased risk of osteoporotic fracture. Observational and interventional human studies sustain the concept of an essential role of protein intake on the IGF-I axis in bone health. Laboratory investigations conducted in reliable animal models of osteoporosis bring strong support to this concept. In this chapter, the main clinical and experimental data that relate the protein intake–IGF-I axis to calcium–phosphate metabolism, bone mineral mass, and fragility fracture are considered.

From: *IGF and Nutrition in Health and Disease*
Edited by: M. S. Houston, J. M. P. Holly, and E. L. Feldman © Humana Press Inc., Totowa, NJ

The strongest evidence for the relationship among protein intake, IGF-I, and osteoporosis has been obtained from observational and then interventional studies in the elderly. Therefore, this aspect is presented first in this review. Then, the role of the protein intake–IGF-I axis in bone health and diseases at earlier adult periods and during childhood and adolescence are discussed.

2. PROTEIN INTAKE, IGF-I, AND OSTEOPOROSIS IN ELDERLY POPULATIONS

Among the determinants of osteoporosis in elderly populations, nutritional deficiencies certainly play a major contributing role *(1–6)*. Indeed, undernutrition is often observed in elderly, and it appears to be more severe in patients with hip fracture than in the general aging population *(7–11)*. Low body mass index, which can be interpreted as a crude "marker" of nutritional state, was found to be a major risk factor in a large prospective study of hip fracture incidence in men aged 50 yr or more living in several countries of southern Europe *(12)*. A variety of evidence also leads to the conclusion that protein intake below the Recommended Dietary Allowance could be particularly detrimental for the conservation of bone integrity with aging *(4,5)*. Indeed, undernutrition can accelerate age-dependent bone loss *(1,2,13,14)*. Protein undernutrition can favor the occurrence of hip fracture by increasing the propensity to fall as a result of muscle weakness, impairment in movement coordination, and/or by affecting protective mechanisms, such as reaction time, muscle strength, and/or by decreasing bone mass *(15–19)*. Furthermore, a reduction in the protective layer of soft tissue padding decreases the force required to fracture an osteoporotic hip *(10,20–23)*.

In association with the progressive age-dependent decrease in both protein intake and bone mass, several reports have documented a decrement in IGF-I plasma levels *(24–27)*. In elderly patients hospitalized for hip fracture a state of undernutrition has been consistently documented on admission *(9,10)*. It is followed by an inadequate food intake during hospital stay that can adversely influence the clinical outcome of hip fracture patients *(10,11)*. In hip fracture patients, in whom a lower femoral neck bone mineral density (BMD) at the level of the proximal femur has been demonstrated *(28)*, a dietary survey based on 50 precise daily measurements of food intake confirmed that nutritional requirements were not met while the patients were in the hospital, although adequate quantities of food were offered *(11)*. Undernutrition includes many nutrients, and the specific role of a low protein intake besides low calorie consumption can be difficult to appraise in the elderly *(16)*. In hip fracture patients, the plasma level of IGF-I was found to be decreased as compared with age-matched controls without fracture *(29)*. Serum IGF-I can be used as a sensitive marker of malnutrition in this population (reviewed in Chapter 4).

3. PROTEIN REPLENISHMENT, IGF-I, AND OSTEOPOROSIS

Intervention studies using supplementary feeding by nasogastric tube or parenteral nutrition *(30)* or even a simple oral dietary preparation that normalizes protein intake *(11)* can improve the clinical outcome after hip fracture. It should be emphasized that in the above-mentioned study *(11)*, a 20-g protein supplement brought the protein intake from low to a level still below the Recommended Daily Allowance (0.8 g/kg body weight). Follow-up showed a significant difference in the clinical course during subsequent rehabilitation hospitalization, with the supplemented patients doing better. Although the mean duration of dietary supplementation did not exceed 30 d, the significantly lower rate of complications (bedsore, severe anemia, undercurrent lung or renal infections, 44% vs 87%), and deaths was still observed at 6 mo (40% vs 74%) *(11)*. The duration of hospital stay of elderly patients with hip fracture is not only determined by the present medical condition but also by domestic and social factors *(10,31,32)*. The total length of stay in the orthopedic ward and convalescent hospital was significantly shorter in supplemented patients than in controls (median: 24 vs 40 d).

After the favorable outcome shown in hip fracture patients receiving a protein-calorie supplement *(11)*, the question as to whether protein represented the key nutrient responsible for the beneficial effect was addressed by comparing the clinical outcome of elderly patients with hip fracture (mean age 82 yr) who received two different dietary supplements that differed only in protein content *(33)*. A specific effect of protein supplements on outcome was demonstrated with 79% in the group receiving protein having a favorable course as compared with 36% in the control group during the stay in the recovery hospital.

In undernourished elderly patients with a recent hip fracture, an increase in the protein intake, from low to normal, can also be beneficial for bone integrity. Indeed, in a double-blind, placebo-controlled study, the effects of protein repletion were investigated in patients with a recent hip fracture *(29)*. Within 1 wk after an osteoporotic hip fracture, 82 patients (80.7 ± 1.2 yr) were randomly allocated to a daily 20-g protein supplement, which nearly corrected protein deficiency, or to an isocaloric placebo, for 6 mo. All were given 200,000 IU vitamin D once at baseline and 550 mg/d of calcium supplementation. As compared with the placebo group, the protein-supplemented patients had significantly greater gains in serum prealbumin, in IGF-I (Fig. 1), and in IgM *(29)*. In agreement with previous results *(11,33)*, protein repletion after hip fracture was associated with a more favorable outcome, including a shorter rehabilitation hospital stay. In a multiple regression analysis, baseline IGF-I concentrations and biceps muscle strength, together with the protein supplements, accounted for more than 30% of the variance in the length of stay in rehabilitation hospitals ($r^2 = 0.312$; $p < 0.0005$). These results support the hypothesis that the beneficial effects of protein repletion after hip fracture could be associated with a stimulation of the IGF-I system in the protein-supplemented patients. Thus, the lower incidence of medical complications observed after such a protein supplement *(11,33)* is also compatible with the hypothesis of IGF-I improving the immune status, as this growth factor can stimulate the proliferation of immunocompetent cells and modulate immunoglobulin secretion *(34)*. Importantly, the proximal femur BMD decrease observed at 1 yr in the placebo group was attenuated by approximately 50% (Fig. 2) *(29)*. These results are compatible with the hypothesis implying that in patients with hip fracture, correction of low protein intake would lead to normalization of IGF-I level, which in turn would increase both bone *(35)* and muscle mass and thus reduce the risk of subsequent osteoporotic fracture while reducing the number of medical complications (Fig. 3).

These results raise the question whether protein repletion of frail elderly could prevent the age-dependent decrease in IGF-I levels and thereby help to prevent falls and to increase bone mass. Indeed, a low IGF-I level has been shown to be a predictor of

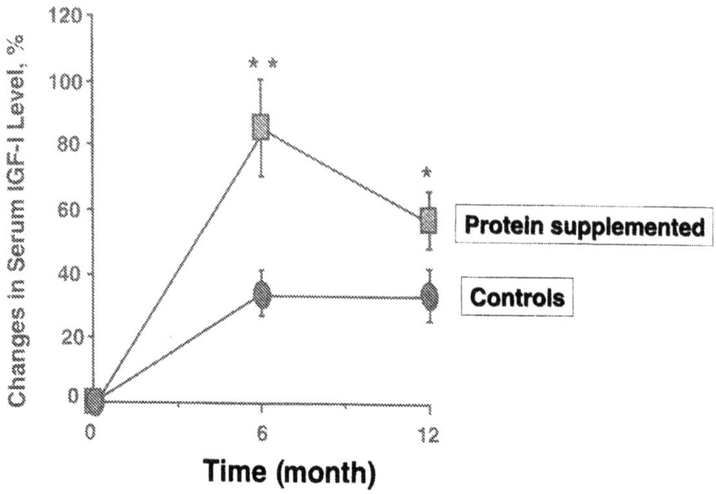

Fig. 1. Effect on plasma IGF-I levels of 20 g/d of milk-derived protein supplement in elderly subjects with a recent hip fracture. The protein supplement was taken over 6 mo. The control group received an isocaloric supplement containing no protein. Both groups were supplemented in calcium and vitamin D. The study was randomized, double blind, and placebo controlled. Mean ±SEM; $*p < 0.06$; $**p < 0.005$. From ref. *29*.

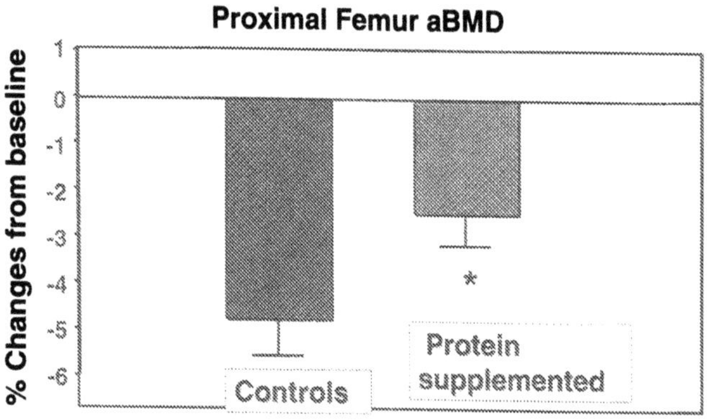

Fig. 2. Effect on change in femoral neck aBMD of 20 g/d of milk-derived protein supplement in elderly subjects with a recent hip fracture. The protein supplement was taken during 6 mo. The control group received an isocaloric supplement containing no protein. Both groups were supplemented in calcium and vitamin D. The study was randomized, double blind, and placebo controlled. Mean ± SEM; $*p < 0.05$. From ref. *29*.

fracture risk *(36)*. Our intervention study *(29)* stresses the impressive bone loss occurring during the months after a hip fracture in the patients who did not receive a protein-containing supplement (Fig. 2). This may explain why patients with osteoporotic fracture have at least a twofold increase in the experience of another fracture, including a second hip fracture *(37–40)*. This prompted our group to set up a dedicated clinical treatment pathway for the management of patients with low trauma fracture *(41)*. This pathway includes a multidisciplinary teaching program for patients and their fam-

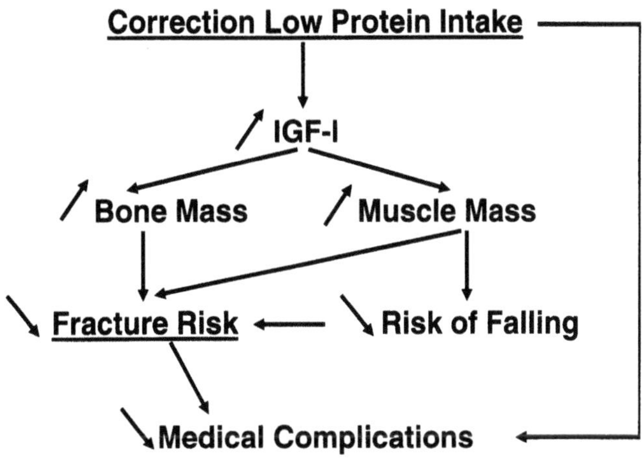

Fig. 3. Implication of the correction of low protein intake on the IGF-I axis in the pathogenesis of osteoporotic hip fracture and its medical complications in elderly.

ilies on physical therapy, daily living activities, and nutrition. Nutritional recommendations include the intake required for calcium, vitamin D, and protein, as well as very practical aspects.

4. EXPERIMENTAL STUDIES ON THE PROTEIN INTAKE–IGF-I–BONE AXIS

To evaluate the early cellular responses to protein deficiency in both cortical and trabecular bone, we submitted adult female rats to a diet with low protein content but isocaloric to the control diet. Histomorphometric and biochemical analyses were performed after 2 wk of protein deficiency, when plasma IGF-I was significantly lower in protein-restricted rats *(42,43)*. Thereafter, to investigate the bone cellular response to IGF-I, we administered a pharmacological dose of rh IGF-I/IGFBP-3 to 15% and 2.5% casein-fed rats for 10 d and evaluated its effects histologically and biochemically *(43)*. After 14 d of protein restriction, significant drops in periosteal formation and mineral apposition rates were observed, indicating a decreased osteoblast recruitment and activity. In rats fed the 15% casein diet, rh IGF/IGFBP-3 increased cancellous and periosteal formation rates, indicating an increased osteoblast recruitment. However, in protein-restricted rats, rh IGF/IGFBP-3 failed to increase cancellous or periosteal bone formation. The early response of bone cells activities to isocaloric low protein intake in adult female rats is envelope specific because short-term dietary protein restriction impairs periosteal bone formation in cortical bone but not in cancellous bone. In addition, dietary protein restriction induces an osteoblastic resistance to IGF-I in both envelopes. This may suggest that low plasma IGF-I and/or osteoblast resistance to IGF-I in response to low protein intake could play an important role in the impairment of periosteal osteoblasts. Moreover, these results suggest that therapeutic administration of IGF-I to subjects with a dietary protein deficiency may be ineffective on bone. This resistance to IGF-I action in states of undernutrition is in agreement with previous experimental studies on body growth *(44)*.

We investigated the influence of IGF-I on BMD in adult rats made osteoporotic by ovariectomy *(45–47)*. BMD was measured by dual-energy X-ray absorptiometry at the levels of lumbar spine, proximal, and total tibia *(48)*. This technique allows a precise and accurate in vivo longitudinal measurement of bone mineral mass, areal BMD (aBMD), and outer bone dimensions in rats, at various skeletal sites characterized by different proportions of cortical and trabecular bone, and thereby by different rates of bone remodeling and responses to dietary or hormonal manipulations. A 6-wk infusion of IGF-I induced a dose-dependent increment of BMD at the three scanned skeletal sites *(45)*. The increase in BMD induced by IGF-I was associated with an increase in the resistance to mechanical strain in relation also with an increase of bone shaft outer dimensions *(45,46)*.

The local production of IGF-I by osteoblastic cells in relation with amino acid concentrations could also play a role. Indeed, the amino acids arginine or lysine increased IGF-I production and collagen synthesis in cultured mice osteoblastic cells, in a time- and concentration-dependent manner *(49)*. This study suggests a possible influence of the local proteins or amino acid environment on IGF-I production by bone cells and suggests a potential role of locally produced IGF-I under the influence of extracellular amino acid concentration in the regulation of osteoblast function.

To address the issue of a specific influence of protein deficiency in the pathogenesis of osteoporosis, an experimental model in adult female or male rats of selective protein deprivation with isocaloric low protein diets supplemented by identical amounts of minerals has been developed *(42,43,50–52)*. This model enables the study of bone mineral mass, bone strength, and remodeling. A decrease of BMD was observed at the level of skeletal sites formed by trabecular or cortical bone only in animals fed 2.5% casein. This was associated with a marked and early decrease in plasma IGF-I by 40%. In this model, sex hormone deficiency or action was also observed, because estrous cycles disappeared under a long-term low protein isocaloric diet. The effects of ovariectomy and protein deficiency were additive, suggesting distinct mechanisms of action. Histomorphometric analysis and biochemical markers of bone remodeling indicate that the low protein intake-induced decrease in bone mineral mass and bone strength was related to an uncoupling between bone formation and resorption *(42,50,51)*. Dietary essential amino acid supplements given to adult rats made osteoporotic by estrogen deficiency and reduced protein intake increase bone strength *(53)*. This beneficial effect was mediated through modifications of BMD, trabecular architecture, and cortical thickness possibly by the associated increase in IGF-I and consecutive stimulation in osteoblastic bone formation *(53)*.

5. OTHER MECHANISMS POTENTIALLY INVOLVED IN PROTEIN-RELATED BONE LOSS

Beside the production and action of the growth hormone-IGF-I system, protein undernutrition can be associated with alterations of cytokine secretion, such as interferon gamma, tumor necrosis factor (TNF)-α, or transforming growth factor beta *(54,55)*. TNF-α and interleukin-6 generally increase with aging *(56)*. In a situation of cachexia, such as in chronic heart failure, an inverse correlation between BMD and TNF-α levels has been found *(57,58)*, further implicating a possible role of uncontrolled cytokines production in bone loss. Increased TNF-α can be a crucial factor in

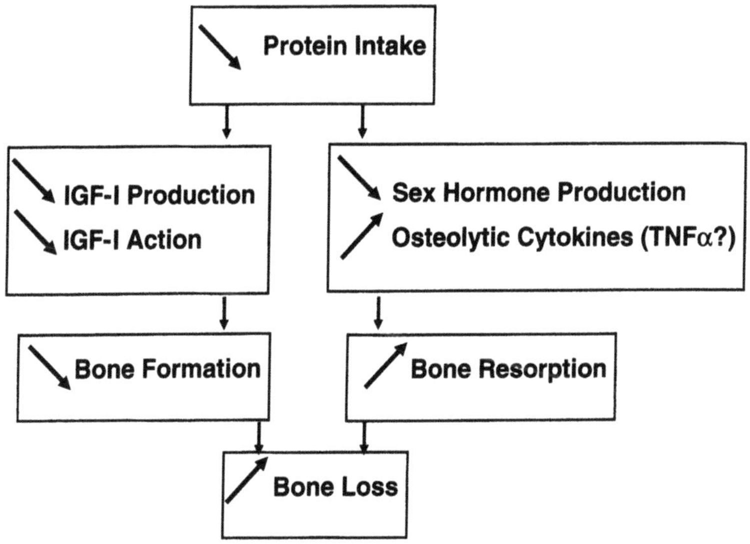

Fig. 4. Mechanisms of accelerated bone loss induced by low protein diet. The decrease in both IGF-I production and action could explain, at least in part, the negative influence of protein deficiency on bone formation. The associated increase in bone resorption appears to be mediated by both sex hormone dependent and independant mechanisms. Studies in transgenic animals suggest that TNF-α could contribute to the increased bone resorption. *See* text for further explanation with references in support of these relationships.

sex hormone deficiency-induced bone loss *(59)*, but it also plays a role in the target organ resistance to insulin and possibly to IGF-I *(60)*. Along the same lines, certain amino acids given to rats fed a low-protein diet can increase the liver protein synthesis response to TNF-α *(61)*. The amino acid oxidation rate is lower in children with kwashiorkor replete with milk as compared with egg white, and protein breakdown and synthesis correlated inversely with TNF-α levels *(62)*. The modulation by nutritional intake of cytokine production and action *(63)* and the strong implication of various cytokines in the regulation of bone remodeling *(64)* suggest a possible role of certain cytokines in the nutrition–bone link. As far as isocaloric protein deficiency-induced bone loss is concerned, the role of TNF-α is supported by studies in female transgenic mice expressing high levels of soluble TNF-α receptor *(65)*. In these transgenic mice, the increased bone resorption resulting in decreased bone mass and strength induced by selective protein under nutrition, was attenuated compared with soluble TNF-α receptor negative littermates. In contrast, the decrease in both IGF-I plasma level and bone formation rate was not affected in the transgenic animals *(65)*.

Figure 4 summarizes the factors (IGF-I, sex hormones, and TNF-α) that appear to mediate the negative uncoupling between bone formation and resorption in response to a selective protein deficiency, that is, without reducing the energy supply.

6. PROTEIN INTAKE AND BONE MASS IN YOUNG ADULTS

A positive correlation between protein intake and bone mass has been found in premenopausal women *(66–68)*. In women maintaining a low-calorie diet, insufficient protein intake could be particularly deleterious for bone mass integrity. In athletes or ballet dancers, intense exercise can lead to hypothalamic dysfunction with delayed menarche and disruption of menstrual cyclicity and bone loss *(69–73)*. Nutritional restriction can play an important role in disturbances of the female reproductive system resulting from intense physical activity. The propensity to nutritional restriction is more common when leanness confers a perceived advantage in athletic performance *(71)*. Insufficient energy intake with respect to energy expenditure supposedly impairs the secretion of gonadotropin-releasing hormone and thereby leads to a state of hypoestrogenism. However, the relative contribution of insufficient protein intake with low IGF-I remains to be assessed because it is frequently associated with reduction in energy intake. As discussed above, bone loss induced by isocaloric protein restriction in adult female rats is mediated by both reduced bone formation and increased bone resorption, which involves both dependent and independent sex-hormone deficiency mechanisms *(42,50,51)*.

Anorexia nervosa is a condition frequently observed in young women. BMD is reduced at several skeletal sites in most women with anorexia nervosa. It is not surprising that young women with anorexia nervosa are at increased risk of fracture later in life *(74)*. Body weight, but not estrogen use, is a significant predictor of BMD in women with anorexia nervosa *(75)*. Abnormally low serum albumin levels (≤36 g/L) and low body weight (≤60% of average body weight) at initial examination both were variables best able to predict a lethal course *(76)*. With estrogen and calcium deficiency, low protein intake very likely contributes to the bone loss observed in anorexia nervosa. Experimental evidence obtained in adult female rats indicates that supplying more carbohydrates cannot compensate for the detrimental effect exerted by a low protein intake on bone mass *(42)*. Surrogate markers of bone formation, serum osteocalcin, and bone specific alkaline phosphatase are significantly reduced *(77)*. Interestingly, IGF-I was the major correlate of bone formation markers in mature adolescents with anorexia nervosa *(77,78)*. Furthermore, IGF-I level changes were dependent on variations in the nutritional state *(78)*.

7. PROTEIN INTAKE AND BONE GROWTH

Several physiological functions influence bone accumulation during growth. Animal studies have identified physiological mechanisms that sustain increased bone mineral demand in relation to variations in growth velocity. In this context, two adaptive mechanisms affecting calcium-phosphate metabolism appear to be particularly important, namely increase in the plasma concentration of 1,25-dihydroxyvitamin D3 (calcitriol), and stimulation of the renal tubular reabsorption of inorganic phosphate (Pi). Elevation in the production and plasma level of calcitriol enhances the capacity of the intestinal epithelium to absorb both calcium and Pi. The increase in tubular reabsorption of Pi results in a rise in its extracellular concentration. Without these two concerted adaptive responses, growth and mineralization cannot be optimal. Note that the increase in tubular Pi reabsorption is not mediated by a rise in renal production or in the plasma level of calcitriol *(79)*.

Analysis of cross-sectional studies suggests that these two adaptive mechanisms could be essential to cope with the increased bone mineral demand during the pubertal growth spurt. An increase in plasma calcitriol concentrations has been reported during pubertal maturation *(80)*. A close relationship exists between the tubular reabsorption of Pi, the plasma Pi level, and growth velocity in children *(81)*. A rise in plasma Pi during puberty has been reported *(82)*.

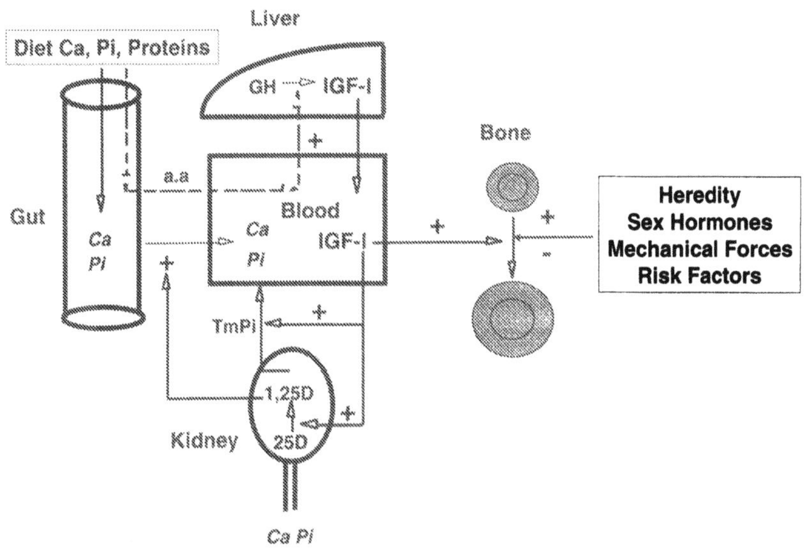

Fig. 5. Role of IGF-I in calcium phosphate metabolism during childhood and pubertal maturation in relation to essential nutrients for bone growth. During the pubertal bone growth spurt there is a rise in circulating IGF-I. The hepatic production of IGF-I is under the positive influence of GH and essential amino acids (aa). IGF-I stimulates bone growth. At the kidney level, IGF-I increases both the 1,25-dihydroxyvitamin D (1,25 D) conversion from 25-hydroxyvitamin D (25D) and the maximal tubular reabsorption of inorganic phosphate (TmPi). By this dual renal action IGF-I favors a positive calcium and phosphate balance as required by the increased bone mineral accrual. Heredity, sex hormones, mechanical forces, and risk factors can either positively or negatively influence the bone response to IGF-I. *See* text for further details.

The mechanism underlying the parallel rise in calcitriol and the tubular reabsorption of Pi has been clarified. One single factor, that is, IGF-I, appears to be responsible for the stimulation of both calcitriol production and tubular Pi reabsorption (TmPi/GFR) in relation to the increased calcium and Pi demand associated with bone growth *(79,83)*. In humans, plasma levels of IGF-I raise transiently during pubertal maturation, reaching a peak during midpuberty, with the maximal level thus occurring at an earlier chronological age in females than in males *(84)*. The role of IGF-I in calcium phosphate metabolism during pubertal maturation in relation with essential nutrients for bone growth is illustrated in Fig. 5. The rise in plasma levels of IGF-I, calcitriol, and Pi are correlated with elevation in indices of the bone appositional rate, such as alkaline phosphatase *(85–88)* and osteocalcin *(87–90)*. Note that the plasma concentrations of gonadal sex hormones, as well as those of adrenal androgens (dehydroepiandrosterone and androstenedione), which increase before and during pubertal maturation, do not seem to accord with the accelerated bone mass gain *(91,92)*. Whether differences in the adaptive responses, which control calcium and phosphate homeostasis, could play a role in the increased variance in lumbar spine or femoral neck BMD/bone mineral content (BMC) remains to be explored. As recently reviewed, the interaction between the growth hormone–IGF I axis and sex steroids is quite complex *(88)*.

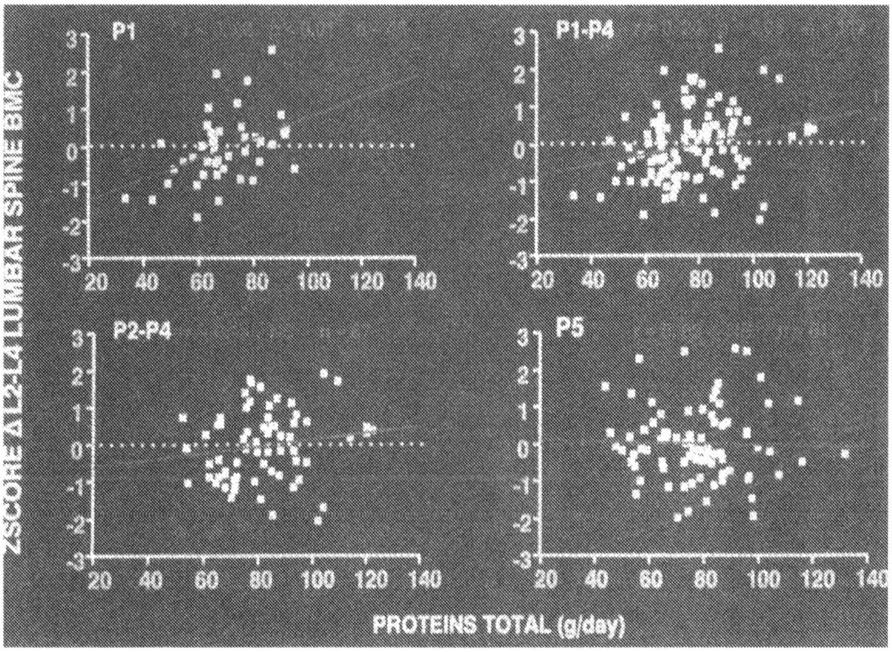

Fig. 6. Relation between protein intake and change in lumbar BMC in pre-, peri-, postpubertal female and male adolescents. The mean protein intake from dairy, vegetable, and mineral sources was recorded in two 5-d diet diaries at a 1-yr interval. A positive correlation was found in prepupertal (P1) but neither in peripubertal (P2–P4) nor in postpubertal (P5) subjects. Each dot corresponds to the change in BMC adjusted for age and gender (Zscore) in 193 subjects aged from 9 to 19 yr. Data are from refs. *99* and *100.*

During growth, undernutrition, including an inadequate supply of energy and protein, can severely impair bone development. Studies in experimental animals indicate that isolated protein deficiency leads to reduced bone mass and strength, that is, to osteoporosis, without histomorphometric evidence of osteomalacia *(3,4)*. Thus, an inadequate supply of protein appears to play a central role in the pathogenesis of the delayed skeletal growth and reduced bone mass observed in undernourished children *(93)*. Dietary proteins play an essential role in the hormonal regulation of mineral metabolism and skeletal growth (Figs. 4 and 5).

This role of dietary proteins should not be considered as merely that of "brick supplier" to the osteogenic cells, thus conferring them the capacity to lay down the organic bone matrix. As discussed for elderly and young adults, the functioning of the endocrine axis (GH–IGF-I), can be markedly impaired by insufficient intake of protein *(5)*. Some amino acids, which remain to be identified, are required for the hepatic production of IGF in response to GH as well as to the action of IGF-I on bone anabolism. Protein restriction also affects nonhepatic IGF-I production *(94)*. As already mentioned, the production of IGF-I by osteogenic cells can also be stimulated by certain amino acids, such as arginine *(49)*. This observation raises the possibility of a defined modulating role of dietary proteins in the paracrine–autocrine regulation of the proliferation-differentiation of osteogenic cells.

In "well"-nourished children and adolescents, the question arises whether or not variations in protein intake within the "normal" range can influence skeletal growth and thereby modulate the influence of genetic factors on peak bone mass attainment *(95–97)*. In the relationship between bone mass gain at the lumbar and femoral levels *(98,99)* and protein intake *(100)*, it is not surprising to find a positive correlation between these two variables. Similar to calcium intake *(99,101)*, the association appears to be particularly significant in prepubertal children *(14)*. Indeed, in healthy prepubertal subjects, a relatively low protein diet, independent of the intake of calcium, is associated with a reduced gain in aBMD or BMC at both femoral and spinal levels (Fig. 6). These results suggest that relatively high protein intakes could favor bone growth accrual during childhood. Nevertheless, these prospective observational results should not be interpreted as evidence for a causal relationship between bone mass gain and protein intake. Indeed, it is quite possible that protein intake, which is related to the overall amount of ingested calories, is to a large extent determined by growth requirements during childhood and adolescence. Only interventional studies testing different levels of protein intakes in otherwise isocaloric diets could eventually determine the quantitative relationship between protein intake and bone mass acquisition during childhood and adolescence. Very recent data from our research group suggest that in healthy prepubertal boys, the response to calcium supplementation can be influenced by the spontaneous protein intake *(102)*. The individual calcium requirement for optimal bone mass accrual could be less at high protein intake. The possible positive interaction between protein and calcium intake deserves to be investigated with the perspective of increasing peak bone mass by modifying bone trophic nutrients.

8. SUMMARY AND CONCLUSIONS

In addition to calcium and vitamin D, protein intake exerts a strong influence on bone metabolism. In elderly, reduced protein intake is associated with lower femoral neck aBMD and poor physical performance. Furthermore, protein malnutrition is present in many elderly women with low femoral neck aBMD and hip fracture. Clinical outcome after hip fracture can be significantly improved by normalizing the protein intake. This effect could be, at least in part, mediated by a positive influence on IGF-I of which the plasma level decreases in both genders with advancing age. As compared with nonfractured controls, patients with hip fractures have a lower IGF-I plasma level, which is associated with reduced proximal femur aBMD, lower plasma levels of prealbumin, albumin, and lower upper extremities muscle strength. In undernourished elderly subjects with hip fracture, a 6-mo intervention of increased protein intake, in the form of milk proteins, induces a significantly greater gain in plasma prealbumin, IGF-I and IgM as compared with an isocaloric placebo. The increased protein intervention also attenuates femoral bone loss and is associated with a shorter rehabilitation hospital stay. To understand the mechanism whereby protein intake influences bone mineral mass, animal models using either adult female or male rats have been developed. In these models isocaloric protein under nutrition mimics osteoporosis observed in elderly in whom both cortical and trabecular skeletal sites are affected with negative uncoupling between bone formation and resorption. Reduced bone formation could be mediated by decreased IGF-I production and action. Increased bone resorption appears to result from both sex hormone deficiency and increased cytokines such as TNF-α. In animal models administration of essential amino acids normalizes IGF-I plasma level, restores bone formation rate, and restores bone mass. In women, a consistent low-calorie, insufficient protein diet could be particularly deleterious for bone mass integrity. With estrogen and calcium deficiency, low protein intake probably contributes to the reduced bone mass observed in some athletes and ballet dancers, and in anorexia nervosa. In healthy prepubertal children, independent of the intake of calcium, a relatively low protein diet is associated with a reduced gain in aBMD at both femoral and spinal levels. Thus, dietary protein, probably by favoring both the production and the anabolic actions of IGF-I, contributes to maintain bone integrity from early childhood to old age. An adequate intake of protein should be recommended in the prevention and treatment of postmenopausal and age-dependent osteoporosis.

REFERENCES

1. Parfitt AM. Dietary risk factors for age-related bone loss and fractures. Lancet 1983;ii:1181–1184.
2. Schaafsma G, Van Beresteyn ECH, Raymakers JA, Duursma SA. Nutritional aspects of osteoporosis. World Rev Nutr Diet 1987;49:121–159.
3. Orwoll ES. The effects of dietary protein insufficiency and excess on skeletal health. Bone 1992;13:343–350.
4. Bonjour JP, Schürch MA, Rizzoli R. Nutritional aspects of hip fractures. Bone 1996;18(Suppl): S139–S144.
5. Bonjour JP, Schürch MA, Chevalley T, Ammann P, Rizzoli R. Protein intake, IGF-I and osteoporosis. Osteoporos Int 1997;7(Suppl 3):S36–S42.
6. Heaney RP. Calcium, dairy product and osteoporosis. J Am Coll Nutr 2000;19(Suppl):83S–99S.
7. Older MWJ, Edwards D, Dickerson JWT. A nutrient survey in elderly women with femoral neck fractures. Br J Surg 1980;67:884–886.
8. Rapin CH, Lagier R, Boivin G, Jung A, MacGee W. Biochemical findings in blood of aged patients with femoral neck fractures: a contribution to the detection of occult osteomalacia. Calcif Tissue Int 1982;34:465–469.
9. Jensen JE, Jensen TG, Smith TK, Johnston DA, Dudrick SJ. Nutrition in orthopaedic surgery. J Bone Joint Surg 1982;64:1263–1272.
10. Bastow MD, Rawlings J, Allison SP. Benefits of supplementary tube feeding after fractured neck of femur: a randomised controlled trial. Br Med J 1983;287:1589–1592.
11. Delmi M, Rapin CH, Bengoa JM, Delmas PD, Vasey H, Bonjour JP. Dietary supplementation in elderly patients with fractured neck of the femur. Lancet 1990;335:1013–1016.
12. Kanis J, Johnell O, Gullberg B, Allander E, Elffors L, Ranstam J, et al. Risk factors for hip fracture in men from Southern Europe: The Medos study. Osteoporos Int 1999;9:45–54.
13. Garn SM, Guzman MA, Wagner B. Subperiostal gain and endosteal loss in protein-calorie malnutrition. Am J Phys Anthropol 1969;30:153–155.
14. Rizzoli R, Bonjour JP. Determinants of peak bone mass and mechanisms of bone loss. Osteoporos Int 1999;9(Suppl. 2):S17–S23.
15. Bell J, Whiting SJ. Elderly women need dietary protein to maintain bone mass. Nutr Rev 2002;60:337–341.
16. Geinoz G, Rapin CH, Rizzoli R, Kraemer R, Buchs B, Slosman D, Michel JP, Bonjour JP. Relationship between bone mineral density and dietary intakes in the elderly. Osteoporos Int 1993;3:242–248.
17. Campbell WW, Barton ML Jr, Cyr-Campbell D, Davey SL, Beard JL, Parise G, Evans WJ. Effects of an omnivorous diet compared with a lactoovovegetarian diet on resistance-training-induced changes in body composition and skeletal muscle in older men. Am J Clin Nutr 1999;70:1032–1039.
18. Evans WJ. Protein nutrition and resistance exercise. Can J Appl Physiol 2001;26(Suppl):S141–S152.
19. Haub MD, Wells AM, Tarnopolsky MA, Campbell WW. Effect of protein source on resistive-training-induced changes in body composition and muscle size in older men. Am J Clin Nutr 2002;76:511–517.

20. Grisso JA, Kelsey JL, Strom BL, Chiu GY, Maislin G, O'Brien LA, Hoffman S, Kaplan F, the Northeast Hip Fracture Study Group. Risk factors for falls as a cause of hip fracture in women. N Engl J Med 1991;324:1326–1331.
21. Vellas B, Baumgartner RN, Wayne SJ, Conceicao J, Lafont C, Albarede JL, Garry PJ. Relationship between malnutrition and falls in the elderly. Nutrition 1992;8:105–108.
22. Vellas BJ, Albarede JL, Garry PJ. Diseases and aging: patterns of morbidity with age: relationship between aging and age-associated diseases. Am J Clin Nutr 1992;55(Suppl 6):1225S–1230S.
23. Schwartz A, Capezuti E, Grisso JA. Falls as risk factors for fractures. In: Osteoporosis. Marcus R, Feldman D, Kelsey J (eds.) .Academic Press, San Diego, 2001, pp. 795–808.
24. Hammerman MR. Insulin-like growth factors and aging. Endocrinol Metab Clin North Am 1987;16:995–1011.
25. Quesada JM, Coopmans W, Ruiz B, Aljama P, Jans I, Bouillon R. Influence of vitamin D on parathyroid function in the elderly. J Clin Endocrinol Metab 1992;75:494–501.
26. Goodman-Gruen D, Barrett-Connor E. Epidemiology of insulin-like growth factor-I in elderly men and women. The Rancho Bernardo Study. Am J Epidemiol 1997;145:970–976.
27. Langlois JA, Rosen CJ, Visser M, Hannan MT, Harris T, Wilson PW F, Kiel DP. Association between insulin-like growth factor I and bone mineral density in older women and men: the Framingham Heart Study. J Clin Endocrinol Metab 1998;83:4257–4262.
28. Chevalley T, Rizzoli R, Nydegger V, Slosman D, Tkatch L, Rapin, C.H., Vasey H, Bonjour JP. Preferential low bone mineral density of the femoral neck in patients with a recent fracture of the proximal femur. Osteoporos Int 1991;1:147–154.
29. Schürch MA, Rizzoli R, Slosman D, Vadas L, Vergnaud P, Bonjour JP. Protein supplements increase serum insulin-like growth factor-I levels and attenuate proximal femur bone loss in patients with recent hip fracture. A randomized, double-blind, placebo-controlled trial. Ann Intern Med 1998;128:801–809.
30. Bastow MD, Rawlings J, Allison SP. Undernutrition, hypothermia, injury in elderly women with fractured femur: an injury response to altered metabolism? Lancet 1983;1:143–146.
31. Sullivan DH, Patch GA, Walls RC, Lipschitz DA. Impact of nutrition status on morbidity in a select population of geriatric rehabilitation patients. Am J Clin Nutr 1990;51:749–758.
32. Schürch MA, Rizzoli R, Mermillod B, Vasey H, Michel JP, Bonjour JP. A prospective study on socioeconomic aspects of fracture of the proximal femur. J. Bone Miner Res 1996;11:1935–1942.
33. Tkatch L, Rapin CH, Rizzoli R, Slosman D, Nydegger V, Vasey H, Bonjour JP. Benefits of oral protein supplement in elderly patients with fracture of the proximal femur. J Am Coll Nutr 1992;11:519–525.
34. Auernhammer CJ, Strasburger CJ. Effects of growth hormone and insulin-like growth factor I on the immune system. Eur J Endocrinol 1995;133:635–645.
35. Rosen CJ. IGF-I and osteoporosis. Clin Lab Med 2000;20:591–602.
36. Garnero P, Sornay-Rendu E, Delmas PD. Low serum IGF-I and occurrence of osteoporotic fractures in postmenopausal women. Lancet 2000;355:898–899.
37. Wasnich RD, Davis J-M, Ross PD. Spine fracture risk is predicted by non-spine fractures. Osteoporos Int 1994;4:1–5.
38. Lindsay R, Silverman SL, Cooper C, Hanley DA, Barton I, Broy SB, et al. Risk of new vertebral fracture in the year following a fracture. JAMA 2001;285:320–323.
39. Kanis J. Diagnosis of osteoporosis and assessment of fracture risk. Lancet 2002;359:1929–1936.
40. Chapurlat RD, Bauer DC, Nevitt M, Stone K, Cummings SR. Incidence and risk factors for a second hip fracture in elderly women. The study of osteoporotic fractures. Osteoporos Int 2003;14:130–136.
41. Chevalley T, Hoffmeyer P, Bonjour JP, Rizzoli R. An osteoporosis clinical path for the medical management of patients with low trauma fracture: a way. Osteoporos Int 2002;13:450–455.
42. Ammann P, Bourrin S, Bonjour JP, Meyer JM, Rizzoli R. Protein undernutrition-induced bone loss is associated with decreased IGF-I levels and estrogen deficiency. J Bone Miner Res 2000;15:683–690.
43. Bourrin S, Ammann P, Bonjour JP, Rizzoli R. Dietary protein restriction lowers plasma insulin-like growth factor I (IGF-I), impairs cortical bone formation, induces osteoblastic resistance to IGF-I in adult female rats. Endocrinology 2000;141:3149–3155.
44. Thissen JP, Ketelslegers JM, Underwood LE. Nutritional regulation of the insulin-like growth factors. Endocr Rev 1994;15:80–101.

45. Ammann P, Rizzoli R, Müller K, Slosman D, Bonjour JP. IGF-I and pamidronate increase bone mineral density in ovariectomized adult rats. Am J Physiol 1993;265:E770–E776.
46. Ammann P, Rizzoli R, Meyer JM, Bonjour JP. Bone density and shape as determinants of bone strength in IGF-I and/or pamidronate-treated ovariectomized rats. Osteoporos Int 1996;6:219–227.
47. Ammann P, Rizzoli R, Caverzasio J, Bonjour JP. Fluoride potentiates the osteogenic effects of IGF-I in aged ovariectomized rats. Bone 1998;22:39–43.
48. Ammann P, Rizzoli R, Slosman D, Bonjour JP. Sequential and precise in vivo measurement of bone mineral density in rats using dual-energy X-ray absorptiometry. J Bone Miner Res 1992;7:311–316.
49. Chevalley T, Rizzoli R, Manen D, Caverzasio J, Bonjour JP. Arginine increases insulin-like growth factor-I production and collagen synthesis in osteoblast-like cells. Bone 1998;23:103–109.
50. Ammann P, Rizzoli R, Bonjour JP. Protein malnutrition-induced bone loss is associated with alteration of growth hormone-IGF-I axis and with estrogen deficiency in adult rats. Osteoporos Int 1998;8(Suppl 3):10.
51. Ammann P, Bourrin S, Bonjour JP, Meyer JM, Rizzoli R. Protein undernutrition-induced bone loss is associated with decreased IGF-I levels and estrogen deficiency. J Bone Miner Res 1999;15:683–690.
52. Bourrin S, Toromanoff A, Ammann P, Bonjour J-P, Rizzoli R. Dietary protein deficiency induces osteoporosis in aged male rats. J Bone Miner Res 2000;15:1555–1563.
53. Ammann P, Laib A, Bonjour JP, Meyer JM, Ruegsegger P, Rizzoli R. Dietary essential amino acid supplements increase bone strength by influencing bone mass and bone microarchitecture in ovariectomized adult rats fed an isocaloric low-protein diet. J Bone Miner Res 2002;17:1264–1272.
54. Chan J, Tian Y, Tanaka KE, Tsang MS, Yu K, Salgame P, et al. Effect of protein calorie malnutrition on tuberculosis in mice. Proc Natl Acad Sci USA 1996;93:14857–14861.
55. Dai G, McMurray DN. Altered cytokine production and impaired antimycobacterial immunity in protein-malnourished guinea pigs. Infect Immunol 1998;66:3562–3568.
56. Spaulding CC, Walford RL, Effros RB. Calorie restriction inhibits the age-related dysregulation of the cytokines TNF-alpha and IL-6 in C3B10RF1 mice. Mech Ageing Dev. 1997;93:87–94.
57. Anker SD, Coats AJ. Cardiac cachexia: A syndrome with impaired survival and immune and neuroendocrine activation. Chest 1999;115:836–847.
58. Anker SD, Clark AL, Teixeira MM, Hellewell PG, Coast AJ. Loss of bone mineral in patients with cachexia due to chronic heart failure. *Am J Cardiol* 1999;83:612–615, A10.
59. Ammann P, Rizzoli R, Bonjour JP, Bourrin S, Meyer JM, Vassalli P, Garcia I. Transgenic mice expressing soluble tumor necrosis factor-receptor are protected against bone loss caused by estrogen deficiency. J Clin Invest 1997;99:1699–1703.
60. Hotamisligil GS. Mechanisms of TNF-alpha-induced insulin resistance. Exp Clin Endocrinol Diabetes 1999;107:119–125.
61. Grimble RF, Jackson AA, Persaud C, Wride MJ, Delers F, Engler R. Cysteine and glycine supplementation modulate the metabolic response to tumor necrosis factor alpha in rats fed a low protein diet. J Nutr 1992;122:2066–2073.
62. Manary MJ, Brewster DR, Broadhead RL, Graham SM, Hart CA, Crowley JR, Fjeld CR, Yarasheski KE. Whole-body protein kinetics in children with kwashiorkor and infection: a comparison of egg white and milk as dietary sources of protein. Am J Clin Nutr 1997;66:643–648.
63. Grimble RF. Nutritional modulation of cytokine biology. Nutrition 1998;14:634–640.
64. Jilka RL. Cytokines, bone remodeling, estrogen deficiency: a 1998 update. Bone 1998;23:75–81.
65. Ammann P, Garcia I, Bonjour J-P, Rizzoli R. Protein undernutrition-induced bone resorption is dependent on tumor necrosis factor alpha (TNF). Osteoporos Int 2002;13(Suppl 1):S5.
66. Hirota T, Nara M, Ohguri M, Manago E, Hirota K. Effect of diet and lifestyle on bone mass in Asian young women. Am J Clin Nutr 1992;55:1168–1173.
67. Cooper C, Atkinson EJ, Hensrud DD, Wahner HW, O'Fallon WM, Riggs BL, Melton LG III. Dietary protein intake and bone mass in women. Calcif Tissue Int 1996;58:320–325.
68. Teegarden D, Lyle RM, McCabe GP, Proulx WR, Michon K, Knight AP, Johnston CC, Weaver CM. Dietary calcium, protein, phosphorus are related to bone mineral density and content in young women. Am J Clin Nutr 1998;68:749–954.
69. Drinkwater BL, K. Nilson CH Chesnut III, W. J. Bremner S Shainholtz, M. B. Southworth. Bone mineral content of amenorrheic and eumenorrheic athletes. N Engl J Med 1984;311:277–281.

70. Marcus R, Cann C, Madvig P, Minkoff J, Goddard M, Bayer M, et al. Menstrual function and bone mass in elite women distance runners. Ann Intern. Med 1985;102:158–163.
71. Warren MP, Perlroth NE. The effects of intense exercise on the female reproductive system J Endocrinol 2001;17:3–11.
72. Gremion G, Rizzoli R, Slosman D, Theintz G, Bonjour J-P. Oligo-amenorrheic long-distance runners may lose more bone in spine than in femur. Med Sci Sports Exerc 2001;33:15–21.
73. Beck BR, Shaw J, Snow CM. Physical activity and osteoporosis. In: Osteoporosis, 2nd ed, vol. 1, chapter 28. Marcus R, Feldman D, Kelsey J (eds.). Academic Press, San Diego, 2001, pp. 701–720, .
74. Lucas AR, Melton LJ 3rd, Crowson CS, O'Fallon WM. Long-term fracture risk among women with anorexia nervosa: a population-based cohort study. Mayo Clin Proc 1999;74:972–977.
75. Grinspoon S, Thomas E, Pitts S, Gross E, Mickley D, Miller K, Herzog D, Klibanski A. Prevalence and predictive factors for regional osteopenia in women with anorexia nervosa. Ann Intern Med 2000;133:790–794.
76. Herzog W, Deter HC, Fiehn W, Petzold E. Medical findings and predictors of long-term physical outcome in anorexia nervosa: a prospective, 12-year follow-up study. Psychol Med 1997;27:269–279.
77. Soyka LA, Grinspoon S, Levitssky LL, Herzog DB, Klibansky A. The effects of anorexia nervosa on bone metabolism in female adolescents. J Clin Endocrinol Metab 1999;84:4489–4496.
78. Soyka LA, Mistra M, Frenchman A, Miller KK, Grinspoon S, Schoenfeld DA, Klibansky A. The effects of anorexia nervosa on bone metabolism in female adolescents. J Clin Endocrinol Metab 2002;87:4177–4185.
79. Bonjour JP, Caverzasio J, Rizzoli R. Homeostasis of inorganic phosphate and the kidney. In: Rickets, Nestlé Nutrition Workshop Serie. Glorieux FH (ed.). Raven Press, New York, vol. 21, 1991, pp. 35–46.
80. Rosen JL, Chesney RW. Circulating calcitriol concentrations in health and disease. J Pediatr 1983;103:1–17.
81. Corvilain J, Abramow M. Growth and renal control of plasma phosphate. J Clin Endocrinol 1972;34:452–459.
82. Round JM, Butcher S, Steele R. Changes in plasma inorganic phosphorus and alkaline phosphatase activity during the adolescent growth spurt. Annu Hum Biol 1979;6:129–136.
83. Caverzasio J, Bonjour JP. IGF-I, a key regulator of renal phosphate transport and 1,25-Dihydroxyvitamine D3 production during growth. News Physiol Sci 1991;6:206–210.
84. Underwood LE, D'Ercole AJ, Van Wyk JJ. Somatomedin C and the assessment of growth. Pediatr Clin North Am 1980;27:771.
85. Krabbe S, Christiansen C, Rodbro P, Transbol I. Pubertal growth as reflected by simultaneous changes in bone mineral content and serum alkaline phosphatase. Acta Pediatr Scand 1980;69:49–52.
86. Krabbe S and Christiansen C. Longitudinal study of calcium metabolism in male puberty. I. Bone mineral content and serum levels of alkaline phosphatase, phosphate and calcium. Acta Pediatr Scand 1984;73:745–749.
87. Riis BJ, Krabbe S, Christiansen C, Catherwood BD, Deftos LJ. Bone turnover in male puberts: a longitudinal study. Calcif Tissue Int 1985;37:213–217.
88. Szulk P, Seeman E, Delmas PD. Biochemical measurements of bone turnover in children and adolescents. Osteoporos Int 2000;11:281–294.
89. Delmas PD, Chatelain P, Malaval L, Bonne G Serum GLA-protein in growth hormone deficient children. J Bone Miner Res 1986;1:333–338.
90. Johansen JS, Giwercman A, Hartwell D, Nielsen CT, Price PA, Christiansen C, Skakkebak NE. Serum bone Gla-protein as a marker of bone growth in children and adolescents: Correlation with age, height, serum insulin-like growth factor I, serum testosterone. J Clin Endocrinol Metab 1988;67:273–278.
91. Van den Brande JL. Régulation endocrinienne de la croissance. In : Endocrinologie Pédiatrique. Bertrand J et al. (eds.). Payot, Lausanne, 1982, pp. 159–181.
92. Krabbe S, Hummer L, Christiansen C. Longitudinal study of calcium metabolism in male puberty II. Relationship between mineralization and serum testosterone. Acta Pediatr Scand 1984;73:750–755.
93. Rizzoli R, Ammann P, Chevalley T, Bonjour JP. Protein intake during childhood and adolescence and attainment of peak bone mass. In Nutrition and Bone Development. Bonjour JP, Tsang RC (eds.). Lippincott-Raven, Philadelphia, 1999, pp. 231–243. (liste B223 - ref. 34 améliorée).

94. Naranjo WM, Yakar S, Sanchez-Gomez M, Perez AU, Setzer J, LERoith D. Protein calorie restriction affects non hepatic IGF-I production and the lymphoid system: studies using the liver-specific IGF-I gene-deleted mouse model. Endocrinology 2002;143:2233–2341.
95. Ferrari S, Rizzoli R, Bonjour JP. Genetic aspects of osteoporosis. Curr Opin Rheumatol 1999 ;11:294–300.
96. Rizzoli R, Bonjour JP, Ferrari SL. Osteoporosis, genetics and hormones. J Mol Endocrinol 2001;26:79–94.
97. Yakar S, Rosen CJ. From mouse to man: redefining the role of insulin-like growth factor-1 in the acquisition of bone mass. Exp Biol Med 2003;228:245–252
98. Bonjour JP, Theintz G, Buchs B, Slosman D, Rizzoli R. Critical years and stages of puberty for spinal and femoral bone mass accumulation during adolescence. J Clin Endocrinol Metab 1991;73:555–563.
99. Theintz G, Buchs B, Rizzoli R, Slosman D, Clavien H, Sizonenko PC, Bonjour J-P. Longitudinal monitoring of bone mass accumulation in healthy adolescents: evidence for a marked reduction after 16 years of age at the levels of lumbar spine and femoral neck in female subjects. J Clin Endocrinol Metab 1992;75:1060–1065.
100. Clavien H, Theintz G, Rizzoli R, Bonjour JP. Does puberty alter dietary habits in adolescents living in a Western society? J. Adolescent Health 19:68–75.
101. Bonjour J-P, Rizzoli R. Bone acquisition in adolescence. In: Osteoporosis, 2nd ed, vol. 1, chapter 25. Marcus R, Feldman D, Kelsey J (eds.). Academic Press, San Diego, 2001, pp. 621–638.
102. Chevalley T, Ferrari S, Hans D, Slosman D, Fueg M, Bonjour J-P, and Rizzoli R. Protein intake modulates the effet of calcium supplementation on bone mass gain in prepubertal boys. J Bone Miner Res 2002;17(Suppl 1):S172.

11 Effect of Insulin-Like Growth Factor Proteins on Skeletal Muscle Protein Metabolism During Normal and Catabolic Conditions

Charles H. Lang and Robert A. Frost

KEY POINTS

- IGF-I increases protein synthesis and decreases protein degradation in skeletal muscle.
- IGF-I-induced increases in muscle protein synthesis are mediated via alterations in translation initiation involving the increased formation of the eIF4E•eIF4G complex.
- IGF-I mRNA and peptide content are consistently decreased in a wide range of catabolic conditions.
- In various catabolic states the decrease in IGF-I in muscle is proportional to the reduction in protein synthesis.
- Increases in IGF binding proteins, particularly IGF binding protein-1, which is elevated in catabolic conditions may decrease the bioavailability and bioactivity of IGF-I thereby exacerbating the reduction in IGF-I and protein synthesis in skeletal muscle.

1. INTRODUCTION

During infection and traumatic injury, the acute loss of skeletal muscle protein may be advantageous to the host. Amino acids derived from muscle protein stores enhance hepatic gluconeogenesis and the synthesis of acute-phase proteins. An enhanced rate of net muscle protein breakdown may also be important in supplying amino acids necessary for various reparative processes and for mounting an optimal immune response. The loss of muscle protein is probably of minor clinical importance when the disease is self-limiting. However, the depletion of muscle protein that is observed during protracted hypermetabolic conditions carries a significant cost to the host and clearly results in not only a loss of muscle function but also an increase in mortality *(1,2)*. The factors that regulate muscle protein balance under

From: *IGF and Nutrition in Health and Disease*
Edited by: M. S. Houston, J. M. P. Holly, and E. L. Feldman © Humana Press Inc., Totowa, NJ

both physiological and pathophysiological conditions are therefore the subject of intense interest.

Many hormones, cytokines, and growth factors impact muscle protein balance. Recent studies suggest that insulin-like growth factor (IGF)-I plays a central role in regulating both muscle protein synthesis and protein degradation. In addition, IGF binding proteins (IGFBPs) provide an additional layer of regulation by altering the stability, transport, and bioactivity of IGF-I. Some IGFBPs may also have IGF-independent effects on muscle protein balance. In this chapter, we summarize studies that address the importance of IGF-I in regulating muscle protein synthesis and, to a lesser extent, protein degradation at the molecular, cellular and organismal level. Studies related to the role of growth hormone *per se* in regulating muscle protein metabolism during health and disease have not been reviewed.

2. EFFECT OF IGF-I ON PROTEIN METABOLISM UNDER NORMAL POSTABSORPTIVE CONDITIONS

2.1. Whole-Body Protein Metabolism

In general, data from early studies indicate that the administration of IGF-I stimulates growth in naive control rats leading to a greater increment in body weight gain *(3–5)*. The IGF-I-induced increase in weight gain apparently results from an increase in food efficiency because the number of calories consumed is not concomitantly increased *(6)*. Moreover, the increase in body weight is a result of an increase in both lean body mass (LBM; i.e., muscle) and the weight of noncarcass tissues *(7,8)*. Furthermore, the anabolic effect is enhanced when an equal amount of LR^3IGF-I, a variant that exhibits weak binding to the IGFBPs, is infused in place of native IGF-I *(6,8)*. These latter data suggest that under normal conditions the prevailing concentrations of the various IGFBPs restrain the ability of IGF-I to stimulate protein accretion. Body protein and nitrogen balance in the healthy subject are maintained within relatively narrow limits. Numerous studies have consistently demonstrated that IGF-I decreases whole-body net protein loss as evidenced by a decrease in urinary nitrogen excretion *(9,10)*. Although these types of nitrogen balance studies are generally considered the "gold standard" for determining the balance between protein synthesis and degradation, they provide little insight into the mechanisms by which protein metabolism has been altered.

Several in vivo approaches have been used to elucidate the dynamic aspects of protein metabolism and the possible mechanisms that may account for IGF-induced changes in nitrogen balance. Essentially all of the early studies regarding the role of IGF-I on protein balance were performed using an acute intravenous (IV) infusion of the growth factor in conjunction with the infusion of isotopically labeled amino acids, particularly leucine. These isotope-dilution studies, performed in a variety of different species, consistently demonstrate that short-term infusion of IGF-I decreases the rate of appearance (Ra) for leucine into the circulation, which provides an estimate of whole-body protein degradation *(9,11–14)*. Furthermore, IGF-I also proportionately decreases the rate of leucine disappearance (Rd). Leucine disappearance from the circulation can have two fates: reincorporation into protein (i.e., protein synthesis) or catabolism. Leucine oxidation is generally used as an index of irreversible amino acid catabolism or degradation, whereas the measurement of nonoxidative leucine disposal (NOLD) is used to estimate the rate of whole-body protein synthesis. In this regard, it is noteworthy that NOLD is not determined directly but instead is calculated as the difference between leucine Ra and leucine oxidation. As a consequence, NOLD and estimates of whole-body protein synthesis often demonstrate large variability. Some studies *(13,14)*, but not all *(12)*, demonstrate that the acute administration of IGF-I also decreases leucine oxidation, and several demonstrate the ability of IGF-I to decrease NOLD (i.e., protein synthesis) *(12,14)*. This latter finding of an IGF-induced decrease in whole-body protein synthesis was, at the time, unexpected. This response is now believed to be a consequence of the ability of IGF-I to reduce the availability of precursors for synthesis of new proteins by reducing protein degradation. Alternatively, or in addition to, the inability of IGF-I to produce a detectable increase in whole-body protein synthesis might be an artifact of the whole-body technique *(15)*.

In contrast, several studies have failed to detect any IGF-induced change in whole body leucine kinetics *(16,17)*. However, in these studies the growth factor was administered as a continuous infusion of IGF-I without a priming dose. It has been speculated that in acute studies the circulating concentration of "free" IGF-I, which is believed to represent the biologically active form of the peptide, is disproportionately increased by the priming dose. In contrast, the primed constant infusion of an equal molar amount of IGF-II has no demonstrative effect on whole-body protein kinetics *(9)*.

The infusion of IGF-I has several metabolic "side effects" that are noteworthy because they may alter the interpretation of the above-mentioned results. First, IGF-I produces hypoglycemia, which, in turn, leads to a compensatory increase in the plasma concentrations of glucagon, catecholamines, and glucocorticoids. Elevations in these various counter-regulatory stress hormones, especially glucocorticoids, can potentially alter protein balance *(7,8,18)*. However, in studies where the plasma glucose concentration is clamped at euglycemic levels, the protein metabolic effect of IGF-I is comparable to that observed under hypoglycemic conditions *(11)*. Thus, these data indicate that the occurrence of hypoglycemia and the concomitant increase in stress hormones do not overtly influence the effect of IGF-I on protein metabolism, at least under acute conditions. A second consequence of IGF-I infusion is a decrease in the circulating concentration of insulin *(11,12,16,19)*, which, based on the plasma C-peptide concentration *(12,16)*, results from a decreased rate of pancreatic insulin secretion. Potentially, the decrease in insulin might be expected to influence protein metabolism. A significant portion of this insulinopenia appears to be mediated by the decrease in plasma amino acids seen after IGF-I infusion because the IGF-induced decrement in insulin is partially attenuated by maintaining normal levels of plasma amino acids via an exogenous infusion *(20,21)*. Finally, acute and chronic administration of IGF-I decreases the plasma concentration of essentially all amino acids *(11,19,22)*, which may be in part related to an increased amino acid uptake by the liver *(22)*. It is now appreciated that this IGF-induced decrease in plasma amino acids represents a major limitation of essentially all early studies where the protein metabolic effects of IGF-I were investigated. This reduction in amino acids markedly reduces substrate availability for protein synthesis. Hence, a dramatically different picture of the effects of IGF-I on whole-body protein metabolism is seen when the plasma amino acids levels are prevented from falling *(23)*. In the study by Russell-Jones et al. *(23)*, where plasma amino acid levels were maintained at normal values, the infusion of IGF-I in healthy humans was shown to increase leucine Rd, leucine oxidation, and NOLD (protein synthesis) but did not significantly change leucine Ra (proteolysis).

2.2. Skeletal Muscle Protein Synthesis

A major limitation of the above-mentioned studies is that the isotope-dilution technique used measures whole-body amino acid flux, which represents a composite picture of protein synthesis and degradation for all tissues in the body. Therefore, despite the fact that skeletal muscle has been estimated to contain approx 50% of all body protein and account for approximately one third of the whole-body protein turnover, such measurements do not accurately estimate protein metabolism in skeletal muscle. To address the role of IGF-I on muscle metabolism *per se* Fryburg *(24)* acutely infused IGF-I intra-arterially into the forearm in postabsorptive humans. Based on phenylalanine balance across the forearm, IGF-I was demonstrated to increase the rate of muscle protein synthesis and decrease the rate of protein degradation. Likewise, based on the incorporation of isotopically labeled phenylalanine into muscle protein, the infusion of IGF-I with amino acid replacement has been shown to increase muscle protein synthesis *(20)*. However, no IGF-induced increase in muscle protein synthesis is evident when plasma amino acid concentrations are not maintained.

Several studies have now also directly demonstrated that IGF-I stimulates protein synthesis under in vivo conditions in heart *(9,19,21,25)* and skeletal muscle *(9,20,24,25)*. The ability of IGF-I to increase protein synthesis occurs rapidly, within 1 h *(25)*, and its effect is greatest in muscles composed predominantly of fast-twitch glycolytic fibers (e.g., gastrocnemius and plantaris) and lesser in slow-twitch oxidative fibers (e.g., soleus). At lower doses of IGF-I, the stimulatory effect of IGF-I on soleus wanes but is still present in the gastrocnemius and heart. This latter observation was confirmed and extended by Young et al. *(21)*, who demonstrated that IV infusion of IGF-I not only increases global cardiac protein synthesis but also increases the synthesis of the contractile proteins myosin and actin. The IGF-I induced increase in protein synthesis appears to be muscle-specific and is not observed in various visceral organs, such as the kidney, liver, spleen, lung, small intestine, colon, and brain *(25)*.

2.3. Potential Mechanisms by Which IGF-I Stimulates Muscle Protein Synthesis

The ability of IGF-I to stimulate muscle protein synthesis dose dependently has been clearly demonstrated using the isolated perfused hindlimb preparation *(26,27)*. Importantly, these studies have begun to address the potential mechanisms whereby IGF-I increases protein synthesis. The perfusion of hindlimb muscles with IGF-I (10 n*M*) for a period of 1 h more than doubles the rate of protein synthesis. Alterations in the number of ribosomes or the efficiency of mRNA translation may increase tissue protein synthesis. Because approx 80% of the RNA in muscle is ribosomal RNA, changes in total RNA content are used to estimate the number of ribosomes. However, there is no significant change in muscle RNA content in response to acute IGF-I treatment *(27)*. Hence, an alteration in the relative abundance of ribosomes is not responsible for the IGF-I-induced increase in muscle protein synthesis. Alternatively, IGF-I might stimulate protein synthesis by increasing the efficiency of translation. Efficiency, calculated by dividing the protein synthetic rate by the total RNA content, provides an index of how rapidly the existing ribosomes are synthesizing protein. Translational efficiency in gastrocnemius muscle is clearly increased in response to the acute administration of IGF-I *(27)*.

The synthesis of protein in eukaryotic cells is achieved through a complex series of discrete reactions (as reviewed in refs. *28* and *29*). The process involves the association of the 40S and 60S ribosomal subunits, mRNA, initiator methionyl-tRNA (met-$tRNA_I$), other amino acyl-tRNAs, cofactors (i.e., GTP, ATP), and protein factors (collectively known as eukaryotic initiation factors [eIFs], elongation factors, and releasing factors) through a series of reactions resulting in the translation of mRNA into proteins. Translation of mRNA on the ribosome consists of three phases: initiation, elongation, and termination. Translational controls most frequently operate during the initiation phase. One of the control points in translation initiation involves the binding of mRNA to the 43S preinitiation complex. This step requires the participation of the three-subunit eIF4F complex, which consists of eIF4A, eIF4E ,and eIF4G *(29)*. eIF4E appears to be the limiting translation initiation factor in muscle. Thus, the availability of eIF4E is important in eIF4F formation and initiation. The binding of eIF4E to eIF4G is controlled in part by the translation repressor protein 4E-BP1. Binding of 4E-BP1 to eIF4E is hypothesized to limit eIF4E availability and formation of the active eIF4E•eIF4G complex. In turn, the binding of 4E-BP1 to eIF4E is downregulated, in part, by the phosphorylation of 4E-BP1 *(30)*. Infusion of IGF-I appears to increase mRNA initiation in muscle by specifically increasing the relative amount of the active eIF4E•eIF4G complex, without concomitant changes in the amount of eIF4E, the formation of the 4E-BP1•eIF4E complex, or the phosphorylation state of 4E-BP1 *(27)*. It is noteworthy that although insulin also increases translational efficiency in muscle, its effect is mediated differently from that of IGF-I. That is, although insulin similarly increases the amount of eIF4E bound to eIF4G, this change is associated with an increased phosphorylation of 4E-BP1 and a concomitant reduction in the amount of the inactive 4E-BP1•eIF4E complex *(31)*.

The direct effect of IGF-I on muscle protein metabolism has also been investigated in vitro using isolated muscle preparations. Under these in vitro conditions, IGF-I consistently increases muscle protein synthesis as well as decreases both total protein breakdown and myofibrillar protein degradation *(32,33)*. The IGF-I-induced changes in protein synthesis and degradation are dependent upon activation of phosphatidylinositol (PI)3-kinase, as evidenced by their reversal in muscles treated with the PI3-kinase inhibitor LY294002 *(32)*. In contrast, treatment of muscles with the p70 S6 kinase inhibitor rapamycin only partially prevents the IGF-I-induced increase in protein synthesis and fails to prevent the decrease in proteolysis, indicating that some of the effects of IGF-I on muscle protein metabolism are independent of p70 S6 kinase activation. Similar observations have been made in human skeletal muscle cells *(34)*.

3. IGF-I ALTERATIONS OF PROTEIN METABOLISM IN CATABOLIC CONDITIONS

3.1. Burn, Sepsis, and Endotoxemia

In response to various types of catabolic conditions, the circulating concentrations of both total and free IGF-I have consistently been reported to be decreased. A marked reduction of IGF-I levels in the blood is observed in hypermetabolic infection *(35)*, sterile peritonitis *(36)*, thermal injury *(37)*, after the administration of endotoxin or inflammatory cytokines *(38–40)*, critical illness *(41)*, AIDS *(42)*, and alcohol intoxication *(43)*. This reduction is not species-specific, having been demonstrated in humans, dogs, pigs, sheep, and rodents. Moreover, many of these catabolic insults also decrease either the content of IGF-I protein and/or IGF-I mRNA in skeletal muscle *per se (35,37–40,43)*. Hence, because of the known anabolic effects of IGF-I, it has been postulated that decreases in blood or tissue IGF-I may in part be responsible for the catabolism of muscle protein *(44)*. This hypothesis is supported, but not proven, by data demonstrating a strong linear relationship between the rate of muscle protein synthesis and the IGF-I content in various catabolic conditions *(35)*. Therefore, there is ample experimental evidence to support the use of IGF-I as an adjunct therapy in reversing or preventing the extensive muscle wasting that accompanies many hypermetabolic conditions.

The treatment of burned rats with IGF-I via a constant infusion *(45)* or via liposome-encapsulated IGF-I cDNA *(46)* enhances body weight gain compared with pair-fed control animals *(47)*. Likewise, treatment of endotoxin-infused rats with IGF-I also improves weight gain. At least a portion of this increase in body weight is attributable to an improvement in overall nitrogen economy. In this regard, a 3-d infusion of IGF-I in burned adults ameliorates the negative nitrogen balance and decreases whole-body protein breakdown based on determinations of ^{15}N-lysine flux *(48)*. Similarly, a 2-d infusion of IGF-I in endotoxin-infused rats also improves whole body nitrogen balance *(47)*.

To circumvent the relatively short half-life of IV-injected IGF-I, several studies also have reported the effectiveness of IGF-I when administered in a complex with IGFBP-3. Injection of the IGF-I/IGFBP-3 binary complex is capable of forming a ternary complex with the acid-labile subunit in vivo, thereby extending the half-life of IGF-I in the circulation. Administration of this binary complex completely reverses the negative phenylalanine net balance across the leg of burned children *(49)* and partially restores leg protein balance in burned adults *(50)* when infused IV for 5 d. In the latter study, the effectiveness of IGF-I appeared most pronounced in the most catabolic patients. In addition, both studies demonstrated the ability of the binary complex to increase protein synthesis in skeletal muscle without producing overt hypoglycemia *(49,50)*.

During a 5-d treatment protocol, the binary complex also effectively reverses the decrease in muscle (gastrocnemius) protein synthesis observed after induction of hypermetabolic infection *(51)*. This improvement is associated with an increase in translational efficiency but not a change in the number of ribosomes. The binary complex-induced increase in muscle protein synthesis is not associated with a change in eIF4E phosphorylation, 4E-BP1 phosphorylation, or the amount of eIF4E bound to the translational repressor molecule 4E-BP1 *(51)*. Given the known effect of IGF-I in the perfused hindlimb *(26)*, it seems likely that the ability of the binary complex to improve muscle protein synthesis in septic rats is caused by the relatively selective increase in the amount of eIF4E bound to eIF4G. These data are consistent with the observation that perfusion of the isolated hindlimb with native IGF-I is capable of increasing muscle protein synthesis, translational efficiency and translation initiation in septic rats to the same extent as control animals *(26)*. Of note, the administration of

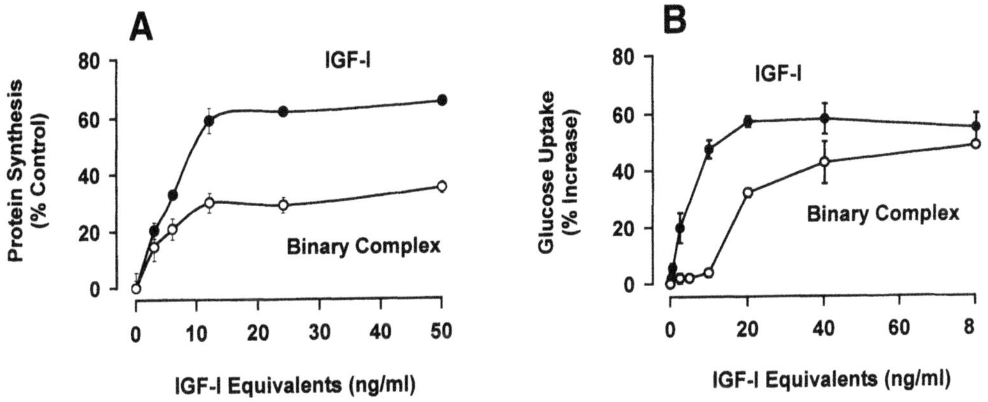

Fig. 1. Effect of native (free) IGF-I and IGF-I in a binary complex with IGFBP-3 to stimulate protein synthesis and glucose uptake in human skeletal muscle cells. Cells were serum deprived in minimal essential media for 24 h and treated with native IGF-I or IGF-I/BP3 binary complex. To determine protein synthesis **(A)**, cells were labeled with [^{3}H]phenylalanine and TCA-precipitable radioactivity determined as previously described *(34,65)*. Glucose uptake **(B)** was determined following the addition of deoxy-D-[^{14}C] glucose *(34)*. Values are means ± SEM.

human binary complex into rats does not appear to exert feedback inhibition of the synthesis and secretion of the native rat IGF-I and does not impair insulin secretion or lower plasma amino acid concentrations, responses that would be expected to impair the anabolic actions of IGF-I *(51)*.

The IGF-I/IGFBP-3 binary complex also stimulates protein synthesis in cultured human skeletal muscle cells (Fig. 1A). At low doses, free IGF-I and an equivalent amount of IGF-I bound to IGFBP-3 show a similar ability to stimulate protein synthesis. Yet the ability of the free peptide and the binary complex to maximally stimulate protein synthesis is considerably different. Free IGF-I stimulates protein synthesis to a level nearly twice that of the binary complex. The free and bound peptides also differ in their ability to stimulate glucose uptake in human skeletal muscle cells (Fig. 1B). Free IGF-I is fourfold more potent than the binary complex at stimulating glucose uptake. This latter response is consistent with the binary complex being a less potent hypoglycemic agent under in vivo conditions.

The ability of IGF-I to modulate muscle protein balance appears to be caused by direct effects of the growth factor. This conclusion is supported by studies in which rats are burned and the extensor digitorum longus muscle is removed and incubated in vitro with IGF-I. Under basal conditions, muscles from burned rats are characterized by a decreased rate of protein synthesis as well as an increased rate of both total and myofibrillar protein degradation *(52,53)*. Incubation of muscles with IGF-I completely prevents the increase in proteolysis and partially reverses the burn-induced decrease in protein synthesis. This partial IGF-induced increase in protein synthesis may be due to the lack of amino acids in the incubation medium in this particular study. Similarly, under basal conditions muscles from septic rats also show an increase in proteolysis and a decrease in protein synthesis compared to muscles from control animals *(54,55)*. Again, when the extensor digitorum longus muscles are isolated and incubated in vitro with IGF-I, the growth factor significantly increased the rate of protein synthesis. In one study IGF-I increased synthesis back to basal control values *(55)*, whereas in a second study IGF-I increased synthesis to the same extent as in control muscles incubated with the growth factor *(54)*. These data clearly demonstrate that sepsis and burn injury do not alter the ability of IGF-I to increase skeletal muscle protein synthesis. However, for sepsis, the available data pertaining to the effect of IGF-I on proteolysis are contradictory. Data from one group of investigators demonstrate that muscle from septic rats is completely unresponsive to the effects of IGF-I on muscle proteolysis *(33,55)*, whereas a separate group demonstrates that IGF-I indeed is able to reverse the sepsis-induced increase in proteolysis back to basal control values *(54)*. It is noteworthy that in this latter study the ability of IGF-I to inhibit sepsis-induced proteolysis is greater than the anabolic effect of insulin *(54)*. These latter data are consistent with reports indicating that IGF-I decreases sepsis- and burn-induced increases in mRNA for ubiquitin and the ubiquitin-conjugating enzyme E2-14 kDa *(52,55)* and suggest that the actions of IGF-I are in part caused by a reduction in proteosome-dependent protein degradation.

Tumor necrosis factor (TNF)-α is a pleiotropic cytokine that when administered to naive animals induces hemodynamic and metabolic changes comparable with those observed in many catabolic states, including a reduction in IGF-I *(39)* and a decrease in muscle protein synthesis *(56)*. In this regard, the acute IV infusion of IGF-I is also capable of decreasing the net protein loss induced by TNF-α *(57,58)*. This response appears to be primarily caused by the inhibition of muscle protein breakdown and less to the stimulation of muscle protein synthesis *(57)*.

3.2. Postsurgery

In contrast to the results from studies on burn, sepsis and endotoxemia, IGF-I has not been demonstrated to have a protein-sparing effect when administered to patients postoperatively *(59,60)*. The reason for this lack of improvement is unclear because the same dosing regime was used as in previous studies demonstrating that IGF-I is capable of increasing whole-body protein synthesis *(17)*. However, because these studies used measurements of whole-body protein flux, it is possible that IGF-I is effective at the level of the muscle, but that the lack of change in other organs and tissues masked the change in muscle. This conclusion is consistent with results from a study demonstrating that IGF-I is efficacious postoperatively at the level of the muscle where it completely reversed the stress-induced increase in the efflux of amino acids from muscle *(61)*.

3.3. Alcohol Ingestion

Excessive alcohol consumption, whether acute intoxication or chronic alcoholism, leads to numerous biochemical, morphological, and functional changes in skeletal muscle, a condition generally referred to as alcoholic myopathy *(62)*. Although there is little consensus at this time regarding the effect of alcohol on muscle protein degradation, several groups have independently demonstrated that alcohol intoxication acutely (<2.5 h) decreases rates of skeletal muscle protein synthesis *(62,63)*. A comparable decrease in muscle protein synthesis is also observed in rats fed a nutritionally complete diet for several weeks in which alcohol constitutes approx 36% of the total caloric intake *(64)*. This decreased rate of muscle protein synthesis appears to be primarily caused by a reduction in translational efficiency and not to a reduction in the number of ribosomes *(64)*. Moreover, both acute and chronic alcohol administration are associated with alterations in peptide-chain initiation. Specifically, muscle from alcohol-treated rats demonstrates an increased phosphorylation of 4E-BP1 that is believed responsible for the concomitant increase in the amount of inactive 4E-BP1•eIF4E complex and the reciprocal decrease in the amount of active eIF4E•eIF4G complex *(63,64)*. Similar protein metabolic changes have been observed in cardiac tissue in response to alcohol *(65)*.

As seen in other catabolic conditions, chronic alcohol consumption decreases the concentration of IGF-I in the blood and skeletal muscle *(43,62)*. For muscle, the alcohol-induced decrease in tissue IGF-I peptide content is accompanied by a proportional reduction in IGF-I mRNA expression *(43)*. It is noteworthy that a strong linear relationship exists between either the IGF-I peptide content or the abundance of IGF-I mRNA and the in vivo rate of protein synthesis and translational efficiency determined in the same muscle *(62)*. Although such relationships do not prove causality, they are consistent with observations that decreases in IGF-I within the physiological range are associated with a reduction in muscle protein synthesis *(66)*.

Ethanol also impairs the responsiveness of cultured cells to the anabolic actions of IGF-I and insulin. When human skeletal muscle cells are incubated with high physiologically relevant concentrations of alcohol the ability of both IGF-I and insulin to stimulate protein synthesis is impaired *(67)*. Likewise, alcohol renders myocytes completely refractory to the ability of IGF-I and insulin to slow protein degradation. Although superficially the effect of alcohol on IGF-I and insulin action appears similar, analysis of the early components of the signaling pathway in this study reveals differences between the two hormones. In this regard, whereas there is no alcohol-induced change in IGF-I stimulation of IGF-I receptor phosphorylation, the ability of insulin to stimulate the phosphorylation of its cognate receptor is markedly attenuated. These alcohol-induced changes could not be attributed to a change in the cellular content of either IGF-I or insulin receptors, or the proportion of insulin receptors that had formed hybrid receptors *(67)*. In addition, it is clear that insulin and IGF-I each use their own cognate receptors to stimulate protein synthesis in human skeletal muscle cells. An antibody (αIR3) that specifically prevents binding to the IGF-I receptor blocks the IGF-I-induced increase in protein synthesis, but has no effect on the ability of insulin to stimulate protein synthesis *(34,67)*. The ability of IGF-I treatment to reverse the catabolic effects of alcohol under in vivo conditions has not been reported.

3.4. Excess Glucocorticoids

Glucocorticoids are potent negative regulators of protein metabolism in muscle and other tissues. The presence of excess glucocorticoids results in a marked reduction in body weight, a negative nitrogen balance, and a decrease in muscle weight *(7,8,68–70)*. The results of several studies using isotope dilution are consistent and indicate that glucocorticoids increase whole-body proteolysis (e.g., leucine Ra) and the irreversible loss of amino acids (e.g., leucine oxidation), but not protein synthesis (e.g., NOLD) *(71)*. However, in other studies where the rate of protein synthesis in muscle is directly assessed, glucocorticoids have been convincingly demonstrated to decrease protein synthesis under in vivo conditions, in the *in situ* perfused muscle, in incubated muscle preparations, and in muscle cell lines *(72–74)*. The glucocorticoid-induced increase in whole-body proteolysis is accompanied by an increase in the urinary excretion of 3-methylhistidine. This amino acid is methylated posttranscriptionally in myofibrillar protein, and hence an increased excretion of the amino acid suggests an enhanced rate of myofibrillar protein breakdown *(8,68)*.

IGF-I clearly has an anabolic response in glucocorticoid-treated subjects. For example, in dexamethasone-treated rats, IGF-I administration prevents or ameliorates the decrease in body weight and markedly improves nitrogen retention *(7,8,68,70)*. In addition, the earlier IGF-I treatment is started relative to the first injection of steroid the more pronounced its anabolic actions *(75)*. However, the ability of IGF-I to improve whole-body protein metabolism is less clear in this particular catabolic condition. That is, two studies failed to detect a significant IGF-I induced change in leucine Ra or oxidation *(76,77)*, whereas a single study demonstrated that IGF-I could partially reverse the increased rate of whole-body proteolysis induced by prednisone *(71)*. Hence, at this time it is unclear as to whether IGF-I significantly affects whole-body determinants of protein metabolism.

Direct measurements of muscle protein synthesis and degradation have yielded more consistent results. Dexamethasone decreases the rate of muscle protein synthesis and increases myofibrillar degradation *(68,75)*. The dexamethasone-induced decrease in muscle protein synthesis results from a decrease in both the capacity of protein synthesis and a reduction in translational efficiency *(68,72)*. The latter defect appears to be the result of a decrease in initiation that is associated with a decrease in 4E-BP1 phosphorylation, an increase in 4E-BP1 binding to eIF4E, and a decrease in the binding of eIF4E with eIF4G *(72)*. Short-term exposure to dexamethasone has also been shown to decrease p70 S6K activity *(78)*. This ability of dexamethasone to impair protein synthesis may be related to its attenuation of p70 S6K activity and hence a decreased phosphorylation of the S6 ribosomal protein *(78)*. The ability of dexamethasone to alter muscle protein synthesis is also preserved when the steroid is administered in vivo and protein metabolism determined in isolated muscles in vitro. Epitrochlearis muscles from dexamethasone-treated rats demonstrate an increase in proteolysis and a decrease in protein synthesis *(79)*.

The in vivo administration of IGF-I attenuates the dexamethasone-induced changes, but rates of protein synthesis and degradation still did not return to basal values seen in control animals *(68)*. Likewise, in isolated epitrochlearis muscles from dexamethasone-treated rats, IGF-I was capable of stimulating protein synthesis and blunting proteolysis but these responses were impaired compared with muscles from control animals *(79)*. In human cultured skeletal muscle cells, dexamethasone decreases basal protein synthesis, and this response can be completely reversed by simultaneous exposure of cells to IGF-I (Fig. 2). This response is consistent with the anabolic effect of IGF-I in glucocorticoid-treated subjects. IGF-I has also been reported to decrease the dexamethasone-induced increase in ubiquitin, E2-14 kDa, and ubiquitin-E2G mRNA in gastrocnemius muscle *(69)*.

4. MODULATION OF IGF-I ACTION BY IGF BINDING PROTEINS

The bioavailability and bioactivity of IGF-I can be modulated by changing the concentration of one or more of the six high-affinity IGFBPs. Early studies demonstrated

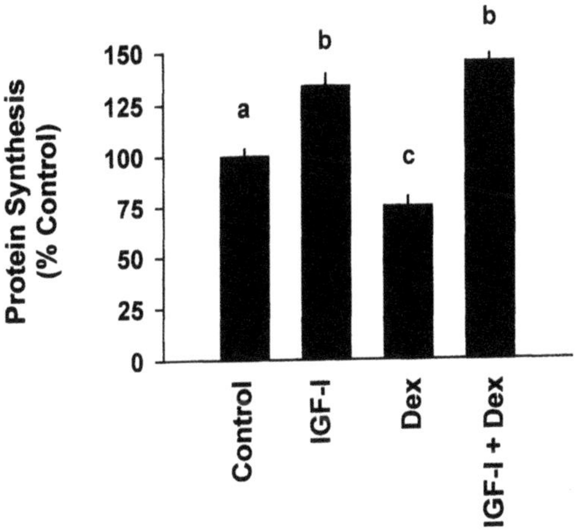

Fig. 2. Effect of IGF-I on dexamethasone-treated human skeletal muscle cells. Cells were incubated with either IGF-I (20 ng/mL), dexamethasone (1 μm), or a combination of the two for 6 h. Protein synthesis was determined as previously described *(34,65)*. Values are means ± SEM and values with different letters (a, b, c) are significantly different ($p < 0.05$).

that desIGF-I and LR^3-IGF-I are both more potent at stimulating weight gain and nitrogen retention in control and glucocorticoid-treated rats than native IGF-I *(6,68)*. Because these IGF-I variants have a reduced affinity for the IGFBPs, these data imply that the IGFBPs normally restrain the protein anabolic effects of IGF-I. This conclusion is supported by in vivo studies in mice where the overexpression of IGFBP-3, acid-labile subunit, IGFBP-2 or IGFBP-1 impairs normal postnatal growth *(80–82)*. However, to date, there are no studies that directly assess the ability of IGFBPs to regulate muscle protein metabolism in the basal state or in conditions where the blood concentrations of the binding proteins are altered.

Data from cell culture experiments support the supposition that IGFBPs compete with the IGF-I receptor for IGF-I and thereby have the potential to regulate protein balance in muscle. For example, serum stimulates protein synthesis in human skeletal muscle cells and its biological activity can be enhanced by an IGF-I analog (Leu^{24} Ala^{31} IGF-I) that displaces IGF-I from IGFBPs but itself has a very low affinity for the IGF-I receptor. Therefore, this analog, in the absence of serum does not stimulate protein synthesis but in the presence of serum presumably releases IGF-I and enhances protein synthesis (Fig. 3A). The IGF-I analog also displaces IGF-I from the IGFBP-3 binary complex. The binary complex itself shows a nominal ability to inhibit protein degradation as measured by [^{3}H]tyrosine release from prelabeled protein. However, when the IGF-I analog is added to the binary complex it displaces sufficient IGF-I to inhibit protein degradation to the same extent as free IGF-I (Fig. 3B).

The ability of increases in IGFBP-1 alone to modulate muscle protein synthesis has generated much interest. The circulating concentration of IGFBP-1 is dramatically increased in a variety of catabolic conditions, including burn, sepsis, endotoxemia, AIDS, and alcoholism *(35–43)*, and this increase appears to result from increases in

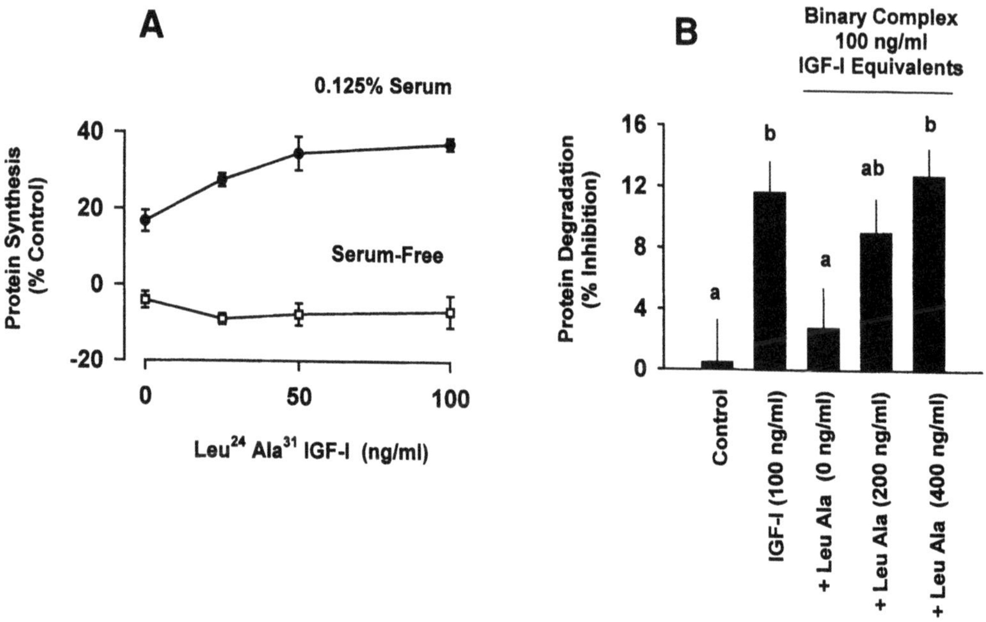

Fig. 3. The effect of Leu^{24} Ala^{31} IGF-I at displacing IGF-I from serum or the IGF-I/BP3 binary complex and altering protein metabolism in human skeletal muscle cells. In **A**, cells were serum-deprived for 24 h and treated with either $Leu^{24}Ala^{31}$ IGF-I alone or in combination with 0.125% serum. Protein synthesis was determined as previously described *(34,65)*. In **B**, cells were prelabeled with [^{3}H]tyrosine for 72 h and subsequently treated with either IGF-I (100 ng/mL) or a binary complex of IGFBP-3 and an equimolar amount of IGF-I. Some cells also received $Leu^{24}Ala^{31}$ IGF-I. Protein degradation was measured as release of [^{3}H]tyrosine into the medium.

various inflammatory cytokines (e.g., interleukin-1 and TNF-α) and glucocorticoids *(39,40,83)*. Moreover, although skeletal muscle does not synthesize IGFBP-1 *per se*, elevated IGFBP-1 protein seems to be sequestered or trapped by muscle during catabolic conditions *(39,40,44)*. Hence, it has been speculated that elevations in IGFBP-1 within the blood or local environment of the muscle might impair the anabolic actions of IGF-I and potentiate the concomitant reduction in IGF-I observed in these conditions. In cultured human skeletal muscle cells, IGFBP-1 dose-dependently decreases the ability of IGF-I to stimulate protein synthesis *(34)*. Conversely, IGFBP-1 fails to form a complex with desIGF-I and consequently IGFBP-1 fails to inhibit the ability of desIGF-I to stimulate protein synthesis. Although phosphorylation of IGFBP-1 is known to increase its affinity for IGF-I and its capacity to inhibit IGF-I action in some cell systems, there is only a small difference in the efficacy of phosphorylated vs nonphosphorylated IGFBP-1 in inhibiting protein synthesis in human myocytes *(34)*. Paradoxically, IGFBP-1 is incapable of preventing IGF-I from inhibiting muscle protein degradation *(34)*. In fact, IGFBP-1 itself has been demonstrated to dose-dependently inhibit muscle protein degradation via an IGF-independent mechanism that involves the β_1-integrin receptor. Comparable results have been obtained using isolated epitrochlearis muscle incubated with IGFBP-1 (Vary and Lang, unpublished observations). Hence, the overall effect of elevations in IGFBP-1 on protein balance in muscle appears multifaceted and not completely defined.

5. SUMMARY AND CONCLUSIONS

It is clear that IGF-I stimulates protein synthesis and inhibits protein degradation in skeletal muscle under conditions where plasma amino acids are not limiting, and this response may not be entirely analogous to that produced by equivalent doses of insulin. The importance of maintaining an adequate substrate supply has potentially important implications in clinical studies when IGF-I is used as an anabolic agent to reverse or minimize the erosion of lean body mass. At the cellular level, the enhancement of muscle protein synthesis by IGF-I is mediated via PI3 kinase and by a stimulation of peptide-chain initiation via alterations in eIF4E availability. Although critical illness appears to depress growth hormone responsiveness, the ability of IGF-I to stimulate muscle protein synthesis in many catabolic conditions is not impaired. In animal and clinical studies, the short-term (e.g., 5 d) exogenous administration of IGF-I, alone or complexed with IGFBP-3, greatly ameliorates the negative nitrogen balance and the decrease in muscle protein synthesis induced by thermal injury or infection, suggesting that IGF-I may be an effective adjunct therapy for severely catabolic critically ill patients.

6. RECOMMENDATIONS AND CHALLENGES FOR THE FUTURE

Traditionally, IGF-I has been considered essential for normal postnatal growth and development. However, it is becoming increasingly evident that IGF-I also plays an important role in the accretion of muscle protein in the adult via its actions on both protein synthesis and protein degradation. Continued research is needed into how signal transduction pathways in the muscle discriminate and differentiate between IGF-I and insulin in regulating in vivo protein metabolism. Moreover, additional studies are necessary to determine whether the trauma- and inflammation-induced decrease in IGF-I is actually causally related to the concomitant impairment in muscle protein balance, and the relative importance of the decrease in IGF-I in blood and muscle in the regulation of tissue metabolism. Intriguing questions remain as to the mechanism by which IGF-I regulates muscle proteolysis, which thus far has only been superficially addressed. Numerous in vitro studies indicate an ability of various IGFBPs to alter IGF-I availability and activity. However, the physiological relevance of changes in circulating levels of IGFBPs, particularly IGFBP-1, in response to catabolic stimuli remains to be elucidated. Finally, the relationship of the IGF system to other determinants of muscle growth and repair, such as satellite cell recruitment and myostatin production, might provide insights into the mechanisms mediating muscle wasting and potential ways to ameliorate this response in critical illness.

ACKNOWLEDGMENTS

Work by the authors and cited in this review was supported in part by grants from the National Institutes of Health GM-28032, AA-11290, and HL-66443.

REFERENCES

1. Windsor JA, Hill GL. Risk factors for postoperative pneumonia. Ann Surg 1988;208:209–214.
2. Kotler DP, Tierney AR, Wang J, Pierson RN. Magnitude of body-cell-mass depletion and the timing of death from wasting in AIDS. Am J Clin Nutr 1989;50:444–447.
3. Hizuka N, Takano K, Shizume K, Asakawa K, Miyakawa M, Tanaka I, Horikawa R. Insulin-like growth factor-I stimulates growth in normal growing rats. Eur J Pharmacol 1986;125:143–146
4. Philipps AF, Persson B, Hall K, Lake M, Skottner A, Sanengen T, Sara VR. The effects of biosynthetic insulin-like growth factor-I supplementation on somatic growth, maturation and erythropoiesis on the neonatal rat. Pediatr Res 1988;23:298–305.
5. Ng EH, Rock CS, Lazarus DD, Stiaino-Coico L, Moldawer LL, Lowry SF. Insulin-like growth factor-I preserves host lean tissue mass in cancer cachexia. Am J Physiol Regul Integr Comp 1992;262:R426–R275.
6. Tomas FM, Knowles SE, Chandler CS, Francis GL, Owens FPC, Ballard FJ. Anabolic effects of insulin-like growth factor-I (IGF-I) and an IGF-I variant in normal female rats. J Endocrinol 1993;137:413–421.
7. Yang H, Grahn M, Schalch DS, Ney DM. Anabolic effects of IGF-I coinfused with total parenteral nutrition in dexamethasone-treated rats. Am J Physiol Endocrinol Metab 1994;266:E69–E698.
8. Tomas FM, Lemmey AB, Read LC, Ballard FJ. Superior potency of infused IGF-I analogues which bind poorly to IGF-binding proteins is maintained when administered by injection. J Endocrinol 1996;150:77–84.
9. Douglas RG, Gluckman PD, Ball K, Breier B, Shaw JHF. The effects of infusion of insulinlike growth factor (IGF) I, IGF-II, and insulin on glucose and protein metabolism in fasted lambs. J Clin Invest 1991;88:614–622.
10. Bagi CM, DeLeon E, Brommage R, Adams S, Rosen D, Sommer A. Systemic administration of rhIGF-I or rhIGF-I/IGFBP-3 increases cortical bone and lean body mass in ovariectomized rats. Bone 1995;16:263S–269S.
11. Jacob R, Barrett E, Plewe G, Fagin KD, Sherwin RS. Acute effects of insulin-like growth factor I on glucose and amino acid metabolism in the awake fasted rat. J Clin Invest 1989;83:1717–1723.
12. Elahi D, McAloon-Dyke M, Fukagawa NF, Sclater AL, Wong GA, Shannon RP, Minaker KL, Miles JM, Rubenstein AH, Vandepol CJ, Guler HP, Good WR, Seaman JJ, Wolfe RR. Effects of recombinant human IGF-I on glucose and leucine kinetics in men. Am J Physiol Endocrinol Metab 1993;265:E831–E838.
13. Turkalj I, Keller U, Ninnis R, Vosmeer S, Stauffacher W. Effect of increasing doses of recombinant human insulin-like growth factor-I on glucose, lipid, and leucine metabolism in man. J Clin Endocrinol Metab 1992;75:1186–1191.
14. Laager R, Ninnis R, Keller U. Comparison of the effects of recombinant human insulin-like growth factor-I and insulin on glucose and leucine kinetics in humans. J Clin Invest 1993;92:1903–1909.
15. Wolfe RR, Volpi E. Insulin and protein metabolism. In: Handbook of Physiology. Section 7. The Endocrine System. Vol. II. The Endocrine Pancreas and Regulation of Metabolism. Jefferson LS, Cherrington Ad (eds.). Oxford University Press, New York, 2001, pp. 735–757.
16. Mauras N, Horber FF, Haymond MW. Low dose recombinant human insulin-like growth factor-I fails to affect protein anabolism but inhibits islet cell secretion in humans. J Clin Endocrinol Metab 1992;75:1192–1197.
17. Mauras N, Martha PM, Quarmby V, Haymond MW. rhIGF-I administration in humans: differential metabolic effects of bolus vs. continuous subcutaneous delivery. Am J Physiol Endocrinol Metab 1997;272:E628–E633.
18. Bessey PG, Lowe KA. Early hormonal changes affect the catabolic response to trauma. Ann Surg 1993;218:476–483.
19. Boulware SD, Tamborlane WV, Matthews LS, Sherwin RS. Diverse effects of insulin-like growth factor I on glucose, lipid, and amino acid metabolism. Am J Physiol Endocrinol Metab 1992;262:E130–E133.
20. Jacob R, Hu X, Niederstock D, Hasan S, McNulty PH, Sherwin RS, Young LH. IGF-I stimulation of muscle protein synthesis in the awake rat: permissive role of insulin and amino acids. Am J Physiol Endocrinol Metab 1996;270:E60–E66.

21. Young LH, Renfu Y, Hu X, Chong S, Hasan S, Jacob R, Sherwin RS. Insulin-like growth factor-I stimulates cardiac myosin heavy chain and actin synthesis in the awake rat. Am J Physiol Endocrinol Metab 1999;276:E143–E150.
22. Roth E, Valentini L, Holzenbein T, Winkler S, Sautner T, Hortnagl H, Karner J. Acute effects of insulin-like growth factor I on inter-organ amino acid flux in protein-catabolic dogs. Biochem J 1993;296:765–769.
23. Russell-Jones DL, Umpleby AM, Hennessy TR, Bowes SB, Shojaee-Moradie F, Hopkins KD, Jackson NC, Kelly JM, Jones RH, Sonksen PH. Use of a leucine clamp to demonstrate that IGF-I actively stimulates protein synthesis in normal humans. Am J Physiol Endocrinol Metab 1994;267:E591–E598.
24. Fryburg DA. Insulin-like growth factor I exerts growth hormone- and insulin-like actions on human muscle protein metabolism. Am J Physiol Endocrinol Metab 1994;267:E331–E336.
25. Bark TH, McNurlan MA, Lang CH, Garlick PJ. Increased protein synthesis after acute IGF-I or insulin infusion is localized to muscle in mice. Am J Physiol Endocrinol Metab 1998;275:E118–E123.
26. Jurasinski CV, Vary TC. Insulin_like growth factor I accelerates protein synthesis in skeletal muscle during sepsis. Am J Physiol Endocrinol Metab 1995;269:E977–E981.
27. Vary TC, Jefferson LS, Kimball SR. Role of eIF4E in stimulation of protein synthesis by IGF-I in perfused rat skeletal muscle. Am J Physiol Endocrinol Metab 2000;278:E58–E64.
28. Young VR, Yu YM. Protein and amino acid metabolism. In: Nutrition and Metabolism in the Surgical Patient. 2nd ed. Fischer JE (ed.). Little, Brown and Company, New York, 1996, pp. 159–201.
29. Pestova TV, Hellen CUT. The structure and function of initiation factors in eukaryotic protein synthesis. Cell Mol Life Sci 2000;57:651–674.
30. Shah OJ, Anthony JC, Kimball SR, Jefferson LS. 4E-BP1 and S6K1: translational integration sites for nutritional and hormonal information in muscle. Am J Physiol Endocrinol Metab 2000;279:E715–E729.
31. Kimball SR, Jurasinski CV, Lawrence JC, Jefferson LS. Insulin stimulates protein synthesis in skeletal muscle by enhancing the association of eIF-4E and eIF-4G. Am J Physiol Endocrinol Metab 1997;272:E754–E759.
32. Dardevet D, Sornet Cl, Vary TC, Grizard J. Phosphatidylinositol 3-kinase and p70 S6 kinase participate in the regulation of protein turnover in skeletal muscle by insulin and insulin-like growth factor I. Endocrinology 1996;137:4087–4094.
33. Hobler SC, Williams AB, Fischer JE, Hasselgren PO. IGF-I stimulates protein synthesis but does not inhibit protein breakdown in muscle from septic rats. Am J Physiol Regulatory Integrative Comp 1998;274:R571–R576.
34. Frost RA, Lang CH. Differential effects of insulin-like growth factor I (IGF-I) and IGF-binding protein-1 on protein metabolism in human skeletal muscle cells. Endocrinology 1999;140:3962–3970.
35. Lang CH, Fan J, Cooney R, Vary TC. Interleukin-1 receptor antagonist attenuates sepsis-induced alterations in the insulin-like growth factor system and protein synthesis. Am J Physiol Endocrinol Metab 1996;270:E430–E437.
36. Fan J, Li YH, Bagby GJ, Lang CH. Modulation of inflammation-induced changes in insulin-like growth factor (IGF)-I and IGF binding protein-1 by anti-TNF antibody. Shock 1995;4:21–26.
37. Lang CH, Liu X, Nystrom GJ, Frost RA. Acute response of IGF-I and IGF binding proteins indued by thermal injury. Am J Physiol Endocrinol Metab 2000;278:E1087–E1096.
38. Lang CH, Frost RA, Jefferson LS, Kimball SR, Vary TC. Endotoxin-induced decrease in muscle protein synthesis is associated with alterations in eIF2B, eIF4e and IGF-I. Am J Physiol Endocrinol Metab 2000;278:E1133–E1143.
39. Fan J, Bagby GJ, Gelato MC, Lang CH. Regulation of insulin-like growth factor I content and IGF-binding proteins by tumor necrosis factor. Am J Physiol Regulatory Integrative Comp 1995;269:R1204–R1212.
40. Fan J, Wojnar WW, Theodorakis M, Lang CH. Regulation of insulin-like growth factor (IGF)-I mRNA and peptide, and IGF binding proteins by interleukin-1. Am J Physiol Regul Integr Comp 1996;270:R621–R629.
41. Wojnar MM, Fan J, Frost RA, Gelato MC, Lang CH. Alterations in the insulin-like growth factor system in trauma patients. Am J Physiol Regul Integr Comp Physiol 1995;268:R970–R977.
42. Frost RA, Fuhrer J, Maruiz, Lang CH, Gelato MC. Wasting in the acquired immune deficiency syndrome is associated with multiple defects in the serum insulin-like growth factor system. Clin Endocrinol 1996;44:501–514.

43. Lang CH, Fan J, Lipton BP, Potter BJ, McDonough KH. Modulation of the IGF system by chronic alcohol feeding. Alcoholism Clin Exp Res 1998;22:823–829.
44. Frost RA, Lang CH. Growth factors in critical illness: regulation and therapeutic aspects. Curr Opin Clin Nutr Metab Care 1998;1:195–204.
45. Strock LL, Singh H, Abdullah A, Miller JA, Herndon DN. The effect of insulin-like growth factor I on postburn hypermetabolism. Surgery 1990;108:161–164.
46. Jeschke MG, Barrow RE, Hawkins HK, Yang K, Hayes RL, Lichtenbelt BJ, Perez-Polo JR, Herndon DN. IGF-I gene transfer in themally injured rats. Gene Ther 1999;6:1015–1020.
47. Dickerson RN, Manzo CB, Charland SL, Settle RG, Stein TP, Kuhl DA, Rajter JJ. The effect of insulin-like growth factor-1 on protein metabolism and hepatic response to endotoxemia in parenterally fed rats. J Surg Res 1995;58:260–266.
48. Cioffi WG, Gore DC, Rue LW, Carrougher G, Guler HP, McNanus WF, Pruitt BA. Insulin-like growth factor-1 lowers protein oxidation in patients with thermal injury. Ann Surg 1994;220:310–319.
49. Herndon DN, Ramzy RI, DebRoy MA, Zheng M, Ferrando AA, Chinkes DL, Barret JP, Wolfe RR, Wolf SE. Muscle protein catabolism after severe burn: effects of IGF-1/IGFBP-3 treatment. Ann Surg 1999;229:713–722.
50. Debroy ME, Wolf ME, Zhang XJ, Chinkes DL, Ferrando AA, Wolfe RR, Herndon DN. Anabolic effects of insulin-like growth factor in combination with insulin-like growth factor binding protein-3 in severely burned adults. J Trauma 1999;47:904–911.
51. Svanberg E, Frost RA, Lang CH, Isgaard J, Jefferson LS, Kimball SR, Vary TC. IGF-I/IGFBP-3 binary complex modulates sepsis-induced inhibition of protein synthesis in skeletal muscle. Am J Physiol Endocrinol Metab 2000;279:E1145–E1158.
52. Fang CH, Li BG, Wang JJ, Fischer JE, Hasselgren PO. Insulin-like growth factor 1 stimulates protein synthesis and inhibits protein breakdown in muscle from burned rats. JPEN 1997;21:245–251.
53. Fang CH, Li BG, Wang JJ, Fischer JE, Hasselgren PO. Treatment of burned rats with insulin-like growth factor I inhibit the catabolic response in skeletal muscle. Am J Physiol Regul Integr Comp 1998;275:R1091–R1098.
54. Vary TC, Dardevet D, Grizard J, Voisin L, Buffiere C, Denis P, Breuille D, Obled C. Differential regulation of skeletal muscle protein turnover by insulin and IGF-I after bacteremia. Am J Physiol Endocrinol Metab 1998;275:E584–E593.
55. Fang CH, Li BG, Sun X, Hasselgren PO. Insulin-like growth factor I reduces ubiquitin and ubiquitin-conjugating enzyme gene expression but does not inhibit muscle proteolysis in septic rats. Endocrinology 2000;141:2743–2751.
56. Lang CH, Frost RA, Narn AC, MacLean DA, Vary TC. TNF" α decreases skeletal muscle and myocardial protein synthesis via alterations in translation initiation but not elongation. Am J Physiol Endocrinol Metab 2002;282:E336–E347.
57. Sakurai Y, Zhang XJ, Wolfe RR. Insulin-like growth factor-I and insulin reduce leucine flux and oxidation in conscious tumor necrosis factor-infused dogs. Surgery 1995;117:305–313.
58. Douglas RG, Gluckman PD, Breier BH, Mccall JL, Parry B, Shaw JHF. Effects of recombinant IGF-I on protein and glucose metabolism in rTNF infused lambs. Am J Physiol Endocrinol Metab 1991;261:E606–E612.
59. Goeters C, Mertes N, Tacke J, Bolder U, Kuhmann M, Lawin P, Lohlein D. Repeated administration of recombinant human insulin-like growth factor-I in patients after gastric surgery. Ann Surg 1995;222:646–653.
60. Leinskold T, Permert J, Olaison G, Larsson J. Effect of postoperative insulin-like growth factor I supplementation on protein metabolism in humans. Br J Surg 1995;82:921–925.
61. Malmlof K, Cortova Z, Saxerholt H, Karlsson E, Arrhenius-Nyberg V, Skottner A. Effects of insulin-like growth factor-I and growth hormone on the net flux of amino acids across the hind limbs in the surgically traumatized pig. Clin Sci 1995;88:285–292.
62. Lang CH, Kimball SR, Frost RA, Vary TC. Alcohol myopathy: impairment of protein synthesis and translation initiation. Int J Biochem Cell Biol 2001;33:457–473.
63. Lang CH, Frost RA, Kumar V, Wu D, Vary TC. Impaired protein synthesis induced by acute alcohol intoxication is associated with changes in eIF4E in muscle and eIF2B in liver. Alcohol Clin Exp Res 2000;24:322–331.

64. Lang CH, Wu D, Frost RA, Jefferson LS, Kimball SR, Vary TC. Inhibition of muscle protein synthesis by alcohol is associated with modulation of eIF2B and eIF4E. Am J Physiol Endocrinol Metab 1999;277:E268–E276.
65. Vary TC, Lynch CJ, Lang CH. Effects of chronic alcohol consumption on regulation of myocardial protein synthesis. Am J Physiol Heart Circulation 2001;281:H1242–H1251.
66. Frost RA, Lang CH, Gelato MC. Transient exposure of human myoblasts to TNF" inhibits serum and IGF-I stimulated protein synthesis. Endocrinology 1997;138:4153–4159.
67. Hong-Brown, LQ, Frost RA, Lang CH. Ethanol impairs protein synthesis and degradation in cultured skeletal muscle cells. Alcohol Clin Exp Res 2001;25:1373–1382.
68. Tomas FM, Knowles SE, Owens PC, Changdler CS, Franscis GL, Read LC, Ballard FJ. Insulin-like growth factor-I (IGF)-I and especially IGF-I variants are anabolic in dexamethasone-treated rats. Biochem J 1992;282:91–97.
69. Chrysis D, Underwood LE. Regulation of components of the ubiquitin system by insulin-like growth factor I and growth hormone in skeletal muscle of rats made catabolic with dexamethasone. Endocrinology 1999;140:5635–5641.
70. Kritsch KR, Huss DJ, Ney DM. Greater potency of IGF-I than IGF-I/BP-3 complex in catabolic parenterally fed rats. Am J Physiol Endocrinol Metab 2000;278:E252–E262.
71. Mauras N, Beaufrere B. Recombinant human insulin-like growth factor-I enhances whole body protein anabolism and significantly diminishes the protein catabolic effects of prednisone in humans without a diabetogenic effect. J Clin Endocrinol Metab 1995;80:869–874.
72. Shah OJ, Kimball SR, Jefferson LS. Acute attenuation of translation initiation and protein synthesis by glucocorticoids in skeletal muscle. Am J Physiol Endocrinol Metab 2000;278:E76–E82.
73. Shoji S, Pennington RJT. The effect of cortisol on protein breakdown and synthesis in rat skeletal muscle. Mol Cell Endocrinol 1977;6:159–169.
74. Rannels SR, Jefferson LS. Effects of glucocorticoids on muscle protein turnover in perfused rat hemicorpus. Am J Physiol Endocrinol Metab 1980;238:E564–E572.
75. Tomas FM. The anti-catabolic efficacy of insulin-like growth factor-I is enhanced by its early administration to rats receiving dexamethasone. J Endocrinol 1998;157:89–97.
76. Oehri M, Ninnis R, Girard J, Frey FJ, Keller U. Effects of growth hormone and IGF-I on glucocorticoid-induced protein catabolism in humans. Am J Physiol Endocrinol Metab 1996;270:E552–E558.
77. Hellstern G, Reijngoud DJ, Stellaard F, Okken A. Insulin-like growth factor-I fails to reverse corticosteroid-induced protein catabolism in growing piglets. Pediatr Res 1996;39:421–426.
78. Shah OJ, Kimball SR, Jefferson LS. Among translational effectors, $p70^{S6k}$ is uniquely sensitive to inhibition by glucocorticoids. Biochem J 2000;347:389–397.
79. Dardevet D, Sornet C, Savary I, Debras E, Patureau-Mirand P, Grizard J. Glucocorticoid effects on insulin- and IGF-I-regulated muscle protein metabolism during aging. J Endocrinol 1998;156:83–89.
80. Rajkumar K, Barron D, Lewitt MS, Murphy LJ. Growth retardation and hyperglycemia in insulin-like growth factor binding protein-1 transgenic mice. Endocrinology 1995;136:4029–4034.
81. Hoeflich A, Nedbal S, Blum WF, Erhard M, Lahm H, Brem G, Kolb HJ, Wanke R, Wolf E. Growth inhibition in giant growth hormone transgenic mice by overexpression of insulin-like growth factor binding protein-2. Endocrinology 2001;142:1889–1898.
82. Silha JV, Gui Y, Modric T, Suwanichkul A, Durham SK, Powell DR, Murphy LJ. Overexpression of the acid-labile subunit of the IGF ternary complex in transgenic mice. Endocrinology 2001;142:4305–4313.
83. Li YH, Fan J, Lang CH. Role of glucocorticoids in mediating endotoxin-induced changes in IGF-I and IGF binding protein-1. Am J Physiol Regul Integr Comp 1997;272:R1970–R1977.

12 Insulin-Like Growth Factors and Nervous System Disorders

Gary Meyer, Aparna Bole, and Eva L. Feldman

KEY POINTS

- Deficits in the IGF system are not a primary cause of neurodegenerative disorders including Parkinson's, Huntington's, or Alzheimer's diseases or amyotrophic lateral sclerosis.
- Systemic decreases of IGF-I in diabetic patients may contribute to diabetic neuropathy.
- Because IGF-I is a potent neuroprotective protein, its use in neurodegenerative diseases is under investigation.
- IGF-I protects neurons from traumatic injury and has proven effective in a clinical trial of head injury.
- IGF-I promotes peripheral nerve regeneration following nerve damage.
- IGF-I promotes the growth of neurons and muscle cells and maintains a healthy interaction between these cell types.
- IGF-I is an important growth factor for muscle development and is a potential treatment of neuromuscular disorders.

1. INTRODUCTION

Insulin-like growth factors (IGFs) are important regulators of neuronal development and survival *(1)*. IGFs-I and -II, both IGF receptors, and the IGF binding proteins (IGF-BPs) are expressed widely in the central and peripheral nervous systems in development, adulthood, and in disease states. IGFs are neurotrophic to a variety of neuronal cells, including cortical *(2)*, hippocampal *(3)*, motor *(4,5)*, sensory *(6)*, and sympathetic *(6,7)* neurons. IGFs also stimulate neurite growth and are the only trophic factors identified thus far that promote regeneration in both sensory and motor neurons *(8)*. The integral involvement of IGFs in the nervous system would suggest that changes in their function and availability could lead to nervous system disease or play a part in endogenous responses to nervous system injury. IGFs have been used as experimental therapies in models of nervous system disease and in several human studies. They represent a promising frontier for the treatment of several disorders for which there are currently few or no effective interventions. Detailed discussions of the signaling mechanisms and developmental roles of IGFs in the nervous system have been published previously

From: *IGF and Nutrition in Health and Disease*
Edited by: M. S. Houston, J. M. P. Holly, and E. L. Feldman © Humana Press Inc., Totowa, NJ

(1,9). This chapter will focus on the impact of nervous system diseases on the IGF system, and the involvement of IGFs in the pathogenesis and treatment of nervous system disease and injury.

2. ALZHEIMER'S DISEASE

2.1. Pathophysiology

Alzheimer's disease (AD) is a frequent cause of dementia, occasionally presenting as early as age 50 and becoming more prevalent after age 65. AD is characterized by loss of cortical, hippocampal, and basal forebrain cholinergic neurons. Histological examination reveals the combination of intraneuronal tangles with high concentrations of phosphorylated tau protein, and extracellular plaques composed of β-amyloid (A-β) protein. Research has been directed at understanding how the formation of tangles and plaques relate to neuronal death and what interventions may abate this process. IGFs have been implicated in the nervous system response to AD. IGF-I is a component of neuritic plaques *(10)*, and IGF-I levels in AD serum relate inversely to cognitive impairment *(11)*.

2.2. Impact on the IGF System

Changes in IGF expression in patients with AD have led to the hypothesis that IGFs are part of a compensatory response to neuronal death. An early study using radioimmunoassays to measure IGF-I in serum from suspected patients with AD found that IGF-I levels were significantly increased compared to normal controls *(12)*. This elevation was confirmed by acid-gel chromatography, which also detected elevated serum IGF-II *(13)*. However, a specific examination of serum IGF-I in patients with the Swedish amyloid precursor protein mutation found decreased IGF-I levels *(14)*. This raises the possibility that one AD etiology may affect the IGF system differently than another. In the cerebral spinal fluid (CSF), IGF-II is elevated in AD compared with normal controls, whereas IGF-I appears to be unchanged *(13,15)*. IGF-I immunoreactivity in AD brain appears to be induced only in some astrocytes in the hippocampus and frontal and temporal cortices *(10,16)*. Despite the elevated levels of IGF-II observed in the CSF, no work has been published characterizing the expression of IGF-II in AD brain tissue.

It is not clear whether expression of the IGF-IR changes in the AD brain. In one study, ^{125}I-IGF-I binding was slightly elevated in membranes prepared from AD frontal cortex *(17,18)*, but a similar technique in another study detected no differences in binding *(10)*. Quantitative autoradiography detects no changes in IGF-IR expression *(19)*.

Two IGFBPs are highly elevated in AD CSF. They are 30 and 33 kDa and are believed to be IGFBP-2 and -6 *(13)*. In AD serum, IGFBP-1 is highly elevated, but IGFBP-3 is decreased *(11)*. The decrease in IGFBP-3 may be related to dysfunction of the hypothalamic–pituitary–adrenal axis in AD. Elevated levels of cortisol lead to decreased IGFBP-3. Dehyroepiandrosterone sulfate has the opposite effect but decreases with aging. Thus, some of the changes seen in the IGF system in patients with AD may be the result of dysfunction of the hypothalamic–pituitary–adrenal axis, rather than compensation for neuronal cell death.

2.3. IGFs in AD Treatment

IGF-I has been implicated in the inactivation of two pathways that contribute to neuronal death in AD (Fig. 1). A-β peptide increases JNK activation in cultured neuroblastoma cells and may induce cell death through the JNK/SAPK pathway *(20)*. IGF-I

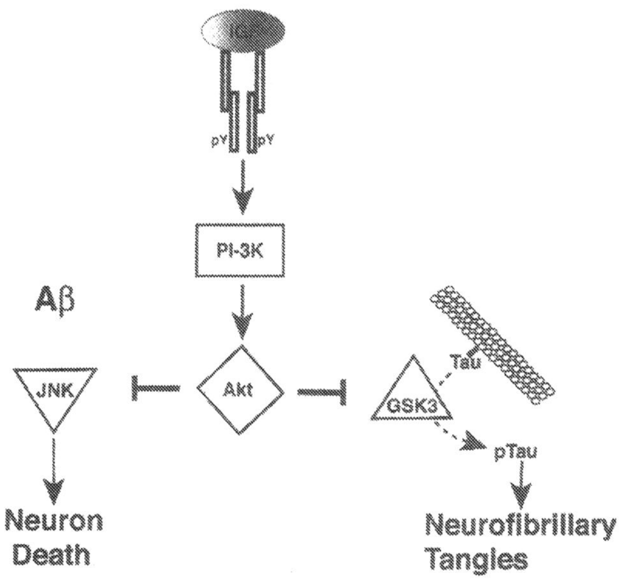

Fig. 1. IGF-I in the treatment of AD. A-β peptide increases JNK activation and may induce cell death through the JNK/SAPK pathway. IGF-I:IGF-IR inhibits JNK activation via PI3K signaling and may provide neuroprotection. Phosphorylated tau has decreased affinity for microtubules and is incorporated into neurofibrillary tangles. IGF-I:IGF:IR decreases tau phosphorylation by inhibiting glycogen synthase kinase-3 (GSK-3) activity via PI3K and Akt signaling and may decrease tangle formation in AD.

inhibits JNK activation via phosphatidyl inositol 3 (PI-3K) signaling *(20)* and protects cultured neuronal cells from A-β-induced death *(20,21)*. IGF-I can protect cultured neurons from a familial mutant of the A-β precursor protein (V642I). Increased expression of IGFBP-3 counters the protective effect of IGF-I *(22)*. IGF-I also decreases tau phosphorylation, by inhibiting glycogen synthase kinase-3 activity via PI-3K and Akt signaling *(23)*. Phosphorylated tau has decreased affinity for microtubules and is incorporated into neurofibrillary tangles.

3. PARKINSON'S DISEASE

Parkinson's disease (PD) results from death of dopaminergic neurons in the substantia nigra. The IGF system has not been implicated in this selective neuronal death, whose cause remains unknown. Dopaminergic regulation of anterior pituitary hormones from the hypothalamus appears to be intact in patients with PD and remains functional after long-term Levodopa therapy *(24)*. As with other conditions of neurodegeneration, neuroprotective growth factors like IGF-I have been suggested as potential agents for preventing the loss of nigrostriatal neurons in PD *(25)*. However, IGFs have not been tested in the treatment of PD.

4. HUNTINGTON'S DISEASE

A single study has identified an interesting function for IGFs in the pathophysiology of Huntington's disease (HD). Expansion of trinucleotide repeats in the huntingtin

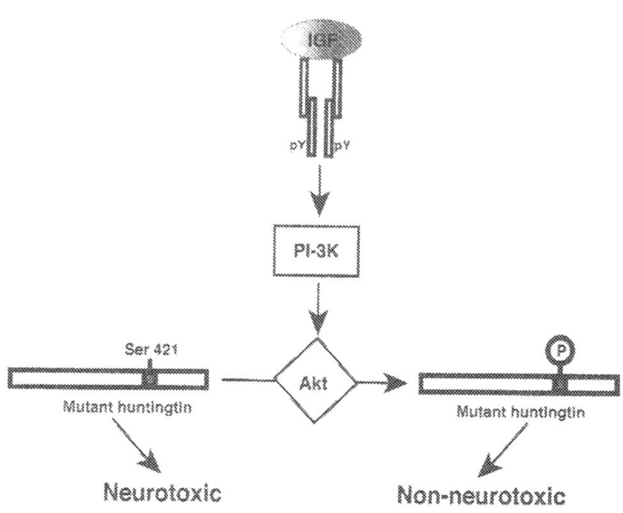

Fig. 2. IGF-I in the Treatment of HD. IGF-I:IGF-IR activates Akt kinase, which phosphorylates the huntingtin protein on serine 421, promoting neuronal survival. Striatal neurons expressing a form of mutant huntingtin lacking this phosphorylation site cannot be rescued by IGF-I.

gene leads to a neurotoxic protein product. IGF-I is protective to cultured neurons expressing mutant huntingtin. IGF-I causes activation of the Akt kinase, which phosphorylates the huntingtin protein on serine 421. Striatal neurons expressing a form of mutant huntingtin lacking this phosphorylation site cannot be rescued by IGF-I. In addition, mutating the phosphorylation site to mimic constitutive phosphorylation decreases the toxicity of the protein *(26)*. This novel mechanism for IGF-mediated neuroprotection could lead to further therapeutic investigations in HD (Fig. 2).

5. CEREBELLAR NEURODEGENERATIVE DISEASES

Numerous conditions, many of genetic etiology, cause selective degeneration of cerebellar neurons. Ataxia-telangiectasia patients have elevated serum IGF-I and IGFBP-2 levels *(27)*. In contrast, patients with olivopontocerebellar atrophy or idiopathic cerebellar cortical atrophy show decreased serum IGF-I and high IGFBP-1 *(28)*. As a treatment for a chemically induced model of cerebellar degeneration in rats, IGF-I administered intraventricularly or subcutaneously was neuroprotective and increased performance on motor tests *(29)*. This effect can be blocked by infusion of an IGF-IR blocker in the ventricles. IGF-I also increased cerebellar neuronal expression of calbindin, glutamate receptor 1, GABA, and bax, which are decreased by the chemical used to induce the cerebellar neurodegeneration *(30)*.

6. MULTIPLE SCLEROSIS

6.1. Pathophysiology

Multiple sclerosis (MS) is a disease of central nervous system demyelination and is presumed to be an autoimmune disorder, although the exact cause of the autoimmune assault remains under investigation. Areas that have been demyelinated become sclerotic from reactive astrocytosis. IGF-IR expression appears to be same across normal, demyelinated, and sclerotic white matter *(31)*. Immunocytochemistry suggests that macrophages and astrocytes and not oligodendrocytes are the primary cell types that express the IGF-IR in MS plaques. Oligodendrocytes and astrocytes in normal white matter express IGFBP-1, whereas macrophages express IGFBP-2 and -3, and IGF-II *(32)*. These results support the idea that IGFs could promote myelin phagocytosis and astrogliosis in MS plaques.

6.2. Impact on the IGF System

Serum and CSF IGF levels have been examined in MS patients. No changes in IGF-I, IGF-II, and IGFBP-1, -2, and -3 have been detected between MS patients and controls *(33,34)*.

6.3. IGFs in MS Treatment

Despite the low receptor expression in oligodendrocytes found in human MS tissue, a large body of evidence has shown that IGFs are potent stimulators of myelination in the central and peripheral nervous systems (for review, *see* ref. *1*). IGFs have been considered as a potential therapy for multiple sclerosis, but the outcomes of several studies have been contradictory. IGF-I has been used to alter the course of the main animal model of MS, experimental autoimmune encephalomyelitis. In some studies, lesion size and number, blood–brain barrier defects, and clinical progression are decreased in animals treated with subcutaneous or intravenous IGF-I *(35–37)*. IGF-I stimulates the proliferation of oligodendrocyte-like cells in lesions *(36,38)* and increases the production of myelin basic protein, proteolipid protein, and 2′,3′-cyclic nucleotide 3′ phosphodiesterase, all components of myelin *(35,38)*. In other studies, however, IGF-I has only transient effects on clinical improvement, remyelination, and progenitor proliferation *(39,40)*. A small trial of IGF-I in humans with MS showed no decrease in lesion frequency over a 24-wk period *(41)*. So, although *in vitro* studies have recorded the importance of IGFs in myelin development, their usefulness for promoting remyelination in the adult central nervous system appears at this time to be limited.

7. CEREBRAL HYPOXIC/ISCHEMIC INJURY

7.1. Pathophysiology

Hypoxia/ischemia (HI) is a major cause of nervous system injury and commonly follows perinatal hypoventilation as well as cerebral hemorrhage or vascular occlusions (stroke). Loss of neurons in HI conditions is selective and delayed and can involve both apoptotic and necrotic mechanisms *(42,43)*.

7.2. Impact on the IGF System

One study examined, in patients suffering acute ischemic stroke, plasma IGF-I and IGFBP-3 levels at timepoints from 1 to 10 d after ischemia. Plasma IGF-I and IGFBP-3 levels were diminished in the stroke patients compared with healthy controls. IGF-I and IGFBP-3 levels were significantly lowered in patients with infarcts greater than 5 cm. Lowered IGF levels may reflect increased demand for trophic factors, central impairment of the growth hormone axis, altered tissue distribution, or altered IGF metabolism *(44)*. Astrocytes in experimentally infarcted brain regions increase expression of IGF-I and IGFBP-3 mRNA *(45)*. IGFBP-2 and IGFBP-5 mRNAs are induced as well in the infarcted region *(46,47)*. IGF-IR binding increases 6 h after ischemia in the CA1 and CA3 regions of the hippocampus and the dentate gyrus *(48)*. IGF-II mRNA is increased, apparently in glial cells in the infarcted regions, 5–7 d after HI *(49)*. IGF-IIR immunoreactivity increases in pyramidal neurons 4–7 d after infarct *(50)*. In sum, the data suggest that IGF system components are upregulated within several days of cerebral HI, particularly in reactive astrocytes and microglia, and may be critical to an endogenous protective response to neuronal injury.

7.3. IGFs in the Treatment of HI

Animal models of HI have been useful in evaluating the effectiveness of IGFs in rescuing neurons. Several studies have found that central administration of IGF-I 1–2 h after carotid artery occlusion in rats reduces loss of neurons and infarct size *(45,51–54)*. One study found that reduction of neuronal apoptosis was partly responsible for this effect *(54)*. Injury from spinal cord ischemia is also abated by IGF-I. IGF-I given 30 min prior to cord ischemia in rabbits led to greater recovery of limb function 48 h after the injury *(55)*. Single doses appear to have beneficial effects on functional outcomes, whereas long-term treatment seems to be necessary to decrease infarct size. For instance, a single dose of IGF-I 2 h after HI injury in rats resulted in improved somatosensation and neuronal survival at 20 d, but infarct size was not affected *(56)*. A 3-d course of intraventricular or subcutaneous IGF-I had positive effects on both functional outcome and infarct size *(57)*. Studies that have tried doses lower than 20 μg/rat have not been successful at decreasing injury *(48,57)*. Most studies have success with an intraventricular delivery of IGF-I, but this would be impractical in human HI patients. Intranasal delivery of IGF-I was tried in a rat HI model and was successful at decreasing impairment and infarct size *(58)*. Although these studies have outlined a role for IGFs in rescuing neurons from HI injury, IGFs remain an exciting but untried possibility for human stroke therapy.

8. AMYOTROPHIC LATERAL SCLEROSIS

8.1. Pathophysiology

Amyotrophic lateral sclerosis (ALS), or Lou Gehrig's disease, is caused by death of upper and lower motor neurons. The cause of this selective neuronal death in most cases is unknown, although a small percentage of cases are familial and linked to mutations of the superoxide dismutase gene. Glutamate neurotoxicity is proposed to be a general mechanism of motor neuron loss in ALS. Because of their neuroprotective functions, the therapeutic potential of IGFs in ALS has been studied extensively.

8.2. Impact on the IGF System

IGF-I levels are not changed in the sera of patients with ALS *(59)*, although one investigation found increased IGF-I expression in the skin (epidermis, dermal blood vessels, and glands) of patients with ALS *(60)*. In the ventral horn of the spinal cord, free IGF-I is decreased, whereas expression of IGFBPs-2, -5, and -6 is increased *(61)*.

Total IGF-I and IGF-II do not appear to differ between patients with ALS and controls *(61,62)*. IGF-IR density, assayed by immunohistochemistry and radioligand binding, is increased in the gray matter of patients with ALS *(63–65)*. NGF receptor expression *(63)* and insulin binding *(65)* were not changed in ALS. Together, these findings suggest that motor-neuron regions of the spinal cord become more capable of specifically binding IGFs in ALS, and are potentially sensitive to endogenous and exogenous sources of IGFs.

8.3. IGFs in the Treatment of ALS

IGFs prevent neuronal death in the wobbler mouse, a model for motor neuron disease *(66)*. The neuroprotective functions of IGFs and the increased availability of binding sites in ALS spinal cords led to clinical trials of IGF-I as a treatment for ALS. Two major placebo-controlled trials produced different results. The North American ALS/IGF-I Study Group found that disease progression slowed and quality of life improved in patients treated with IGF-I daily for 9 mo *(67)*. However, no measurable benefit from IGF therapy was found in the European ALS/IGF Study Group's trials *(68)*. A study of these trials found trends, although not significant, suggesting that IGFs benefit patients with ALS *(69)*.

Because there seems to be some positive effect of IGFs on ALS patients, they may be useful in a combination therapy for ALS. IGF-I administered with glycosaminoglycans was even more effective at preventing neuronal death in the wobbler mouse *(70)*. A glutamate-toxicity model of ALS was treated with both IGF-I and GDNF. The two growth factors together were additively neuroprotective *(71)*. Although combination paradigms have not yet been investigated in humans, a rat study combining IGF-I with the glutamate-release inhibitor Riluzole, currently in use to treat patients with ALS, did not find any significant additive effect *(72)*. More study is needed to determine the therapeutic potential of IGFs in the treatment of motor neuron disease.

9. DIABETIC NEUROPATHY

9.1. Pathogenesis

Neuropathy is a complication of poorly controlled diabetes. Painful sensory neuropathies are common, and autonomic neuropathies, leading to critical autonomic dysfunction, may occur. The cause of neuropathy in diabetes has been the focus of much investigation but remains elusive. Mechanisms that may contribute to the pathogenesis of diabetic neuropathy include damaged nerve microvasculature, neuronal apoptosis precipitated by high glucose, and impaired nerve regeneration. Studies suggest that the IGF system may be depressed in diabetic neuropathy, leading to compromised peripheral nerve health.

9.2. Impact on the IGF System

Both IGF-I and IGF-II mRNAs are decreased in the peripheral nerves of rats with experimental insulin-dependent diabetes (IDDM) *(73)*. This deficiency is not unique to peripheral nerves—decreased IGF mRNA can also be found in the liver, adrenal glands, and spinal cord in this model *(74)*. IGF-II in the brain is reduced in rat models of both IDDM and noninsulin-dependent diabetes (NIDDM) *(75)*. Insulin therapy in the IDDM model partially restores the levels of IGF mRNA in all these tissues. NIDDM rats have diminished IGF-II mRNA in the peripheral nerves and spinal cord, but IGF-I mRNA appears normal *(76)*. IDDM rats' dorsal root ganglia neurons have reduced expression of IGF-I and the IGF-IR *(77)*. IGF-I and IGF-IR expression is also reduced in the superior cervical ganglia of these rats; expression can be partially restored with insulin therapy *(78)*.

Diabetic humans with neuropathy have significantly lower circulating levels of IGF-I than non-neuropathic diabetic and normal controls *(79,80)*. IGFBP-1 levels, conversely, are increased in diabetics with neuropathy *(81)*. These findings support a relationship between peripheral nerve damage in diabetic neuropathy and decreased IGF availability.

9.3. IGFs in the Treatment of Diabetic Neuropathy

Several studies in rat models of diabetes have found that insulin therapy partially restores IGF levels *(73,74)*. Investigations in human diabetics have found a positive relationship between insulin levels and IGF-I levels and a negative relationship between IGF-I levels and neuropathy *(80,81)*. Thus, good insulin maintenance may lead to normal availability of IGFs and better nerve function.

A number of studies have examined the therapeutic potential of direct administration of IGFs to diabetic rats. IDDM rats subjected to sciatic nerve crush received IGF-I locally via a miniosmotic pump at the injury site or systemically by subcutaneous injection. Nerve regeneration was improved in IGF-treated animals, regardless of the glycemic state of the animal, suggesting that IGFs have a direct effect on nerve regeneration *(82)*. Subcutaneous IGF-I or IGF-II for 2 wk led to decreased hyperalgesia and better nerve regeneration in IDDM rats *(83)*. IGF-I protects against the development of autonomic neuropathy in IDDM rats, as measured by the degree of neuroaxonal dystrophy of the superior mesenteric ganglion and ileal mesenteric nerve *(84)*. IGFs may benefit autonomic neurons by preventing apoptosis in response to high glucose and by promoting neurite growth, which is inhibited by high glucose *(85)*. IGF-IR distribution in the autonomic neurite is abnormal in hyperglycemia and can be restored to normal with IGF-I treatment. These studies indicate that the neurotrophic effects of IGFs could be helpful in ameliorating diabetic neuropathy by promoting neuronal survival and neurite growth.

10. TRAUMATIC BRAIN AND NERVE INJURY

The neuroprotective and neurite regenerative effects of IGF-I have been tested in models of traumatic nervous system injury. IGF-I promotes nerve regeneration in crushed sciatic nerves of rats *(86)*. IGF-II has similar effects on the frog sciatic nerve *(87)*. IGF-I improves motor neuron survival and functional re-innervation of skeletal muscle following sciatic transection in rats *(4)*. Motor and cognitive functions are improved when rats with traumatic brain injury are treated with IGF-I *(88)*. The benefit of IGF-I for humans with head trauma has been examined in only one clinical trial thus far. A 14-d continuous intravenous infusion of IGF-I was given to patients with severe isolated brain trauma. Six months after treatment, 8 of 11 patients who achieved high levels of serum IGF-I had moderate-to-strong improvement, whereas only one of the five patients with low serum IGF-I showed similar improvement *(89)*. These promising results warrant further investigation of the therapeutic potential of IGFs in traumatic nervous system injury.

11. MUSCLE DISEASES

Muscular dystrophies are characterized by defective muscle growth and development. IGFs promote muscle growth and development and may be involved in the pathogenesis and treatment of muscular dystrophies. A study of serum IGF-I and IGFBP-3 in patients with Duchenne's muscular dystrophy (DMD) found no abnormalities *(90)*, but an in vitro study of fibroblasts and myocytes from DMD patients suggests that abnormalities of IGFBP expression may contribute to failure of muscle cell growth. IGFBP-5 message and secretion were increased in DMD fibroblasts, whereas IGFBP-3 message was decreased. DMD myocytes cultured with DMD fibroblasts or with conditioned media from the same fibroblasts showed defective growth. Blocking fibroblast IGFBP-5 expression with antisense oligonucleotides, or neutralizing IGFBP-5 with an antibody, removed the inhibitory effect of the conditioned media on DMD myocytes *(91)*. How the genetic abnormality in DMD would cause altered IGFBP expression in fibroblasts is unclear, but this study identifies a mechanism that can potentially be manipulated therapeutically to promote muscle cell growth.

Myocytes express both IGF-I and a unique splice variant of IGF-I, called mechanogrowth factor (MGF) *(92)*. Proper structural and mechanical function of myocytes leads to autocrine release of IGFs. MGF and IGF-I expression levels are increased after muscle stretching. MGF and IGF-I expression are decreased in the mdx mouse, a genetic model for DMD *(93)*. This apparently depressed IGF function has prompted examination of the effects of exogenous IGFs on dystrophic muscle. In the mdx mouse, an 8-wk course of IGF-I improves diaphragm force, endurance, and oxidative capabilities, and in addition increases the proportion of type IIa fibers *(94)*. Finally, IGF-I promotes glucose uptake in human myotonic dystrophy muscle cells, which are typically resistant to insulin *(95)*. The results from these studies extend the beneficial functions of IGF-I to include improvement of the metabolic functioning of dystrophic muscle.

Steroid myopathy is a common outcome of long-term glucocorticoid therapy (*see* Chapter 11). This myopathy is characterized by type II fiber atrophy and an increase in urine creatine excretion. Rat studies indicate that high-dose steroids decrease IGF-I and -II expression in the liver and muscle *(96)* and may contribute to the pathogenesis of myopathy. Further, hepatocytes exhibit increased IGFBP-1 expression, which could also limit the availability of circulating IGF-I. Dexamethasone inhibits IGF-I signaling to PI-3K and Akt, an important pathway for maintaining cell viability in the face of a variety of stressors *(97)*. IGF-I was given to rats simultaneously with triamcinolone to see if exogenous IGFs could prevent myopathy. Compared with controls, IGF-I helped maintain muscle cell diameter and decreased urine creatine excretion *(98)*. Further studies are needed to determine whether IGFs can reverse pre-existing steroid myopathy.

Muscle wasting and malnutrition are common problems in a number of critical illnesses, including cancer and AIDS (*see* Chapter 3). IGF-I has been tried, sometimes in conjunction with GH, in the treatment of muscle wasting from cancer *(99)*, osteoporosis *(100)*, renal failure *(101)*, severe burns *(102)*, and chronic obstructive pulmonary disease *(103)*. These have shown some success at increasing muscle mass and strength.

IGF-I and GH, however, did not affect muscle wasting in AIDS patients. Adequate nutritional support is needed to permit a response to GH and/or IGF administration *(103)*. Initial studies suggest that coadministration of IGF-I and IGFBP-3 may lead to even more improvement in muscle growth and to fewer side-effects *(105)*. A mouse model of cancer muscle wasting showed better muscle protein synthesis when IGF-I and IGFBP-3 were given together *(106)*.

12. SUMMARY AND CONCLUSIONS

The IGF system is likely involved in the development of some nervous system diseases and in the endogenous response to nervous system disease. IGF expression is lowered in patients with diabetic neuropathy and in myocytes with the DMD mutation, potentially contributing to defective axon and muscle growth. IGFs may stimulate reactive astrocytosis in multiple sclerosis. IGF, IGF-IR, and IGFBP expression are altered locally or systemically in AD, hypoxia/ischemia, and ALS, suggesting that upregulation of IGF availability or sensitivity is part of an endogenous protection of injured neurons.

Effective treatment of nervous system disease remains a formidable challenge. Understanding the factors that prevent neuronal death and restore functional neuronal processes may lead to successful treatments of several nervous system diseases. The neuroprotective and neurite-stimulating effects of IGFs make them strong candidates for the treatment of nervous system disease. They have been used successfully in culture and animal models of AD, HD, MS, stroke, ALS, trauma, and neuropathy. IGFs have been used in human trials of trauma, ALS, and critical-illness muscle wasting. Although these trials show promise for effectiveness, much more work is needed to understand how IGFs can be used to combat these diseases.

13. FUTURE CHALLENGES

Despite advances in understanding the involvement of IGFs in nervous system development and health, there has been little direct investigation of the impact of nutrition on IGF function in the nervous system. There are nervous system diseases caused by improper nutrition, including various neuropathies and Wernicke–Korsakoff syndrome. For a number of these conditions, a specific insult—such as a vitamin deficiency—has been identified. However, the impact of these deficiencies on the IGF system in these diseases is unknown. Critical illness can certainly have a negative impact on nutrition status, and whether poor nutrition from severe nervous system disease affects the IGF system awaits investigation.

ACKNOWLEDGMENTS

This work was supported by the National Institutes of Health (NS38849 and NS36778), the Juvenile Diabetes Research Foundation and the Program for Understanding Neurological Diseases (PFUND).

REFERENCES

1. Leinninger GM, Meyer GE, Feldman EL. IGFs and the Nervous System. In: Insulin-Like Growth Factors. LeRoith D, Zumkeller W, Baxter R (eds.). http://www.eurekah.com/chapter.php?chapid=975&bookid=34&catid=19: Eurekah.com, 2003.

2. Wilkins A, Chandran S, Compston A. A role for oligodendrocyte-derived IGF-1 in trophic support of cortical neurons. Glia 2001;36:48–57.
3. Zhang Y, Tatsuno T, Carney JM, et al. Basic FGF, NGF, and IGFs protect hippocampal and cortical neurons against iron-induced degeneration. J Cereb Blood Flow Metab 1993;13:378–388.
4. Vergani L, Di Giulio AM, Losa M, et al. Systemic administration of insulin-like growth factor decreases motor neuron cell death and promotes muscle reinnervation. J Neurosci Res 1998;54:840–847.
5. Pu SF, Zhuang HX, Marsh DJ, et al. Insulin-like growth factor-II increases and IGF is required for postnatal rat spinal motoneuron survival following sciatic nerve axotomy. J Neurosci Res 1999;55:9–16.
6. Ishii DN, Glazner GW, Pu S-F. Role of insulin-like growth factors in peripheral nerve regeneration. Pharmacol Ther 1994;62:125–144.
7. Zackenfels K, Oppenheim RW, Rohrer H. Evidence for an important role of IGF-I and IGF-II for the early development of chick sympathetic neurons. Neuron 1995;14:731–741.
8. Vincent AM, Feldman EL. Control of cell survival by IGF signaling pathways. Growth Hormone IGF Res 2002;12:193.
9. Bondy CA, Lee W-H, Cheng CM. IGF1 and brain development. In: LeRoith D, Zumkeller W, Baxter R eds. Insulin-Like Growth Factors. http:www.eurekah.com, 2003.
10. Jafferali S, Dumont Y, Sotty F, et al. Insulin-like growth factor-I and its receptor in the frontal cortex, hippocampus, and cerebellum of normal human and Alzheimer disease brains. Synapse 2000;38:450–459.
11. Murialdo G, Barreca A, Nobili F, et al. Relationships between cortisol, dehydroepiandrosterone sulphate and insulin-like growth factor-I system in dementia. J Endocrinol Invest 2001;24:139–146.
12. Sara VR, Hall K, Enzell K, et al. Somatomedins in aging and dementia disorders of the Alzheimer type. Neurobiol Aging 1982;3:117–120.
13. Tham A, Nordberg A, Grissom FE, et al. Insulin-like growth factors and insulin-like growth factor binding proteins in cerebrospinal fluid and serum of patients with dementia of the Alzheimer type. J Neural Transm Park Dis Dement Sect 1993;5:165–176.
14. Mustafa A, Lannfelt L, Lilius L, et al. Decreased plasma insulin-like growth factor-I level in familial Alzheimer's disease patients carrying the Swedish APP 670/671 mutation. Dement Geriatr Cogn Disord 1999;10:446–451.
15. Tham A, Sparring K, Bowen D, et al. Insulin-like growth factors and somatomedin B in the cerebrospinal fluid of patients with dementia of the Alzheimer type. Acta Psychiatr Scand 1988;77:719–723.
16. Connor B, Beilharz EJ, Williams C, et al. Insulin-like growth factor-I (IGF-I) immunoreactivity in the Alzheimer's disease temporal cortex and hippocampus. Brain Res Mol Brain Res 1997;49:283–290.
17. Crews FT, McElhaney R, Freund G, et al. Binding of [125I]-insulin-like growth factor-1 (IGF-1) in brains of Alzheimer's and alcoholic patients. Adv Exp Med Biol 1991;293:483–492.
18. Crews FT, McElhaney R, Freund G, et al. Insulin-like growth factor I receptor binding in brains of Alzheimer's and alcoholic patients. J Neurochem 1992;58:1205–1210.
19. De Keyser J, Wilczak N, Goossens A. Insulin-like growth factor-I receptor densities in human frontal cortex and white matter during aging, in Alzheimer's disease, and in Huntington's disease. Neurosci Lett 1994;172:93–96.
20. Wei W, Wang X, Kusiak JW. Signaling events in amyloid beta-peptide-induced neuronal death and insulin-like growth factor I protection. J Biol Chem 2002;277:17649–17656.
21. Dore S, Bastianetto S, Kar, S et al. Protective and rescuing abilities of IGF-I and some putative free radical scavengers against beta-amyloid-inducing toxicity in neurons. Ann N Y Acad Sci 1999;890:356–364.
22. Niikura T, Hashimoto Y, Okamoto T, et al. Insulin-like growth factor I (IGF-I) protects cells from apoptosis by Alzheimer's V642I mutant amyloid precursor protein through IGF-I receptor in an IGF-binding protein-sensitive manner. J Neurosci 2001;21:1902–1910.
23. Hong M, Lee VM. Insulin and insulin-like growth factor-1 regulate tau phosphorylation in cultured human neurons. J Biol Chem 1997;272:19547–19553.
24. Martignoni E, Horowski R, Liuzzi A, et al. Effects of terguride on anterior pituitary function in parkinsonian patients treated with L-dopa: a double-blind study versus placebo. Clin Neuropharmacol 1996;19:72–80.

25. Unsicker K. Growth factors in Parkinson's disease. Prog Growth Factor Res 1994;5:73–87.
26. Humbert S, Bryson EA, Cordelieres FP, et al. The IGF-1/Akt pathway is neuroprotective in Huntington's disease and involves Huntingtin phosphorylation by Akt. Dev Cell 2002;2:831–837.
27. Busiguina S, Fernandez AM, Barrios V, et al. Neurodegeneration is associated to changes in serum insulin-like growth factors. Neurobiol Dis 2000;7:657–665.
28. Torres-Aleman I, Barrios V, Lledo A, et al. The insulin-like growth factor I system in cerebellar degeneration. Ann Neurol 1996;39:335–342.
29. Fernandez AM, de la Vega AG, Torres-Aleman I. Insulin-like growth factor I restores motor coordination in a rat model of cerebellar ataxia. Proc Natl Acad Sci USA 1998;95:1253–1258.
30. Fernandez AM, Gonzalez de la Vega AG, Planas B, et al. Neuroprotective actions of peripherally administered insulin-like growth factor I in the injured olivo-cerebellar pathway. Eur J Neurosci 1999;11:2019–2030.
31. Wilczak N, De Keyser J. Insulin-like growth factor-I receptors in normal appearing white matter and chronic plaques in multiple sclerosis. Brain Res 1997;772:243–246.
32. Gveric D, Cuzner ML, Newcombe J. Insulin-like growth factors and binding proteins in multiple sclerosis plaques. Neuropathol Appl Neurobiol 1999;25:215–225.
33. Wilczak N, Schaaf M, Bredewold R et al. Insulin-like growth factor system in serum and cerebrospinal fluid in patients with multiple sclerosis. Neurosci Lett 1998;257:168–170.
34. Torres-Aleman I, Barrios V, Berciano J. The peripheral insulin-like growth factor system in amyotrophic lateral sclerosis and in multiple sclerosis. Neurology 1998;50:772–776.
35. Yao DL, Liu X, Hudson LD, et al. Insulin-like growth factor-I given subcutaneously reduces clinical deficits, decreases lesion severity and upregulates synthesis of myelin proteins in experimental autoimmune encephalomyelitis. Life Sci 1996;58:1301–1306.
36. Liu X, Yao DL, Webster J. Insulin-like growth factor I treatment reduces clinical deficits and lesion severity in acute demyelinating autoimmune encephalomyelitis. Mult Scler 1995;1:2–9.
37. Li W, Quigley L, Yao D-L, et al. Chronic relapsing experimental autoimmune encephalomyelitis: effects of insulin-like growth factor-I treatment on clinical deficits, lesion severity, glial responses, and blood brain barrier defects. J Neuropathol Exp Neurol 1998;57:426–438.
38. Yao D-L, Liu X, Hudson LD, et al. Insulin-like growth factor I treatment reduces demyelination and up-regulates gene expression of myelin-related proteins in experimental autoimmune encephalomyelitis. Proc Natl Acad Sci USA 1995;92:6190–6194.
39. Cannella B, Pitt D, Capello E, et al. Insulin-like growth factor-1 fails to enhance central nervous system myelin repair during autoimmune demyelination. Am J Pathol 2000;157:933–943.
40. Lovett-Racke AE, Bittner P, Cross AH, et al. Regulation of experimental autoimmune encephalomyelitis with insulin-like growth factor (IGF-1) and IGF-1/IGF-binding protein-3 complex (IGF-1/IGFBP3). J Clin Invest 1998;101:1797–1804.
41. Frank JA, Richert N, Lewis B, et al. A pilot study of recombinant insulin-like growth factor-1 in seven multiple sclerosis patients. Mult Scler 2002;8:24–29.
42. Scott RJ, Hegyi L. Cell death in perinatal hypoxic ischemic brain injury. Neuropathol Appl Neurobiol 1997;23:307–314.
43. Johnson EM, Greenlund LJ, Akins PT, et al. Neuronal apoptosis: current understanding of molecular mechanisms and potential role in ischemic brain injury. J Neurotrauma 1995;12:843–852.
44. Schwab S, Spranger M, Krempien S, et al. Plasma insulin-like growth factor I and IGF binding protein 3 levels in patients with acute cerebral ischemic injury. Stroke 1997;28:1744–1748.
45. Gluckman P, Klempt N, Guan J, et al. A role for IGF-1 in the rescue of CNS neurons following hypoxic-ischemic injury. Biochem Biophys Res Commun 1992;182:593–599.
46. Klempt ND, Klempt M, Gunn AJ, et al. Expression of insulin-like growth factor-binding protein 2 (IGF-BP 2) following transient hypoxia-ischemia in the infant rat brain. Brain Res Mol Brain Res 1992;15:55–61.
47. Beilharz EJ, Klempt ND, Klempt M, et al. Differential expression of insulin-like growth factor binding proteins (IGFBP) 4 and 5 mRNA in the rat brain after transient hypoxic-ischemic injury. Brain Res Mol Brain Res 1993;18:209–215.
48. Bergstedt K, Wieloch T. Changes in insulin-like growth factor 1 receptor density after transient cerebral ischemia in the rat. Lack of protection against ischemic brain damage following injection of insulin-like growth factor 1. J Cereb Blood Flow Metab 1993;13:895–898.

49. Beilharz EJ, Bassett NS, Sirimanne ES, et al. Insulin-like growth factor II is induced during wound repair following hypoxic-ischemic injury in the developing rat brain. Brain Res Mol Brain Res 1995;29:81–91.
50. Stephenson DT, Rash K, Clemens JA. Increase in insulin-like growth factor II receptor within ischemic neurons following focal cerebral infarction. J Cereb Blood Flow Metab 1995;15:1022–1031.
51. Guan J, Williams CE, Skinner SJM, et al. The effects of insulin-like growth factor (IGF)-1, IGF-2, and des-IGF-1 on neuronal loss after hypoxic-ischemic brain injury in adult rats: Evidence for a role for IGF binding proteins. Endocrinology 1996;137:893–898.
52. Guan J, Williams C, Gunning M, et al. The effects of IGF-1 treatment after hypoxic-ischemic brain injury in adult rats. J Cereb Blood Flow Metab 1993;13:609–616.
53. Zhu CZ, Auer RN. Intraventricular administration of insulin and IGF-1 in transient forebrain ischemia. J Cereb Blood Flow Metab 1994;14:237–242.
54. Tagami M, Ikeda K, Fujino H, et al. Insulin-like growth factor-1 attenuates apoptosis in hippocampal neurons caused by cerebral ischemia and reperfusion in stroke-prone spontaneously hypertensive rats. Lab Invest 1997;76:613–617.
55. Nakao Y, Otani H, Yamamura T, et al. Insulin-like growth factor 1 prevents neuronal cell death and paraplegia in the rabbit model of spinal cord ischemia. J Thorac Cardiovasc Surg 2001;122:136–143.
56. Guan J, Miller OT, Waugh KM, et al. Insulin-like growth factor-1 improves somatosensory function and reduces the extent of cortical infarction and ongoing neuronal loss after hypoxia-ischemia in rats. Neuroscience 1902;105:299–306.
57. Schabitz WR, Hoffmann TT, Heiland S, et al. Delayed neuroprotective effect of insulin-like growth factor-i after experimental transient focal cerebral ischemia monitored with mri. Stroke 2001;32:1226–1233.
58. Liu XF, Fawcett JR, Thorne RG, et al. Intranasal administration of insulin-like growth factor-I bypasses the blood-brain barrier and protects against focal cerebral ischemic damage. J Neurol Sci 2001;187:91–97.
59. Braunstein GD, Reviczky AL. Serum insulin-like growth factor-I levels in amyotrophic lateral sclerosis. J Neurol Neurosurg Psychiatry 1987;50:792–794.
60. Ono S, Hu J, Imai T, et al. Increased expression of insulin-like growth factor I in skin in amyotrophic lateral sclerosis. J Neurol Neurosurg Psychiatry 2000;69:199–203.
61. Wilczak N, de Vos RA, De Keyser J. Free insulin-like growth factor (IGF)-I and IGF binding proteins 2, 5, and 6 in spinal motor neurons in amyotrophic lateral sclerosis. Lancet 2003;361:1007–1011.
62. Kerkhoff H, Hassan SM, Troost D, et al. Insulin-like and fibroblast growth factors in spinal cords, nerve roots and skeletal muscle of human controls and patients with amyotrophic lateral sclerosis. Acta Neuropathol 1994;87:411–421.
63. Adem A, Ekblom J, Gillberg P-G. Growth factor receptors in amyotrophic lateral sclerosis. Mol Neurobiol 1994;9:225–231.
64. Adem A, Ekblom J, Gillberg P-G, et al. Insulin-like growth factor-1 receptors in human spinal cord: Changes in amyotrophic lateral sclerosis. J Neural Transm 1994;97:73–84.
65. Doré S, Krieger C, Kar S, et al. Distribution and levels of insulin-like growth factor (IGF-I and IGF-II) and insulin receptor binding sites in the spinal cords of amyotrophic lateral sclerosis (ALS) patients. Brain Res Mol Brain Res 1996;41:128–133.
66. Vaught JL, Contreras PC, Glicksman MA, et al. Potential utility of rhIGF-1 in neuromuscular and/or degenerative disease. CIBA Found Symp 1996;196:18–27.
67. Lai EC, Felice KJ, Festoff BW, et al. Effect of recombinant human insulin-like growth factor-I on progression of ALS. A placebo-controlled study. The North America ALS/IGF-I Study Group. Neurology 1997;49:1621–1630.
68. Borasio GD, Robberecht W, Leigh PN, et al. A placebo-controlled trial of insulin-like growth factor-I in amyotrophic lateral sclerosis. European ALS/IGF-I Study Group. Neurology 1998;51:583–586.
69. Mitchell JD, Wokke JH, Borasio GD. Recombinant human insulin-like growth factor I (rhIGF-I) for amyotrophic lateral sclerosis/motor neuron disease. Cochrane Database Syst Rev 2002; CD002064.
70. Gorio A, Lesma E, Madaschi L, et al. Co-administration of IGF-I and glycosaminoglycans greatly delays motor neurone disease and affects IGF-I expression in the wobbler mouse: a long-term study. J Neurochem 2002;81:194–202.

71. Bilak MM, Corse AM, Kuncl RW. Additivity and potentiation of IGF-I and GDNF in the complete rescue of postnatal motor neurons. Amyotroph Lateral Scler Other Motor Neuron Disord 2001;2:83–91.
72. Iwasaki Y, Ikeda K. Prevention by insulin-like growth factor-I and riluzole in motor neuron death after neonatal axotomy. J Neurol Sci 1999;169:148–155.
73. Wuarin L, Guertin DM, Ishii DN. Early reduction in insulin-like growth factor gene expression in diabetic nerve. Exp Neurol 1994;130:106–114.
74. Ishii DN, Guertin DM, Whalen LR. Reduced insulin-like growth factor-I mRNA content in liver, adrenal glands and spinal cord of diabetic rats. Diabetologia 1994;37:1037–1081.
75. Wuarin L, Namdev R, Burns JG, et al. Brain insulin-like growth Factor-II mRNA content is reduced in insulin-dependent and non-insulin-dependent diabetes Mellitus. J Neurochem 1996;67:742–751.
76. Zhuang HX, Wuarin L, Fei ZJ, et al. Insulin-like growth factor (IGF) gene expression is reduced in neural tissues and liver from rats with non-insulin-dependent diabetes mellitus, and IGF treatment ameliorates diabetic neuropathy. J Pharmacol Exp Ther 1997;283:366–374.
77. Craner MJ, Klein JP, Black JA, et al. Preferential expression of IGF-I in small DRG neurons and down-regulation following injury. Neuroreport 2002;13:1649–1652.
78. Bitar MS, Pilcher CW, Khan I, et al. Diabetes-induced suppression of IGF-1 and its receptor mRNA levels in rat superior cervical ganglia. Diabetes Res Clin Pract 1997;38:73–80.
79. Guo H, Yang Y, Geng Z, et al. The change of insulin-like growth factor-1 in diabetic patients with neuropathy. Chin Med J (Engl) 1999;112:76–79.
80. Migdalis IN, Kalogeropoulou K, Kalantzis L, et al. Insulin-like growth factor-I and IGF-I receptors in diabetic patients with neuropathy. Diabet Med 1995;12:823–827.
81. Crosby SR, Tsigos C, Anderton CD, et al. Elevated plasma insulin-like growth factor binding protein-1 levels in Type 1 (insulin-dependent) diabetic patients with peripheral neuropathy. Diabetologia 1992;35:868–872.
82. Ishii DN, Lupien SB. Insulin-like growth factors protect against diabetic neuropathy: Effects on sensory nerve regeneration in rats. J Neurosci Res 1995;40:138–144.
83. Zhuang HX, Synder CK, Pu SF, et al. Insulin-like growth factors reverse or arrest diabetic neuropathy: Effects on hyperalgesia and impaired nerve regeneration in rats. Exp Neurol 1996;140:198–205.
84. Schmidt RE, Dorsey DA, Beaudet LN, et al. Insulin-like growth factor I reverses experimental diabetic autonomic neuropathy. Am J Pathol 1999;155:1651–1660.
85. Russell JW, Feldman EL. Insulin-like growth factor-I prevents apoptosis in sympathetic neurons exposed to high glucose. Horm Metab Res 1999;31:90–96.
86. Kanje M, Skottner A, Sjoberg J, et al. Insulin-like growth factor I (IGF-I) stimulates regeneration of the rat sciatic nerve. Brain Res 1989;486:396–398.
87. Edbladh M, Fex-Svenningsen Å, Ekström PA, et al. Insulin and IGF-II, but not IGF-I, stimulate the in vitro regeneration of adult frog sciatic sensory axons. Brain Res 1994;641:76–82.
88. Saatman KE, Contreras PC, Smith DH, et al. Insulin-like growth factor-1 (IGF-1) improves both neurological motor and cognitive outcome following experimental brain injury. Exp Neurol 1997;147:418–427.
89. Hatton J, Rapp RP, Kudsk KA, et al. Intravenous insulin-like growth factor-I (IGF-I) in moderate-to-severe head injury: a Phase II safety and efficacy trial. J Neurosurg 1997;86:779–786.
90. Nagel BH, Mortier W, Elmlinger M, et al. Short stature in Duchenne muscular dystrophy: a study of 34 patients. Acta Paediatr 1999;88:62–65.
91. Melone MA, Peluso G, Galderisi U, et al. Increased expression of IGF-binding protein-5 in Duchenne muscular dystrophy (DMD) fibroblasts correlates with the fibroblast-induced downregulation of DMD myoblast growth: an in vitro analysis. J Cell Physiol 2000;185:143–153.
92. Yang S, Alnaqeeb M, Simpson H, et al. Cloning and characterization of an IGF-1 isoform expressed in skeletal muscle subjected to stretch. J Muscle Res Cell Motil 1996;17:487–495.
93. Goldspink G. Changes in muscle mass and phenotype and the expression of autocrine and systemic growth factors by muscle in response to stretch and overload. J Anat 1999;194:323–334.
94. Gregorevic P, Plant DR, Leeding KS, et al. Improved contractile function of the mdx dystrophic mouse diaphragm muscle after insulin-like growth factor-I administration. Am J Pathol 2002;161:2263–2272.
95. Furling D, Marette A, Puymirat J. Insulin-like growth factor I circumvents defective insulin action in human myotonic dystrophy skeletal muscle cells. Endocrinology 1999;140:4244–4250.

96. Gayan-Ramirez G, Vanderhoydonc F, Verhoeven G, et al. Acute treatment with corticosteroids decreases IGF-1 and IGF-2 expression in the rat diaphragm and gastrocnemius. Am J Respir Crit Care Med 1999;159:283–289.
97. Singleton JR, Baker BL, Thorburn A. Dexamethasone inhibits insulin-like growth factor signaling and potentiates myoblast apoptosis. Endocrinology 2000;141:2945–2950.
98. Kanda F, Takatani K, Okuda S, et al. Preventive effects of insulinlike growth factor-I on steroid-induced muscle atrophy. Muscle Nerve 1999;22:213–217.
99. Ng E-H, Rock CS, Lazarus DD, et al. Insulin-like growth factor I preserves host lean tissue mass in cancer cachexia. Am J Physiol 1992;262:R426–R431.
100. Sugimoto T, Nakaoka D, Nasu M, et al. Effect of recombinant human growth hormone in elderly osteoporotic women. Clin Endocrinol (Oxf) 1999;51:715–724.
101. Johannsson G, Bengtsson BA, Ahlmen J. Double-blind, placebo-controlled study of growth hormone treatment in elderly patients undergoing chronic hemodialysis: anabolic effect and functional improvement. Am J Kidney Dis 1999;33:709–717.
102. Fang CH, Li BG, Wang JJ, et al. Treatment of burned rats with insulin-like growth factor I inhibits the catabolic response in skeletal muscle. Am J Physiol 1998;275:R1091–R1098.
103. Clemmons DR, Underwood LE. Role of insulin-like growth factors and growth hormone in reversing catabolic states. Horm Res 1992;38(Suppl)2:37–40.
104. Lee PD, Pivarnik JM, Bukar JG, et al. A randomized, placebo-controlled trial of combined insulin-like growth factor I and low dose growth hormone therapy for wasting associated with human immunodeficiency virus infection. J Clin Endocrinol Metab 1996;81:2968–2975.
105. Clemmons DR, Moses AC, McKay MJ, et al. The combination of insulin-like growth factor I and insulin-like growth factor-binding protein-3 reduces insulin requirements in insulin-dependent type 1 diabetes: evidence for in vivo biological activity. J Clin Endocrinol Metab 2000;85:1518–1524.
106. Wang W, Iresjo BM, Karlsson L, et al. Provision of rhIGF-I/IGFBP-3 complex attenuated development of cancer cachexia in an experimental tumor model. Clin Nutr 2000;19:127–132.

13 The Kidney and the Insulin-Like Growth Factor System in Health and Disease

Ralph Rabkin, Steven S. Guest, and Franz Schaefer

KEY POINTS

- Given the complexity of renal structure it is not surprising that the expression of the IGF-I axis within the kidney is anatomically heterogeneous. As in other tissues, the local kidney IGF-I system is nutrient sensitive.
- IGF-I stimulates renal growth, increases renal blood flow and glomerular filtration rate and modifies several tubular processes including the transport of phosphate and sodium.
- Potassium depletion, metabolic acidosis and diabetes are conditions in which renal hypertrophy, growth retardation and muscle wasting occur simultaneously and in which local and systemic changes in IGF-I levels are thought to play an important role.
- A number of studies have implicated GH/IGF-I in the development and progression of kidney disease.
- An important area that merits further study is the resistance of IGF-I and GH that develops in uremia.

1.INTRODUCTION

Insulin-like growth factor-I (IGF-I) is produced in tissues throughout the body under the influence of growth hormone (GH), and this system is highly sensitive to nutrients *(1–4)*. The liver is the main source of circulating IGF-I, and the kidney is a major endocrine target for this growth factor. IGF-I stimulates renal growth, increases renal blood flow and glomerular filtration rate (GFR), and modifies several tubular processes, including the transport of phosphate and sodium *(1)*. IGF-I mediates most but not all of the renal actions attributed to GH. Circulating IGF-I is mostly bound to high affinity insulin-like growth factor binding proteins (IGFBPs), especially IGFBP-3, that together with an acid-labile subunit forms a 150-kDa complex *(5)*. Lesser amounts of IGF-I circulates bound to the lower molecular weight IGFBPs, namely IGFBP-1, -2, -4, -5, and -6, forming smaller complexes, and typically less than 2% of the serum IGF-I circulates in the freely bioavailable unbound form *(5)*. In general IGF-

From: *IGF and Nutrition in Health and Disease*
Edited by: M. S. Houston, J. M. P. Holly, and E. L. Feldman © Humana Press Inc., Totowa, NJ

BPs have an inhibitory effect on IGF-I action; however, some IGFBPs may actually enhance IGF-I activity in certain cells. Some of the circulating lower molecular weight IGF-I/IGFBP complexes are preferentially delivered to the kidney. The locally expressed renal IGF-I system consists of IGF-I, IGF-I receptors, GH receptors, and six IGFBPs *(1)*. Although the IGF-I receptors are expressed throughout the kidney, the other components of the IGF-I system are expressed in anatomically heterogeneous manner. Local IGF-I and circulating IGF-I have a major impact on kidney structure and function both in health and disease and these effects are modulated by nutrients *(1,2)*. In turn, loss of renal function has a negative impact on the IGF-I system. For example, reduced IGF-I generation and bioavailability appears to play a key role in the growth retardation that occurs in kidney failure *(6)*.

In this chapter, we review the physiology of the renal IGF-I system and the impact of nutrients thereon, the potential role of IGF-I in the pathogenesis of kidney disease with emphasis on nutrient related disease processes, and the impact of renal failure on the extra-renal IGF-I system. Finally, we will briefly review the role of nutrition, IGF-I, and GH in the management of renal failure.

2. BACKGROUND

2.1. The Intrarenal IGF-I Axis

The kidney is a heterogeneous structure consisting of a vascular network from which the glomerulus and peritubular vessels arise, an interstitial compartment, and tubules composed of various cell types and functions delivering a modified glomerular ultrafiltrate into a collecting system that terminates in the kidney pelvis. Given this complexity of renal structure, it is not surprising that the expression of the IGF-I axis within the kidney is anatomically heterogeneous (Fig. 1.) This has made it difficult to evaluate the specific renal actions of the various components of this axis.

In the glomerulus, the mRNAs for the IGF-I and IGF-II receptors, IGF-I and IGFBP-2, -4, and -5 are present *(7–10)*. In the proximal tubule, the mRNAs for the GH and IGF-I receptors, and IGFBP-4 and -5 are expressed *(7,8,11)*. IGF-I is transiently expressed in the proximal tubule after acute tubular necrosis but is undetectable in the uninjured tubule *(12)*. In contrast IGF-I peptide is detectable along the luminal and antiluminal poles of the proximal tubule reflecting trapping by the abundant IGF-I receptors and possibly by IGFBPs *(12–15)*. The IGF-I receptor, present throughout the kidney, is far more abundant in the antiluminal plasma membranes than in the luminal membranes. The thick ascending limb of Henle in the rat expresses all the most important components of the IGF-I axis, namely the mRNA for the GH and IGF-I receptors, IGF-I and IGFBP-1 *(7,8,11)*. IGF-I mRNA has not been detected in the human loop of Henle. The distal tubule expresses the IGF-I and IGF-II receptor mRNAs, in the rat the mRNAs for IGFBP-1, -2, and -4, and in humans IGFBP-2. Although the IGF-I peptide is detectable at this site *(16)*, it is controversial whether IGF-I is actually synthesized here. In the rat renal interstitium, there is expression of the mRNAs for IGFBP-2 through IGFBP-5, and in the human kidney, IGF-II mRNA and peptide are detectable *(11,17,18)*.

Given the complexity and anatomical heterogeneity of the renal IGF-I system, it is difficult to envisage how the various components interact and mediate their respective actions. The presence of IGF-I receptors throughout the kidney is consistent with the

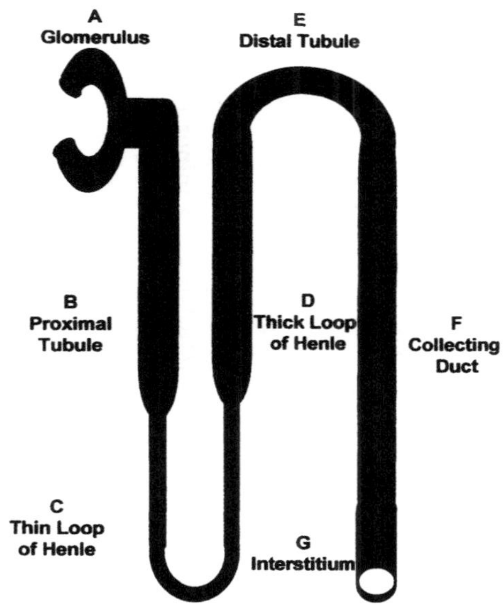

	A	B	C	D	E	F	G
IGF - I			+	+	+	+	
IGF - II						+	
IGF - I Rec	+	+		+	+	+	+
IGF - II Rec	+	+	+			+	+
IGFBP - I	+		+	+	+	+	
IGFBP - 2	+		+		+	+	+
IGFBP - 3	+						+
IGFBP - 4	+	+				+	+
IGFBP - 5	+	+			+		+
GH Rec				+			

Fig. 1. Expression of the IGF-I system in the kidney. Note the marked anatomical variation in expression. Rec, receptor.

multifunctional nature of this growth factor. The colocalization of the GH receptor and IGF-I receptor, IGF-I, and IGFBP-1 in the loop of Henle suggests that this nephron segment is a major site of GH-induced renal IGF-I production and that IGFBP-I is a major modulator of IGF-I action at this site. In addition to GH, IGF-I production is stimulated by EGF *(19)*, and this effect is affected by nutrient intake.

2.2. Renal Uptake and Excretion of IGF-I and IGFBPs

Insulin-like growth factor-1 has a molecular weight of 7.5 kDa. Proteins of this size usually pass through the glomerular filtration barrier with little restriction, followed by nearly complete absorption in the proximal tubule with urinary excretion of the balance *(20)*. Absorption occurs by a process of receptor-mediated endocytosis in the proximal tubule and intracellular transport of IGF-I to the lysosomes where it is degraded *(15)*. A small amount of IGF-I may be delivered to the nucleus *(21)*. IGF-I is also removed from the peritubular circulation to be taken up through the antiluminal tubular cell membrane by receptor-mediated endocytosis *(15)*. Because of the normally high rate of renal blood flow (approx 25% of the cardiac output) and glomerular filtration (180 L of plasma water filtered per day), the kidney is a major site of low molecular weight protein clearance from the circulation *(20)*. However, the renal handling of IGF-I is complicated because of the binding of IGF-I to the IGFBPs with the formation of approx 45- and 150-kDa complexes that restrict the passage of the bound IGF-I through the filtration barrier *(5)*. Most of the bound IGF-I circulates complexed to IGFBP-3, that together with an acid-labile subunit forming a 150-kDa complex. A lesser amount of IGF-I circulates bound to IGFBP-1, -2, -4, and -6. Because normally less than 2% of the circulating IGF-I is not bound to protein and relatively freely filtered, the role of the kidney in its clearance is limited. This has been confirmed in human studies that found similar serum clearance of IGF-I in patients with advanced chronic renal failure and normal controls *(22)*.

IGFBPs also undergo glomerular filtration and appear in the urine in small amounts. Reflecting their higher circulating levels, the filtered IGF binding proteins are composed predominantly of IGFBP-1, IGFBP-2, and IGFBP-3, with IGFBP-2 and IGFBP-3 being the predominant binding proteins found in the urine *(1)*. The excretion of IGF-I in the urine tends to be higher in the young, reflecting their higher serum levels, and falls with age. It is increased several fold in acromegalics and also in patients with severe proteinuria, as discussed later.

2.3. Insulin-Like Growth Factors and Nephrogenesis

During fetal life, IGF-II is a major endocrine, paracrine, and autocrine regulator of tissue growth and differentiation, whereas IGF-I plays a minor role in fetal growth and organogenesis. IGF-II mRNA is strongly expressed in the fetal human kidney *(24–26)*. IGF-II expression is localized to interstitial cells, the renovascular system, glomerular epithelium, undifferentiated but not mature tubular epithelium, and pelvic urothelium *(26)*. IGF-I is expressed with lower abundance than IGF-II in the rat and hardly detectable in the human fetal kidney *(24,27,28)*. Acting via IGF receptors expressed in the metanephroi with a peak in early gestation *(29,30)*, IGF-II and (at least in the rat) IGF-I promote the formation and growth of nephrons *(28)*. Whereas renal IGF-II expression is downregulated with progressive differentiation of the nephrogenic zone *(25,31)*, renal IGF-I mRNA levels are constant during intrauterine life and increase only after birth *(32–34)*. The tissue actions of IGF-II are also regulated by the IGF-II/mannose receptor, a clearance receptor that is highly expressed in fetal tissues, including the developing kidney *(35)*. In experimental maternal diabetes, altered nephrogenesis is associated with increased IGF-II/mannose receptor expression in the metanephroi *(36)*.

The expression of IGF-binding proteins in the kidney emerges with increasing differentiation of renal cell types. IGFBP-2 is the most abundantly expressed binding protein in the fetal kidney *(31,33,37)*. In human kidneys, IGFBP-2 is mainly expressed by differentiating glomerular epithelial cells *(31)*. Although the local, developmentally regulated IGF-II expression and impaired metanephroi development of cultured organs exposed to neutralizing IGF-II antibodies suggest an important growth promoting role of IGF-II in the nephrogenic zone *(28)*, it is still unclear whether IGF-II is an indispensable mediator of nephrogenesis. Mice lacking the IGF-II gene are small but their kidneys are of normal morphology and function *(38)*. In the neonatal rat with urinary tract obstruction, treatment with IGF-I attenuates the tubulointerstitial fibrosis but does not affect the impaired nephrogenesis caused by the obstruction *(39)*.

3. MODULATING EFFECTS OF IGF-I AND IGF BINDING PROTEINS ON KIDNEY STRUCTURE AND FUNCTION

3.1. Effect of IGF-I on Normal Kidney Structure and Function

IGF-I is a potent promoter of renal growth. When administered to rats, it causes renal hypertrophy by inducing both cellular hypertrophy and hyperplasia *(40,41)*. Mice transgenic for IGF-I have enlarged kidneys, as do GH transgenic mice *(42,43)*. Renal enlargement with increased renal blood flow and GFR is also seen in humans with acromegaly and this regresses after treatment of the condition and the secondary fall in IGF-I levels *(44–46)*. The growth-promoting effect of IGF-I differs somewhat from that of GH. GH causes a general increase in body growth with a proportional increase in organ size, whereas IGF-I produces a disproportional increase in kidney, spleen, and adrenal size and a lesser increase in body growth *(47)*. Because the response to these two growth promoters differs somewhat, it is not clear as to what extent the renotropic action of GH is mediated through IGF-I or via a direct action of GH. The presence of GH receptors in nephron segments, such as the proximal tubule, which normally do not express the IGF-I mRNA, suggests that some of the GH-induced renotropic effects are directly mediated by GH. However, as will be discussed later, the renal actions of GH are predominantly mediated through IGF-I.

Renal blood flow and glomerular filtration rate increase markedly within minutes to hours after the administration of IGF-I *(48–50)*. In humans IGF-I causes a 20–30% increase in RBF and GFR, which is sustained as long as IGF-I is administered. In contrast, it takes several days of GH treatment to induce a similar response, which correlates with the rise in serum IGF-I levels *(51–54)*, indicating that the renal hemodynamic effects of GH are mediated by IGF-I. Administration of IGF-I to GH-deficient rats or to Laron-type dwarfs (patients with mutated nonfunctional GH receptors) normalizes the low GFR *(55,56)*. In sophisticated physiologic studies, Hirschberg et al. *(57)* showed that these effects of IGF-I were mediated by inducing glomerular arteriolar vasodilatation with a fall in afferent and efferent arteriolar resistance and by increasing the glomerular ultrafiltration coefficient. The arteriolar vasodilation appeared to be caused by metabolites of cyclooxygenase activity and the generation of nitrous oxide *(58,59)*.

IGF-I also modulates renal tubular function. Most striking is its effect on tubular phosphate reabsorption, which it stimulates by activating a specific sodium-phosphate co-transporter in the brush border membrane of the proximal tubular cell *(60)*. It appears that GH-induced phosphate reabsorption is entirely mediated by IGF-I, for exposure of isolated proximal tubules to IGF-I either on its luminal or antiluminal aspect stimulates phosphate transport whereas GH exposure does not *(61)*. IGF-I also stimulates tubular sodium reabsorption, most likely through the activation of amiloride-sensitive sodium channels located in the distal tubule *(61,62)*. The attendant sodium and water reabsorption that follows high-dose IGF-I treatment in humans is usually modest in extent but can lead to edema formation *(63,64)*. IGF-I may also increase sodium and water reabsorption indirectly by stimulating renin release and suppressing atrial natriuretic peptide secretion *(64)*.

3.2. Effect of Insulin-Like Growth Factor Binding Proteins on the Kidney

Circulating and locally produced IGFBPs have profound effects on the delivery and action of IGF-I on the kidney as well as possessing some limited IGF-I-independent actions *(5,65)*. Because of the high affinity of IGFBPs for IGF-I, relatively tight IGFBP-IGF complexes are formed and this generally limits the bioactivity of IGF-I. However, there are instances when selected IGFBPs actually enhance the bioactivity of IGF-I or even exhibit IGF-I-independent actions.

In renal diseases, there are often profound changes in the circulating and local kidney IGFBP profile, as described in later sections. However, it has been difficult to understand what impact these various changes have on the action of IGF-I on the kidney. This is largely because of the heterogeneity of cell types within the kidney and the variable changes in renal expression of the individual IGFBPs within the kidney. There are studies that indicate that IGFBP-1 can affect renal growth. When this binding protein is infused into GH-deficient dwarf mice, renal but not body growth is stimulated *(66,67)*. However, transgenic mice overexpressing IGFBP-1, show reduced nephron number and glomerulosclerosis *(68,69)*. In various conditions that cause renal hypertrophy, such as diabetes, K depletion, and compensatory renal growth, renal IGFBP-1 expression is elevated and it has been suggested that this results in trapping of IGF-I within the kidney, which then promotes cellular growth *(70–72)*.

IGFBP-3 may also play a role in modulating the action of IGF-I on the kidney. Infusions of IGFBP-3 complexed with IGF-I into rodents increase the amount of IGF-I localized to the glomerulus, although the biological effects thereof are unknown *(73)*. When IGFBP-3 and IGF-I are incubated together with cultured kidney tubular cells, IGF-I receptor binding and internalization is inhibited, and the action of IGF-I is depressed *(74)*. IGFBP-3 may also inhibit DNA synthesis in cultured kidney tubular cells independently of IGF-I *(74)*. IGFBP-5 is another IGFBP that exhibits IGF-I-independent actions. When incubated with cultured mesangial cells in the absence of IGF-I, cell migration is activated by binding of IGFBP-5 to a serine-kinase receptor *(75)*.

4. EFFECT OF NUTRIENTS ON THE RENAL IGF-I SYSTEM AND RENAL STRUCTURE AND FUNCTION

4.1. Starvation and Protein Energy Malnutrition

As in other tissues, the IGF-I system in the kidney is nutrient sensitive. Large variations in dietary intake or composition also affect renal structure and function and some of these changes may be mediated by changes in the renal IGF-I system. For example, starvation or protein calorie malnutrition reduces kidney IGF-I gene expression as it does in liver and muscle, and renal mass decreases as does renal blood flow and GFR *(2,58,76)*. It has been suggested that the fall in IGF-I levels, both circulating and intrarenal, accounts for the changes in kidney mass and function. Because similar changes occur when the GH-deficient rat is exposed to these diets, it appears that the nutrient regulation of renal mass and function is GH independent *(76)*.

4.2. Dietary Protein Loading

Conversely to the effects of reduced food intake, dietary protein loading leads to renal hypertrophy and an increase in renal blood flow, intraglomerular pressure and GFR *(77)*. Because of these renal hemodynamic effects, a high-protein diet can accelerate the progression of underlying kidney disease, and this is one of the rationales for selectively restricting protein intake in patients with chronic renal failure. Hepatic, whole kidney, and glomerular IGF-I levels increase in rats fed with a high-protein diet *(78)*. The expression of IGF-I mRNA increases in the medullary thick ascending limb of Henle whereas the IGFBP-1 levels fall. This is the converse of what occurs when dietary protein intake falls *(79)*. Whether the increase in kidney IGF-I levels induced by high protein feeding contributes to the progression of kidney disease remains to be established. In a recent study it was noted that when soy protein was substituted for casein in the diet of rats with polycystic kidney disease, kidney IGF-I levels fell and the progression of the kidney disease was slowed, supporting the role of IGF-I in progressive renal damage *(80)*.

4.3. Potassium Depletion

Potassium depletion results in profound changes in kidney structure and function, and IGF-I has been implicated as a potential mediator of these changes *(72,81,82)*. In the growing animal, K deficiency is followed by a substantial increase in renal mass as a result of tubular cell proliferation and hypertrophy, whereas glomerular volume remains unchanged *(72,83,84)*. Unlike most other states of renal hypertrophy, renal blood flow and GFR fall. There is central polydipsia and vasopressin-resistant polyuria and increased renal ammoniagenesis. Paradoxically, body growth is attenuated, and there is muscle wasting *(83)*. Infants and young children with Bartter's syndrome, a renal tubular K wasting disorder, have severe growth retardation *(72)*. If K deficiency persists, cellular infiltrates appear in the renal interstitium, and this eventually leads to tubulointerstitial fibrosis and kidney failure *(85)*. Kidney cysts may also develop in chronically hypokalemic patients, although this is not a uniform finding *(86)*. In K-deficient rats total kidney IGF-I levels are elevated for a few days after the intake of K is restricted, whereas IGF-I mRNA levels fall. This increase in kidney IGF-I content has been suggested to be one of the causes of the renal hypertrophy and appears to be the result of increased local trapping of IGF-I by local IGFBP-1 *(83)*. Kidney IGF-I levels may also be elevated because of decreased renal IGF-I degradation and enhanced renal delivery of circulating IGF-I bound to the elevated serum low molecular weight IGFBPs. Interestingly, in muscle there is a fall in GH receptor and IGF-I gene expression and IGF-I peptide levels are low and this may account, in part, for the lack of muscle growth *(83)*. With prolonged hypokalemia, total kidney IGF-I mRNA and peptide levels fall but there is an increase in IGF-I peptide in the hyperplastic collecting ducts and hypertrophied thick ascending limbs of Henle where IGFBP-1 levels are increased *(84)*. This suggests that local trapping of IGF-I occurs and that this contributes to the progressive tubular cell hypertrophy, hyperplasia and possibly the cellular interstitial infiltrates. There is also evidence for the role of several other factors in the genesis of hypokalemic nephropathy including ammonia, angiotensin II, vasopressin, aldosterone, and pituitary hormones *(72)*.

4.4. Metabolic Acidosis

Metabolic acidosis is another condition in which renal hypertrophy, muscle wasting, and growth retardation occurs simultaneously *(87)*. Kidney IGF-I peptide levels increase as early as 4 h after the induction of acidosis returning to baseline within 4 d. This occurs without an increase in mRNA levels. However, the mRNA levels of several IGFBPs, especially IGFBP-1 and -4, are elevated in the kidney. Thus the increase in IGF-I likely results from increased local trapping and may play a role in inducing renal hypertrophy.

5. IMPACT OF RENAL FAILURE ON THE IGF-I SYSTEM

Chronic renal failure induces a state of GH/IGF-I resistance *(88)*. Children with renal failure have stunted growth and adults often develop muscle wasting. Because GH is largely cleared from the circulation through the kidneys, its metabolic clearance rate is reduced in renal failure, and this largely accounts for the prolonged half-life and the normal or elevated plasma GH levels *(89)*. Several mechanisms have been proposed to explain the resistance to GH in uremia, which include diminished GH receptor number, impaired GH-mediated signal transduction with reduced IGF-I expression, and resistance to the action of IGF-I. In adult uremic patients serum IGF-I levels are reduced in those that are malnourished *(2)*. In children with advanced chronic renal failure (CRF), normal or low serum IGF-I levels may also be present *(90)*. In animals with experimental CRF, IGF-I mRNA levels are reduced in liver, muscle, and long bone growth plate, and this can be partly attributed to impaired food intake *(91)*.

With respect to the GH receptor, there is some evidence to suggest that the levels are decreased in uremia. Some studies in uremic rats have shown reduced hepatic and growth plate GH receptor levels *(91–93)*. Other animal studies have suggested that the receptor levels are unaltered by uremia *per se* but that reduced food intake is the cause of the GH receptor changes *(94,95)*. In humans GHBP levels have been taken as surrogate indicators of GH receptor number since in humans GHBP is generated by proteolytic cleavage of the GHR with release of the soluble extracellular domain into the circulation. Although most clinical studies have shown low serum GHPB concentrations, suggesting reduced receptor number *(6,96)*, a recent study of children with end-stage renal disease (ESRD) failed to show any alteration in GHBP profile *(97)*. Clearly further work is required to resolve these discrepancies and to determine whether serum GHBP levels are a valid marker of tissue GHR levels.

Another potential cause of GH resistance is a defect in the post-receptor signaling pathway at one or more sites. In a recent study of rats with CRF, a defect in the hepatic GH-stimulated JAK/STAT pathway was identified *(98)*. Although GH receptor binding and the abundance of the downstream signaling proteins, namely JAK2, STAT5, STAT3, and STAT1 were normal, tyrosine phosphorylation of these proteins was depressed. Because activation of STAT5 is required for normal growth, it was concluded that this defect in JAK-STAT phosphorylation contributed to the GH resistance. It was also noted that the expression of inhibitors of JAK/STAT signaling known as suppressors of cytokine signaling (SOCS)-2 and -3, were elevated in the uremic rats. This provides one potential explanation for the depressed signal transduction. An acquired defect in GH receptor-JAK-2/STAT signaling with upregulation of SOCS expression has also been described in inflammatory conditions. This may be relevant to the GH resistance in renal failure because patients with ESRD and malnutrition often have underlying subclinical chronic inflammation *(99)*.

Resistance to GH also arises because of changes affecting the sensitivity to IGF-I, the mediator of most GH actions. Resistance to IGF-I in uremia has been mainly attributed to the accumulation of circulating IGFBPs that form high affinity complexes with IGF-I and thus reduce the bioavailability of IGF-I *(6,88)*. In children with chronic renal failure serum concentrations of the binding proteins are inversely related to growth rates, supporting an important role of IGFBP excess in the pathogenesis of clinical GH/IGF-I insensitivity in uremia *(98)*. Of the IGF binding proteins studied, IGFBP-1, IGFBP-2, IGFBP-4, and IGFBP-6 are elevated in renal failure *(90,100,101)*. The IGF-BPs accumulate largely because of reduced renal clearance: elevation of their serum levels is inversely related to glomerular filtration rate *(102)*. Lower molecular weight fragments of IGFBP-3 also accumulate in CRF and these fragments are capable of binding to IGF-I, albeit with reduced affinity *(102)*. In addition, there is some evidence to suggest that production of IGFBP-1 is augmented in uremia *(6,100)*. Because of the accumulation in IGFBPs in the vascular compartment, the distribution volume of IGF-I is decreased in renal failure. Thus when exogenous IGF-I is administered, higher serum levels are achieved in subjects with CRF than in normals, even though the metabolic clearance rate of IGF-I is unaltered in CRF *(22)*. Despite the higher serum levels achieved, the metabolic response to IGF-I is impaired in uremic subjects *(103)*. Animal studies indicate that IGF-I resistance in uremia may also be caused by end organ insensitivity caused by a postreceptor signaling defect *(104)*, although the location of the defect is controversial *(105)*. Tissue resistance may also arise because of altered local IGFBP production and accumulation.

Renal failure is often complicated by chronic metabolic acidosis *(106)*. Apart from the effects of acidosis on kidney growth as discussed earlier, acidosis causes systemic changes including alterations in the GH/IGF-I axis *(106,107)*. Acidosis induces negative nitrogen balance, protein catabolism, bone demineralization, and growth retardation. Acidosis induces growth retardation by blunting secretion of GH, depressing hepatic IGF-I gene expression resulting in reduced serum IGF-I levels *(87,107,108)*. In growth plate chondrocytes, acidosis depresses IGF-I and GH receptor density and increases expression of IGFBP-2 and IGFBP-4, which further reduces IGF-I bioactivity *(109)*. All of these effects may worsen GH resistance in uremia.

6. THE INSULIN-LIKE GROWTH FACTOR SYSTEM IN KIDNEY DISEASE

6.1. Diabetes Mellitus

Several studies have suggested that GH and IGF-I may play a role in the development of diabetic nephropathy *(70,71,81)*. In early diabetes, the kidney enlarges, and renal blood flow and GFR increase. In those patients who develop diabetic nephropathy, typical structural changes occur and renal function declines with time. In rats during the first few days of diabetes, but before the kidney hypertrophies, kidney IGF-I content increases *(81)*. In most reports this occurs in the absence of an increase in IGF-I mRNA levels, and the increase in IGF-I peptide likely reflects increased trapping by IGFBPs and IGF-I receptor binding *(9,70,71,110,111)*. Cell culture studies have demonstrated that mesangial cells from nonobese diabetic mice secrete increased amounts of IGF-I and exhibit constitutive activation of the IGF-I signaling pathways *(112)*, whereas mesangial cells from db/db mice have an increase in IGF-I receptor number *(113)*. Exposing mesangial cells to IGF-I increases cell proliferation and matrix production while inhibiting matrix degradation and mesangial cell motility *(114)*. Furthermore, high glucose levels increase the sensitivity of mesangial cells to IGF-I possibly by decreasing mesangial cell IGFBP-2 secretion *(115)*. Taken together these findings suggest that local IGF-I activity may participate in the development and progression of diabetic glomerular disease. Indeed administration of an IGF-I receptor antagonist inhibits renal hypertrophy in diabetic rats *(116)*.

Another way in which IGF-I may participate in the pathogenesis of diabetic nephropathy is through the increase in filtration of IGF-I complexed to IGFBPs through the altered glomerulus. As proteinuria develops the tubular cells are exposed to higher levels of IGF-I, and it has been suggested that this may contribute to the sodium retention and progressive tubulointerstitial disease present in diabetic nephropathy *(117,118)*.

A role for GH in the pathogenesis of diabetic nephropathy is strongly supported by animal studies. For example, administration of a GHR antagonist or somatostatin or an analog thereof to diabetic mice reduces the glomerular hypertrophy, the elevated GFR and the proteinuria *(119,120)*. Also mice homozygous for a disrupted GH receptor/binding protein gene are protected against diabetic kidney disease, which develops in heterozygotes and normal controls after the induction of diabetes *(121)*. Conversely, chronic exposure to exogenous GH in canines *(122)* or to endogenous GH in GH transgenic mice *(43)* results in increased kidney weight, mesangial matrix, glomerular hypertrophy, and diffuse glomerular sclerosis, findings similar to early human diabetic nephropathy. Finally, a recent study demonstrated increased GH receptor-mediated signal transduction in the kidneys of streptozotocin diabetic rats *(123)*. In regards to human studies, the data available is less compelling but do suggest that GH may participate in the genesis of diabetic nephropathy. For example, when poorly controlled diabetes is tightly controlled the elevated plasma GH levels normalize, whereas glomerular hyperfiltration declines in parallel *(124)*. Furthermore, the administration of a somatostatin analog to diabetic subjects reduces renal hypertrophy and glomerular hyperfiltration in the absence of a change in glycemic control *(125)*. Taken together with the animal studies, these results suggest a potential role for GH in the development of diabetic nephropathy and offer the hope that GH receptor antagonists may have clinical utility in blocking the development of diabetic nephropathy *(126)*.

6.2. Compensatory Renal Growth

In a variety of renal diseases, the kidney compensates for loss of functioning tissue by growth and hypertrophy of nonaffected segments and it has been suggested that the GH/IGF-I axis may play a role in inducing this compensatory renal growth (CRG) *(81)*. In animal models, renal growth after uninephrectomy varies by species, gender, and age *(127–129)*. In mature male rats, growth occurs mainly by cellular hypertrophy whereas in the immature rat and in the adult female rat, cellular hyperplasia predominates *(127,128)*. In adult male rodents, renal growth is GH dependent *(129)*, whereas in adult females and in immature rats there is no requirement for GH *(127)*. Thus, it appears that the presence or absence of GH dependence plays a role in determining whether CRG involves a predominantly hyperplastic or hypertrophic growth response. Interestingly, adult female rats and immature rats exhibit an early increase in both IGF-I receptor and gene expression *(127,130)*. In males IGF-I receptor expression is unchanged early after loss of renal mass, but when measured 1 mo later, the IGF-I receptor levels are increased *(131)*.

A role for IGF-I in CRG has been most clearly demonstrated in experiments where a single kidney has been surgically removed or obstructed *(81,132,133)*. In the adult rat after a uninephrectomy, there is an early increase in IGF-I levels in the remaining kidney that returns to basal levels after 4 d *(81)*. Furthermore, administration of an IGF-I receptor antagonist prevents the CRG *(116)*. Surprisingly most although not all, studies have failed to show an increase in IGF-I gene expression to account for the increase in IGF-I peptide *(81,134–136)*. It has been suggested that the source of the increase in IGF-I peptide is the serum and that it accumulates in the kidney because of increased trapping to local IGFBPs and IGF-I receptors *(81)*.

6.3. Nephrotic Syndrome

The nephrotic syndrome occurs in patients with extensive glomerular damage. It is caused by increased permeability of proteins through the glomerular filtration barrier and characterized by heavy proteinuria, hypercholesterolemia, hypoalbuminemia, and clinical edema. In these patients and in animal models, filtration of the smaller IGF1-IGFBP complexes increases and a larger amount of IGF-I is excreted in the urine *(137–140)*. Urinary IGFBP-1, -2, and -3, and acid labile subunit excretion is also increased *(137,139)*. It has been suggested that the greater exposure of the tubular cells to filtered IGF-I may play a role in the progressive tubulointerstitial disease that occurs in most glomerular diseases causing the nephrotic syndrome *(117,118)*. Another feature of the nephrotic syndrome is reduced serum IGF-I levels. This is mostly the result of the protein malnutrition caused by the proteinuria; however, the excessive urinary loss of IGF-I may also contribute *(137,138)*.

Serum IGFBP levels are also altered in the nephrotic syndrome *(137–139)*. Immunoreactive IGFBP-3 levels are increased, but this is caused by the accumulation of IGFBP-3 fragments; intact IGFBP-3 levels are reduced, as are the 150-kDa ternary complexes. The reduced IGFBP-3 levels may in part be caused by increased losses into the glomerular ultrafiltrate, although an animal study suggests that increased serum proteolysis of IGFBP-3 may contribute *(140)*. In contrast to the low serum IGFBP-3 levels, serum IGFBP-2 levels are elevated *(137)*. This may reflect a compensatory increase in hepatic production, possibly a response to protein malnutrition *(140)*. The net effect of these changes in IGFBP levels is to increase the proportion of IGF-I bound to IGFBP-2, which is more readily filtered than the larger MW IGF-I/IGFBP-3/acid labile subunit complex.

6.4. Progression of Kidney Failure

Regardless of the underlying cause of renal insufficiency, many factors may contribute to the progression of renal damage. These include increased systemic and intraglomerular blood pressure, increased angiotensin and aldosterone production, overexpression of paracrine fibrogenic growth factors, and exposure of tubular cells to the excessive amounts of filtered proteins and growth factors in heavy proteinuric states *(77,117,118)*. A number of studies have implicated GH/IGF-I in the development and progression of kidney disease *(141)*. For example, GH transgenic mice develop glomerulosclerosis *(42,43)*, and GH treatment accelerates the progression of kidney disease in several animal models *(142,143)*. Furthermore as discussed earlier, GHR or GH blockade prevents the development of experimental diabetic kidney disease *(120,144)*. However, extended GH treatment has no detrimental effects on kidney disease progression in children with CRF *(145,146)*. It has also been suggested that in proteinuric states, the large amounts of filtered IGF-I may activate a tubulointerstitial reaction that contributes to progression *(118)*. However, IGF-I transgenic mice do not develop glomerulosclerosis *(43)*, and short-term IGF-I treatment does not cause a decline in kidney function in adults with advanced CRF *(63,147)*.

7. RECOMBINANT IGF-I AND NUTRITION IN THE MANAGEMENT OF RENAL FAILURE

7.1. Protein Energy Malnutrition

Protein energy malnutrition manifests as loss of muscle mass and reduced serum albumin and is quite common in patients with severe acute renal failure or advanced CRF. It occurs in 20–50% of patients with ESRD and is associated with an increase in morbidity and mortality *(148,149)*. The causes of the malnourished state generally fall into two major categories that usually overlap *(149,150)*. These categories include inadequate food intake, usually the result of anorexia, and increased catabolism, often with impaired protein synthesis. Chronic subclinical infection with cytokine release is a frequent cause of the increased catabolism *(99)*. Even when kidney function is normal, malnutrition depresses GH and IGF-I production, resulting in low serum IGF-I levels *(2–4)*. The GH-IGF-I axis is also depressed by acidosis *(106)*, which is common in advanced kidney failure *(150)*. Other endocrine abnormalities that occur with declining renal function further aggravate tissue catabolism. These include altered hormone production, secretion, and metabolism and resistance to their action *(88)*.

Because malnutrition adversely affects outcome in patients with advanced renal failure, there has been considerable interest in developing new therapeutic strategies to improve the nutritional state of these patients *(149,151)*. One approach is the use of recombinant GH or IGF-I. Several clinical studies have been conducted and although they are limited in regard to patient number, study duration, and the presence or absence of malnutrition or inflammation, it has been shown that short-term therapy with GH or IGF-I does induce a positive anabolic response in adult ESRD patients *(152–154)*. Although these results are encouraging, it is important to keep in mind that the mainstay of management of malnutrition in kidney failure is nutritional. This includes ensuring that the patient receives and ingests the nutrients required to improve lean body mass. An aggressive approach, even including tube feeding or parenteral nutrition, may be required. In addition, it is essential to correct acidosis when present, to eliminate any source of chronic inflammation, and to make sure that the patient with ESRD receives optimal dialysis therapy. The use of IGF proteins as markers of nutritional status in renal and other diseases is reviewed in chapter 4.

7.2. Growth Retardation

It is well established that administration of recombinant GH to children who are growth retarded because of CRF induces significant catch-up body growth, and with long-term treatment, most attain normal adult height *(155,156)*. Side effects of this treatment have been relatively minor. There have been concerns that GH might accelerate the progression of renal disease, increase the rate of graft rejection or induce diabetes, but there is no evidence that such ill effects occur *(145,146,157)*. However, hyperinsulinemia occurs commonly during GH therapy and needs to be followed over the long term for potential adverse effects on the cardiovascular system *(146,158)*.

7.3. Acute Renal Failure

Several investigators have shown that IGF-I therapy accelerates recovery from experimental acute renal failure in rats *(159–161)*. This is thought to be mediated through the renal hemodynamic, proliferative, and antiapoptotic actions of IGF-I. Stimulated by the successful preclinical studies, a multicenter placebo-controlled study of 72 patients with severe acute renal failure was conducted recently. Unfortunately, IGF-I failed to modify the course of the illness *(162)*. The reason for this failure despite successful animal studies remains unresolved and merits further study.

7.4. Kidney Function in Chronic Renal Failure

Both recombinant GH and IGF-I have been administered to adults with advanced CRF with the aim of increasing glomerular filtration rate. Although GH treatment did not alter renal function in adults or children with advanced renal failure *(51,146)*, several small studies in adults have shown that recombinant IGF-I causes a modest increase in GFR *(63,147)*. However, large-scale studies are required to determine whether IGF-I can effectively and safely induce a sustained increase in renal function in patients with advanced CRF and thus delay the need for renal replacement therapy.

8. SUMMARY AND CONCLUSIONS

Insulin-like growth factor-I plays a role in promoting renal growth and modulating renal blood flow, GFR, and renal transport function. Within the kidney IGF-I, IGFBPs, and the GH receptor are expressed in an anatomically heterogenous and limited manner, whereas the IGF-I receptor is expressed throughout the kidney. IGF-I production within the kidney is modulated by GH and is nutrient sensitive. However, the level of IGF-I within the kidney depends not only on local IGF-I production, but also on the rate of delivery of IGF-I to the kidney which is influenced by the serum IGFBP levels, the level of intrarenal IGF-I receptor and IGFBP expression, and finally by the local IGF-I degrading activity.

Recent work has shown that IGF-I plays an important role in the initiation of compensatory renal growth and renal hypertrophy in several renal diseases and may contribute to the progression of kidney damage. In turn, kidney failure leads to profound alterations in the extrarenal GH/IGF-I system. These may in part be caused by the malnutrition and metabolic acidosis commonly present in advanced kidney failure. Advanced kidney failure also compromises the cellular response to GH and IGF-I. GH and IGF-I resistance manifest as impaired body growth in children and as muscle wasting in adults. Resistance can be overcome by administering pharmacologic doses of the recombinant growth factors. GH is widely used in the management of growth retardation in children with CRF. Early studies indicate that GH may also be effective in treating wasting in adults with CRF.

9. RECOMMENDATIONS AND CHALLENGES

A major challenge to the physician caring for the patient with significant kidney damage is to arrest progressive kidney destruction. Because several studies have suggested that IGF-I/GH may contribute to this complex process and thus there is a need to further characterize the true role of IGF-I and GH in mediating progression. In the long term, this may well lead to the development of therapeutic strategies to halt the progression of kidney failure, possibly by blocking renal IGF-I production or action. Another important area that merits further study is the resistance to IGF-I and GH that develops in uremia. Understanding the mechanisms causing resistance could potentially lead to the development of therapies to restore normal sensitivity to the endogenous growth factor or low doses of the recombinant moiety and thus avoid the risk of adverse side effects that may occur with high dose therapy. Finally, although initial studies suggest that IGF-I has the potential to enhance renal function in patients with advanced chronic renal failure, large-scale controlled studies are required to establish the efficacy and safety of this form of treatment before it enters into clinical usage.

ACKNOWLEDGMENTS

Support was provided in part by funds from the Research Service Department of Veterans Affairs.

REFERENCES

1. Feld S, Hirschberg R. Growth hormone, the insulin-like growth factor system, and the kidney. Endocr Rev 1996;17:423–480.
2. Rabkin R. Nutrient regulation of insulin-like growth factor I. Min Electrolyte Metabo 1997;23:157–160.
3. Thissen JP, Ketelslegers JM, Underwood LE. Nutritional regulation of the insulin-like growth factors. Endocr Rev 1994;15:80–101.
4. Thissen JP, Underwood LE, Ketelslegers JM. Regulation of insulin-like growth factor-I in starvation and injury. Nutr Rev 1999;57:167–176.

5. Baxter RC. Insulin-like growth factor (IGF)-binding proteins: interactions with IGFs and intrinsic bioactivities. Am J Physiol Endocrinol Metab 2000;278:E967–E976.
6. Tonshoff B, Blum WF, Mehls O. Derangements of the somatotropic hormone axis in chronic renal failure. Kidney Int Suppl 1997;58:S106-S113.
7. Chin E, Zhou J, Bondy CA. Renal growth hormone receptor gene expression: relationship to renal insulin-like growth factor system. Endocrinology 1992:3061–3066.
8. Chin E, Zhou J, Bondy C. Anatomical relationship in the patterns of insulin-like growth factor (IGF)-I, IGF binding protein-1, and IGF-I receptor gene expression in the rat kidney. Endocrinology 1992;130:3237–3245.
9. Landau D, Chin E, Bondy C, et al. Expression of insulin-like growth factor binding proteins in the rat kidney: effects of long-term diabetes. Endocrinology 1995;136:1835–1842.
10. Nakamura T, Fukui M, Ebihara I, Osada S, Nagaoka I, Tomino Y, Koide H. mRNA expression of growth factors in glomeruli from diabetic rats. Diabetes 1993;42:450–456.
11. Rabkin R, Brody M, Lu L, et al. Expression of genes encoding the rat renal insulin-like growth factor-I system. J Am Soc Nephrol 1995;6:1511–1518.
12. Matejka GL, Jennische E. IGF-I binding and IGF-I mRNA expression in the post-ischemic regenerating rat kidney. Kidney Int 1992;42:1113–1123.
13. Matejka GL, Eriksson PS, Carlsson B, et al. Distribution of IGF-I mRNA and IGF-I binding sites in the rat kidney. Histochemistry 1992;97:173–180.
14. Kobayashi S, Clemmons DR, Venkatachalam MA. Colocalization of insulin-like growth factor-binding protein with insulin-like growth factor I. Am J Physiol 1991;261:F22–F28.
15. Flyvbjerg A, Nielsen S, Sheikh MI, et al. Luminal and basolateral uptake and receptor binding of IGF-I in rabbit renal proximal tubules. Am J Physiol 1993;265:F624–F633.
16. Bortz JD, Rotwein P, DeVol D, et al. Focal expression of insulin-like growth factor I in rat kiney collecting duct. J Cell Biol 1988;107:811–819.
17. Chin E, Zhou J, Dai J, et al. Cellular localization and regulation of gene expression for components of the insulin-like growth factor ternary binding protein complex. Endocrinology 1994;134:2498–2504.
18. Chin E, Michels K, Bondy CA. Partition of insulin-like growth factor (IGF)-binding sites between the IGF-I and IGF-II receptors and IGF-binding proteins in the human kidney. J Clin Endocrinol Metab 1994;78:156–164.
19. Rogers SA, Miller SB, Hammerman MR. Insulin-like growth factor I gene expression in isolated rat renal collecting duct is stimulated by epidermal growth factor. J Clin Invest 1991;87:347–351.
20. Rabkin R, Haussman M: Renal metabolism of hormones. In: Principles and Practice of Endocrinology and Metabolism. Becker KL (ed.). Lippincott, Philadelphia, 2000. p. 1895–1901.
21. Li W, Fawcett J, Widmer HR, et al. Nuclear transport of insulin-like growth factor-I and insulin-like growth factor binding protein-3 in opossum kidney cells. Endocrinology 1997;138:1763–1766.
22. Rabkin R, Fervenza FC, Maidment H, et al. Pharmacokinetics of insulin-like growth factor-1 in advanced chronic renal failure. Kidney Int 1996;49:1134–1140.
23. Hammerman MR. The growth hormone-insulin-like growth factor axis in kidney re-revisited. Nephrol Dial Transplant 1999;14:1853–1860.
24. Han VK, Lund PK, Lee DC, D'Ercole AJ. Expression of somatomedin/insulin-like growth factor messenger ribonucleic acids in the human fetus: identification, characterization, and tissue distribution. J Clin Endocrinol Metab 1988;66:422–429.
25. Brice AL, Cheetham JE, Bolton VN, Hill NC, Schofield PN. Temporal changes in the expression of the insulin-like growth factor II gene associated with tissue maturation in the human fetus. Development 1989;106:543–554.
26. Birnbacher R, Amann G, Breitschopf H, Lassmann H, Suchanek G, Heinz-Erian P. Cellular localization of insulin-like growth factor II mRNA in the human fetus and the placenta: detection with a digoxigenin-labeled cRNA probe and immunocytochemistry. Pediatr Res 1998;43:614–620.
27. Chin E, Bondy C. Insulin-like growth factor system gene expression in the human kidney. J Clin Endocrinol Metab 1992;75:962–968.
28. Rogers SA, Ryan G, Hammerman MR. Insulin-like growth factors I and II are produced in the metanephros and are required for growth and development in vitro. J Cell Biol 1991;113:1447–1453.
29. Grone HJ, Neumann P, Fuchs E. Localization and characterization of IGF-I receptors in fetal and adult human kidneys. Miner Electrolyte Metab 1992;18:256–263.

30. Liu ZZ, Wada J, Alvares K, Kumar A, Wallner EI, Kanwar YS. Distribution and relevance of insulin-like growth factor-I receptor in metanephric development. Kidney Int 1993;44:1242–1250.
31. Matsell DG, Bennett T. Evaluation of metanephric maturation in a human fetal kidney explant model. In Vitro Cell Dev Biol Anim 1998;34:138–148.
32. Adamo M, Lowe WL Jr, LeRoith D, Roberts CT Jr. Insulin-like growth factor I messenger ribonucleic acids with alternative 5′-untranslated regions are differentially expressed during development of the rat. Endocrinology 1989;124:2737–2744.
33. Lindenbergh-Kortleve DJ, Rosato RR, van Neck JW, Nauta J, van Kleffens M, Groffen C, Zwarthoff EC, Drop SL. Gene expression of the insulin-like growth factor system during mouse kidney development. Mol Cell Endocrinol 1997;132:81–91.
34. Shoba L, An MR, Frank SJ, Lowe WL Jr. Developmental regulation of insulin-like growth factor-I and growth hormone receptor gene expression. Mol Cell Endocrinol 1999;152:125–136.
35. Ballesteros M, Scott CD, Baxter RC. Developmental regulation of insulin-like growth factor-II/mannose 6-phosphate receptor mRNA in the rat. Biochem Biophys Res Commun 1990;172:775–779.
36. Amri K, Freund N, Van Huyen JP, Merlet-Benichou C, Lelievre-Pegorier M. Altered nephrogenesis due to maternal diabetes is associated with increased expression of IGF-II/mannose-6-phosphate receptor in the fetal kidney. Diabetes 2001;50:1069–1075.
37. Peng M, Pelletier G, Palin MF, Veronneau S, LeBel D, Abribat T. Ontogeny of IGFs and IGFBPs mRNA levels and tissue concentrations in liver, kidney and skeletal muscle of pig. Growth Dev Aging 1996;60: 171–187.
38. DeChiara TM, Robertson EJ, Efstratiadis A. Parental imprinting of the mouse insulin-like growth factor II gene. Cell 1991;64:849–859.
39. Chevalier RL, Goyal S, Kim A, Chang AY, Landau D, LeRoith D. Renal tubulointerstitial injury from ureteral obstruction in the neonatal rat is attenuated by IGF-I. Kidney Int 2000;57:882–890.
40. Ritz E, Tonshoff B, Worgall S, et al. Influence of growth hormone and insulin-like growth factor-I on kidney function and kidney growth. Pediatr Nephrol 1991;5:509–512.
41. Mehls O, Irzynjec T, Ritz E, et al. Effects of rhGH and rhIGF-I on renal growth and morphology. Kidney Int 1993;44:1251–1258.
42. Doi T, Striker LJ, Quaife C, et al. Progressive glomerulosclerosis develops in transgenetic mice chronically expressing growth hormone and growth hormone releasing factor but not in those expressing insulin-like growth factor-1. Am J Pathol 1988;131:398–403.
43. Doi T, Striker LJ, Gibson CC, et al. Glomerular lesions in mice transgenetic for growth hormone and insulin-like growth factor-I. Relationship between increased glomerular size and mesangial sclerosis. Am J Pathol 1990;137:541–552.
44. Gershberg H, Heinemann H, Stumpf H. Renal function studies and autopsy report in a patient with gigantism and acromegaly. J Clin Endocrinol Metab 1957;17:377–385.
45. Dullaart RP, Meijer S, Marbach P, et al. Effect of a somatostatin analogue, octreotide, on renal haemodynamics and albuminuria in acromegalic patients. Eur J Clin Invest 1992;22:494–502.
46. Ikkos D, Ljunggren H, Luft R. Glomerular filtration rate and renal plasma flow in acromegaly. Acta Endocrinol 1956;21:226–236.
47. Skottner A, Clark RG, Fryklund L, Robinson IC. Growth responses in a mutant dwarf rat to human growth hormone and recombinant human insulin-like growth factor. Endocrinology 1989;124:2519–2526.
48. Hirschberg R, Brunori G, Kopple DJ, et al. Effects of insulin-like growth factor I on renal function in normal men. Kidney Int 1993;43:387–397.
49. Guler HP, Eckardt KU, Zapf J, et al. Insulin-like growth factor I increase glomerular filtration rate and renal plasma flow in man. Acta Endocrinol 1989;121:101–106.
50. Guler HP, Schmid C, Zapf J, et al. Effects of recombinant insulin-like growth factor I on insulin secretion and renal function in normal human subjects. Proc Natl Acad Sci USA 1989;86:2868–2872.
51. Haffner D, Zacharewicz S, Mehls O, et al. The acute effect of growth hormone on GFR is obliterated in chronic renal failure. Clin Nephrol 1989;32:266–269.
52. Parving H, Noer I, Mogensen C, et al. Kidney function in normal man during short-term growth hormone infusion. Acta Endocrinol 1978;89:796–800.

53. Christiansen JS, Gammelgaard J, Orskov H, et al. Kidney function and size in normal subjects before and during growth hormone administration for one week. Eur J Clin Invest 1981;11:487–490.
54. Hirschberg RR, Kopple JD. Increase in renal plasma flow and glomerular filtration rate during growth hormone treatment may be mediated by insulin-like growth factor I. Am J Nephrol 1988;8:249–254.
55. Hirschberg R. Effects of growth hormone and IGF-I on glomerular ultrafiltration in growth hormone-deficient rats. Regul Pept 1993;48:241–250.
56. Laron Z, Klinger B. IGF-I treatment of adult patients with Laron syndrome: preliminary factor I on glomerular dynamics in the rat. J Clin Invest 1991;87:1200–1206.
57. Hirschberg R, Kopple JD, Blantz RC, Tucker BJ. Effects of recombinant human insulin-like growth factor I on glomerular dynamics in the rat. J Clin Invest 1991;87:1200–1206.
58. Hirschberg R, Kopple JD. Evidence that insulin-like growth factor I increases renal plasma flow and glomerular filtration rate in fasted rats J Clin Invest 1989;83:326–330.
59. Baumann U, Eisenhauer T, Hartmann H. Increase of glomerular filtration rate and renal plasma flow by insulin-like growth factor-I during euglycaemic clamping in anaesthetized rats. Eur J Clin Invest 1992;22:204–209.
60. Caverzasio J, Bonjour J-P. Growth factors and renal regulation of phosphate transport. Pediatr Nephrol 1993;7:802–806.
61. Quigley R, Baum M. Effects of growth hormone and insulin-like growth factor I on rabbit proximal convoluted tubule transport. J Clin Invest 1991;88:368–374.
62. Gesek FA, Schoolwerth AC. Insulin increases Na(+)-H+ exchange activity in proximal tubules from normotensive and hypertensive rats. Am J Physiol 1991;260:F695-F703.
63. Ike JO, Fervenza FC, Hoffman AR, et al. Early experience with extended use of insulin-like growth factor-1 in advanced chronic renal failure. Kidney Int 1997;51:840–849.
64. Moller J, Jorgensen JO, Marqversen J, et al. Insulin-like growth factor I administration induces fluid and sodium retention in healthy adults: possible involvement of renin and atrial natriuretic factor. Clin Endocrinol 2000;52:181–186.
65. Baxter RC. Signalling pathways involved in antiproliferative effects of IGFBP-3: a review. Mol Pathol 2001;54:145–148.
66. Van Buul-Offers SC, Van Kleffens M, Koster JG, et al. Human insulin-like growth factor (IGF) binding protein-1 inhibits IGF-I-stimulated body growth but stimulates growth of the kidney in snell dwarf mice. Endocrinology 2000;141:1493–1499.
67. Van Kleffens M, Lindenbergh-Kortleve DJ, Koster JG, et al. The role of the IGF axis in IGFBP-1 and IGF-I induced renal enlargement in Snell dwarf mice. J Endocrinol 2001;170:333–346.
68. Doublier S, Seurin D, Fouquerary B, et al. Glomerulosclerosis in mice transgenic for human insulin-like growth factor-binding protein-1. Kidney Int 2000;57:2299–2307.
69. Doublier S, Amri K, Seurin D, et al. Overexpression of human insulin-like growth factor binding protein-1 in the mouse leads to nephron deficit. Pediatr Res 2001;49:660–666.
70. Flyvbjerg A. Putative pathophysiological role of growth factors and cytokines in experimental dia betic kidney disease. Diabetologia 2000;43:1205–1223.
71. Rabkin R, Fervenza FC. Renal hypertrophy and kidney disease in diabetes. Diabetes Metab Rev 1996;12:217–241.
72. Fervenza FC, Rabkin R. The role of growth factors and ammonia in the genesis of hypokalemic nephropathy.J Ren Nutr 2002;12:151–159.
73. Sandra A, Boes M, Dake BL, et al. Infused IGF-I/IGFBP-3 complex causes glomerular localization of IGF-I in the rat kidney. Am J Physiol 1998;275:E32–E37.
74. Yap J, Tsao T, Fawcett J, et al. Effect of insulin-like growth factor binding proteins on the response of proximal tubular cells to insulin-like growth factor-I. Kidney Int 1997;52:1216–1223.
75. Berfield AK, Andress DL, Abrass CK. IGFBP-5(201–218) stimulates Cdc42GAP aggregation and filopodia formation in migrating mesangial cells. Kidney Int 2000;57:1991–2003.
76. Kobayashi S, Nogami H, Ikeda T. Growth hormone and nutrition interact to regulate expressions of kidney IGF-I and IGFBP mRNAs. Kidney Int 1995;48:65–71.
77. Hostetter TH, Meyer TW, Rennke HG, Brenner BM. Chronic effects of dietary protein in the rat with intact and reduced renalmass. Kidney Int. 1986;30:509–517.

78. Murray BM, Campos SP, Schoenl M, MacGillivray MH. Effect of dietary protein intake on renal growth: possible role of insulin-like growth factor-I. J Lab Clin Med 1993;122:677–685.
79. Chin E, Bondy CA. Dietary protein-induced renal growth: correlation between renal IGF-I synthesis and hyperplasia. Am J Physiol 1994;266:C1037–C1045.
80. Aukema HM, Housini I. Dietary soy protein effects on disease and IGF-I in male and female Han:SPRD-cy rats. Kidney Int 2001;59:52–61.
81. Flyvbjerg A, Orskov H, Nyborg K, et al. Kidney IGF-I accumulation occurs in four different conditions with rapid initial kidney growth in rats. In: Modern Concepts of Insulin-like Growth Factors. Spencer EM (ed.). Elsevier Science Publishing Co, New York, 1991. p. 207–217.
82. Dorup I. Magnesium and potassium deficiency. Its diagnosis, occurrence and treatment in diuretic therapy and its consequences for growth, protein synthesis and growth factors. Acta Physiol Scand Suppl 1994;618:1–55.
83. Hsu FW, Tsao T, Rabkin R. The IGF-I axis in kidney and skeletal muscle of potassium deficient rats. Kidney Int 1997;52:363–370.
84. Tsao T, Fawcett J, Fervenza FC, et al. Expression of insulin-like growth factor-I and transforming growth factor-beta in hypokalemic nephropathy in the rat. Kidney Int 2001;96–105.
85. Schwartz WB, Relman AS: Effects of electrolyte disordes on renal structure and function. N Engl J Med 1967;276:383–389.
86. Torres VE, Young, Jr WF, Offord KP, et al. Association of hypokalemia, aldosteronism, and renal cysts. N Engl J Med 1990;322:345–351.
87. Fawcett J, Hsu FW, Tsao T, et al. Effect of metabolic acidosis on the insulin-like growth factor-I system and cathepsins B and L gene expression in the kidney. J Lab Clin Med 2000;136:475.
88. Rabkin R. Growth factor insensitivity in renal failure. Renal Failure 2001;23:291–300.
89. Haffner D, Schaefer F, Girard J, et al. Metabolic clearance of recombinant human growth hormone in health and chronic renal failure. J Clin Invest 1994;93:1163–1171.
90. Tönshoff B, Blum WF, Wingen AM, et al. Serum insulin-like growth factors (IGFs) and IGF binding proteins 1,2 and 3 in children with chronic renal failure: relationship to height and glomerular filtration rate. J Clin Endocrinol Metab 1995;80:2684–2691.
91. Chan W, Valerie KC, Chan JCM. Expression of insulin-like growth factor-1 in uremic rats: Growth hormone resistance and nutritional intake. Kidney Int 1993;43:790–795.
92. Tönshoff B, Eden S, Weiser E, et al. Reduced hepatic growth hormone (GH) receptor gene expression and increase in plasma GH binding protein in experimental uremia. Kidney Int 1994;45:1085–1092.
93. Edmondson SR, Baker NL, Oh J, et al. Growth hormone receptor abundance in tibial growth plates of uremic rats: GH/IGF-I treatment. Kidney Int 2000;58:62–70.
94. Villares SM, Goujon L, Maniar S, et al. Reduced food intake is the main cause of low growth hormone receptor expression in uremic rats. Mol Cell Endocrinol 1994;106:51–56.
95. Mart'nez V, Balb'n M, Ord—nez FA, et al. Hepatic expression of growth hormone receptor/binding protein and insulin-like growth factor I genes in uremic rats. Influence of nutritional deficit. Growth Horm IGF Res 1999;9:61–68.
96. Baumann G. Growth hormone binding protein 2001. J Pediatr Endocrinol Metab 2001;14:355–375.
97. Powell D, Liu F, Baker B et al. Modulation of growth factors by growth hormone in children with chronic renal failure. Kidney Int 1997;51:1970–1979.
98. Schaefer F, Chen Y, Tsao T, et al. Impaired JAK-STAT signal transduction contributes to growth hormone resistance in chronic uremia. J Clin Invest 2001;108:467–475.
99. Kaysen GA. The microinflammatory state in uremia: causes and potential consequences. J Am Soc Nephrol. 2001;12:1549–1557.
100. Powell DR, Liu F, Baker BK, et al. Effect of chronic renal failure and growth hormone therapy on the insulin-like growth factors and their binding proteins. Pediatr Nephrol 2000;14:579–583.
101. Ulinski T, Mohan S, Kiepe D, et al. Serum insulin-like growth factor binding protein (IGFBP)-4 and IGFBP-5 in children with chronic renal failure: Relationship to growth and glomerular filtration rate. Pediatr Nephrol 2000;14:589–597.
102. Frystyk J, Ivarsen P, Skjaerbaek C, et al. Serum-free insulin-like growth factor 1 correlates with clearance in patients with chronic renal failure. Kidney Int 1999;56:2076–2084.
103. Fouque D, Peng SC, Kopple JD. Impaired metabolic response to recombinant insulin-like growth factor-1 in dialysis patients. Kidney Int 1995;47:876–883.

104. Ding H, Gao XL, Hirschberg R, et al. Impaired actions of insulin-like growth factor 1 on protein synthesis and degradation in skeletal muscle of rats with chronic renal failure. Evidence for a postreceptor defect. J Clin Invest 1996;97:1064–1075.
105. Tsao T, Fervenza FC, Friedlaender M, et al. Effect of prolonged uremia on insulin-like growth factor-I receptor autophosphorylation and tyrosine kinase activity in kidney and muscle. Exp Nephrol 2002;10:285–292.
106. Franch HA, Mitch WE. Catabolism in uremia: the impact of metabolic acidosis. J Am Soc Nephrol 1998;9:S78–S81.
107. Kuemmerle N, Krieg RJ Jr, Latta K, Challa A, Hanna JD, Chan JC. Growth hormone and insulin-like growth factor in non-uremic acidosis and uremic acidosis. Kidney Int Suppl 1997;58:S102–S105.
108. Brungger M, Hulter HN, Krapf R. Effect of chronic metabolic acidosis on the growth hormone/IGF-I endocrine axis: new cause of growth hormone insensitivity in humans. Kidney Int 1997;51:216–221.
109. Green J, Maor G. Effect of metabolic acidosis on the growth hormone/IGF-I endocrine axis in skeletal growth centers. Kidney Int 2000;57:2258–2267.
110. Fervenza FC, Tsao T, Hoffman AR, et al. Regional changes in the intrarenal insulin-like growth factor-I axis in diabetes. Kidney Int 1997;51:811–818.
111. Segev Y, Landau D, Marbach M, et al. Renal hypertrophy in hyperglycemic non-obese diabetic mice is associated with persistent renal accumulation of insulin-like growth factor-1. J Am Soc Nephrol 1997;8:436–444.
112. Tack I, Elliot SJ, Potier M, et al. Autocrine activation of the IGF-I signaling pathway in mesangial cells isolated from diabetic NOD mice. Diabetes 2002;51:182–188.
113. Oemer BS, Foellmer HG, Hodgdon-Anandant L, et al. Regulation of insulin-like growth factor I receptors in diabetic mesangial cells. J Biol Chem 1991;266:2369–2373.
114. Schreiber B, Hughes M, Groggel G. Insulin-like growth factor-1 stimulates production of mesangial cell matrix components. Clin Nephrol 1995;43:368–374.
115. Horney M, Shirley D, Kurtz D, et al. Elevated glucose increases mesangial cell sensitivity to insulin-like growth factor 1. Am J Physiol 1998;274:F1045–1053.
116. Haylor J, Hickling H, El Eter E, et al. JB3, an IGF-I receptor antagonist, inhibits early renal growth in diabetic and uninephrectomized rats. J Am Soc Nephrol 2000;11:2027–2035.
117. Wang S, LaPage J, Hirschberg R. Glomerular ultrafiltration and apical tubular action of IGF-I, TGF-Œ≤, and HGF in nephrotic syndrome. Kidney Int 1999;56:1247–1251.
118. Hirschberg R: Bioactivity of glomerular ultrafiltrate during heavy proteinuria may contribute to renal tubulo-interstitial lesions: Evidence for a role for insulin-like growth factor I. J Clin Invest 1996;97:116–124.
119. Landau D, Sergev Y, Afargan M, et al. A novel somatostatin analogue prevents early renal complications in the nonobese diabetic mouse. Kidney Int 2001;60:505–512.
120. Sergev Y, Landau D, Rasch R, et al. Growth hormone receptor antagonism prevents early renal changes in nonobese diabetic mice. J Am Soc Nephrol 1999;10:2374–2381.
121. Bellush L, Douplier S, Holland A, et al. Protection against diabetes – induced nephropathy and growth hormone receptor/binding protein gene-disrupted mice. Endocrinology 2000;141:163–168.
122. Molon-Noblot S, Laroque P, Prahalada S, et al. Morphological changes in the kidney of dogs chronically exposed to exogenous growth hormone. Toxicology Pathology 2000;28:510–517.
123. Thirone AC, Scarlett JA, Gasparetti AL, et al. Modulation of growth hormone signal transduction in kidneys of streptozotocin-induced diabetic animals: effect of a growth hormone receptor antagonist. Diabetes 2002;51:2270–2281.
124. Hansen AP, Mogensen CE. Growth hormone secretion and kidney function during normalization of the metabolic state in newly diagnosed juvenile diabetes. Horm Metab Res 1972;4:11–15.
125. Serri O, Beauregard H, Brazeau P, et al. Somatostatin analogue, octreotide, reduces increased glomerular filtration rate and kidney size in insulin-dependent diabetes. JAMA 1991;265:888–892.
126. Flyvbjerg A. Potential use of growth hormone receptor antagonist in the treatment of diabetic kidney disease. Growth Horm IGF Res 2001;11(suppl A):S115-S119.
127. Mulroney SE, Pesce C. Early hyperplastic renal growth after uninephrectomy in adult female rats. Endocrinology 2000;141:932–937.
128. Mulroney SE, Woda C, Johnson M, et al. Gender differences in renal growth and function after uninephrectomy in adult rats. Kidney Int 1999;56:944–953.

129. Haramati A, Lumpkin MD, Mulroney SE. Early increase in pulsatile growth hormone release after unilateral nephrectomy in adult rats. Am J Physiol 1994;266:F628–F632.
130. Mulroney SE, Lumpkin MD, Roberts CT, et al. Effect of a growth hormone-releasing factor antagonist on compensatory renal growth, insulin-like growth factor-I and IGF-I receptor gene expression after unilateral nephrectomy in immature rats. Endocrinology 1992;130:2697–2702.
131. Hise MK, Lahn JS, Shao ZM, et al. Insulin-like growth factor-I receptor and binding proteins in rat kidney after nephron loss. J Am Soc Nephrol 1993;4:62–68.
132. Stiles AD, Sosenko RS, D'Ercole AJ, et al. Relation to kidney tissue somatomedin C/insulin-like growth factor I to postnephrectomy renal growth in the rat. Endocrinology 1985;117:2397–2401.
133. Serel T, Savas C, Delibas N, et al. Free insulin-like growth factor 1 and unilateral complete ureteral obstruction in the rat. Urology 2000;56:863–866.
134. Fagin JA, Melmed S. Relative increase in insulin-like growth factor I messenger ribonucleic acid levels in compensatory renal hypertrophy. Endocrinology 1987;120:718–724.
135. Hise MK, Li L, Mantzouris N, et al. Differential mRNA expression of insulin-like growth factor system during renal injury and hypertrophy. Am J Physiol 1995;269:F817-F824.
136. Fervenza FC, Tsao T, Hsu F, Rabkin R. Intrarenal insulin-like growth factor-1 axis after unilateral nephrectomy in rat. J Am Soc Nephrol 1999;10:43–50.
137. Haffner D, Tonshoff B, Blum WF, et al. Insulin-like growth factors (IGFs) and IGF binding proteins, serum acid-labile subunit and growth hormone binding protein in nephrotic children. Kidney Int 1997;52:802–810.
138. Lee DY, Park SK, Kim JS. Insulin-like growth factor-I (IGF-I) and IGF-binding proteins in children with nephrotic syndrome. J Clin Endocrinol Metab 1996;81:1856–1860.
139. Zhou X, Loke KY, Pillai CC, et al. IGFs and IGF-binding proteins in short children with steroid-dependent nephrotic syndrome on chronic glucocorticoids: changes with 1 year exogenous GH. Eur J Endocrinol 2001;144:237–243.
140. Hirschberg R, Kaysen GA. Insulin-like growth factor I and its binding proteins in the experimental nephrotic syndrome. Endocrinology 1995;136:1565–1571.
141. Hirschberg R, Adler S. Insulin-like growth factor system and the kidney: physiology, pathophysiology, and therapeutic implications. Am J Kidney Dis 1998;31:901–919.
142. Allen DB, Fogo A, el-Hayek R, et al. Effects of prolonged growth hormone adminstration in rats with chronic renal insufficiency. Pediatr Res 1992;31:406–410.
143. Trachtman H, Futterweit S, Schwob N, et al. Recombinant human growth hormone exacerbates chronic puromycin aminonucleoside nephropathy in rats. Kidney Int 1993;44:1281–1288.
144. Yoshida H, Mitarai T, Kitamura M, et al. The effect of selective growth hormone defect in the progression of glomerulosclerosis. Am J Kidney Dis 1994;23:302–312.
145. Haffner D, Nissel R, Wuhl E, et al. Metabolic effects of long-term growth hormone treatment in prepubertal children with chronic renal failure and after kidney transplantation. The German Study Group for Growth Hormone Treatment in Chronic Renal Failure. Pediatr Res 1998;43:209–215.
146. Tönshoff B, Tönshoff C, Mehls O, et al. Growth hormone treatment over one year in children with preterminal chronic renal failure: no adverse effect on glomerular filtration rate. Eur J Pediatr 1992;151:601–607.
147. Vijayan A, Franklin SC, Behrend T, et al. Insulin-like growth factor I improves renal function in patients with end-stage chronic renal failure. Am J Physiol 1999;276:R929-R934.
148. Riella MC. Malnutrition in dialysis: malnourishment or uremic inflammatory response? Kidney Int 2000;57:1211–1232.
149. Rabkin R: Therapeutic use of growth factors in renal disease. In: Nutritional Management of Renal Disease. Kopple JD, Massry SG (eds.). Lippincott, William and Wilkins, 2003, in press.
150. Mitch WE. Insights into the abnormalities of chronic renal disease attributed to malnutrition. J Am Soc Nephrol 2002;13(Suppl 1):S22–S27.
151. Chen Y, Fervenza FC, Rabkin R. Growth factors in the treatment of wasting in kidney failure. J Ren Nutr 2001;11:62–66.
152. Ziegler TR, Lazarus JM, Young LS, et al. Effects of recombinant human growth hormone in adults receiving maintenance hemodialysis. J Am Soc Nephrol 1991;2:1130–1135.

153. Ikizler TA, Wingard RL, Hakim RM. Interventions to treat malnutrition in dialysis patients: the role of the dose of dialysis, intradialytic parenteral nutrition, and growth hormone. Am J Kidney Dis 1995;26:256–265.
154. Fouque D, Peng SC, Shamir E, Kopple JD. Recombinant human insulin-like growth factor-1 induces an anabolic response in malnourished CAPD patients. Kidney Int 2000;57:646–654.
155. Haffner D, Schaefer F, Nissel R, et al. Effect of growth hormone treatment on adult height of children with chronic renal failure. N Engl J Med 2000;343:923–930.
156. Roelfsema V, Clark RG. The growth hormone and insulin-like growth factor axis: its manipulation for the benefit of growth disorders in renal failure. J Am Soc Nephrol 2001;12:1297–1306.
157. Fine RM. Growth hormone treatment of children with chronic renal insufficiency and end-stage renal disease following renal transplantation. J Pediatr Endocrinol Metab 1997;10:361–370.
158. Anonymous. Critical evaluation of the safety of recombinant human growth hormone administration: Statement from the Growth Hormone Research Society. J Clin Endocrinol Metab 2001;86:1868–1870.
159. Ding H, Kopple DJ, Cohen A, et al. Recombinant human insulin-like growth factor-I accelerates recovery and reduces catabolism in rats with ischemic acute renal failure. J Clin Invest 1993;91:2281–2287.
160. Miller SB, Martin DR, Kissane J, et al. Insulin-like growth factor I accelerates recovery from ischemic acute tubular necrosis in the rat. Proc Natl Acad Sci USA 1992;89:11876–11880.
161. Clark R, Mortensen D, Rabkin R. Recovery from acute ischaemic renal failure is accelerated by des-(1–3)-insulin-like growth factor-1. Clin Sci 1994;86:709–714.
162. Hirschberg R, Kopple J, Lipsett P, et al. Multicenter clinical trial of recombinant human insulin-like growth factor I in patients with acute renal failure. Kidney Int 1999;55:2424–2432.

V IGF in Disease States

14 The IGF and IGFBP System in Insulin Resistance and Diabetes Mellitus

Kerstin Brismar and Moira S. Lewitt

KEY POINTS

- The IGF system and insulin play complementary roles in the maintenance of glucose homeostasis.
- The IGFs are important beta cell survival factors.
- IGFBP-1 is a marker of hepatic insulin action.
- Low levels of IGFBP-1 are associated with insulin resistance and cardiovascular disease risk.
- High IGFBP-1 levels indicate the need for increased insulin replacement in diabetes.

1. INTRODUCTION

Insulin resistance and diabetes mellitus are important public health issues, and their management represents an enormous economic burden worldwide. The prevalence of these disorders is increasing, particularly in the developing world, because of changes in nutrition and increasing age of population. Insulin resistance is a fundamental defect in the metabolic syndrome (also known as syndrome X), and is associated with an adverse lipid profile, hypertension, and impaired glucose tolerance *(1,2)*. The metabolic syndrome is a major risk factor and target for the preventative management of cardiovascular disease *(2)* and diabetes mellitus *(3)*.

Nutritional disturbances are important in the pathophysiology of insulin resistance and diabetes mellitus. This is reflected in changes in the insulin-like growth factor (IGF) system, which, as we will discuss, can be used under certain conditions as markers of these disorders, for preventative care.

2. SCOPE AND AIM

In this chapter, we outline the importance of the IGF system, in relation to nutrition; in the pathogenesis, prevention, and treatment of insulin resistance and diabetes mellitus; and their related complications. The physiology of the IGF system is covered in detail in other chapters. Here, we focus on the specific role of the IGF system in the

From: *IGF and Nutrition in Health and Disease*
Edited by: M. S. Houston, J. M. P. Holly, and E. L. Feldman © Humana Press Inc., Totowa, NJ

regulation of insulin sensitivity and glucose homeostasis. We then describe the changes in the IGF system in insulin resistance, type 1 and type 2 diabetes mellitus. Among the IGF binding proteins (IGFBPs), we concentrate largely on IGFBP-1, for which insulin is a dominant regulator. After reviewing each of these conditions we will discuss in more detail three issues of topical interest: (1) conditions associated with "inappropriately" high IGFBP-1 concentrations; (2) the use of components of the IGF system in the prediction and management of disease; and (3) the use of IGFs and IGFBPs in the treatment of insulin resistance and diabetes mellitus.

3. PHYSIOLOGY

3.1. Role of the IGF System in Normal Glucose Homeostasis

Although the endocrine regulation of blood glucose is achieved by insulin, which promotes glucose disposal, and by the opposing actions of several counter-regulatory hormones, there is also strong evidence of a complementary role for the IGF system in its regulation *(4)*. It was recognized very early that serum contained a fraction of "non-suppressible insulin-like activity," the action of which could not be blocked by the use of insulin antiserum *(5)*. It is now known that this is caused by IGF-I and -II, which share structural similarity with insulin and have similar metabolic actions and receptor cross-reactivity. The IGFs stimulate glucose uptake and use in muscle, with a potency that is approx 5% of insulin when administered intravenously *(6)*. There are differences in the spectrum and potency of biologic activities between insulin and IGFs caused in part by differential distribution of receptors and the occurrence of heteroreceptor complexes as well as intrinsic differences in signal transduction (*see* Chapter 1). Studies in vivo show that, in the short-term, IGF-I decreases insulin secretion, probably as a response to hypoglycemia *(6)* and, in the long-term, there is an increase in tissue sensitivity to insulin *(7)*. The IGFs are important pancreatic β-cell survival factors, preventing apoptosis *(8)*. Insulin itself is a positive regulator of IGF-I in vivo *(9)* and in vitro *(10)*. Thus, in addition to being subject to the positive effect of GH, IGF-I is under nutritional control (discussed in Chapter 2).

In contrast to insulin, which is synthesized, stored, and secreted by pancreatic β-cells, IGFs are synthesized and secreted by a wide variety of tissues and have paracrine activity. Unlike insulin, they associate with a family of six specific IGF-binding proteins that are important in determining IGF availability and activity *(11)*. When the IGFs associate with IGFBP-3 or, to a lesser extent, IGFBP-5, these binary complexes can associate with a third, acid labile subunit. These ternary complexes form a stable circulating storage pool showing little diurnal variation and, in this way, block most of the hypoglycemic potential of the IGFs. Binary complexes between the IGFs and IGFBP-1 to -6, unbound IGFs, and unbound IGFBPs are able to cross the capillary membrane rapidly to reach the tissues. Posttranslational modifications of IGFBPs may alter their association with IGFs *(12)* and thus may modify IGF action in glucose homeostasis. Phosphorylation of IGFBP-1, for example, is likely to promote the inhibitory effect of IGFBP-1 on IGF actions, whereas proteolysis of IGFBP-3 and other IGFBPs is likely to promote IGF availability.

The concentrations of IGF-I and IGF-II in the human circulation represent at least 50 times the hypoglycemic potential of insulin *(4)*. Although most of this is inhibited,

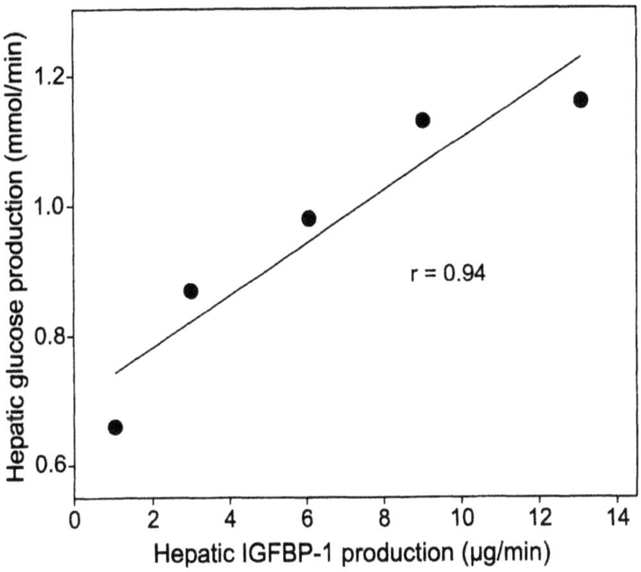

Fig. 1. Correlation between hepatic IGFBP-1 secretion and glucose production in normal individuals. Blood samples were taken from the hepatic vein and brachial artery in five healthy men after an overnight fast and used to calculate the splanchnic production of IGFBP-1 and glucose *(19)*.

even 1% availability to the tissues would represent a significant activity. Estimates of steady-state free IGF levels support this concept and studies in rodents suggest that this activity can be blocked by IGFBP administration or overexpression *(13,14)*. Assays have recently been developed for the "free" IGF fraction. In this review we use the term "free" IGF for those assays that use ultrafiltration under near-physiological conditions and "readily dissociable" IGF for values from immunoradiometric assays which do not have an ultrafiltration step and which result in somewhat higher concentrations *(15)*.The patterns of regulation of the IGFBPs also suggest that they may play specific roles in glucose homeostasis. IGFBP-1, with its characteristic diurnal rhythm *(16,17)* associated with food intake, and a classical pattern of response after insulin-induced hypoglycemia *(18)*, appears to play a role as a glucose counter-regulatory hormone, blocking the availability of IGFs *(4)*. Hepatic IGFBP-1 secretion is inhibited by insulin *(9,19)*, and under normal conditions circulating concentrations are inversely related to insulin or C-peptide levels *(20)*, accounting for the response to food intake. After the induction of hypoglycemia, IGFBP-1 concentrations increase dramatically *(18,21)*. This may be caused in part by falling insulin concentrations *(21)* with a contribution from the stimulatory effect of glucose counter-regulatory hormones *(22–24)*. IGFBP-1 has a similar pattern of regulation to phosphoenol pyruvate carboxykinase, and this is reflected in the close relationship between hepatic IGFBP-1 production and hepatic glucose production *(19)*, which is also illustrated in Fig. 1.

Circulating concentrations of IGFBP-2, which binds IGF-II with a higher affinity than IGF-I, are increased in fasting and in tumour hypoglycemia *(25)*, and it is speculated that it might target IGF-II to the tissues in these situations. Endocrine IGF-II may thus have particular importance as a metabolic hormone, although there may be species differences in this role. In rodents circulating IGF-II levels decrease after birth and are absent in the adult circulation, whereas in humans circulating IGF-II concentrations are high throughout the lifespan. It appears that IGF-II may have a separate paracrine role in the developing pancreas where it co-localizes with insulin in β cells both in humans and in rats *(26)*.

3.2. Glucose Homeostasis in IGF System Transgenic and Knockout Mice

Transgenic and knockout mice have been used specifically in the investigation of the role of the IGF system, and the resulting phenotypes support a role for "available" IGFs in glucose homeostasis. Transgenic mice with a dominant-negative insulin-like growth factor-I receptor targeted to skeletal muscle have hybrid receptors that are inactive. These animals develop insulin resistance and pancreatic β cell dysfunction at an early age *(27)*. Mice with liver-specific knockout of the *IGF-I* gene also have insulin insensitivity, attributed to the loss of feedback on, and therefore increase in, GH levels *(28)*. When the liver IGF-I knockout is combined with a knockout of acid labile subunit, which alone has normal fasting insulin concentrations, GH and insulin concentrations increase to levels above that of the hepatic IGF-I knockout alone *(29)*.

IGF-II-deficient mice have reduced glycogen stores and fasting hypoglycemia postnatally *(30)*, indicating a role for IGF-II in glycogen metabolism at this developmental stage, at least in the mouse. Mice overexpressing hepatic IGF-II from 3–4 wk of age have increased basal and insulin-stimulated glucose disposal *(31)*, again supporting a metabolic role in adult life for IGF-II. However, mice overexpressing IGF-II in β-cells develop reduced apoptosis and islet cell hyperplasia *(32)*, which may be associated with hyperinsulinemia, mild hyperglycemia, fatty liver, and obesity *(33)*.

Further evidence for a role of the IGF system in glucose homeostasis comes from IGFBP transgenic mice *(34)*. It has been clearly shown that transgenic mice overexpressing rat IGFBP-1 have increased fasting blood glucose *(14)*, perhaps because of enhanced gluconeogenesis and hepatic insulin resistance *(35)*. They also have evidence of inhibition of IGF-I action in adipose tissue *(36)*. One strain of mice overexpressing human IGFBP-1 exhibited little change in glucose tolerance *(37)*, a difference that may be caused by the inability of mouse kinase activity to phosphorylate the human isoform *(38)*. Overexpression of human IGFBP-1, along with its regulatory sequences, so that its inverse relationship to insulin is maintained, develop glucose intolerance in later life, particularly in males, accompanied by a blunted hypoglycemic response to IGF-I *(39)*. IGFBP-3 transgenic mice also have impaired glucose homeostasis, with marked peripheral insulin resistance *(40)*. A possible role of muscle IGFBP-3 transgene expression in determining this response has not yet been clarified.

IGFBP-1 *(14)*, IGFBP-2 *(41)*, and IGFBP-3 *(42)* transgenic mice are all growth retarded. However, in contrast to IGFBP-1 and -3, IGFBP-2 transgenic mice tend to have reduced fasting glucose concentrations *(41)*. Glucose homeostasis in these animals has not been studied in detail; however, it has been noted that IGFBP-2 expression is highest in the pancreas, where it may have an impact on local IGF activity and therefore insulin secretion, in addition to endocrine effects on IGF availability for growth.

4. THE IGF SYSTEM IN INSULIN RESISTANCE

Insulin resistance is a heterogeneous disorder that may be present in up to 20% of the population and in which peripheral insulin resistance (reduced insulin-mediated glucose uptake in peripheral tissues) and hepatic insulin resistance (reduced insulin-mediated suppression of hepatic glucose production) are present to varying degrees. Insulin resistance, along with other components of the metabolic syndrome, predicts the development of type 2 diabetes *(3)*. Plasma insulin concentrations increase to maintain normoglycemia and fasting levels may be used, along with glucose concentrations, in the Homeostasis Assessment Model, which is a mathematical model allowing for both insulin sensitivity and β-cell-function. The Homeostasis Assessment Model is simple, gives an estimate of basal insulin resistance, and is convenient for large epidemiological studies *(43)*. The euglycemic clamp technique determines resistance under insulin-stimulated conditions and is appropriate for smaller physiological studies. Isotope studies under euglycemic clamp conditions are needed to properly determine hepatic insulin resistance. Unfortunately, early studies of the role of the IGF system have not clearly discriminated between peripheral and hepatic resistance, and most of the following comments apply to whole body or predominantly peripheral insulin resistance. Hepatic insulin resistance is discussed in greater detail (*see* Section 6). States of severe insulin resistance are usually characterized by diabetes and are covered in Section 5.3.

4.1. Changes in the IGF System in Insulin Resistance

The most profound change in the IGF system in insulin resistance is suppression of IGFBP-1. Because IGFBP-1 is inhibited by insulin, it reflects hepatic insulin action and, therefore, under conditions of preserved hepatic insulin sensitivity, the prevailing insulin concentrations. Under these conditions it is good a marker of peripheral insulin sensitivity. Animal models with peripheral insulin resistance, such as Zucker diabetic fatty rats have decreased IGFBP-1 concentrations *(44)*. In human obesity associated with hyperinsulinemia, circulating IGFBP-1 concentrations are low *(45–47)*, and lifestyle interventions (diet and exercise) in middle-aged men with the metabolic syndrome result in an IGFBP-1 increase *(48)*. Total IGF-I concentrations may be normal, and IGFBP-3 and IGF-II even increased, in obesity *(49)*. In obese children low levels of IGFBP-1 may be seen even in the presence of normal peripheral insulin levels *(50)*. This suggests that IGFBP-1 is a sensitive marker of portal insulin action and may be a predictor of the later development of frank insulin resistance. IGFBP-2 has been observed to decrease in adolescent obesity *(51)*.

IGFBP-1 is also decreased in endocrinopathies associated with insulin resistance and hyperinsulinemia, such as GH excess *(52)* and Cushing's disease *(52,54)* or glucocorticoid administration *(55,56)*. In HIV lipodystrophy, severe insulin resistance is associated with reduced IGFBP-1 levels although there is a blunted response to hyperinsulinemia *(57)*.

Patients with acromegaly may experience marked improvement in symptoms during nutritional deprivation, even in the presence of sustained, high GH levels. A case study is described in Fig, 2. In this patient insulin sensitivity and glucose tolerance improved during caloric restriction and IGF-I levels fell by 50%. As insulin sensitivity improved, there was clinical improvement and a normal diurnal response for IGFBP-1 was seen, with clear falls in IGFBP-1 levels in relation to the small meals consumed (approx 30 kcal, in the form of carbohydrate drinks).

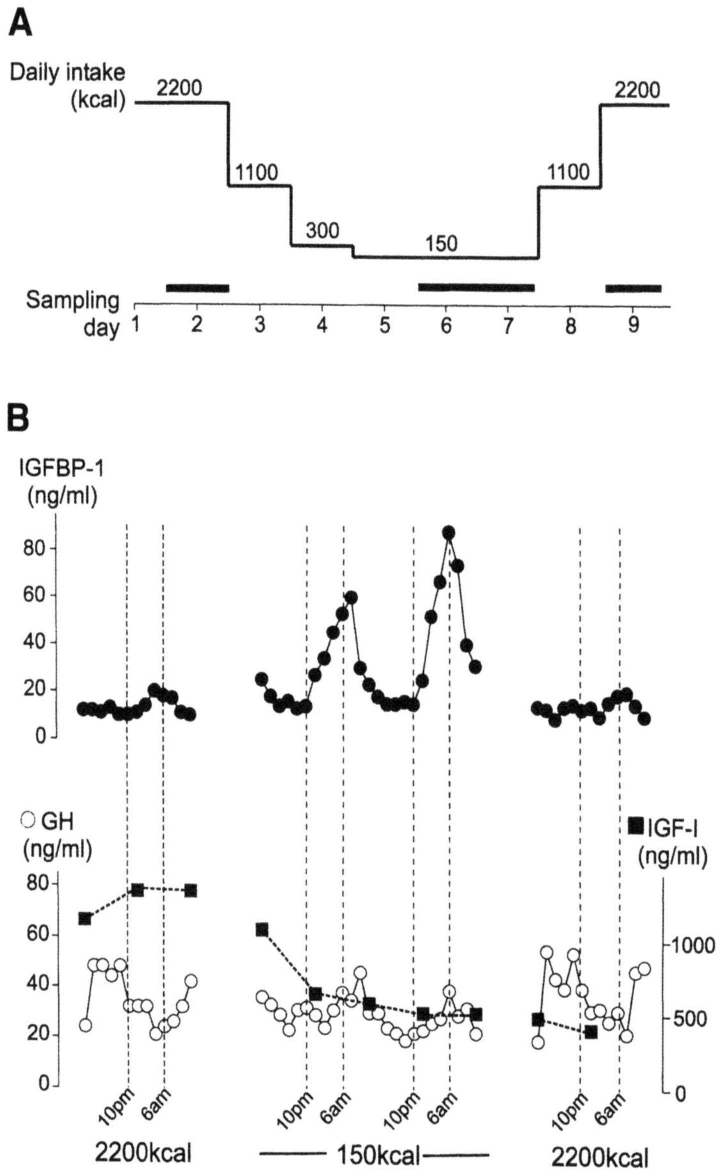

Fig. 2. Response to nutritional deprivation in acromegaly. A 47-yr-old woman with acromegaly was assessed with 2-h sampling during a period of nutritional deprivation (**A**). Throughout the study meals or snacks were consumed at 0800 h, 1200 h, 1400 h, 1700 h, and 1930 h. She reported a marked improvement in sweating and arthralgias while on 150 kcal/d. IGFBP-1, GH, and IGF-I concentrations, measured by radioimmunoassay, are shown in **B**. Solid lines indicate periods of sampling. The mean blood glucose was 6.8, 3.9, and 5.7 mmol/L during each these study periods and the mean insulin, 85, 16, and 237 pmol/L, respectively.

4.2. The IGF System and the Pathophysiology of Insulin Resistance

Genetic and environmental factors contribute to the pathogenesis of insulin resistance. Nutritional factors play an important role and, during the normal lifespan hormonal changes, contribute to the relative insulin resistance that occurs during puberty and pregnancy. Genetic variations at the IGF-II and IGFBP-1 loci have been implicated in insulin resistance *(58)*, although a larger cohort study has not yet been reported.

It is proposed that low IGFBP-1 is responsible for the observed increase in "free" IGF-I in obesity *(49)*. "Readily dissociable" IGF-I also tends to increase in obesity *(51)*. Reduced GH concentrations may be a direct response to increased feedback inhibition by IGF-I *(51)*. An increase in available IGF-I would explain normal growth in obese children despite the low levels of GH. The potential contribution of relative GH deficiency to reduced insulin sensitivity *(59)* is entirely speculative.

Insulin resistance is characteristic of the polycystic ovarian syndrome, and IGFBP-1 is decreased in this disorder *(60,61)*. It has been proposed that this results in increased ovarian IGF activity and may contribute to the pathogenesis.

5. THE IGF SYSTEM IN DIABETES MELLITUS

Diabetes mellitus is a group of disorders characterized by hyperglycemia. The American Diabetes Association recommends that diabetes be diagnosed on the basis of (1) classical symptoms plus a random plasma glucose of ≥11.1mmol/L or (2) a fasting plasma glucose of ≥7.0 mmol/L or (3) a 2-h plasma glucose after a 75-g oral glucose load of ≥11.1mmol/L *(62)*. There are a number of pathogenic processes involved in the development of diabetes mellitus. The American Diabetes Association has established a useful etiological classification, dividing the disorder into four groups *(62)*. Type 1 diabetes refers to the outcome of β-cell destruction, which is usually caused by an autoimmune process, so that individuals are insulin deficient and prone to ketoacidosis. Type 2 diabetes is the most prevalent form and represents a spectrum from predominantly insulin resistance with relative insulin deficiency to a predominant insulin secretory defect with insulin resistance. Fat distribution and nutritional factors may contribute to this variability. Other specific types of diabetes include genetic defects of β-cell function and insulin action, endocrinopathies, and diseases of the exocrine pancreas. One disease of the exocrine pancreas, fibrocalculous pancreatopathy, results in diabetes and is caused by both genetic and environmental factors, including nutritional factors.

5.1. The IGF System in Type 1 Diabetes Mellitus

In poorly controlled type 1 diabetes IGF-I, IGF-II, and IGFBP-3 concentrations are decreased *(63)*, whereas IGFBP-1 is increased *(63–67)* because of high hepatic production and not to a decreased clearance rate *(9)*. The responses are thus similar to those seen in nutritional deprivation. Very high concentrations of phosphorylated IGFBP-1 are seen in severe ketoacidosis *(68)*. There are many facets of the IGF system that are yet to be explored; for example, the report of increased urinary IGFBP protease activity *(69)*. Animal models of type 1 diabetes, such as streptozotocin-induced insulin deficiency, are useful models for the IGF system in this disease *(70)*.

In response to insulin treatment, total IGF-I increases, independently of a change in GH levels *(63)*. A reduction in IGFBP-1 *(63)* and increase in "free" IGF-I *(71)* also is observed. The most effective suppression of IGFBP-1 is seen during intensive insulin therapy *(72,73)* and particularly when insulin is delivered via the peritoneal or portal route *(67,74)*. Withdrawal of insulin results in a dramatic increase in IGFBP-1 levels 1 h later (*see* Fig. 3).

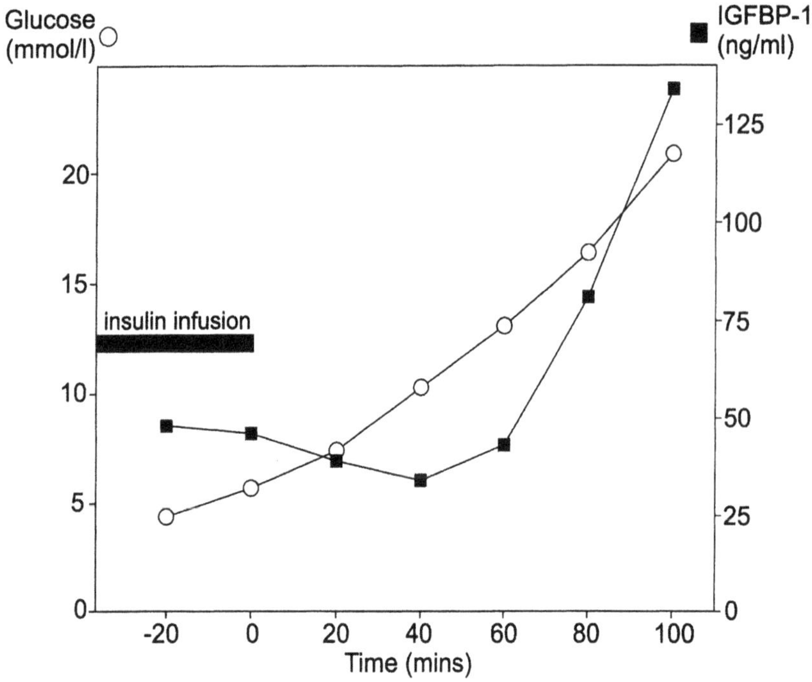

Fig. 3. IGFBP-1 response to cessation of an insulin infusion in type 1 diabetes mellitus. Insulin was infused intravenously in a 30-yr-old woman for 20 h, the rate adjusted to maintain euglycemia.

It is speculated that elevated IGFBP-1 levels have a detrimental effect on metabolic control *(75–78)*, as well on growth *(78,79)*. The increased IGFBP-1, by decreasing IGF bioavailability, may contribute to the elevated GH concentrations, insulin resistance, and hyperglycemia *(77)*.

The IGF system has been shown to influence β-cell function in animal models (*see* Section 3.2.), and it has been reported that IGF-I treatment delays the onset of obesity in nonobese diabetic mice *(80)*. However, the role of the IGF system in the pathogenesis of type 1 diabetes in humans has not been investigated.

5.2. The IGF System in Type 2 Diabetes Mellitus

There is marked phenotypic heterogeneity in type 2 diabetes mellitus. The changes in IGFBP-1 levels reflect this, being variably reported from low *(66)* to high *(72,81)*. It has been suggested that the method of treatment may also affect it secretion. Patients on sulfonylurea therapy have increased proinsulin and low IGFBP-1, and those on multiple insulin injcctions have increased concentrations *(82)*. There are few animal models of type 2 diabetes in which the IGF system has been characterized. We have found, in the Goto-Kakizaki rat, that IGFBP-1 clearly increases and there is no relationship to circulating insulin, suggesting that there is significant hepatic insulin resistance in these lean animals (unpublished data). IGFBP-3 proteolysis, speculated to be related to insulin resistance, has been documented in human type 2 diabetes *(83)*.

Insulin resistance often precedes type 2 diabetes, and individuals with the metabolic syndrome are at increased risk of impaired glucose tolerance. This is also true for the group of individuals born small-for gestational age *(84)*. In individuals who are small for gestational age, in which changes in the IGF system such as low IGF-I in early childhood and low IGFBP-1 in later childhood, have been observed, it has been speculated that the IGF system is involved in the pathogenesis of later insulin resistance and cardiovascular consequences.

5.3. Other Types of Diabetes Mellitus and the IGF System

Severe insulin-resistant states are characterized by acanthosis nigricans, acromegaloid features, and ovarian hyperandrogenism, in addition to hyperinsulinemia and diabetes. In a small series of women with congenital partial lipodystrophy decreases in total and "readily available" IGF-I, and IGFBP-1 were observed, although the ratio of "readily available" IGF-I to IGFBP-1 was increased *(85)*. It is speculated that IGF-I is responsible for the development of acromegaloid and other features in this disorder.

5.4. The Role of the IGF System in Diabetes Complications

Although a direct effect on macrovascular complications is yet to be proven, IGF-I and IGFBP-1 are clearly markers of cardiovascular risk and disease (*see* Section 7). Growth factors, including IGFs, are more strongly implicated directly in the development of microvascular disease *(86)*. In humans, studies are limited to observations on the circulating IGF system, which may not precisely reflect changes in individual tissues.

Changes in the expression of various components of the IGF system occur early in animal models of kidney disease *(87)* and are discussed in greater detail in Chapter 13. The IGF system may participate in diabetic nephropathy by mediating increases in mesangial extracellular matrix production *(88,89)*.

Despite an early report linking IGF-I to retinopathy *(90)*, there are few studies that determine the precise role of the IGF system in this disorder. The few studies performed report either no change, an increase or a decrease in circulating IGF-I levels *(91)*. IGFBP-1 is present in the vitreous of patients with diabetic retinopathy, with no correlation with serum levels *(92)*, and may relate to a nonspecific increase in intravitreal proteins *(93)*.

Animal studies support a potential role for IGF-I in diabetic neuropathy *(86)*. One clinical study in a group of type 1 diabetic patients failed to demonstrate a difference in circulating IGF-I compared to matched control group *(94)*. However, in this study, IGFBP-1 levels were reported to be elevated.

6. CONDITIONS ASSOCIATED WITH INAPPROPRIATELY ELEVATED IGFBP-1 LEVELS

In healthy individuals, fasting IGFBP-1 and insulin concentrations are closely inversely related *(95)*. However, in type 1 diabetes IGFBP-1 is elevated in relation to the peripheral insulin levels *(95)*. The fact that these peripheral levels of exogenous insulin are much lower than the endogenous portal insulin concentrations that would normally be present may contribute to this observation. Elevated levels of IGFBP-1 in relation to insulin can also be seen in type 2 diabetes *(81,82)* when endogenous insulin production fails to further increase with increasing insulin resistance. When no change in glucose homeostasis is observed, this is consistent with the concept that predominantly hepatic insulin resistance has developed. However reduced hepatic insulin extraction may also result in inappropriate elevations of IGFBP-1 in relation to insulin, and in this situation C-peptide levels may more reliably reflect portal insulin secretion *(96)*. Another possible explanation for the relative high IGFBP-1 in some patients with type 1 or type 2 diabetes is impaired renal clearance due to reduced glomerular filtration rate.

An elevated IGFBP-1 in relation to insulin is a characteristic of catabolic states *(97)*. In these conditions there is increased secretion of glucose counter-regulatory hormones and cytokines, both of which increase IGFBP-1. Cytokines may themselves induce hepatic insulin resistance. Intensive care patients are a group with severe peripheral and hepatic insulin resistance, in whom elevated IGFBP-1 is a marker of poor outcome and resistance to insulin therapy *(98)*. It is speculated that, in these critically ill patients, hypoxia may play a role in the development of hepatic insulin resistance. IGFBP-1 is also stimulated by hypoxia *(99)*. Thus, in severe catabolic stress, hepatic insulin resistance and factors (e.g., cytokines, glucose counter-regulatory hormones, and hypoxia), which are direct stimulators of IGFBP-1, coexist, suggesting that IGFBP-1 cannot be used as an independent marker of either parameter. Rodents may not be ideal experimental models for dissecting out the relative contributions of hepatic insulin resistance and these stimulators. Glucocorticoids, for example, stimulate IGFBP-1 potently in vivo in rodents *(100)*, whereas no elevation in IGFBP-1 is seen in dexamethasone-treated humans *(55,56)*. One study in obese rats has demonstrated that the decrease in insulin levels after surgical removal of visceral fat *(101)* is associated with a decrease in IGFBP-1; however, weight loss in humans with central adiposity is associated with an increase IGFBP-1 (K. Brismar, unpublished observations).

7. THE IGF PROTEINS AS CLINICAL MARKERS IN INSULIN RESISTANCE AND DIABETES

In subjects with normal pancreatic β-cell function, a low IGFBP-1 level is a sensitive marker of portal insulin levels and therefore may be a valuable diagnostic tool for whole body insulin resistance. Low levels of IGFBP-1 are a common finding in all conditions with hyperinsulinemia. Moreover, even in healthy nonobese subjects with normal oral glucose tolerance, the basal IGFBP-1 can be used to predict the insulin and C-peptide response to glucose infusion, more reliably than the fasting insulin concentrations *(55)*. We believe that the stability of IGFBP-1 in serum and blood, and less rapid response to environmental stimuli, give this measurement an advantage over currently available insulin and C-peptide methods.

Low levels of IGFBP-1 have been shown to be associated with impaired glucose tolerance *(102)*, and cardiovascular disease risk both in healthy individuals *(102–104)* and in those with type 2 diabetes *(105,106)*. In one study a predictive role of IGFBP-1 for impaired glucose tolerance was found to be dependent on the presence of low IGF-I levels *(107)*. Low total IGF-I levels predict worsening of insulin-mediated glucose uptake over a 1-yr period in older (55–80 y) individuals *(108)* and low "readily dissociable" IGF-I has been associated with signs of cardiovascular disease *(103)*.

In type 1 diabetes, where there is no endogenous insulin secretion, IGFBP-1 cannot be used as a marker of insulin sensitivity *(109)*; however, we recommend that high IGFBP-1 levels can be used to detect inadequate insulin replacement. Circulating IGF-

I concentrations are low in poorly controlled type 1 diabetes and can be used to reflect inadequate nutrition as well as insulin deficiency. In patients with type 2 diabetes on oral hypoglycemic agents, increasing circulating concentrations of IGFBP-1 indicate an inadequate insulin response to overcome the insulin resistance. Conversely, decreasing IGFBP-1 levels may be a useful indicator of improved insulin sensitivity in response to therapeutic intervention.

8. THE IGF SYSTEM IN THERAPEUTICS

The effects of recombinant human IGF-I administration in normal individuals and its potential use in catabolic disease, bone, and neurological diseases are discussed in detail in other chapters. Therefore we will limit our discussion here to the clinical use of IGF-I in diabetes and insulin resistant states.

8.1. Type 1 Diabetes Mellitus

In 1992, intravenous IGF-I was reported to rapidly reverse hyperglycemia and ketoacidosis in an adolescent with type 1 diabetes and severe insulin resistance *(110)*. In a group of adolescents a single subcutaneous injection of 40 μg/kg was found to reduce overnight GH concentrations and insulin requirements *(111)*. When, in a placebo-controlled trial, 20–40 μg/kg IGF-I was given daily in addition to multiple-injection insulin therapy, HbA1c decreased at 12 wk; however, this was not seen at 24 wk *(112)*. There are two reports of randomized, double-blind, placebo-controlled studies in young adults with type 1 diabetes that show that 1-wk therapy with 40 μg/kg/d in combination with insulin therapy reduces mean overnight GH concentrations *(113,114)*, improves peripheral insulin sensitivity *(114)*, and decreases hepatic glucose production *(113)*.

8.2. Type 2 Diabetes Mellitus

Despite the observation that individuals with type 2 diabetes mellitus may have IGF-I resistance in peripheral tissues *(115)*, treatment with IGF-I results in improved glucose and lipid metabolism *(116)*. Improvements in muscle as well as hepatic insulin sensitivity can be demonstrated *(117)*. The use of IGF-I in type 2 diabetes may result in changes in IGFBP-1, -2, and -3, which may alter the tissue bioavailability of IGFs *(118)*.

8.3. Insulin Resistance

Rats with a metabolic syndrome caused by maternal malnutrition respond to IGF-I therapy with a reduction in food intake, obesity, and hypertension *(119)*. Although IGF-I has not been used in this circumstance in humans, it has been used in high doses with metabolic improvement in patients with severe insulin resistance, such insulin receptor mutations and congenital generalized lipodystrophy *(120–123)*, although at least two studies fail to demonstrate significant glucose lowering response *(124,125)*. In some of the individuals studied, there was an improvement in acanthosis nigricans and hirsutism *(121)*.

8.4. Side Effects

High-dose IGF-I infusion is associated with acute symptomatic hypophosphatemia *(110)*. IGF-I treatment may induce changes in the profile of circulating IGFBPs that may affect its bioavailability *(25)*. Chronic low-dose subcutaneous therapy has been associated with an unacceptable rate of adverse events, including facial and hand edema, bilateral jaw tenderness, arthralgias, tachycardia, and flushing *(126)*. The combination of IGF-I and IGFBP-3 is more promising. Continuous subcutaneous infusion of this combination or placebo for 2 wk reduced mean GH levels, insulin requirements, and blood glucose in young adults with type 1 diabetes with no reported side effects *(127)*.

9. SUMMARY AND CONCLUSIONS

IGF-I, IGF-II, and insulin have homology in structure and in their receptors. Although they can partially replace each other, they have distinct roles in whole body metabolism. The IGFs play a more long-term role, whereas insulin regulates meal-related responses. The two systems are closely linked, with insulin regulating IGFBP-1, and IGFs being important in pancreatic β-cell survival.

IGFBP-1 is marker of insulin production and action and has been used as a marker for failure of insulin production, as well as insulin resistance. A low IGFBP-1 is an early marker of insulin resistance and is emerging as useful predictor of those individuals who are at risk of developing cardiovascular disease and type 2 diabetes. Although, theoretically, IGFBP-1 levels that are high in relation to insulin may reflect significant hepatic insulin resistance, the clinical conditions in which this is seen are also accompanied by increased hormones and cytokines which themselves promote insulin resistance but also directly stimulate hepatic IGFBP-1 secretion.

The low IGF-I and high IGFBP-1 levels seen in poorly controlled type 1 diabetes are likely to contribute to short stature in children and may also have detrimental effects on metabolic control.

The measurement of IGF-I is well established in the clinic as a marker of GH secretion. IGFBP-1, alongside IGF-I, has now emerged as an even more valuable tool in determining nutritional status and in the choice of treatment in both type 1 and type 2 diabetes mellitus. IGFs, in combination with IGFBPs, may also play a future role in therapeutic regimens for diabetes mellitus associated with insulin resistance.

10. RECOMMENDATIONS AND CHALLENGES FOR THE FUTURE

Although it is clear that components of the IGF system are altered, sometimes profoundly, in insulin-resistant states and in both type 1 and type 2 diabetes mellitus, their role in the pathophysiology of these disorders is not yet clearly defined. Interventions that might restore these responses to normal have important implications in the management of a group of disorders that are a growing social and economic burden.

10.1. What Are the Changes to the IGF System at the Tissue Level in Insulin Resistance and Diabetes Mellitus?

We should be cautious in interpreting IGF activity at the tissue level from circulating concentrations. In addition to the circulating IGFBP profile, protease activity in the circulation and tissues, and interaction with IGFBPs at the tissue level will influence the final effect of the IGFs on glucose homeostasis. This is particularly important when considering the role of the IGF system in diabetes complications. We propose that the use of knockout and transgenic mice for components of the IGF system, including IGFBP proteases, generally and in specific tissues, in combination with the induction of diabetes along with its complications is an experimental approach that could be explored.

10.2. What Is the Predictive Value of a Low IGFBP-1 for the Long-Term Risk of Type 2 Diabetes?

Although low circulating IGFBP-1 concentrations are related to diabetes mellitus in cross-sectional studies, it's role as a predictive marker is unclear. One study suggests that it is useful only when combined with a low IGF-I level *(107)*. Large prospective studies are indicated to clarify its potential role in predicting this condition with its associated morbidity and mortality.

10.3. What Is the Cause of the Early Postprandial Rise in IGFBP-1?

Some studies have demonstrated rapid meal-related rises in IGFBP-1, prior to the fall due to rising insulin concentrations *(82)*. This is more pronounced in patients with type 2 diabetes. The reason is not immediately clear and requires careful study. We speculate the role of altered blood flow and of IGFBP-1 degradation and clearance in this phenomenon.

10.4. What Is the Outcome of a Low IGFBP-1 in Insulin Resistance?

The possibility of a direct effect of IGFBP-1 on IGF actions in the ovary in polycystic ovarian syndrome *(60,61)*, and in the pituitary to reduce GH secretion in obesity *(51)* has been proposed. There is also the theoretical possibility of a role in increased cancer risk seen in obesity *(128)*. The pathophysiological consequences of low hepatic IGFBP-1, independent of its effect on IGF activity, should be also considered, including loss of the protective effect of IGFBP-1 on hepatic apoptosis *(129)*. If low IGFBP-1 concentrations are detrimental, should IGFBP-1 be replaced if other therapeutic approaches, for example, diet and weight loss, are unsuccessful?

10.5. Can IGFBP-1 Be Used as a Marker of Hepatic Insulin Resistance?

There are a number of conditions, for example, catabolic states, where IGFBP-1 is inappropriately elevated and hepatic insulin resistance is present. What is the cause of the elevated IGFBP-1 in these circumstances? Is it a marker of hepatic insulin resistance alone, or does it reflect more precisely other aspects of the catabolic response, such as cytokine secretion and the presence of oxidative stress? These questions are yet to be answered by carefully designed clinical studies.

10.6. What Is the Outcome of Inappropriately Elevated IGFBP-1?

When circulating IGFBP-1 is high in relation to insulin, what are the metabolic consequences? What are the consequences of suppressing or blocking this "inappropriate" activity? It has recently been observed that inhibitors of glycogen synthase kinase-3 are able to reduce IGFBP-1 in the presence of insulin resistance in vitro *(130)* and this indicates a possible approach to this question for future in vivo studies.

ACKNOWLEDGMENTS

The authors wish to thank Professor Kerstin Hall for many helpful discussions. We acknowledge the support of the Swedish Research Council (#04224), Novo Nordisk Foundation, Swedish Diabetes Association and the Persson Family Foundation.

REFERENCES

1. Reaven GM. Role of insulin resistance in human disease. Diabetes 1988;37:15951–607.
2. 2001 Executive summary of the third report of the national cholesterol education program (NCEP) expert panel on detection, evaluation, and treatment of high blood cholesterol in adults (adult treatment panel III). JAMA 285:2486–2497.
3. Laaksonen DE, Lakka H-M, Niskanen LK, Kaplan GA, Salonen JT, Lakka TA. Metabolic syndrome and development of diabetes mellitus: Application and validation of recently suggested definitions of the metabolic syndrome in a prospective cohort study. Am J Epidemiol 2002;156:1070–1077.
4. Lewitt MS. Role of the insulin-like growth factors in the endocrine control of glucose homeostasis. Diab Res Clin Pract 1994;23:3–15.
5. Froesch ER, Bürgi H, Ramseier EB, Bally P, Labhart A. Antibody-suppressible and nonsuppressible insulin-like activities in human serum and their physiologic significance. An insulin assay with adipose tissue of increased precision and specificity. J Clin Invest 1963;42:1816–1834.
6. Guler H-P, Zapf J, Froesch ER. Short-term metabolic effects of recombinant human insulin-like growth factor I in healthy adults. N Engl J Med 1987;317:137–140.
7. Moses AC, Young SCJ, Morrow LA, Obrien M, Clemmons DR. Recombinant human insulin-like growth factor I increases insulin sensitivity and improves glycemic control in type II diabetes. Diabetes 1996;45:91–100.
8. Mabley JG, Belin V, John N, Green IC. Insulin-like growth factor I reverses interleukin-1-beta inhibition of insulin secretion, induction of nitric oxide synthase and cytokine-mediated apoptosis in rat islets of Langerhans. FEBS Lett 1997;417:235–238.
9. Brismar K, Fernqvist-Forbes E, Wahren J, Hall K. Effect of insulin on the hepatic production of insulin-like growth factor-binding protein-1 (IGFBP-1), IGFBP-3, and IGF-I in insulin-dependent diabetes. J Clin Endocrinol Metab 1994;79:872–878.
10. Johnson TR, Blossey BK, Denko CW, Ilan J. Expression of insulin-like growth factor I in cultured rat hepatocytes: effects of insulin and growth hormone. Mol Endocrinol 1989;3:580–587.
11. Baxter RC. Insulin-like growth factor (IGF)-binding proteins: interactions with IGFs and intrinsic bioactivities. Am J Physiol Endocrinol Metab 2000;278:E967–E76.
12. Firth SM, Baxter RC. Cellular actions of the insulin-like growth factor binding proteins. Endocr Rev 2002;23:824–854.
13. Lewitt MS, Denyer GS, Cooney GJ, Baxter RC. Insulin-like growth factor-binding protein-1 modulates blood glucose levels. Endocrinology 1991;129:2254–2256.
14. Rajkumar K, Barron D, Lewitt MS, Murphy LJ. Growth retardation and hyperglycemia in insulin-like growth factor binding protein-1 transgenic mice. Endocrinology 1995;136:4029–4034.
15. Frystyk J, Ivarsen P, Stoving RK, Dall R, Bek T, Hagen C, Ørskov H. Determination of free insulin-like growth factor-I in human serum: comparison of ultrafiltration and direct immunoradiometric assay. Growth Horm IGF Res 2001;11:117–127.
16. Rutanen E-M, Seppälä M, Pietila R, Bohn H. Placental protein 12 (PP12): Factors affecting levels in late pregnancy. Placenta 1984;5:243–248.
17. Baxter RC, Cowell CT. Diurnal rhythm of growth hormone-independent binding protein for insulin-like growth factors in human plasma. J Clin Endocrinol Metab 1987;65:432–440.
18. Yeoh S-I, Baxter RC. Metabolic regulation of the growth hormone independent insulin-like growth factor binding protein in human plasma. Acta Endocrinol (Copenh) 1988;119:465–473.
19. Fernqvist-Forbes E, Ekberg K, Lingren B, Brismar K. Splanchnic exchange of insulin-like growth factor binding protein-1 (IGFBP-1), IGF-I and acid-labile subunit (ALS) during normo- and hyper-insulinaemia in healthy subjects. Clin Endocrinol 1999;51:327–332.

20. Suikkari A-M, Koivisto VA, Koistinen R, Seppälä M, Yki-Järvinen H. Dose-response characteristics for suppression of low molecular weight plasma insulin-like growth factor-binding protein by insulin. J Clin Endocrinol Metab 1989;68:135–140.
21. Cotterill AM, Holly JMP, Amiel S, Wass JAH. Suppression of endogenous insulin secretion regulates the rapid rise of insulin-like growth factor binding protein (IGFBP)-1 levels following acute hypoglycaemia. Clin Endocrinol 1993;38:633–639.
22. Hilding A, Brismar K, Thorén M, Hall K. Glucagon stimulates insulin-like growth factor binding protein-1 secretion in healthy subjects, patients with pituitary insufficiency, and patients with insulin-dependent diabetes mellitus. J Clin Endocrinol Metab 1993;77:1142–1147.
23. Conover CA, Divertie GD, Lee PDK. Cortisol increases plasma insulin-like growth factor binding protein-1 in humans. Acta Endocrinol 1993;128:140–143.
24. Fernqvist-Forbes E, Hilding A, Ekberg K, Brismar K. Influence of circulating epinephrine and norepinephrine on insulin-like growth factor binding protein-1 in humans. J Clin Endocrinol Metab 1997;82:2677–2680.
25. Zapf J, Schmid C, Guler HP, Waldvogel M, Hauri C, Futo E, Hossenlopp P, Binoux M, Froesch ER. Regulation of binding proteins for insulin-like growth factors (IGF) in humans. Increased expression of IGF binding protein 2 during IGF-I treatment of healthy adults and in patients with extrapancreatic tumor hypoglycemia. J Clin Invest 1990;86:952–961.
26. Maake C, Reinecke M. Immunohistochemical localization of insulin-like growth factor 1 and 2 in the endocrine pancreas of rat, dog, and man, and their coexistence with classical islet hormones. Cell Tissue Res 1993;273:249–259.
27. Fernandez AM, Kim JK, Yakar S, Dupont J, Hernandez-Sanchez C, Castle AL, et al. Functional inactivation of the IGF-I and insulin receptors in skeletal muscle causes type 2 diabetes. Genes Dev 2001;15:1926–1934.
28. Yakar S, Liu JL, Fernandez AM, Wu Y, Schally AV, Frystyk J, et al. Liver-specific IGF-1 gene deletion leads to muscle insulin insensitivity. Diabetes 2001;50:1110–1118.
29. Yakar S, Rosen CJ, Beamer WG, Ackert-Bicknell CL, Wu Y, Liu JL, et al. Circulating levels of IGF-1 directly regulate bone growth and density. J Clin Invest 2002;110:771–781.
30. Lopez MF, Dikkes P, Zurakowski D, Villa-Komaroff L, Majzoub JA. Regulation of hepatic glycogen in the insulin-like growth factor II-deficient mouse. Endocrinology 1999;140:1442–1448.
31. Rossetti L, Barzilai N, Chen W, Harris T, Yang D, Rogler CE. Hepatic overexpression of insulin-like growth factor-II in adulthood increases basal and insulin-stimulated glucose disposal in conscious mice. J Biol Chem 1996;271:203–208.
32. Petrik J, Pell JM, Arany E, McDonald TJ, Dean WL, Reik W, Hill DJ. Overexpression of insulin-like growth factor-II in transgenic mice is associated with pancreatic islet cell hyperplasia. Endocrinology 1999;140:2353–2363.
33. Devedjian JC, George M, Casellas A, Pujol A, Visa J, Pelegrin M, Gros L, Bosch F. Transgenic mice overexpressing insulin-like growth factor-II in beta cells develop type 2 diabetes. J Clin Invest 2000;105:731–740.
34. Silha JV, Murphy LJ. Insights from insulin-like growth factor binding protein transgenic mice. Endocrinology 2002;143:3711–3714.
35. Rajkumar K, Murphy LJ. Enhanced gluconeogenesis and hepatic insulin resistance in insulin-like growth factor binding protein-1 transgenic mice. Biochim Biophys Acta 1999;1426:491–497.
36. Rajkumar K, Modric T, Murphy LJ. Impaired adipogenesis in insulin-like growth factor binding protein-1 transgenic mice. J Endocrinol 1999;162:457–465.
37. Gay E, Seurin D, Babajko S, Doublier S, Cazillis M, Binoux M. Liver-specific expression of human insulin-like growth factor binding protein-1 in transgenic mice - repercussions on reproduction, ante- and perinatal mortality and postnatal growth. Endocrinology 1997;138:2937–2947.
38. Sakai K, D'Ercole AJ, Murphy LJ, Clemmons DR. Physiological differences in insulin-like growth factor binding protein- 1 (IGFBP-1) phosphorylation in IGFBP-1 transgenic mice. Diabetes 2001;50:32–38.
39. Crossey PA, Jones JS, Miell JP. Dysregulation of the insulin/IGF binding protein-1 axis in transgenic mice is associated with hyperinsulinemia and glucose intolerance. Diabetes 2000;49:457–465.
40. Silha JV, Gui Y, Murphy LJ. Impaired glucose homeostasis in insulin-like growth factor-binding protein-3-transgenic mice. Am J Physiol 2002;283:E937–E945.

41. Hoeflich A, Wu M, Mohan S, Foll J, Wanke R, Froehlich T, et al. Overexpression of insulin-like growth factor-binding protein-2 in transgenic mice reduces postnatal body weight gain. Endocrinology 1999; 140:5488–5496.
42. Modric T, Silha JV, Shi Z, Gui Y, Suwanichkul A, Durham SK, et al. Phenotypic manifestations of insulin-like growth factor-binding protein- 3 overexpression in transgenic mice. Endocrinology 2001;142:1958–1967.
43. Wallace TM, Matthews DR. The assessment of insulin resistance in man. Diabet Med 2002;19:527–534.
44. Lewitt MS, Saunders H, Phuyal JL, Baxter RC. Regulation of insulin-like growth factor-binding protein-1 in rat serum. Diabetes 1994;43:232–239.
45. Weaver JU, Holly JMP, Kopelman PG, Noonan K, Giadom CG, White N, et al. Decreased sex hormone binding globulin (SHBG) and insulin-like growth factor binding protein (IGFBP-1) in extreme obesity. Clin Endocrinol 1990;33:415–422.
46. Ricart W, Fernandez-Real JM. No decrease in free IGF-I with increasing insulin in obesity-related insulin resistance. Obes Res 2001;9:631–636.
47. Conover CA, Lee PDK, Kanaley JA, Clarkson JT, Jenson MD. Insulin regulation of insulin-like growth factor binding protein-1 in obese and nonobese humans. J Clin Endocrinol Metab 1992;74:1355–1360.
48. Hellenius M, Brismar KE, Berglund BH, Defaire UH. Effects on glucose tolerance, insulin secretion, insulin-like growth factor 1 and its binding protein, IGFBP-1, in a randomized controlled diet and exercise study in healthy, middle-aged men. J Intern Med 1995;238:121–130.
49. Frystyk J, Vestbo E, Skjaerbaek C, Mogensen CE, Ørskov H. Free insulin-like growth factors in human obesity. Metabolism 1995;10(Suppl 4):37–44.
50. Saitoh H, Kamoda T, Nakahara S, Hirano T, Nakamura N. Serum concentrations of insulin, insulin-like growth factor(IGF)-I, IGF binding protein (IGFBP)-1 and -3 and growth hormone binding protein in obese children: fasting IGFBP-1 is suppressed in normoinsulinaemic obese children. Clin Endocrinol 1998;48:487–492.
51. Attia N, Tamborlane WV, Heptulla R, Maggs D, Grozman A, Sherwin RS, et al. The metabolic syndrome and insulin-like growth factor I regulation in adolescent obesity. J Clin Endocrinol Metab 1998;83:1467–1471.
52. Hall K, Lundin G, Povoa G. Serum levels of the low molecular weight form of insulin-like growth factor binding protein in healthy subjects and in patients with growth hormone deficiency, acromegaly and anorexia nervosa. Acta Endocrinol 1988;118:321–326.
53. Degerblad M, Povoa G, Thorén M, Wivall I-L, Hall K. Lack of diurnal rhythm of low molecular weight insulin-like growth factor binding protein in patients with Cushing's disease. Acta Endocrinol (Copenh) 1989;120:195–200.
54. Bang P, Degerblad M, Thoren M, Schwander J, Blum W, Hall K. Insulin-like growth factor (IGF) I and -II and IGF binding protein (IGFBP) 1, 2 and 3 in serum from patients with Cushings syndrome. Acta Endocrinol 1993;128:397–404.
55. Brismar K, Grill V, Efendic S, Hall K. The insulin-like growth factor binding protein-1 in low and high insulin responders before and during dexamethasone treatment. Metabolism 1991;40:728–732.
56. Miell JP, Taylor AM, Jones J, Holly JMP, Gaillard RC, Pralong FP, et al. The effects of dexamethasone treatment on immunoreactive and bioactive insulin-like growth factors (IGFs) and IGF-binding proteins in normal male volunteers. J Endocrinol 1993;136:525–533.
57. Mynarcik DC, McNurlan MA, Steigbigel RT, Fuhrer J, Gelato MC. Association of severe insulin resistance with both loss of limb fat and elevated serum tumor necrosis factor receptor levels in HIV lipodystrophy. J Acquir Immune Defic Syndr 2000;25:312–321.
58. Ukkola O, Sun G, Bouchard C. Insulin-like growth factor 2 (IGF2) and IGF-binding protein 1 (IGFBP1) gene variants are associated with overfeeding-induced metabolic changes. Diabetologia 2001;44:2231–2236.
59. McCallum RW, Petrie JR, Dominiczak AF, Connell MC. Growth hormone deficiency and vascular risk. Clin Endocrinol 2002;57:11–24.
60. Pekonen F, Laatikainen T, Buyalos R, Rutanen E-M. Decreased 34K insulin-like growth factor binding protein in polycystic ovarian disease. Fertil Steril 1989;51:972–975.
61. Homburg R, Pariente C, Lunenfeld B, Jacobs HS. The role of insulin-like growth factor-1 (IGF-1) and IGF binding protein-1 (IGFBP-1) in the pathogenesis of polycystic ovary syndrome. Hum Reprod 1992;7:1379–1383.

62. Association AD. Clinical practice recommendations. Report of the expert committee on the diagnosis and classification of diabetes mellitus. Diabetes Care 2002;25(Suppl 1):S5–S20.
63. Bereket A, Lang CH, Blethen SL, Gelato MC, Fan J, Frost RA, Wilson TA. Effect of insulin on the insulin-like growth factor system in children with new-onset insulin-dependent diabetes mellitus. J Clin Endocrinol Metab 1995;80:1312–1317.
64. Suikkari A-M, Koivisto VA, Rutanen E-M, Yki-Järvinen H, Karonen S-L, Seppälä M. Insulin regulates the serum levels of low molecular weight insulin-like growth factor-binding protein. J Clin Endocrinol Metab 1988;66:266–272.
65. Holly JMP, Biddlecombe RA, Dunger DB, Edge JA, Amiel SA, Howell R, et al. Circadian variation of GH-independent IGF-binding protein in diabetes mellitus. A new role for insulin? Clin Endocrinol 1988;29:667–675.
66. Brismar K, Gutniak M, Povoa G, Werner S, Hall K. Insulin regulates the 35 kDa IGF binding protein in patients with diabetes mellitus. J Endocrinol Invest 1988;11:599–602.
67. Shishko PI, Dreval AV, Abugova IA, Zajarny IU, Goncharov VC. Insulin-like growth factors and binding proteins in patients with recent-onset type 1 (insulin-dependent) diabetes mellitus—influence of diabetes control and intraportal insulin infusion. Diab Res Clin Pract 1994;25:1–12.
68. Frost RA, Bereket A, Wilson TA, Wojnar MM, Lang CH, Gelato MC. Phosphorylation of insulin-like growth factor binding protein-1 in patients with insulin-dependent diabetes mellitus and severe trauma. J Clin Endocrinol Metab 1994;78:1533–1535.
69. Akinci A, Copeland KC, Garmong A, Clemmons DR. Insulin-like growth factor binding proteins (IGFBPs) in serum and urine and IGFBP-2 protease activity in patients with insulin-dependent diabetes mellitus. Metabolism 2000;49:626–633.
70. Bach LA, Rechler MM. Insulin-like growth factors and diabetes. Diabetes Metab Rev 1992;8:229–257.
71. Bereket A, Lang CH, Blethen SL, Ng LC, Wilson TA. Insulin-treatment normalizes reduced free insulin-like growth-factor-I concentrations in diabetic children. Clin Endocrinol 1996;45:321–326.
72. Suikkari A-M, Rutanen E-M, Seppälä M. Circulating levels of immunoreactive insulin-like growth factor-binding protein in non-pregnant women. Hum Reprod 1987;2:297–300.
73. Hall K, Johansson BL, Povoa G, Thalme B. Serum levels of insulin-like growth factors (IGF) I, II and IGF binding protein in diabetic adolescents treated with continuous subcutaneous insulin infusion. J Intern Med 1989;225:273–278.
74. Hopkins KD, Russelljones DL, Lehmann ED, Wheeler MJ, Sonksen PH. Intraperitoneal insulin affects insulin-like growth factor binding protein-1 in a well-controlled type-1 diabetic patient. Diabetes Care 1993;16:1404–1405.
75. Cotterill AM, Daly F, Holly JMP, Hughes SC, Camacho-Hübner C, Abdulla AF, et al. The 'dawn phenomenon' in adolescents with insulin dependent diabetes mellitus: possible contribution of insulin-like growth factor binding protein-1. Clin Endocrinol 1995;43:567–574.
76. Batch JA, Baxter RC, Werther G. Abnormal regulation of insulin-like growth factor binding proteins in adolescents with insulin-dependent diabetes. J Clin Endocrinol Metab 1991;73:964–968.
77. Halldin MU, Tylleskar K, Hagenas L, Tuvemo T, Gustafsson J. Is growth hormone hypersecretion in diabetic adolescent girls also a daytime problem? Clin Endocrinol 1998;48:785–794.
78. Halldin MU, Hagenäs L, Tuvemo T, Gustafsson J. Profound changes in the GH-IGF-I system in adolescent girls with IDDM: can IGFBP1 be used to reflect overall glucose regulation. Pediatr Diabetes 2000;1:121–130.
79. Taylor AM, Dunger DB, Preece MA, Holly JMP, Smith CP, Wass JAH, et al. The growth hormone independent insulin-like growth factor-I binding protein BP-28 is associated with serum insulin-like growth factor-I inhibitory bioactivity in adolescent insulin-dependent diabetics. Clin Endocrinol 1990;32:229–239.
80. Kaino Y, Hirai H, Ito T, Kida K. Insulin-like growth-factor-I (IGF-I) delays the onset of diabetes in nonobese diabetic (NOD) mice. Diabetes Res Clin Pract 1996;34:7–11.
81. Clauson PG, Brismar K, Hall K, Linnarsson R, Grill V. Insulin-like growth factor-I and insulin-like growth factor binding protein-1 in a representative population of type 2 diabetic patients in Sweden. Scand J Clin Lab Invest 1998;58:353–360.
82. Gibson JM, Westwood M, Crosby SR, Gordon C, Holly JMP, Fraser W, et al. Choice of treatment affects plasma levels of insulin-like growth factor-binding protein-1 in noninsulin-dependent diabetes mellitus. J Clin Endocrinol Metab 1995;80:1369–1375.

83. Bang P, Brismar K, Rosenfeld RG. Increased proteolysis of insulin-like growth factor-binding protein-3 (IGFBP-3) in noninsulin-dependent diabetes mellitus serum, with elevation of a 29-kilodalton (kDa) glycosylated IGFBP-3 fragment contained in the approximately 130- to 150-kDa ternary complex. J Clin Endocrinol Metab 1994;78:1119–1127.
84. Woods KA, van Helvoirt M, Ong KK, Mohn A, Levy J, de Zegher F, Dunger DB. The somatotropic axis in short children born small for gestational age: relation to insulin resistance. Pediatr Res 2002;51:76–80.
85. Janssen JA, Hoogerbrugge N, van Neck JW, Uitterlinden P, Lamberts SW. The IGF-I/IGFBP system in congenital partial lipodystrophy. Clin Endocrinol 1998;49:465–73.
86. Chiarelli F, Santilli F, Mohn A. Role of growth factors in the development of diabetic complications. Horm Res 2000;53:53–67.
87. Flyvbjerg A. Putative pathophysiological role of growth factors and cytokines in experimental diabetic kidney disease. Diabetologia 2000;43:1205–1223.
88. Pugliese G, Pricci F, Locuratolo N, Romeo G, Romano G, Giannini S, et al. Increased activity of the insulin-like growth factor system in mesangial cells cultured in high glucose conditions. Relation to glucose-enhanced extracellular matrix production. Diabetologia 1996;39:775–784.
89. Tack I, Elliot SJ, Potier M, Rivera A, Striker GE, Striker LJ. Autocrine activation of the IGF-I signaling pathway in mesangial cells isolated from diabetic NOD mice. Diabetes 2002;51:182–188.
90. Merimee TJ, Zapf J, Froesch ER. Insulin-like growth factors. Studies in diabetics with and without retinopathy. N Engl J Med 1983;309:527–530.
91. Janssen JAMJL, Lamberts SWJ. Circulating IGF-I and its protective role in the pathogenesis of diabetic angiopathy. Clin Endocrinol 2000;52:1–9.
92. Hopkins KD, Brart DO, Russelljones DL, Chignell AH, Sonksen PH. Insulin-like growth factor binding protein-1 levels in diabetic proliferative retinopathy. Horm Metab Res 1993;25:331–332.
93. Burgos R, Mateo C, Canton A, Hernandez C, Mesa J, Simo R. Vitreous levels of IGF-I, IGF binding protein 1, and IGF binding protein 3 in proliferative diabetic retinopathy: a case-control study. Diabetes Care 2000;23:80–83.
94. Crosby SR, Tsigos C, Anderton CD, Gordon C, Young RJ, White A. Elevated plasma insulin-like growth factor binding protein-1 levels in type-1 (insulin-dependent) diabetic patients with peripheral neuropathy. Diabetologia 1992;35:868–872.
95. Hilding A, Brismar K, Degerblad M, Thorén M, Hall K. Altered relation between circulating levels of insulin-like growth factor-binding protein-1 and insulin in growth hormone-deficient patients and insulin-dependent diabetic patients compared to that in healthy subjects. J Clin Endocrinol Metab 1995;80:2646–2652.
96. Brismar K, Hilding A, Lindgren B. Regulation of IGFBP-1 in humans. Prog Growth Factor Res 1995;6:449–456.
97. Cotterill AM, Mendel P, Holly JMP, Timmins AG, Camachohubner C, Hughes SC, et al. The differential regulation of the circulating levels of the insulin-like growth factors and their binding proteins (IGFBP)1, 2 and 3 after elective abdominal surgery. Clin Endocrinol 1996;44:91–101.
98. Mesotten D, Delhanty PJ, Vanderhoydonc F, Hardman KV, Weekers F, Baxter RC, et al. Regulation of insulin-like growth factor binding protein-1 during protracted critical illness. J Clin Endocrinol Metab 2002;87:5516–5523.
99. Tazuke SI, Mazure NM, Sugawara J, Carland G, Faessen GH, Suen LF, et al. Hypoxia stimulates insulin-like growth factor binding protein 1 (IGFBP-1) gene expression in HepG2 cells: a possible model for IGFBP-1 expression in fetal hypoxia. Proc Natl Acad Sci USA 1998;95:10188–10193.
100. Luo J, Reid RE, Murphy LJ. Dexamethasone increases hepatic insulin-like growth factor binding protein-1 (IGFBP-1) mRNA and serum IGFBP-1 concentrations in the rat. Endocrinology 1990;127:1456–1462.
101. Barzilai N, She L, Liu BQ, Vuguin P, Cohen P, Wang J-, et al. Surgical removal of visceral fat reverses hepatic insulin resistance. Diabetes 1999;48:94–98.
102. Heald AH, Cruickshank JK, Riste LK, Cade JE, Anderson S, Greenhalgh A, et al. Close relation of fasting insulin-like growth factor binding protein-1 (IGFBP-1) with glucose tolerance and cardiovascular risk in two populations. Diabetologia 2001;44:333–339.
103. Janssen JAMJL, Stolk RP, Pols H, Grobbee DE, Lamberts SWJ. Serum total IGF-I, free IGF-I, and IGFBP-1 levels in an elderly population—relation to cardiovascular risk factors and disease. Arter Thromb Vasc Biol 1998;18:277–282.

104. Harrela M, Koistinen R, Tuomilehto J, Nissinen A, Seppälä M. Low serum insulin-like growth factor-binding protein-1 is associated with an unfavourable cardiovascular risk profile in elderly men. Ann Med 2000;32:424–428.
105. Gibson JM, Westwood M, Young RJ, White A. Reduced insulin-like growth factor binding protein-1 (IGFBP-1) levels correlate with increased cardiovascular risk in noninsulin dependent diabetes mellitus (NIDDM). J Clin Endocrinol Metab 1996;81:860–863
106. Heald AH, Siddals KW, Fraser W, Taylor W, Kaushal K, Morris J, et al. Low circulating levels of insulin-like growth factor binding protein-1 (IGFBP-1) are closely associated with the presence of macrovascular disease and hypertension in type 2 diabetes. Diabetes 2002;51:2629–2636.
107. Sandhu MS, Heald AH, Gibson JM, Cruickshank JK, Dunger DB, Wareham NJ. Circulating concentrations of insulin-like growth factor-I and development of glucose intolerance: a prospective observational study. Lancet 2002;359:1740–1745.
108. Paolisso G, Tagliamonte MR, Rizzo MR, Carella C, Gambardella A, Barbieri M, et al. Low plasma insulin-like growth factor-1 concentrations predict worsening of insulin-mediated glucose uptake in older people. J Am Ger Soc 1999;47:1312–1318.
109. Yki-Järvinen H, Makimattila S, Utriainen T, Rutanen EM. Portal insulin concentrations rather than insulin sensitivity regulate serum sex hormone-binding globulin and insulin-like growth factor binding protein 1 in vivo. J Clin Endocrinol Metab 1995;80:3227–3232.
110. Usala A-L, Madigan T, Burgurera B, Sinha MK, Caro JF, Cunningham P, et al. Treatment of insulin-resistant diabetic ketoacidosis with insulin-like growth factor I in an adolescent with insulin-dependent diabetes. N Engl J Med 1992;327:853–857.
111. Cheetham TD, Jones J, Taylor AM, Holly J, Matthews DR, Dunger DB. The effects of recombinant insulin-like growth factor-I administration on growth hormone levels and insulin requirements in adolescents with type-1 (insulin-dependent) diabetes-mellitus. Diabetologia 1993;36:678–681.
112. Acerini CL, Patton CM, Savage MO, Kernell A, Westphal O, Dunger DB. Randomised placebo-controlled trial of human recombinant insulin-like growth factor I plus intensive insulin therapy in adolescents with insulin-dependent diabetes mellitus. Lancet 1997;350:1199–1204.
113. Acerini CL, Harris DA, Matyka KA, Watts AP, Umpleby AM, Russell-Jones DL, et al. Effects of low-dose recombinant human insulin-like growth factor-I on insulin sensitivity, growth hormone and glucagon levels in young adults with insulin-dependent diabetes mellitus. Metab Clin Exp 1998;47:1481–1489.
114. Carroll PV, Christ ER, Umpleby AM, Gowrie I, Jackson N, Bowes SB, et al. IGF-I treatment in adults with type 1 diabetes: Effects on glucose and protein metabolism in the fasting state and during a hyperinsulinemic-euglycemic amino acid clamp. Diabetes 2000;49:789–796.
115. Pratipanawatr T, Pratipanawatr W, Rosen C, Berria R, Bajaj M, Cusi K, et al. Effect of IGF-I on FFA and glucose metabolism in control and type 2 diabetic subjects. Am J Physiol Endocrinol Metab 2002;282:E1360–E1368.
116. Zenobi PD, Jaeggigroisman SE, Riesen WF, Roder ME, Rudolffroesch E. Insulin-like growth factor-I improves glucose and lipid metabolism in type-2 diabetes mellitus. J Clin Invest 1992;90:2234–2241.
117. Cusi K, DeFronzo R. Recombinant human insulin-like growth factor I treatment for 1 week improves metabolic control in type 2 diabetes by ameliorating hepatic and muscle insulin resistance. J Clin Endocrinol Metab 2000;85:3077–3084.
118. Young SCJ, Clemmons DR. Changes in insulin-like growth factor (IGF)-binding proteins after IGF-I injections in noninsulin-dependent diabetics. J Clin Endocrinol Metab 1994;78:609–614.
119. Vickers MH, Ikenasio BA, Breier BH. IGF-I treatment reduces hyperphagia, obesity, and hypertension in metabolic disorders induced by fetal programming. Endocrinology 2001;142:3964–3973.
120. Schoenle EJ, Zenobi PD, Torresani T, Werder EA, Zachmann M, Froesch ER. Recombinant human insulin-like growth factor I (rhIGF -I) reduces hyperglycaemia in patients with extreme insulin resistance. Diabetologia 1991;34:675–679.
121. Kuzuya H, Matsuura N, Sakamoto M, Makino H, Sakamoto Y, Kadowaki T, et al. Trial of insulinlike growth factor-I therapy for patients with extreme insulin resistance syndromes. Diabetes 1993;42:696–705.
122. Morrow LA, O'Brien MB, Moller DE, Flier JS, Moses AC. Recombinant human insulin-like growth factor-I therapy improves glycemic control and insulin action in the type A syndrome of severe insulin resistance. J Clin Endocrinol Metab 1994;79:205–210.

123. Nakae J, Kato M, Murashita M, Shinohara N, Tajima T, Fujieda K. Long-term effect of recombinant human insulin-like growth factor I on metabolic and growth control in a patient with Leprechaunism. J Clin Endocrinol Metab 1998;83:542–549.
124. Backeljauw PF, Alves C, Eidson M, Cleveland W, Underwood LE, Davenport ML. Effect of intravenous insulin-like growth factor I in two patients with leprechaunism. Pediatr Res 1994;36:749–754.
125. Longo N, Singh R, Griffin LD, Langley SD, Parks JS, Elsas LJ. Impaired growth in Rabson-Mendenhall syndrome: lack of effect of growth hormone and insulin-like growth factor-I. J Clin Endocrinol Metab 1994;79:799–805.
126. Jabri N, Schalch DS, Schwartz SL, Fischer JS, Kipnes MS, Radnik BJ, et al. Adverse effects of recombinant human insulin-like growth factor I in obese insulin-resistant type II diabetic patients. Diabetes 1994;43:369–374.
127. Clemmons DR, Moses AC, McKay MJ, Sommer A, Rosen DM, Ruckle J. The combination of insulin-like growth factor I and insulin-like growth factor-binding protein-3 reduces insulin requirements in insulin- dependent type 1 diabetes: evidence for in vivo biological activity. J Clin Endocrinol Metab 2000;85:1518–1524.
128. Bianchini F, Kaaks R, Vainio H. Overweight, obesity and cancer risk. Lancet Oncol 2002;3:565–574.
129. Leu JI, Crissey MA, Taub R. Massive hepatic apoptosis associated with TGF-beta1 activation after Fas ligand treatment of IGF binding protein-1-deficient mice. J Clin Invest 2003;111:129–139.
130. Lewitt MS, Brismar K, Ohlson J, Hartman J. Lithium chloride inhibits the expression and secretion of insulin-like growth factor-binding protein-1. J Endocrinol 2001;171:R11–R15.

15 Insulin-Like Growth Factors in Relation to Gastrointestinal Diseases and Parenteral Nutrition

Denise M. Ney

KEY POINTS

- IGF-I is an intestinal mitogen that stimulates bowel growth via systemic or endocrine actions as well as autocrine/paracrine actions of locally expressed IGFs in bowel.
- Studies in transgenic mice suggest that GH promotes differentiated function of the enterocytes whereas IGF-I exerts primarily mitogenic and anti-apoptotic actions in the small intestine.
- The intestinal mucosa is resistant to the mitogenic effects of GH-stimulated endogenous IGF-I during parenteral nutrition at the postreceptor level.
- Greater knowledge is needed regarding how local expression of IGFBP-3 and -5 modulate IGF-I action in order to fully understand the role of IGF-I in intestinal adaptation and its potential to treat intestinal failure due to short bowel syndrome.
- A complete understanding of IGF-I action in the GI tract will require characterization of the mechanisms of IGF interactions with other hormones and cytokines during normal physiology and disease.

1. INTRODUCTION

The gastrointestinal (GI) tract is a major target organ for the insulin-like growth factor (IGF)-I system. However, a thorough understanding of the role of the IGF system in proliferation, apoptosis, differentiation, and development of the GI tract is just beginning to emerge. Growth hormone (GH) and IGF-I act on the GI tract in an endocrine manner *(1,2)*. In addition, IGFs expressed locally in the bowel have autocrine or paracrine effects on specific cell types within the bowel *(3)*. IGF-I is thought to mediate many of the actions of GH although unique effects of each growth factor have been noted in the GI tract *(1,4)*. Evidence that systemically administered IGF-I stimulates hyperplasia of the small intestinal epithelium suggests that the IGF-I system may have therapeutic benefits in patients with GI disease. This chapter discusses current understanding of the role of the IGF-I system in normal physiology of the GI tract and in conditions of intestinal adaptation including parenteral nutrition, intestinal resection, and inflammatory bowel disease.

From: *IGF and Nutrition in Health and Disease*
Edited by: M. S. Houston, J. M. P. Holly, and E. L. Feldman © Humana Press Inc., Totowa, NJ

2. BACKGROUND

This section provides a brief review of the structure of the intestinal wall, turnover of the epithelial cell layer that composes the mucosal lining of the intestine, and the process of intestinal adaptation.

2.1. Structure of the Intestinal Wall

The structure of the intestinal wall consists of an epithelial cell layer that faces the lumen of the bowel, the underlying lamina propria, a thin layer of smooth muscle called the submucosa or muscularis mucosa composed of fibroblasts and collagen, and enteric smooth muscle called the muscularis externa (Figs. 1 and 2) *(1)*. Epithelial cells are separated by a basement membrane from a layer of mesenchymal cells (fibroblasts/myofibroblasts) in the lamina propria where local IGF-I synthesis occurs, as discussed in the next section (Figs. 1 and 2). The lamina propria also contains capillaries, immune cells, and smooth muscle cells. Interactions between epithelial cells and adjacent mesenchymal cells are integral to normal development, differentiation, and morphogenesis of the intestinal epithelial lining *(1,5)*.

The mucosal lining of the intestine or intestinal mucosa plays an essential role in digestion and absorption of nutrients by producing electrolytes, digestive enzymes, and transport proteins. Coordinated contraction of enteric smooth muscle provides mixing of ingested foods to facilitate digestion and absorption. Moreover, the GI tract is the largest immune organ in the body. The intestinal mucosa provides a barrier to prevent entry of ingested microorganisms and toxins into the body and the lamina propria contains a variety of immune cells that are central to gut mucosal immune function.

The small intestinal epithelium is organized into a crypt-villus axis (Figs. 1 and 3), and the colon is organized into crypts and surface epithelium (Figs. 2 and 3). In the small intestine, cells migrate from the crypts onto the villi, and five to seven- crypts feed onto one villus *(6)*. The crypts in both the small intestine and colon contain a compartment of continuously proliferating cells. As cells exit the crypts, they undergo terminal differentiation into one of three types of epithelial cells *(1,5)*: (1) columnar epithelial cells that express proteins involved in electrolyte secretion, nutrient digestion, and nutrient absorption; (2) goblet cells that secrete mucus; or (3) enteroendocrine cells that secrete a wide range of bioactive hormones and peptides that control gut function and metabolism. There are distinct populations and proportions of particular epithelial cell types along the length of the small intestine and colon. In the small intestine, columnar epithelial cells and goblet cells migrate up the villus until they are sloughed off at the villus tips. In the colon, migrating surface colonic enterocytes are sloughed off into the lumen. The mechanisms underlying loss of enterocytes in the small intestine and colon include programmed senescence that involves loss of cell adhesion factors and possibly programmed cell death or apoptosis *(7)*.

2.2. Turnover of the Mucosal Epithelial Layer

The epithelial lining of the small intestine and colon undergoes constant renewal and has one of the fastest rates of cell turnover among tissues in the body. The intestinal epithelial layer is completely replaced within 2 to 3 d in mice and rats and within 3 to 6 d in humans *(8)*. Maintenance of a steady-state functional mass of intestinal epithelium requires a balance between the rates of cell proliferation and cell loss (Fig. 3). Cell differ-

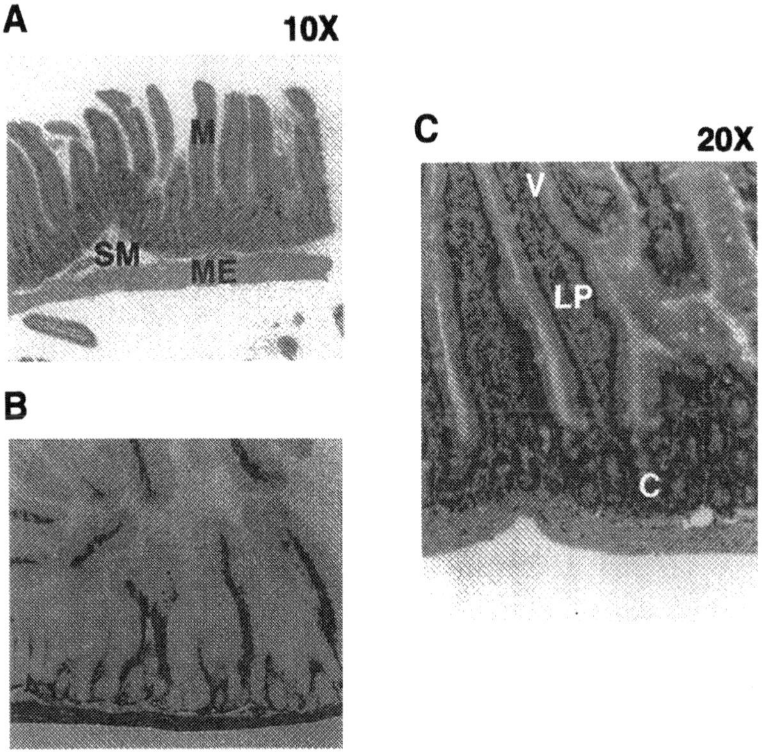

Fig. 1. Photomicrographs illustrating the microanatomy of the small intestine. **(A)** Low-power photomicrograph of a section through the wall of the small intestine. M, mucosa; SM, submucosa; ME, muscularis externa. **(B)** Localization of mesenchymal cells that show positive immunostaining for α smooth muscle actin illustrates positively stained pericryptal myofibroblasts, a core of positive-stained cells within the villi, a thin layer of positively stained smooth muscle cells separating the mucosa and submucosa (musclaris mucosa), and the intensely stained muscularis externa. **(C)** High-power photomicrograph to illustrate crypts (C), villi (V), and lamina propria (LP). Reprinted with permission from ref. *1*.

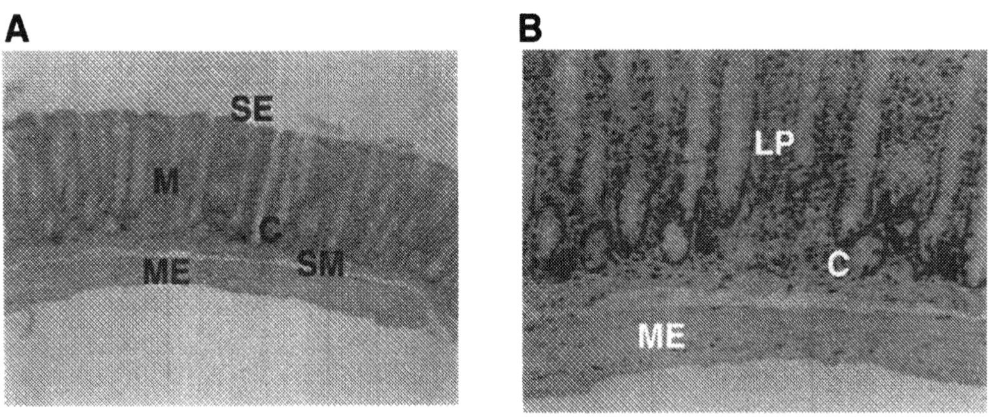

Fig. 2. Low- **(A)** and high- **(B)** power photomicrographs illustrating the microanatomy of the colon. SE, surface epithelial cells; L, lamina propria; SM, submucosa; ME, muscularis externa. Reprinted with permission from ref. *1*.

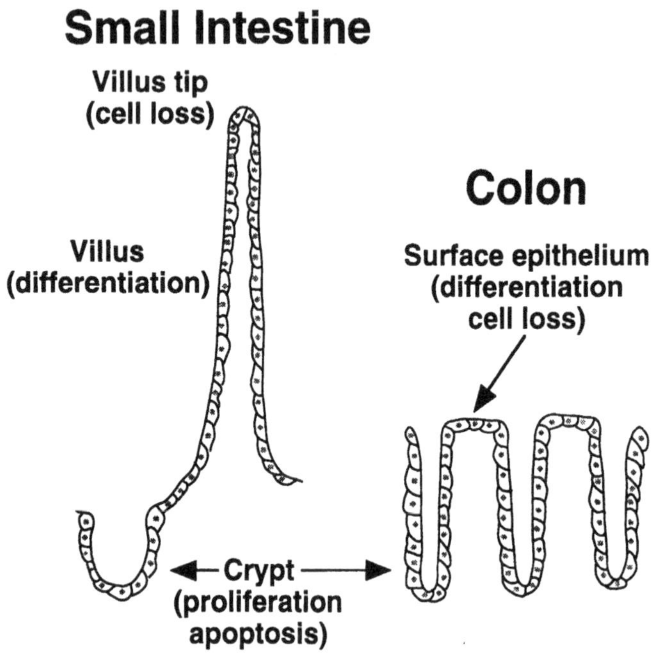

Fig. 3. Schematic of the small intestine and colon showing the location of proliferating crypt cells, differentiated cells, and cells that undergo spontaneous apoptosis in the crypts.

entiation is also tightly regulated to maintain the normal array of different epithelial cell types within a specific intestinal segment. Cells in the crypt undergo spontaneous apoptosis in response to excessive cell proliferation or exposure to the toxic environment of the intestinal lumen *(7)*. This provides a mechanism to dispose of genetically damaged crypt progenitor cells that may protect the GI tract from cancer *(7)*. IGF-I decreases apoptosis in the crypt stem cell zone, thus mediating a net increase in epithelial cell mass; however, excess IGF-I may also increase the risk of tumorigenesis in the GI tract *(9,10)*.

2.3. Intestinal Adaptation

Intestinal adaptation is defined as the process by which the small intestine, and to a lesser degree the large intestine, adjust structural mass and functional capabilities to meet physiologic needs *(8,11)*. This process has been studied extensively in rodent models using experimental designs that use fasting-refeeding, parenteral nutrition, and intestinal resection as discussed in subsequent sections of this chapter. Limited data suggest that small intestinal adaptation occurs in humans *(11,12)*. Despite extensive research, the regulation of intestinal adaptation by factors, including luminal nutrients *(13)*, hormones such as IGF, pancreaticobiliary secretions, and the enteric nervous system, remains poorly defined *(11)*. Defining the mechanisms that regulate intestinal adaptation may lead to improved treatments for a variety of diseases of the GI tract *(1)*.

3. IGF-I AND NORMAL INTESTINAL PHYSIOLOGY

IGF-I and/or IGF-II are expressed throughout human and rodent small intestine *(14,15)*. In rats, IGF-II predominates in intestine during embryonic development whereas IGF-I predominates postnatally *(14)*. Limited evidence in humans suggests that, unlike the rat, significant levels of IGF-II mRNA are present in adult human intestine *(1)*. The IGF system stimulates intestinal growth by endocrine actions through binding to specific GH and IGF-I receptors in the small and large intestine *(2,16)* as well as through local IGF-I synthesis and autocrine/paracrine actions. The major sites of local IGF-I or IGF-II synthesis in normal small intestine in vivo are mesenchymal cells (fibroblasts, myofibroblasts, or smooth muscle cells) scattered within the pericryptal regions and the lamina propria *(1,17–19)*. Increased local IGF-I expression during adaptive growth of intestinal epithelium in adult rat and a recent report in transgenic mice *(3)* indicate that IGF-I is an important mesenchymal cell-derived growth factor that exerts paracrine/autocrine actions in the GI tract *(1,3)*.

3.1. IGF-I Is an Intestinal Mitogen That Improves Transport Function

A number of lines of evidence demonstrate that IGF-I is an intestinal mitogen. IGF-I stimulates proliferation of cultured intestinal epithelial cells, fibroblasts, myofibroblasts, and smooth muscle cells *(3,20,21)*. Subcutaneous administration of IGF-I increases intestinal weight, length, villus height, and crypt cell proliferation in orally fed, normal adult rats *(22)* and in suckling rats *(23)* in a dose-dependent manner. Increased crypt cell proliferation is observed within 3 d of IGF-I treatment *(24)*. In animal models of intestinal adaptation, including parenteral nutrition *(4,10)*, intestinal resection *(25–28)*, and dexamethasone-induced stress *(29)* administration of IGF-I induces selective increases in small intestinal mass, villus height, and crypt depth that is correlated with increased enterocyte proliferation. Oral administration of IGF-I does not consistently induce mucosal growth perhaps due to degradation of IGF-I by gastric acid and digestive enzymes *(30–33)*.

IGF-I administration also improves intestinal transport function. Subcutaneous administration of IGF-I increases galactose transport in the intestine of cirrhotic rats compared with controls *(34)*. Intravenous administration of IGF-I normalizes aberrations in intestinal ion transport induced by parenteral nutrition in conjunction with attenuation of TPN-induced mucosal hypoplasia *(35)*. Oral administration of IGF-I increases sodium absorption, sodium-dependent nutrient absorption, and disaccharidase activity per unit mass in neonatal piglets who do not show mucosal growth in response to oral administration of IGF-I *(30)*. Improved intestinal disaccharidase activity and lactase processing were noted in piglets consuming formula containing IGF-I *(36,37)*.

3.2. IGF Binding Proteins Modulate IGF-I Action in the GI Tract

The IGF binding proteins (IGFBPs) modulate IGF-I action in the GI tract based on both systemic and local interactions with IGF-I. Subcutaneous administration of IGF analogs with reduced affinity for IGFBPs have more potent enterotropic effects than native IGF-I *(23,24)*. Continuous intravenous administration of an IGF-I analog prebound to IGFBP-3 shows reduced clearance and greater serum total IGF-I concentrations but has reduced enterotropic potency compared with continuous infusion of free IGF-I *(38)*. These observations support the notion that circulating complexes of IGF-I, IGFBP-3, and the acid labile subunit prolong the half life of IGF-I and decrease its bioavailability to IGF-I receptors in the gut *(38,39)*. These studies with systemic infusion of IGF-I analogs suggest that the serum concentration of free IGF-I determines the enterotropic potency of IGF-I *(23,38)*.

The major IGFBPs found in the intestine of normal adult rats and mice, and in humans include IGFBP-3, IGFBP-4 and IGFBP-5 *(1)*. Evidence suggests that IGFBP-3 and IGFBP-5 act in a paracrine manner to modulate IGF-I bioavailability and anabolic action on neighboring intestinal epithelial cells *(1,17,18)*. Evidence for paracrine effects of IGFBP-4 on IGF-I is limited *(27,40)*. IGFBP-3 mRNA is expressed primarily in the lamina propria of the normal intestine of the rat *(17,18)* and mouse *(41)* based on *in situ* hybridization. In vitro, IGFBP-3 can inhibit or potentiate IGF-I action, depending on the cell system *(39,42)*. Expression of IGFBP-3 is reduced in the lamina propria of small intestine during adaptive hyperplasia of the mucosa in association with proximal small bowel resection *(43)*, fasting followed by refeeding *(18)* and myenteric denervation *(1)*.

IGFBP-5 mRNA is expressed primarily in the muscularis propria of normal rat *(17)* and human small intestine *(44)*. IGFBP-5 appears to potentiate the anabolic effects of IGF-I in cultured smooth muscle cells derived from the intestine *(45)*. Systemic administration of IGF-I increases the expression of both IGFBP-3 and IGFBP-5 in rat small intestine *(17)* and colon *(46)*. Induction of IGFBP-5 mRNA in the pericryptal regions of the lamina propria by systemic administration of IGF-I is linked with the enterotropic effects of IGF-I on the small intestinal epithelium in humans *(44)* and in the rat *(17,46,47)*.

3.3. Insights From Transgenic Mice

Transgenic mice with overexpression of GH and IGF-I genes have helped to elucidate the role of the IGF-I system in proliferation, apoptosis, differentiation, and development of the normal intestine. Publications describing the enterotropic effects of three IGF system transgenic mouse models are available from the laboratory of Dr. P. Kay Lund: (1) metallothionein-1 promoter driven expression of the bovine GH transgene (MT-bGH) *(48)*, which shows elevated levels of GH and IGF-I; (2) metallothionein-1 promoter driven expression of human IGF-I cDNA (MT-hIGF-I) *(41)*, which shows elevated levels of serum IGF-I but undetectable levels of serum GH; and (3) overexpression of IGF-I in mesenchymal cells via an α smooth muscle actin promoter (SMP8-IGF-I) *(3)* that shows normal levels of serum IGF-I but elevated IGF-I transgene expression in smooth muscle in the small intestine and other tissues *(49)*. A discussion of information gained regarding IGF-I system action in the GI tract using these three models follows.

A comparison of the MT-bGH and MT-hIGF-I transgenic mouse models provides insights regarding the interrelated and unique enterotropic actions of GH and IGF-I *(1)*. Both models show similar elevated circulating levels of IGF-I; however, the MT-hIGF-I mice show a much higher level of local IGF-I expression in the small intestine compared with the MT-bGH mice. Overall, a comparison of the MT-bGH and MT-hIGF-I trangenics indicates that the intestine is particularly responsive to excess IGF-I and that IGF-I can mediate most but not all of the enterotropic effects of GH, even in the absence of detectable GH in the circulation. For example, both models showed significant increases in mass and length of the bowel although the MT-hIGF-I transgenics showed a 44% increase in small bowel length compared with a 20% increase in MT-bGH transgenics. This selective lengthening of the intestine in MT-hIGF-I transgenics is especially dramatic when expressed relative to body weight because the MT-bGH transgenics showed a twofold greater increase in body weight than the MT-hIGF-I transgenics *(1)*.

Relative enterotropic effects observed in the MT-bGH and MT-hIGF-I transgenics suggest that GH may promote differentiated function of the enterocytes whereas IGF-I may exert primarily mitogenic and anti-apoptotic actions in the small intestine *(1)*. MT-bGH transgenics show increased activity of sucrase, a marker of villus cell differentiation, and MT-hIGF-I transgenics do not *(41,48)*. Moreover, MT-bGH transgenics do not show sustained increases in crypt cell proliferation or alterations in crypt cell apoptosis whereas and MT-hIGF-I transgenics show sustained increases in crypt cell proliferation *(41)*.

Information about the effects of GH and IGF-I on apoptosis in the intestine is important to understanding the potential risk of cancer associated with therapeutic use of these growth factors. There is limited information about GH effects on apoptosis whereas in vitro studies *(50)* and recent in vivo reports *(9,10)* indicate that IGF-I has antiapoptotic actions in the intestine. MT-hIGF-I transgenics show reduction of spontaneous and irradiation-induced apoptosis and reduced effects of irradiation to arrest enterocyte proliferation in the small intestine crypt stem cell compartment *(9)*. IGF-I preferentially promotes survival of crypt stem cells *(9,10)*, in part, by decreasing the accumulation of Bax protein expression *(9)*.

The SMP8-IGF-I transgenic mouse model provides insights regarding the endocrine and local actions of IGF-I in the intestine. This model has been used to test the hypothesis that IGF-I overexpressed in intestinal mesenchymal cells in vivo, in the absence of altered circulating IGF-I, exerts paracrine actions on growth or function of the mucosal epithelium *(3)*. SMP8-IGF-I transgenics showed mucosal growth in ileum, but not jejunum or colon, and muscularis growth throughout the small intestine and colon providing definitive evidence for autocrine and paracrine actions of mesenchymal cell-derived IGF-I on intestinal smooth muscle and epithelium *(3)*. Upregulation of IGFBP-5 mRNA in ileal lamina propria is associated with preferential paracrine effects of IGF-I in mesenchymal cells to stimulate ileal mucosal growth and sucrase activity. This study suggests that upregulation of locally expressed IGF-I has distinct actions on expression of IGFBP-3 and -5 in bowel compared with systemic administration of IGF-I, possibly because of differences in blood supply to the intestinal mucosa *(3)*.

The transgenic mouse models provide useful insights regarding the consequences of a single genetic perturbation of the IGF-I system on intestinal growth. However, these models have limitations in interpretation to normal in vivo conditions because sites of transcript expression may differ compared to normal physiology. For example, the MT-hIGF-I transgenics show increased expression of the IGF-transgene within the mucosal epithelial cells whereas endogenous IGF-I is expressed in intestinal mesenchymal cells. Systemic administration of IGF-I and GH, as discussed in the next section on parenteral nutrition provide a useful complement to data from the transgenic models to understand IGF-I action in the GI tract.

4. PARENTERAL NUTRITION

Enteral nutrition or the presence of exogenous luminal nutrients in the GI tract provides growth-promoting signals that regulate functional mass of the intestine and continuous renewal of the mucosal epithelium *(8,11)*. Total parenteral nutrition (TPN) consists of infusion of all nutrients directly into the circulatory system thus bypassing the GI tract. This feeding technique plays a vital role in the management of many gas-

Table 1
Coinfusion of IGF-I With TPN Solution Stimulates Body Weight Gain and Reverses TPN Mucosal Hypoplasia in Association With Increased Enterocyte Proliferation and Reduced Apoptosis in Growing Rats Maintained With TPN for 7 d[a]

Treatment	*Weight gain (g body weight gain/7 d)*	*Serum IGF-I (µg/L)*	*Jejunal mucosa (mg dry mass/cm)*	*Villus (apoptotic cells/ villus, n)[b]*	*Crypt (Apoptotic cells/crypt, n)[b]*	*Crypt Mitotic cells/ crypt, n)[b]*
Oral	28 ± 4[a]	392 ± 28[b]	7.1 ± 0.4[a]	0.03 ± 0.02[b]	0.06 ± 0.02[b]	1.06 ± 0.10[a]
TPN	13 ± 2[b]	337 ± 23[b]	4.5 ± 0.5[b]	0.30 ± 0.11[a]	0.24 ± 0.07[a]	0.67 ± 0.06[b]
TPN+IGF-I	30 ± 2[a]	857 ± 43[a]	7.1 ± 0.4[a]	0.20 ± 0.06[a]	0.06 ± 0.03[b]	0.92 ± 0.05[a]

[a]Values are means ± SE, n = 6–9. Means in a column with different superscripts differ, $p < 0.05$. Adapted from ref. *10.*

[b]Defined as he number of apoptotic cells per villus column or the nmber of apoptotic or mitotic cells per crypt column, one side of a villus or crypt in a longitudinal cross-section.

trointestinal and surgical conditions where patients cannot tolerate enteral feeding. The experimental model of TPN provides a physiologic tool to examine how the absence of exogenous luminal nutrients affects gut structure and function without the confounding factor of malnutrition due to food deprivation. Insights can also be gained regarding the role of the endogenous IGF-I system in mediating the enterotropic effects of luminal nutrients. Moreover, systemic administration of IGF-I or GH in the TPN model provides a sensitive system for evaluating the enterotropic actions of these growth factors because the magnitude of the mucosal growth response to IGF-I in the TPN model is greater than that observed with oral feeding *(22)*.

4.1. IGF-I Reverses TPN Mucosal Hypoplasia and Improves Transport Function

TPN induces hypoplasia of the small intestine mucosal epithelium in association with a one-third reduction in enterocyte proliferation and increases in apoptosis in growing rats maintained exclusively with TPN for 7 d (Table 1) *(10)*. Pigs *(51)* and rabbits *(52)* also show similar reductions in jejunal epithelial proliferation rates after 6–10 d of parenteral nutrition. Moreover, decreased levels of total thymidine incorporation into DNA were observed in small bowel biopsies from human patients receiving one month of TPN for inflammatory bowel disease *(53)*. Coinfusion of IGF-I with TPN solution reverses the TPN mucosal hypoplasia, based on significant increases in mucosal protein and DNA, in association with increased enterocyte proliferation and decreased apoptosis (Table 1). The ability of IGF-I to stimulate mucosal hyperplasia is correlated with increased IGFBP-5 expression in both the lamina propria and muscularis *(17,46,47)* leading to the hypothesis that IGFBP-5 enhances IGF-I action in the small intestine.

IGF-I treatment normalizes the dramatic increases in apoptosis in the crypt and villus compartments that are induced by TPN in the rat *(10)*. Apoptosis is increased approximately fourfold in the crypt compartment and is distributed throughout the

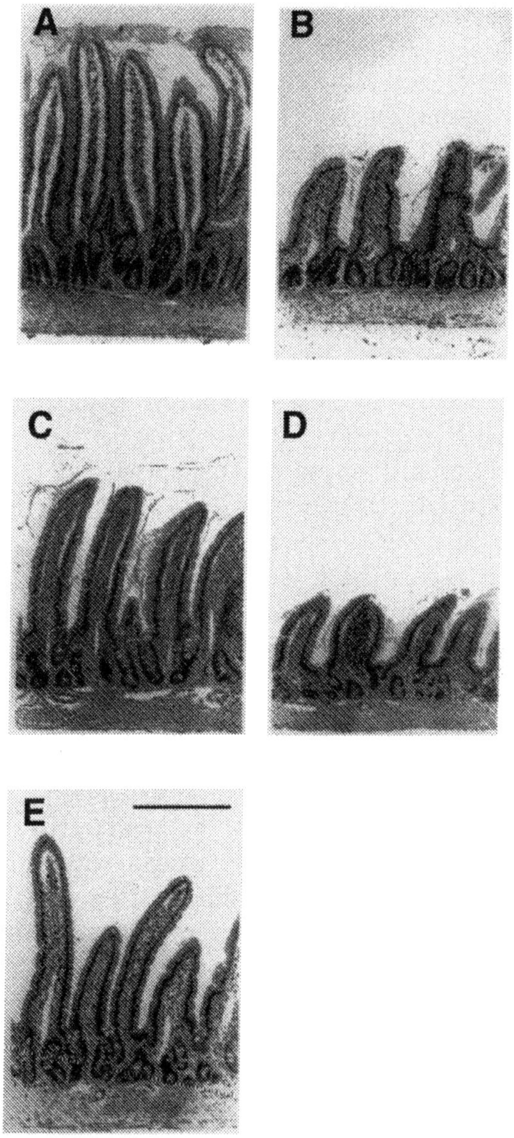

Fig. 4. Photomicrographs of jejunum of ad libitum-fed rat (**A**), TPN-fed animal given TPN alone (**B**), or TPN supplemented with GH (**C**), ***IGF-I*** *(D)*, or GH + IGF-I (**E**). Note the mucosal atrophy and hypoplasia induced by TPN and reversal of this effect by IGF-I alone or GH + IGF-I but not GH alone. Reprinted with permission from ref. *1*.

length of the crypt with TPN rather than being concentrated in the stem cell zone as occurs with oral feeding *(10)*. IGF-I treatment reduces apoptosis specifically in the crypt stem cell zone, similar to that reported in transgenic mice with chronic IGF-I excess *(9)*. TPN-induced mucosal hypoplasia is characterized by villus atrophy, reflected in villi that are 36% shorter compared with orally fed rats (Fig. 4A,B), and a decrease in the rate of enterocyte migration *(4)*. The TPN villus atrophy is associated with a 7- to 13-fold increase in apoptosis in the villus, an effect that is not altered by IGF-I treatment (Table 1). Thus, decreased enterocyte proliferation and increased apoptosis appear to mediate the mucosal hypoplasia that accompanies TPN in rats *(10)* and pigs *(51)* and occurs to a lesser degree in humans *(54,55)*. IGF-I acts to reverse TPN mucosal atrophy by increasing enterocyte proliferation and decreasing apoptosis specifically in the crypt stem cell zone.

TPN mucosal atrophy is associated with aberrations in intestinal ion transport function in the rat *(35)* and intestinal dysfunction in humans requiring TPN as they transition to enteral feeding *(56)*. Interestingly, the transport characteristics of the jejunum of TPN rats resemble those of fasted animals *(57)*. The jejunum of TPN rats has increased ionic permeability or is "leakier" than that of orally fed rats and shows abnormal increases in ion transport responses to secretory and absorptive agents in Ussing chambers *(35)*. Coinfusion of IGF-I with TPN solution reverses the aberrations in ion transport induced by TPN and improves ionic permeability in association with IGF-induced mucosal growth *(35)*.

Given that IGF-I attenuates the mucosal hypoplasia induced by TPN, it is tempting to speculate that TPN mucosal hypoplasia is caused by a deficiency of circulating IGF-I or local expression of IGF-I in the gut. This is not the case as circulating IGF-I (Table 1) and hepatic expression of IGF-I are not altered by TPN *(2,17,47)* with the exception of excessive provision of parenteral energy that induces hepatic steatosis and reduces abundance of hepatic IGF-I mRNA in the rat *(58)*. Neonatal piglets do show a decrease in circulating IGF-I with parenteral compared with enteral feeding *(59)* and children with gut resection receiving partial parenteral nutrition also show reduced serum IGF-I *(60)*. Local expression of IGF-I mRNA in jejunum is also not reduced by TPN in parallel with the mucosal hypoplasia *(17)*. This contrasts with fasting followed by refeeding, where both circulating IGF-I and jejunal IGF-I are reduced by fasting and then increased in association with mucosal growth induced by refeeding *(18)*. The overall state of systemic nutrition, rather than the presence of exogenous luminal nutrients in the gut, appears to regulate expression of both hepatic and jejunal IGF-I mRNA.

4.2. GH Elevates Serum IGF-I Levels But Does Not Alter TPN Mucosal Hypoplasia

Using a TPN rat model of surgical stress and bowel disease *(61)*, Lo et al. confirm that simultaneous treatment with GH and IGF-I additively increases serum IGF-I levels and whole-body anabolism as noted in humans *(62)*. GH and IGF-I show unique tissue-specific anabolic effects in that GH selectively increases skeletal muscle mass and protein synthesis in skeletal muscle and jejunal muscularis and IGF-I increases jejunal mucosal mass and protein synthesis in jejunal mucosa and muscularis *(63)*. Thus, IGF-I but not GH reverses TPN mucosal atrophy but both peptides stimulate protein synthesis in the jejunal muscularis layer (Fig. 4). These findings indicate that the intestinal mucosa is resistant to the proliferative effects of GH-stimulated endogenous IGF-I during TPN *(17,64)*, similar to that noted in transgenic mice that overexpress GH and show increased circulating endogenous IGF-I *(48)*. The resistance to GH action is specific to mucosal growth because GH increases protein synthesis in the jejunal muscularis *(63)* and modulates ion transport and sucrase activity within the mucosa 4. Studies in human subjects, similar to the animal evidence, have shown mixed results regarding the ability of GH to stimulate intestinal growth *(65–67)*.

Previous studies have tested several possible theories to explain the selective resistance to the anabolic action of GH in the intestinal mucosa. Reduced expression of IGFBP-5 in GH compared with IGF-I-treated rats may play a role but is unlikely to fully explain the striking differences in the enterotropic effects of GH and IGF-I *(17)*. Differences in expression of the GH receptor or GH binding activity also cannot explain the GH resistance *(47,64)*. This has led to the current hypothesis that a state of postreceptor resistance to GH action is responsible for the inability of GH to stimulate mucosal hyperplasia during TPN *(64)*. An elevated level of an intracellular inhibitor of GH action, suppressor of cytokine signaling-2 (SOCS-2), may play a key role in the resistance to GH action as a feedback inhibitor of the trophic actions of GH *(68)*.

A better understanding of GH and IGF-I action in the small intestine is needed to fully define the potential benefit of GH or IGF-I therapy for patients with GI disease, especially those individuals who require TPN because of intestinal failure because of massive bowel resection as discussed in the next section.

5. INTESTINAL RESECTION

Partial intestinal resection provides a strong stimulus for adaptive growth of intestine that ultimately results in increases in length and functional mass of the residual bowel in animal models and in some humans *(11,12)*. Partial intestinal resection is the strongest known stimulus to increase enterocyte proliferation and mucosal mass in animal models, although the mechanisms underlying this adaptive growth are incompletely understood. Resection-induced growth of the intestine is the most extensively studied and clinically relevant example of intestinal adaptation.

5.1. Short Bowel Syndrome

Short bowel syndrome is a form of intestinal failure defined as clinically significant lack of absorption of nutrients and water after massive intestinal resection. Surgical resection of the intestine is required for a variety of clinical situations including mesenteric infarction, Crohn's disease, ulcerative colitis, neoplasia, congenital disorders, and necrotizing enterocolitis. Failure of the intestine to adapt after massive intestinal resection in humans may be the result of a lack of endogenous enterotropic growth factors. For example, the presence of residual ileum and/or colon, the primary sites of synthesis and secretion of the enterotropic hormone glucagon-like peptide-2, appears to determine whether resection-induced adaptation occurs in both animals *(13,28)* and humans *(69)*. The presence of nutrients in the gastrointestinal tract indirectly stimulates endogenous production of enterotropic growth factors *(59)*; however, luminal nutrients are not essential for resection-induced adaptation when residual ileum and colon are present *(13)*.

Patients who do not show sufficient intestinal adaptation after bowel resection are dependent on parenteral nutrition to sustain nutritional status and life. In patients with less than 100 cm of residual intestinal length, 45% require lifelong parenteral nutrition to maintain their nutritional status with a 5-yr mortality rate of approximately 25% *(70)*. In the United States, it is estimated that 20,000 adult patients with intestinal disease are currently maintained on home parenteral nutrition at an average annual cost of $150,000 per patient *(71)*. Moreover, there are increasing numbers of children with intestinal disease who require parenteral nutrition and the incidence of short bowel syndrome is increasing in premature infants who develop necrotizing enterocolitis and require massive intestinal resection.

5.2. Role of the IGF System in Intestinal Adaptation to Resection

Evidence in laboratory rodents suggests that IGF-I promotes resection-induced intestinal growth both as an endogenously synthesized and an exogenously administered growth factor. With respect to endogenous paracrine effects of IGF-I, increased expression of IGF-I mRNA in residual small intestine *(27,40)* and colon *(46,72)*, and decreased expression of IGFBP-3 mRNA *(27)* have been noted in association with resection-induced adaptive growth in rats. However, increased intestinal IGF-I mRNA in resected rats did not result in increased intestinal IGF-I protein suggesting posttranscriptional processing of IGF-I message *(46)*. In addition, IGF-I receptor binding capacity is increased in jejunal and colonic membranes after resection, suggesting increased responsiveness of the residual intestine to IGF-I *(46)*. Resection-induced adaptive growth in colon occurs in association with local increases in both IGF-I and IGFBP-5 mRNA, supporting the notion that IGFBP-5 positively modulates local IGF-I action in the colon *(46)*. Overall, resection upregulates the local IGF-I system in residual bowel of rats fed enterally or parenterally.

Systemic growth factors play an important role in mediating intestinal adaptation to resection *(73)*. Systemic administration of glucagon-like peptide-2 *(74)*, epidermal growth factor *(75)*, and IGF-I *(25,26)* augment resection-induced adaptation in the rat. The ability of GH to augment intestinal adaptation is unclear; studies have shown both positive *(76)* and neutral effects *(77)* regarding the ability of GH to stimulate intestinal growth after intestinal resection in rats.

In a rat model of human short bowel syndrome where minimal adaptation of the proximal intestine occurs and prolonged diarrhea, malabsorption and weight loss accompany enteral feeding, coinfusion of IGF-I with TPN solution induces structural and functional adaptation of the jejunum that otherwise does not occur *(28)*. This jejunal adaptation includes increased jejunal mucosal mass, enterocyte proliferation and migration rates, and improved intestinal barrier function *(28)*. Moreover, acute IGF-I treatment in this model produces increases in serum IGF-I concentration, body weight and jejunal mucosal cellularity that are sustained after cessation of IGF-I treatment and transition to oral feeding *(78)*. These studies in rat models of intestinal resection support the therapeutic use of enterotropic growth factors, such as IGF-I, to improve intestinal adaptation in humans with short bowel syndrome.

5.3. Treatment of Short Bowel Syndrome

Improved treatments for short bowel syndrome, such as bowel transplantation, bowel lengthening procedures, and/or use of enterotropic hormones, are needed. Thus, there has been considerable interest in studying the potential for hormones, such as glucagon-like peptide-2, GH, or IGF-I, to stimulate intestinal adaptation in patients with short bowel syndrome so that they can transition from parenteral to enteral feeding. Ideal use of enterotropic hormones would be acute treatment that produces sustained effects so that long-term therapy with these mitogenic hormones and the associated risk of cancer could be minimized *(78)*. Treatment with glucagon-like peptide -2 for 35 d in patients with short bowel syndrome improves intestinal absorption of energy and wet weight, resulting in an increase in body weight, lean body, and bone mass *(69)*.

Treatment with GH alone or in combination with a high carbohydrate diet and glutamine has shown controversial results in humans with short bowel syndrome *(65,66,79)*. However, positive effects of GH in humans with parenteral nutrition-dependent short bowel syndrome were recently observed in a placebo-controlled, crossover study with a threefold lower dose of GH than previously used combined with an ad libitum western hyperphagic diet with no glutamine supplementation *(67)*. Three weeks of treatment with low-dose GH increased intestinal absorption of energy by 15%, and increased lean body mass and serum concentrations of IGF-I and IGFBP-3, without any major adverse effect. The authors suggest that a hyperphagic diet and the absence of malnutrition are needed for an optimal enterotropic response to low dose GH *(67)*.

IGF-I has not been tested in humans with short bowel syndrome, but it has been shown to promote whole body anabolism in humans without surgical stress *(62)* and after large bowel resection *(80)*. Treatment with IGF-I may be particularly useful for children with short bowel syndrome who demonstrate growth failure, low serum IGF-I levels, and appear to be resistant to GH induction of hepatic IGF-I synthesis *(60)*. Determining the optimum dose of glucagon-like peptide-2, GH and/or IGF-I will be an important factor in assessing their efficacy in improving intestinal absorption and allowing successful weaning from parenteral nutrition to oral feeding.

6. INFLAMMATORY BOWEL DISEASE

Inflammatory bowel disease includes the immunologically mediated conditions of ulcerative colitis and Crohn's disease. Ulcerative colitis is limited to the colon and is characterized by acute and chronic inflammation of the lamina propria with or without epithelial cell destruction, epithelial ulceration, and crypt abscesses *(81)*. Crohn's disease differs from ulcerative colitis in that it may affect any region of the GI tract and is characterized by transmural inflammation and fibrosis *(82)*. Fibrosis involves disorganized hyperplasia and collagen deposition throughout the bowel wall that can lead to stricture formation and bowel obstruction. Intestinal resection is a frequent complication of Crohn's disease that often results in short bowel syndrome.

Growth factors, such as GH and IGF-I, may have both positive and negative effects during inflammatory bowel disease. They could protect against mucosal damage during active inflammation or facilitate repair of damaged mucosa during disease remission by promoting mesenchymal cell proliferation and collagen deposition *(1)*. In contrast, growth factors may exacerbate inflammation by chemotactic or mitogenic effects on immune cells or by stimulating the production of proinflammatory cytokines. In excess, growth factors could promote aberrant proliferation of mucosal cells and enhance susceptibility to colon cancer, a particular problem in inflammatory bowel disease *(81)*.

6.1. Altered IGF-I Expression Is Associated With Bowel Inflammation and Fibrosis

Given the ability of GH and IGF-I to regulate immune function it is not surprising that altered IGF-I production in the bowel is associated with the chronic inflammation that characterizes these conditions *(1,82)*. IGF-I expression is increased in rats with experimentally induced colitis *(83)* or Crohn's disease *(84)*. Patients with Crohn's disease show increased IGF-I and IGFBP-5 mRNAs in inflamed and strictured segments of resected bowel; IGF-I mRNA is most highly expressed in fibroblast-like cells in the submucosa and muscularis externa *(44)*. In contrast, levels of IGF-I mRNA are not altered in patients with ulcerative colitis who do not show fibrosis of the bowel *(1)*.

IGF-I has potent fibrogenic actions as evidenced by its ability to induce proliferation of fibroblasts, myofibroblasts, and smooth muscle cells and to increase collagen synthesis by these cells *(21,85)*. In vitro studies support the hypothesis that proinflammatory cytokines, such as interleukin-1 and tumor necrosis factor-α, induce IGF-I expression in intestinal mesenchymal cells during chronic inflammation *(1)*. Interestingly, fasting inhibits experimentally induced murine colitis and prevents the increase in interleukin-1 and IGF-I expression *(86)*. Overall, these data suggest that locally produced IGF-I may promote tissue fibrosis during intestinal inflammation, in particular during Crohn's disease. It will be important to understand the relative effects of locally produced IGF-I compared to circulating IGF-I on intestinal fibrosis when considering treatment with GH or IGF-I in patients with inflammatory bowel disease.

6.2. Treatment of Inflammatory Bowel Disease

Treatment of inflammatory bowel disease is aimed at reducing inflammation and inducing remission through the use of immunosuppressive and antiinflammatory drugs. Unfortunately, many of the drugs have severe side effects and may exacerbate tissue catabolism in conjunction with the malabsorption and malnutrition that often accompany inflammatory bowel disease. The use of high-protein diets has been partially successful in treating the symptoms of Crohn's disease in children *(87)*. Nutritional therapy that normalizes concentrations of circulating IGF-I appears to reverse growth failure in children with inflammatory bowel disease *(88)*. Results from a rat model of acute colitis indicate that systemic IGF-I may reduce epithelial damage and/or submucosal inflammation *(89)*. Thus, administration of an anabolic hormone such as GH or IGF-I in conjunction with nutritional therapy may promote remission, mucosal repair and an increase in lean body mass in patients with inflammatory bowel disease.

The ability of GH administration to counteract the catabolic process of Crohn's disease and reduce morbidity has recently been tested *(90)*. In a placebo-controlled pilot study, Slonim et al. reported a significant decrease in scores on the Crohn's Disease Activity Index, with improvements in terms of stool frequency, abdominal pain, and well-being, among 19 patients with moderate-to-severe Crohn's disease who received subcutaneous GH for 4 mo in conjunction with a high-protein diet. The beneficial effects of GH in this study did not appear to be caused by IGF-I action because the degree of clinical improvement in individual patients did not correlate with their circulating levels of IGF-I *(90)*. Additional studies are needed to confirm these results and to address many issues including optimal dosing of GH and long- term side effects such as fibrogenic complications in patients with Crohn's disease.

7. SUMMARY AND CONCLUSIONS

IGF-I action in the GI tract is characterized by stimulation of proliferation or differentiated cell function in a physiological or pathophysiological context that includes synergy with other hormones and cytokines *(1)*. A complete understanding of the role of the IGF-I system in the GI tract will require characterization of the mechanisms of IGF interactions with other hormones and cytokines during normal physiology and disease. A better understanding of the relative effects of circulating IGF-I and local expression of the IGF system, in particular the role of IGFBP-3 and -5, on intestinal adaptation is needed. Evidence clearly indicates that the IGF system holds promise for the treatment of GI disease in children and adults. Comprehensive knowledge of the effects of the IGF system on apoptosis in the bowel is needed to appreciate the potential risks of tumorigenesis associated with administration of GH or IGF-I *(91)*.

ACKNOWLEDGMENTS

The author's work is supported by NIH Grants R01-DK-42835 and T32-DK-07665, a USDA National Needs Graduate Fellowship, and by funds from the College of Agriculture and Life Sciences, University of Wisconsin-Madison. The author wishes to thank Dr. P. Kay Lund for sharing unpublished data and providing Figs. 1, 2, and 3 during the preparation of this chapter. The author also extends thanks to those past and current members of her laboratory who have conducted some of the work reviewed here including: Huan Yang, Catherine Peterson, Paula Lo, Pamela Hinton, Karen Kritsch, Melanie Gillingham, Elizabeth Dahly, David Huss, Mike Grahn, and Sangita Murali.

REFERENCES

1. Lund PK. IGFs and the digestive tract. In: Contemporary Endocrinology: The IGF System. Rosenfeld R, Roberts C Jr (eds.). Humana Press, Totowa, NJ, 1999. p. 517–544.
2. Ney DM, Huss DJ, Gillingham MB, et al. Investigation of insulin-like growth factor (IGF)-I and insulin receptor binding and expression in jejunum of parenterally fed rats treated with IGF-I or growth hormone. Endocrinology 1999;140:4850–4860.
3. Williams KL, Fuller CR, Fagin J, Lund PK. Mesenchymal IGF-I overexpression: paracrine effects in the intestine, distinct from endocrine actions. Am J Physiol 2002;283:G875–G885.
4. Peterson CA, Carey HV, Hinton PL, Lo HC, Ney DM. GH elevates serum IGF-I levels but does not alter mucosal atrophy in parenterally fed rats. Am J Physiol 1997;272:G1100–G1108.
5. Louvard D, Kedinger M, Hauri HP. The differentiating intestinal epithelial cell: establishment and maintenance of functions through interactions between cellular structures. Annu Rev Cell Biol 1992;8:157–195.
6. Potten C. The significance of spontaneous and induced apoptosis in the gastrointestinal tract of mice. Cancer Metastasis Rev 1992;11:179–195.
7. Potten C, Wilson J, Booth C. Regulation and significance of apoptosis in the stem cells of the gastrointestinal epithelium. Stem Cells 1997;15:82–93.
8. Williamson R, Chir M. Intestinal adaptation: structural, functional and cytokinetic changes. New Eng J Med 1978;298:1393–1402.
9. Wilkins HR, Ohneda K, Keku TO, et al. Reduction of spontaneous and irradiation-induced apoptosis in small intestine of IGF-I transgenic mice. Am J Physiol 2002;283:G457–G464.
10. Dahly E, Ziwen G, Ney D. Alterations in enterocyte proliferation and apoptosis accompany TPN-induced mucosal hypoplasia and IGF-I-induced hyperplasia in rats. J Nutr 2002;132:2010–2014.
11. Jenkins AP, Thompson RP. Mechanisms of small intestinal adaptation. Dig Dis 1994;12:15–27.
12. Tavakkolizadeh A, Whang EE. Understanding and augmenting human intestinal adaptation: a call for more clinical research. JPEN 2002;26:251–255.
13. Dahly EM, Gillingham MB, Guo Z, et al. Role of luminal nutrients and endogenous GLP-2 in intestinal adaptation to mid-small bowel resection. Am J Physiol Gastrointest Liver Physiol 2003;284:G670–G682.
14. Lund PK, Moats-Staats BM, Hynes MA, et al. Somatomedin-C/insulin-like growth factor-I and insulin-like growth factor-II mRNAs in rat fetal and adult tissues. J Biol Chem 1986;261:14539–14544.

15. Han VK, D'Ercole AJ, Lund PK. Cellular localization of somatomedin (insulin-like growth factor) messenger RNA in the human fetus. Science 1987;236:193–197.
16. Rouyer-Fessard C, Gammeltoft S, Laburthe M. Expression of two types of receptor for insulinlike growth factors in human colonic epithelium. Gastroenterology 1990;98:703–707.
17. Peterson CA, Gillingham MB, Mohapatra NK, et al. Enterotrophic effect of Insulin-like growth factor-I but not growth hormone and localized expression of insulin-like growth factor-I, Insulin-like Growth Factor Binding Protein-3 and -5 mRNAs in jejunum of parenterally-fed rats. JPEN 2000;24:288–295.
18. Winesett DE, Ulshen MH, Hoyt EC, Mohapatra NK, Fuller CR, Lund PK. Regulation and localization of the insulin-like growth factor system in small bowel during altered nutrient status. Am J Physiol 1995;268:G631–G640.
19. Pucilowska JB, McNaughton KK, Mohapatra NK, et al. IGF-I and procollagen alpha1 (I) are coexpressed in a subset of mesenchymal cells in active Crohn's disease. Am J Physiol 2000;279:G1307–G1322.
20. Simmons JG, Pucilowska JB, Lund PK. Autocrine and paracrine actions of intestinal fibroblast-derived insulin-like growth factors. Am J Physiol 1999;276:G817–G827.
21. Zimmermann EM, Li L, Hou YT, Cannon M, Christman GM, Bitar KN. IGF-I induces collagen and IGFBP-5 mRNA in rat intestinal smooth muscle. Am J Physiol 1997;273:G875–G882.
22. Steeb CB, Trahair JF, Tomas FM, Read LC. Prolonged administration of IGF peptides enhances growth of gastrointestinal tissues in normal rats. Am J Physiol 1994;266:G1090–G1098.
23. Steeb CB, Shoubridge CA, Tivey DR, Read LC. Systemic infusion of IGF-I or LR(3)IGF-I stimulates visceral organ growth and proliferation of gut tissues in suckling rats. Am J Physiol 1997;272:G522–G533.
24. Steeb CB, Trahair JF, Read LC. Administration of insulin-like growth factor-I (IGF-I) peptides for three days stimulates proliferation of the small intestinal epithelium in rats. Gut 1995;37:630–638.
25. Lemmey AB, Martin AA, Read LC, Tomas FM, Owens PC, Ballard FJ. IGF-I and the truncated analogue des-(1–3)IGF-I enhance growth in rats after gut resection. Am J Physiol 1991;260:E213–E219.
26. Vanderhoof JA, McCusker RH, Clark R, et al. Truncated and native insulinlike growth factor I enhance mucosal adaptation after jejunoileal resection. Gastroenterology 1992;102:1949–1956.
27. Ziegler TR, Mantell MP, Chow JC, Rombeau JL, Smith RJ. Intestinal adaptation after extensive small bowel resection: differential changes in growth and insulin-like growth factor system messenger ribonucleic acids in jejunum and ileum. Endocrinology 1998;139:3119–3126.
28. Gillingham MB, Dahly EM, Carey HV, Clark MD, Kritsch KR, Ney DM. Differential jejunal and colonic adaptation due to resection and IGF-I in parenterally fed rats. Am J Physiol Gastrointest Liver Physiol 2000;278:G700–G709.
29. Read LC, Tomas FM, Howarth GS, et al. Insulin-like growth factor-I and its N-terminal modified analogues induce marked gut growth in dexamethasone-treated rats. J Endocrinol 1992;133:421–431.
30. Alexander AN, Carey HV. Oral IGF-I enhances nutrient and electrolyte absorption in neonatal piglet intestine. Am J Physiol 1999;277:G619–G625.
31. Burrin DG, Wester TJ, Davis TA, Amick S, Heath JP. Orally administered IGF-I increases intestinal mucosal growth in formula-fed neonatal pigs. Am J Physiol 1996;270:R1085–R1091.
32. Fholenhag K, Arrhenius-Nyberg V, Sjogren I, Malmlof K. Effects of insulin-like growth factor I (IGF-I) on the small intestine: a comparison between oral and subcutaneous administration in the weaned rat. Growth Factors 1997;14:81–88.
33. Xian CJ, Shoubridge CA, Read LC. Degradation of IGF-I in the adult gastrointestinal tract is limited by a specific antiserum or the dietary protein casein. J Endocrinol 1995;146:215–225.
34. Castilla-Cortazar I, Prieto J, Urdaneta E, et al. Impaired intestinal sugar transport in cirrhotic rats: correction by low doses of insulin-like growth factor I. Gastroenterology 1997;113:1180–1187.
35. Peterson CA, Ney DM, Hinton PS, Carey HV. Beneficial effects of insulin-like growth factor I on epithelial structure and function in parenterally fed rat jejunum. Gastroenterology 1996;111:1501–1508.
36. Houle VM, Park YK, Laswell SC, Freund GG, Dudley MA, Donovan SM. Investigation of three doses of oral insulin-like growth factor-I on jejunal lactase phlorizin hydrolase activity and gene expression and enterocyte proliferation and migration in piglets. Pediatr Res 2000;48:497–503.
37. Burrin DG, Stoll B, Fan MZ, Dudley MA, Donovan SM, Reeds PJ. Oral IGF-I alters the posttranslational processing but not the activity of lactase-phlorizin hydrolase in formula-fed neonatal pigs. J Nutr 2001;131:2235–2241.

38. Kritsch KR, Huss DJ, Ney DM. Greater potency of IGF-I than IGF-I/BP-3 complex in catabolic parenterally fed rats. Am J Physiol Endocrinol Metab 2000;278:E252–E262.
39. Baxter RC. Insulin-like growth factor (IGF)-binding proteins: interactions with IGFs and intrinsic bioactivities. Am J Physiol 2000;278:E967–E976.
40. Ziegler TR, Mantell MP, Chow JC, Rombeau JL, Smith RJ. Gut adaptation and the insulin-like growth factor system: regulation by glutamine and IGF-I administration. Am J Physiol 1996;271:G866–G875.
41. Ohneda K, Ulshen MH, Fuller CR, D'Ercole AJ, Lund PK. Enhanced growth of small bowel in transgenic mice expressing human insulin-like growth factor I. Gastroenterology 1997;112:444–454.
42. Collett-Solberg PF, Cohen P. Genetics, chemistry, and function of the IGF/IGFBP system. Endocrine 2000;12:121–136.
43. Albiston AL, Taylor RG, Herington AC, Beveridge DJ, Fuller PJ. Divergent ileal IGF-I and IGFBP-3 gene expression after small bowel resection: a novel mechanism to amplify IGF action? Mol Cell Endocrinol 1992;83:R17–R20.
44. Zimmerman EM, Li L, Hou YT, Mohapatra NK, Pucilowska JB. Insulin-like growth factor I and insulin-like growth factor binding protein 5 in Crohn's disease. Am J Physiol 2001;280:G1022–G1029.
45. Parker A, Rees C, Clarke J, Busby WH, Jr., Clemmons DR. Binding of insulin-like growth factor (IGF)-binding protein-5 to smooth- muscle cell extracellular matrix is a major determinant of the cellular response to IGF-I. Mol Biol Cell 1998;9:2383–2392.
46. Gillingham MB, Kritsch KR, Murali SG, Lund PK, Ney DM. Resection upregulates the IGF-I system of parenterally fed rats with jejunocolic anastomosis. Am J Physiol Gastrointest Liver Physiol 2001;281:G1158–G1168.
47. Yang H, Ney DM, Peterson CA, Lo HC, Carey HV, Adamo ML. Stimulation of intestinal growth is associated with increased insulin- like growth factor-binding protein 5 mRNA in the jejunal mucosa of insulin-like growth factor-I-treated parenterally fed rats. Proc Soc Exp Biol Med 1997;216:438–445.
48. Ulshen MH, Dowling RH, Fuller CR, Zimmermann EM, Lund PK. Enhanced growth of small bowel in transgenic mice overexpressing bovine growth hormone [see comments]. Gastroenterology 1993;104:973–980.
49. Wang J, Niu W, Nikiforov Y, et al. Targeted overexpression of IGF-I evokes distinct patterns of organ remodeling in smooth muscle cell tissue beds of transgenic mice. J Clin Invest 1997;100:1425–1439.
50. Parrizas M, LeRoith D. Insulin-like growth factor-1 inhibition of apoptosis is associated with increased expression of the bcl-xL gene product. Endocrinology 1997;138:1355–1358.
51. Burrin DG, Stoll B, Jiang R, et al. GLP-2 stimulates intestinal growth in premature TPN-fed pigs by suppressing proteolysis and apoptosis. Am J Physiol Gastrointest Liver Physiol 2000;279:G1249–G1256.
52. Eastwood GL. Small bowel morphology and epithelial proliferation in intravenously alimented rabbits. Surgery 1977;82:613–620.
53. Rossi TM, Lee PC, Young C, Tjota A. Small intestinal mucosa changes, including epithelial cell proliferative activity, of children receiving total parenteral nutrition (TPN). Dig Dis Sci 1993;38:1608–1613.
54. Buchman AL, Moukarzel AA, Ament ME, et al. Effects of total parenteral nutrition on intestinal morphology and function in humans. Transplant Proc 1994;26:1457.
55. Groos S, Hunefeld G, Luciano L. Parenteral versus enteral nutrition: morphological changes in human adult intestinal mucosa. J Submicrosc Cytol Pathol 1996;28:61–74.
56. Biasco G, Callegari C, Lami F, Minarini A, Miglioli M, Barbara L. Intestinal morphological changes during oral refeeding in a patient previously treated with total parenteral nutrition for small bowel resection. Am J Gastroenterol 1984;79:585–588.
57. Carey HV, Hayden UL, Tucker KE. Fasting alters basal and stimulated ion transport in piglet jejunum. Am J Physiol 1994;267:R156–R163.
58. Ney DM, Yang H, Smith SM, Unterman TG. High-calorie total parenteral nutrition reduces hepatic insulin-like growth factor-I mRNA and alters serum levels of insulin-like growth factor-binding protein-1, -3, -5, and -6 in the rat. Metabolism 1995;44:152–160.
59. Burrin DG, Stoll B, Jiang R, et al. Minimal enteral nutrient requirements for intestinal growth in neonatal piglets: how much is enough? Am J Clin Nutr 2000;71:1603–1610.
60. Barksdale EM, Jr., Koehler AN, Yaworski JA, Gardner M, Reyes J. Insulinlike growth factor 1 and insulinlike growth factor 3: indices of intestinal failure in children. J Pediatr Surg 1999;34:655–661; discussion 661–662.

16 Impact of Critical Illness on the Growth Hormone/Insulin Growth Factor System in Relation to Other Endocrine Responses

Greta Van den Berghe

KEY POINTS

- Pronounced changes in the GH/IGF/IGFBP axis occur immediately and uniformly in response to all types of severe illnesses, independent of its cause.
- Prolonged critical illness, in which the onset of recovery does not occur within a few days, reflects a novel pathophysiological condition characterized by a peculiar type of hypercatabolism which occurs despite adequate parenteral and/or enteral nutrition.
- Low circulating levels of IGF-I and alterations in IGFBPs mark the hypercatabolic state of critical illness. The origin of these changes appears differently during the first hours to days after onset than in prolonged critical illness.
- Immediately after the onset of severe illness or injury, acute peripheral GH resistance is indicated by low serum concentrations of IGF-I, IGFBP-3 and ALS in the presence of activated GH secretion. Increased IGFBP-3 protease activity in serum, as well as increased circulating levels of IGFBP-1, may alter IGF-1 tissue availability.
- In prolonged critical illness, GH secretion is no longer elevated, becomes erratic and almost nonpulsatilve, and occurs with low pulsative TSH and LH. The reduced pulsatile component of GH secretion likely contributes to inadequate generation of IGF-I and IGF-BPs and to impaired anabolism.
- High IGFBP-1 and low insulin levels predict a fatal outcome for prolonged critical illness.
- Treatment with releasing factors (GH secretagogues, TRH, and GnRH) takes advantage of active feedback inhibition loops and may be safer and more effective than administration of high-dose GH and/or IGF-I to counter the catabolic state in prolonged critical illness.

1. INTRODUCTION

By definition, critical illness is any condition requiring support of failing vital organ functions, either with mechanical aids (e.g., mechanical ventilation, hemodialysis or filtration, or cardiac assist devices) or pharmacological agents (such as inotropes or vasopressors), without which death would ensue *(1)*. According to this definition, critical

From: *IGF and Nutrition in Health and Disease*
Edited by: M. S. Houston, J. M. P. Holly, and E. L. Feldman © Humana Press Inc., Totowa, NJ

releasing peptides (GHRPs) and nonpeptide analogs have been developed that potently release GH through a specific G protein-coupled receptor located in the hypothalamus and the pituitary *(17,18)*. It now appears that there exists at least one highly conserved endogenous ligand for this receptor *(19)*, named "ghrelin," which originates in peripheral tissues such as the stomach as well as in the hypothalamic arcuate nucleus and which seems to be another key factor in the complex physiological regulation of pulsatile GH secretion. As originally shown in rodents *(20)*, there is now also evidence that in the human *(21)*, the pulsatile nature of GH secretion is important for its metabolic effects *(4,22)*. In the acute phase of stress, as after surgery, trauma, or onset of sepsis, circulating GH levels become elevated and the normal GH profile, consisting of peaks alternating with virtually undetectable troughs, is altered: peak GH levels and especially the interpulse concentrations are high, and the GH pulse frequency is elevated (Fig. 1) *(10,23,24)*. It is still unclear which factor ultimately controls the stimulation of GH release in response to stress. As in starvation *(25)*, more frequent withdrawal of the inhibitory somatostatin and/or an increased availability of stimulatory (hypothalamic and/or peripheral) GH-releasing factors could hypothetically be involved. The constellation of low circulating levels of IGF-I, IGFBP-3, and ALS and amplified GH secretion, as uniformly occurs in experimental human and animal models of acute stress and in acutely ill patients, is therefore a classical example of acquired peripheral GH resistance *(11,23)*. This is most likely brought about by the effects of cytokines such as tumor necrosis factor-α, interleukin-1, and interleukin-6. The role of cytokines in critical illness is discussed further in Chapter 3. It has been hypothesized, but remains unproved, that the primary events in acute illness are cytokine and/or starvation-induced reduced GH receptor expression and impairment of GH signaling at the intracellular level *(13)* and hence low circulating IGF-I levels which, in turn, through reduced negative feedback inhibition, drive the abundant release of GH. The large amounts of GH may then exert direct (IGF-I-independent) lipolytic, insulin-antagonizing and immune-stimulatory actions, whereas the indirect IGF-I-mediated somatotropic effects may be attenuated *(26,27)*. This phenomenon would make sense in stressful conditions. Indeed, the set of alterations within the GH–IGF-I axis could contribute to the provision of metabolic substrates (glucose, free fatty acids, amino-acids such as glutamine) for vital organs, such as the brain and the heart and for host defense and thus could be conceived as adaptive and beneficial for survival. However, the adaptive nature of low IGF availability is merely a theoretical concept as it has never been proven. An alternative interpretation could be that increased IGFBP-3 protease activity in plasma, also reported in acute illnesses *(11,28)*, results in facilitated dissociation of IGF-I from the ternary complex, which could theoretically be an adaptive escape mechanism to secure IGF-I activity at the tissue level *(28)*. Once more, proof for such a phenomenon is thus far lacking.

Circulating levels of the small, binary complex IGF-binding proteins, such as IGFBP-1 and IGFBP-2, have been reported to be elevated in the acute phase of critical illness *(11,29)*. It is unclear whether the changes in these IGF-binding proteins enhance or reduce the tissue effects of IGF-I. A high serum IGFBP-1 level on ICU admission has been found to be associated with a more negative nitrogen balance during the first 2 d of intensive care *(11)*. Part of this association can be explained by the effects of relative starvation, which is uniformly present in all models of acute stress, including acute critical illness in the ICU. Indeed, when patients are starved on admission to the ICU, they will lose more lean tissue over the next few days.

3. CHANGES WITHIN THE IGF SYSTEM IN THE CHRONIC PHASE OF CRITICAL ILLNESS

In prolonged critical illness, the changes observed within the somatotropic axis are different than the initial phases of critical illness. First, the pattern of GH secretion becomes very chaotic and the amount of GH that is released in pulses is now much more reduced compared with the acute phase (Fig. 1) *(5,30,31)*. Moreover, although the non-pulsatile fraction is still somewhat elevated and the number of pulses is still high, mean nocturnal GH serum concentrations are hardly elevated when compared with the healthy, nonstressed condition and substantially lower than in the acute phase of stress *(10)*. We observed that when intensive care patients are studied from 7–10 d of illness onward in the absence of drugs known to exert profound effects on GH secretion, such as dopamine *(32,33)*, calcium entry blockers, or glucocorticoids (to name but a few), they present uniformly with mean nocturnal GH levels of about 1 μg/L, trough (interpulse) levels that are easily detectable and thus still elevated, and peak GH levels that hardly ever exceed 2 μg/L. This, surprisingly, is independent of the patient's age, body composition, and type of underlying disease *(4,10)*. Second, the pulsatile component of GH secretion, which is substantially reduced, has been found to correlate positively with circulating levels of IGF-I, IGFBP-3, and ALS, which are all low *(5,30,31)*. In other words, the more the pulsatile GH secretion is suppressed, the lower the circulating levels of the GH-dependent IGF-I and ternary complex binding proteins become. This is not what one would expect if GH resistance were the primary cause of the low IGF-I levels, which would result in an inverse correlation or no correlation between GH secretion and circulating IGF-I. The recently documented elevated serum levels of GH-binding protein *(4)*, assumed to reflect GH receptor expression in peripheral tissues, in prolonged critically ill patients compared with those measured in a matched control group are in line with recovery of GH responsiveness with time during severe illness *(4,5)*. It seems that the lack of pulsatile GH secretion in the condition of prolonged stress is contributing to the low circulating levels of IGF-I and ternary complex binding proteins. Moreover, it was demonstrated that these low serum levels of GH-dependent IGF-I and binding proteins (IGFBP-3, ALS, IGFBP-5) are tightly related to biochemical markers of impaired anabolism, such as low serum osteocalcin and leptin concentrations during prolonged critical illness *(5)*. Together, these findings suggest that a relative hyposomatotropism, as demonstrated by a lack of pulsatile GH secretion, participates in the pathogenesis of the particular lean tissue wasting condition distinctively occurring in the chronic phase of critical illness. In line with a higher risk for adverse outcome associated with male gender *(4)*, men appear to do worse than women in the sense that they lose more of the pulsatility and regularity within the GH-secretory pattern when critical illness progresses (despite indistinguishable total GH output) and concomitantly reveal even lower IGF-I and ALS levels than their female counterparts (Fig. 2) *(4)*. It remains unclear whether this sexual dimorphism within the GH/IGF-I axis is causally related to the gender difference in outcome of prolonged critical illness or merely reflects a casual association.

Serum concentrations of the small binding proteins IGFBP-2, IGFBP-4, and IGFBP-6 are clearly elevated in prolonged critical illness *(5,6)*, the cause of which

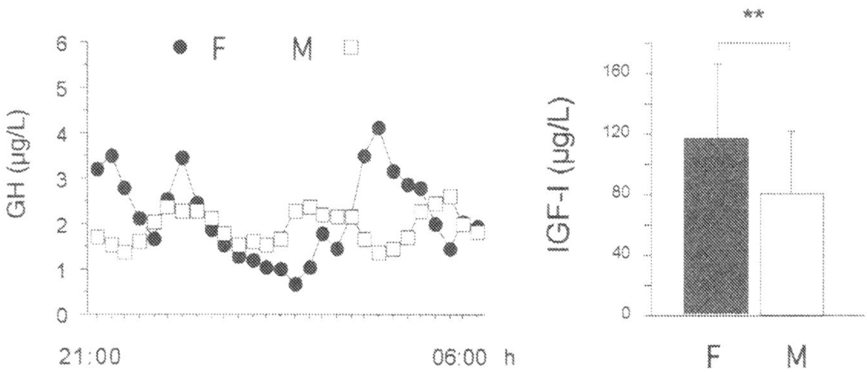

Fig. 2. The more "feminized" pattern of GH secretion (more irregular and less pulsatile GH secretory pattern for an identical mean nocturnal GH level) in prolonged critically ill men compared to women is illustrated by the representative nocturnal (21:00–06:00 h) GH serum concentration series (sampling every 20 min) obtained in a male (squares) and a matched female (circles) patient. Concomitantly, protracted critically ill men have lower circulating levels of IGF-I than female patients. IGF-I results are presented as mean ± SD. $^{**}p < 0.01$. Adapted with permission from ref. *4*.

still remains unclear. Also, the consequences of these changes for metabolism are not known. Serum IGFBP-1 concentrations in the chronic phase of critical illness are much lower than those observed in the acute phase, which is probably caused by the effect of feeding. Indeed, parenteral and/or enteral feeding is built up over the first few days of intensive care to a maintenance level of about 25 kcal/kg bodyweight per 24 h, composed of normal and equilibrated amounts of glucose, protein, and lipids. However, serum IGFBP-1 levels in prolonged critical illness still appears to correlate with lean tissue wasting, which occurs despite feeding *(4,5,10)*. In patients who subsequently won't survive, serum IGFBP-1 concentrations increase again when deterioration starts, a noticeable distinction between survivors and nonsurvivors that is present several weeks before death. Indeed, a high serum IGFBP-1 concentration in the chronic phase of critical illness, in the fed state, seems to predict an adverse outcome of chronic critical illness (Fig. 3) (ref. *5* and Van den Berghe, unpublished observations). IGFBP-1 is distinct among the members of the IGFBP family in being acutely regulated by metabolic stimuli *(34)*. Studies with cultured human liver explants suggest that the major regulatory influences on IGFBP-1 production are insulin, which is inhibitory, and hepatic substrate deprivation, which is stimulatory, acting through a cyclic AMP-dependent mechanism *(35,36)*. Moreover, an inverse correlation of IGFBP-1 with IGF-I and the GH-dependent proteins ALS and IGFBP-3 during critical illness is consistent with its inverse regulation by GH, as previously suggested *(37–39)*. The higher IGFBP-1 levels observed in prolonged critically ill patients who did not survive coincide with lower insulin concentrations compared with survivors, for the same range of blood glucose level; a surprising finding considering that these patients are thought to be insulin resistant (Fig. 3). Whether or not this indicates that also insulin secretion is becoming impaired in the long-stay intensive care patients remains unclear. It is clear, however, that in unfavorable metabolic

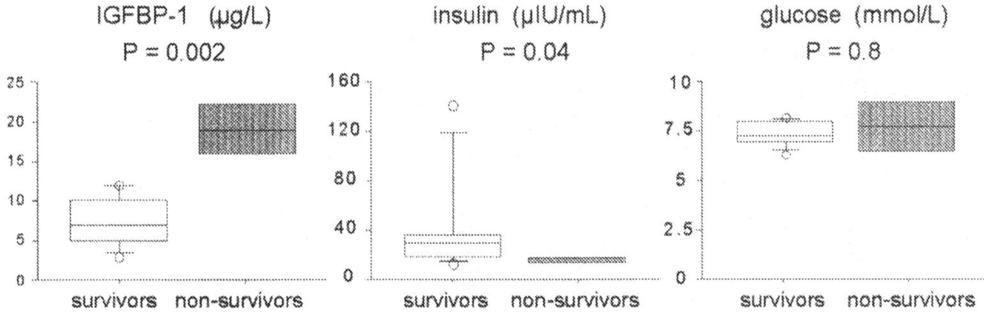

Fig. 3. Serum IGFBP-1 concentrations were found to be higher in nonsurvivors compared with survivors in prolonged critical illness. With permission from ref. *1*. Concomitantly, nonsurvivors revealed lower serum insulin levels for the same blood glucose level. Box plots represent medians, P25-P75 and P10-P90 and circles represent the absolute values for outliers.

conditions, the hepatocyte alters its production of IGF-regulatory proteins, for which the trigger might be reduced hepatocyte substrate availability (theoretically caused by either hepatic hypoperfusion or hypoxia, hypoglycemia, relative insulin deficiency, or hepatic insulin resistance), leading to increased cyclic AMP production, which would both suppress IGF-I and ALS *(40)* and stimulate IGFBP-1 *(35)*. It is unclear to what extent loss of GH pulsatility may contribute to this switch, but recent data *(35)* suggest that activation of hepatic IGF-I and ALS expression may require pulsatile GH. Animal studies similarly suggest that suppression of hepatic IGFBP-1 expression by insulin requires acute, rather than prolonged or nonpulsatile, GH action *(41)*. Further exploration of the apparent link among serum IGFBP-1 levels, insulin, and outcome of prolonged critical illness will shed new light on the pathophysiological processes crucial for recovery and survival. We recently showed that intensive insulin therapy to strictly maintain normoglycemia indeed substantially reduces the morbidity and mortality of intensive care-dependent critical illness *(42)*.

4. PATHOPHYSIOLOGY OF CHRONIC CHANGES

Because impaired pulsatile GH secretion in the chronic phase of critical illness seems to contribute to the low IGF-I and GH-dependent IGFBPs; the ensuing question is, what is its cause? Is the pituitary taking part in the "multiple organ failure syndrome," becoming unable to synthesize and secrete GH? Or, alternatively, is the lack of pulsatile GH secretion caused by increased somatostatin tone and/or to a reduced stimulation by the endogenous releasing factors, such as GHRH and/or ghrelin? Studying GH responses to administration of GH secretagogues (GHRH and GHRP), in a dose that is known to evoke a maximal GH response in healthy volunteers, enables, to a certain extent, differentiation between a primarily pituitary and a hypothalamic origin of the relatively impaired GH release in critically ill patients. Indeed, the combined administration of GHRH and GHRP appears to be the most powerful stimulus for pituitary GH release in humans *(43)*. A low GH response in critical illness would thus be compatible with pituitary dysfunction and/or a high

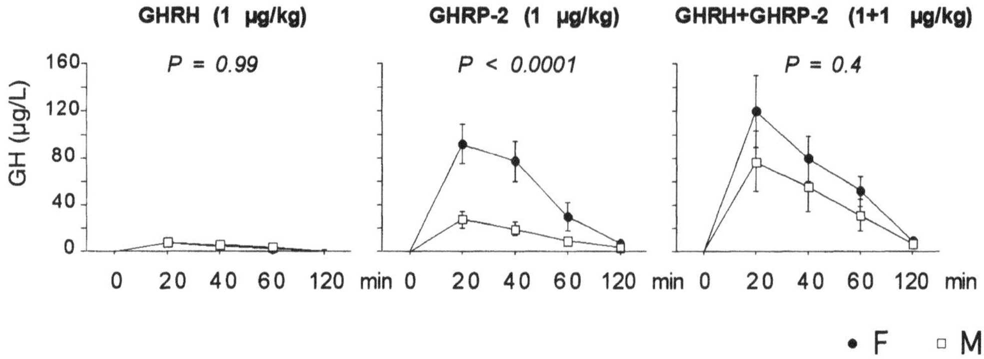

Fig. 4. Responses (increments above baseline) of GH obtained 20, 40, 60, and 120 min after intravenous bolus administration of GHRH (1 µg/kg), GHRP-2 (1 µg/kg), and GHRH + GHRP-2 (1 + 1 µg/kg) in matched male and female protracted critically ill patients. Five men and five women were randomly allocated to each secretagogue group. Results are presented as mean ± SEM. Circles depict results from female and squares from male patients. *p* values were obtained using repeated measures analysis of variance. Adapted with permission from ref. *4*.

somatostatin tone, whereas a high GH response would indicate reduced (hypothalamic) stimulation of the somatotropes.

We found that GH responses to a bolus injection of GHRP are high in long-stay intensive care patients and several-fold higher than the response to GHRH, the latter being normal or often subnormal *(44)*. GHRH plus GHRP evokes a clear synergistic response in this condition, revealing the highest GH responses ever reported in a human study *(44)*. The exuberant GH responses to secretagogues exclude the possibility that the relatively impaired pulsatile GH secretion during protracted critical illness is caused by a lack of pituitary capacity to synthesize GH or by accentuated somatostatin-induced suppression of GH release. Inferentially, one of the mechanisms that could be involved is reduced availability of ghrelin or another putative endogenous ligand for the GHRP receptor. Ultimately, the combination of low availability of somatostatin and of an endogenous GHRP-like ligand emerges as a plausible mechanism that clarifies (1) the reduced GH burst amplitude, (2) the increased frequency of spontaneous GH secretory bursts, and (3) the elevated interpulse levels as well as (4) the striking responsiveness to GHRP alone or in combination with GHRH, and this without markedly increased responsiveness to GHRH alone. Female patients with prolonged critical illness have a markedly higher response to a bolus of GHRP compared with male patients, a difference that is lost when GHRH is injected together with GHRP (Fig. 4) *(4)*. Less endogenous GHRH action in prolonged critically ill men, possibly because of the concomitant profound hypoandrogenism *(4)* accompanying loss of action of an endogenous GHRP-like ligand with prolonged stress in both genders, may explain this finding.

5. EFFECTS OF GH-RELEASING FACTORS ON THE IGF SYSTEM AND ON METABOLISM IN THE CHRONIC PHASE OF CRITICAL ILLNESS

The hypothesis of reduced endogenous stimulation of GH secretion and recovery of peripheral GH sensitivity in patients who are critically ill for a prolonged duration was

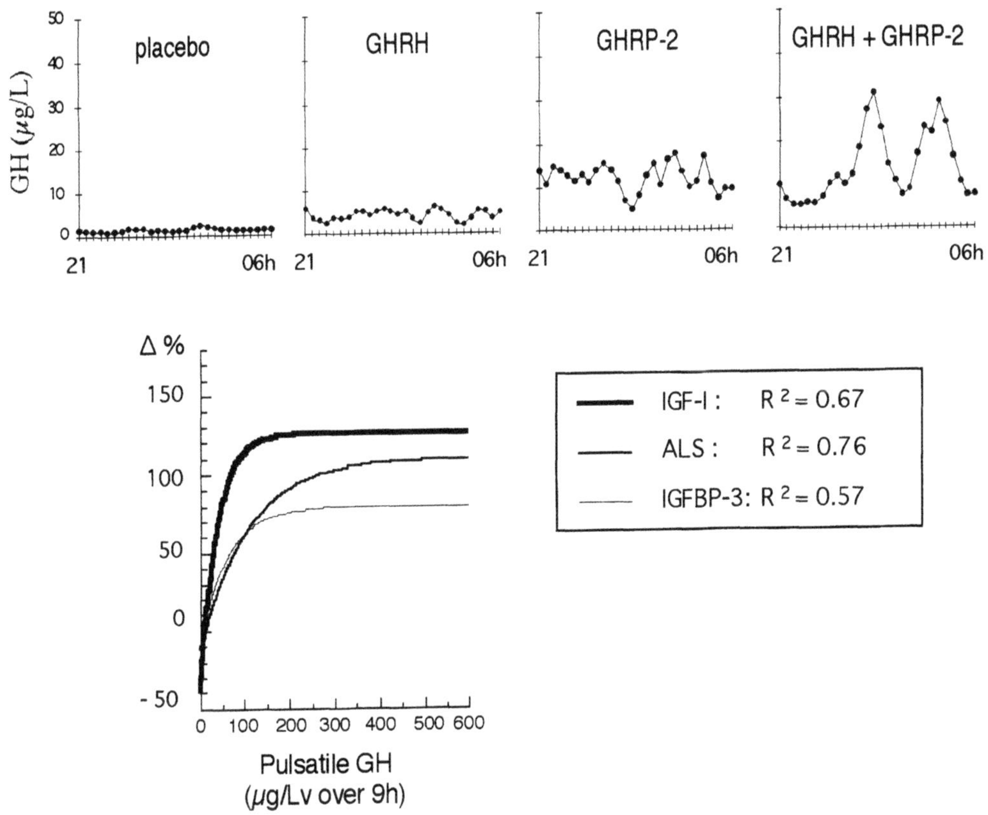

Fig. 5. Nocturnal serum GH profiles in the prolonged phase of illness illustrating the effects of continuous infusion of placebo, GHRH (1 µg/kg/h), GHRP-2 (1 µg/kg/h), or GHRH+GHRP-2 (1 + 1 µg/kg/h). Exponential regression lines have been reported between pulsatile GH secretion and the changes in circulating IGF-I, ALS, and IGFBP-3 obtained with 45-h infusion of either placebo, GHRP-2, or GHRH+GHRP-2. They indicate that the parameters of GH responsiveness increase in proportion to GH secretion up to a certain point, beyond which further increase of GH secretion has apparently little or no additional effect. It is noteworthy that the latter point corresponds to a pulsatile GH secretion of approx 200 µg/Lv over 9 h, or less, a value that can usually be evoked by the infusion of GHRP-2 alone. In the chronic, nonthriving phase of critical illness, GH sensitivity is clearly present, in contrast to the acute phase of illness, which is thought to be primarily a condition of GH resistance. From ref. *10* with permission.

further explored by examining the effects of continuous infusion of GHRP with or without GHRH. Continuously infusing GHRP (1 µg/kg/h) alone, and even more so the combination of GHRH and GHRP (1+1 µg/kg/h), for up to 2 d was found to substantially amplify pulsatile GH secretion (>6-fold and >10-fold, respectively) in this condition, without altering the relatively high burst frequency (Fig. 5) *(30,31)*. Reactivated pulsatile GH secretion was accompanied by a proportionate rise in serum IGF-I (66% and 106%, respectively), IGFBP-3 (50% and 56%), and ALS (65% and 97%), indicating peripheral GH-responsiveness (Fig. 5) *(5,31)*. The presence of considerable responsiveness to reactivated pulsatile GH secretion in these patients and the high serum levels of GH binding protein clearly delineate the distinct pathophysiological paradigm

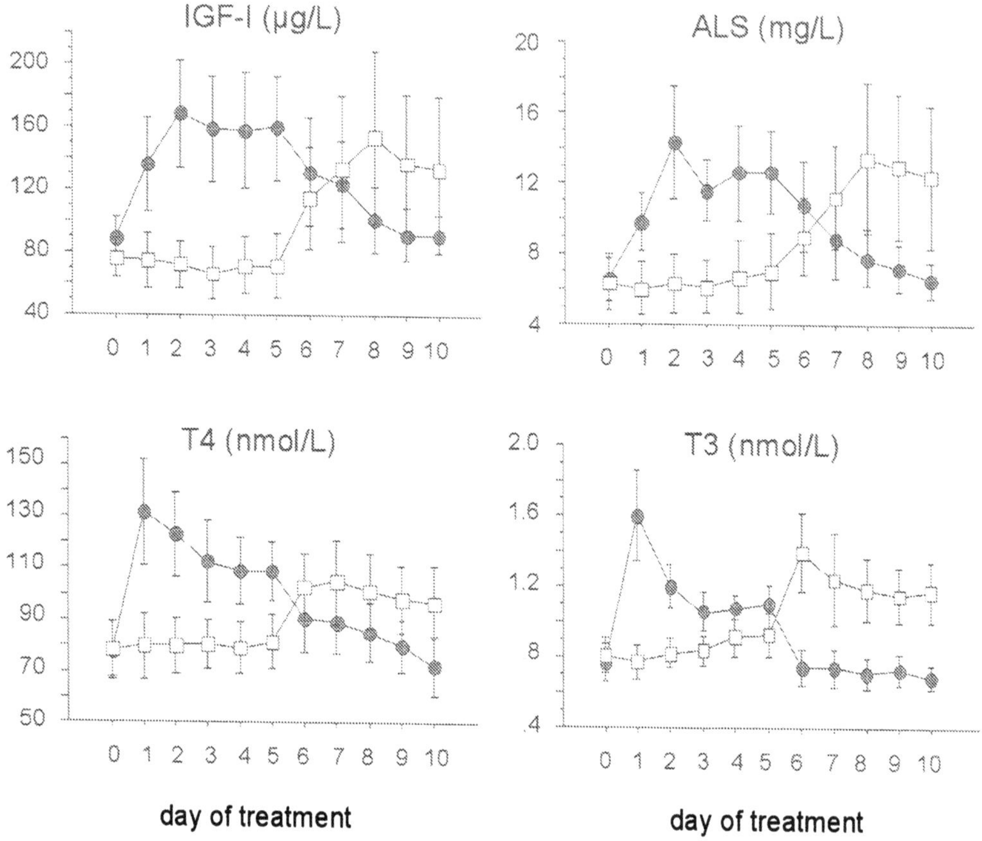

Fig. 6. Serum concentrations (mean ± SEM) of IGF-I, ALS, T4, and T3 in response to a randomized treatment with either 5 d GHRP-2 + TRH infusion (1 + 1 μg/kg/h) followed by 5 d placebo (filled symbols) or 5 d placebo followed by 5 d GHRP-2 + TRH infusion (1 + 1 μg/kg/h) (open symbols) in a group of 10 male and 4 female prolonged critically ill patients. All $p < 0.0001$ with analysis of variance. The mean age of the patients was 68 yr. The mean intensive care stay at the time of study start was 40 d. Adapted with permission from ref. *1*.

present in the chronic phase of critical illness as opposed to the acute phase, which is thought to be primarily a condition of GH-resistance. After 2 d of treatment with GHRP, (near) normal levels of IGF-I, IGFBP-3, IGFBP-5, and ALS are reached and, as shown in a subsequent study, maintained for at least up to 5 d (Fig. 6) *(5)*. GH secretion after 5 d of treatment with GH secretagogues was found to be lower than after 2 d, suggesting active feedback inhibition loops that prevented overtreatment *(5,31)*. In this study in which GHRP was infused together with thyrotropin-releasing hormone (TRH) for 5 d (*see* Section 6), the self-limited endocrine responses induced a shift towards anabolism at the level of several peripheral tissues, as indicated by a rise in serum levels of osteocalcin, insulin, and leptin and a decrease in urea production *(5)*.

Usually, infusion of GHRP without GHRH suffices to reactivate pulsatile GH secretion sufficiently in the prolonged critically ill patient and to elicit the IGF-I and IGFBP responses in prolonged critical illness. However, in critically ill men, particularly those men who are being treated in the intensive care unit for a very long time (several weeks), it may be necessary to add a low dose of GHRH (0.1 μg/kg/h) (ref. *1*; Van den Berghe G, unpublished observations) because of the simultaneous lack of endogenous GHRH activity accompanying the reduced availability of the GHRP-like ligand *(4)*.

6. INTERACTION OF THE IGF SYSTEM WITH THE THYROID AND GONADAL AXES DURING CRITICAL ILLNESS

The acute and prolonged phase of critical illness is also characterized by distinct changes within the thyroid axis and the gonadal axis. Within 2 h after onset of severe physical stress, such as surgery or trauma, serum levels of T3 decrease, whereas T4 and thyroid-stimulating hormone (TSH) briefly rise *(45)*. Apparently, low T3 levels at that stage are mainly caused by a decreased peripheral conversion of T4 to T3 *(46)*. Subsequently, circulating TSH and T4 levels often return to "normal" whereas T3 levels remain low. Although mean serum TSH concentrations are indistinguishable from normal values at that time point, the normal nocturnal TSH surge has been shown to be absent *(47,48)*. The decrease in serum T3 during the first 24 h has been found to reflect severity of illness *(49,50)*. Although cytokines are capable of mimicking the acute stress-induced alterations in thyroid status, cytokine antagonism in sick mice failed to restore normal thyroid function *(51)*. Low concentrations of binding proteins and inhibition of hormone binding, transport, and metabolism by elevated levels of free fatty acids and bilirubin have been proposed as factors contributing to the low T3 syndrome at the tissue level *(52)*. Teleologically, the acute changes in the thyroid axis have been interpreted as an attempt to reduce energy expenditure at least when they occur during starvation *(53)* and thus as an appropriate response that does not warrant intervention. Whether this is also applicable to other acute stress conditions, such as surgery, infection, or the initial phase of critical illness, is still a matter of controversy *(54–56)*.

Patients treated in intensive care units for several weeks, however, present with a different set of changes within the thyroid axis. A single sample usually reveals low or low-normal TSH values and low T4 and T3 serum concentrations *(57)*. However, overnight repeated sampling revealed that, essentially, the pulsatility in the TSH secretory pattern is dramatically diminished and that, as for the GH axis, it is the loss of TSH pulse amplitude which is related to low serum levels of thyroid hormone *(57)*. Moreover, Fliers and co-workers elegantly provided evidence for reduced expression of the TRH gene in hypothalamic paraventricular nuclei in the chronic phase of illness *(58)*. Together, these findings point to reduced hypothalamic stimulation of the thyrotrophs, leading to reduced drive of the thyroid gland in this phase. A rise of TSH marking onset of recovery from severe illness *(59)* is in line with this concept. Because circulating cytokine levels are usually much lower at that stage *(60)*, other mechanisms operational within the central nervous system are presumably involved. Endogenous dopamine and prolonged hypercortisolism may each play a role because exogenous dopamine as well as glucocorticoids are known to provoke or severely aggravate hypothyroidism in critical illness *(61,62)*. Low thyroid hormone levels in protracted critical illness correlate inversely with urea production and bone degradation which could reflect either an adaptive, protective mechanism against hypercatabolism or its cause *(5)*. However, restoring physiological levels of thyroid hormones by continuously infusing TRH (together with a GH secretagogue) (Fig. 7) was found to reduce

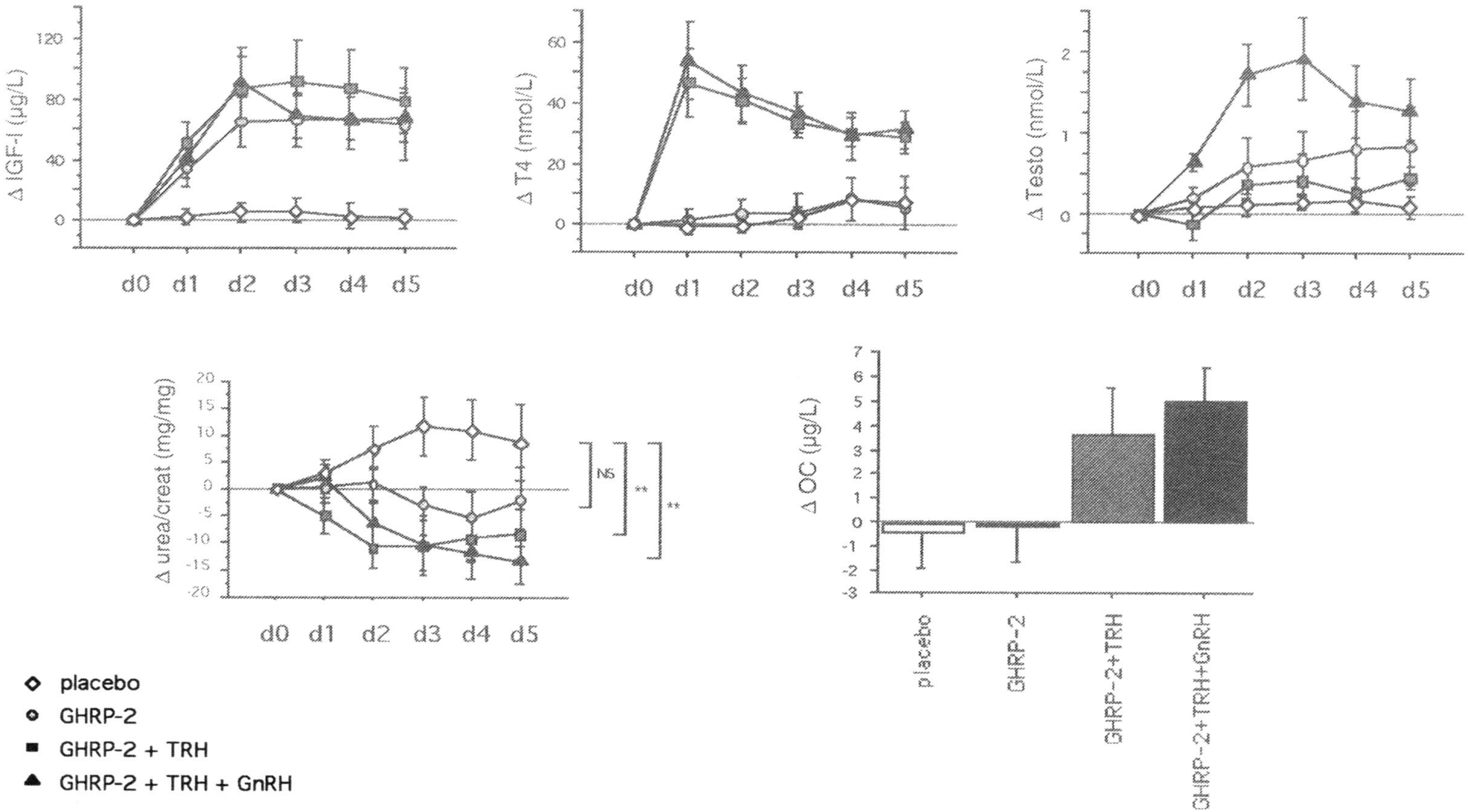

Fig. 7. Results of a prospective, randomized study of 32 men with prolonged critical illness who were treated for 5 d with either placebo, continuous GHRP-2 infusion (1 μg/kg/h), continuous GHRP-2 + TRH infusion (1 + 1 μg/kg/h), or continuous GHRP-2 + TRH infusion (1 + 1 μg/kg/h) + GnRH pulses of 0.1 μg/kg every 90 min. Serum IGF-I concentrations increased equally in all groups who had GHRP-2 in the treatment schedule; serum T4 concentrations rose equally in the two groups who received TRH and serum testosterone rose only in the group who also received GnRH pulses. Anabolic tissue responses, such as reduced protein breakdown in skeletal muscle and new bone formation, occurred only in the groups treated with GHRP-2 + TRH and with GHRP-2 + TRH + GnRH, but not with GHRP-2 alone, as reflected by the studied biochemical markers. This indicates that tissue "IGF-I-resistance" in critical illness may be partly explained by the concomitant suppression of the thyroid axis and the gonadal axis. Adapted, with permission from ref. *69*.

rather than increase hypercatabolism *(5,63)*, an effect that was related only to thyroid hormone changes. During TRH infusion in prolonged critical illness, the negative feedback exerted by thyroid hormones upon the thyrotrophs was found to be maintained, thus precluding overstimulation of the thyroid axis *(31)*. This self-limitation may be extremely important during critical illness in order to avoid hyperthyroidism, which would inadvertently aggravate catabolism. The coinfusion of TRH and GH-releasing factors appears a better strategy than the infusion of TRH alone because the combination, but not TRH alone, avoids a rise in circulating reverse T3 *(31)*. The latter may point to the effect of GH on the activity of type I deiodinase and eventually to other important interactions among different anterior pituitary axes for optimal peripheral responses *(5)*. It remains controversial, however, whether correction of the low serum and tissue concentrations of T3 by either T4 or T3 administration is required to improve clinical problems distinctively associated with prolonged critical illness *(64–68)*. In contrast to treatment with thyroid hormones, infusing TRH allows for peripheral shifts in thyroid hormone metabolism during intercurrent events and, accordingly, permits the body to elaborate appropriate concentrations of thyroid hormones in the circulation and at tissue level, thus setting the scene for a safer treatment than the administration of T3 *(5,31)*.

Also the peripheral tissue responses to the normalization of serum concentrations of IGF-I and binding proteins as evoked by GHRP infusion seem to depend on the coinfusion of TRH and the concomitant normalization of the thyroid axis. Indeed, GHRP-2 infused alone evokes identical increments in serum concentrations of IGF-I, IGFBP-3, and ALS but is devoid of the anabolic tissue responses that are present with the combined infusion of GHRP and TRH (Fig. 7) *(69)*. Outcome benefit of TRH infusion alone or in combination with growth hormone-secretagogues in prolonged critical illness is yet to be studied.

For luteinizing hormone (LH), too, the pulsatility in the secretory pattern is important for its bioactivity *(70,71)*. Because testosterone is the most important endogenous anabolic steroid, changes within the LH/testosterone axis in the male could be relevant for the catabolic state of critical illness. A variety of catabolic states are indeed accompanied by low serum testosterone levels in men. These conditions include starvation *(72,73)*, the postoperative phase *(74)*, myocardial infarction *(75,76)*, burn injury *(8,77)*, psychological and physical stress *(79,80)*, and prolonged critical illness *(69,81,82)*.

The low serum testosterone concentrations despite elevated LH levels documented during the acute stress of surgery or myocardial infarction *(74,76)* suggest an immediate stress-induced Leydig cell suppression, the exact cause of which remains obscure. A role for inflammatory cytokines (interleukin-1 and interleukin-2) is possible, as suggested by experimental studies *(83,84)*. It may be considered appropriate that the secretion of anabolic androgens be switched off in circumstances of acute stress to reduce the consumption of energy and substrates for, at that time at least, less vital functions. When a severe stress condition, like critical illness, becomes prolonged, hypogonadotrophism is present *(77,85)*. Concomitantly, circulating levels of testosterone become extremely low (often undetectable) in men. Total estradiol levels also appear somewhat low but in view of suppressed levels of sex hormone binding globulin, it can be inferred that bioavailable estradiol levels are maintained. This points to increased aromatization of androgens *(82)*. The progressive decrease of serum gonadotrophin levels appears to lag behind the rapid decline in serum testosterone *(75,76,86)*. In prolonged critically ill men, a preserved LH pulse frequency with an abnormally low LH pulse amplitude has been observed *(81)*, which was interpreted as an impaired compensatory LH hypersecretion in response to the very low serum testosterone levels. Endogenous dopamine, opiates, and in particular the maintained bioactive estradiol levels *(82)* could be involved in the pathogenesis of hypogonadotrophism *(69,81,82,87)*. Animal data suggest that prolonged exposure of the brain to interleukin-1 may also play a role through the suppression of gonadotropin-releasing hormone (GnRH) synthesis *(83)*. Pioneering studies evaluating the effects of androgen treatment in prolonged critical illness failed to demonstrate conclusive clinical benefit *(88)*. In view of the secretory characteristics of the other anterior pituitary hormones, we recently investigated the therapeutic potential of GnRH pulses in prolonged critically ill men, alone *(82)* and together with GHRP-2 and TRH *(69)*. GnRH alone appears only partially and transiently effective *(82)*. However, when GnRH pulses were given together with GHRP-2 and TRH infusion, superior target organ responses and anabolic effects followed (Fig. 7) that were far more pronounced than with either of the compounds separately. These data underline the importance of correcting all the hypothalamic/pituitary defects instead of applying a single hormone treatment.

7. SUMMARY AND CONCLUSIONS

Low circulating levels of IGF-I and alterations in IGFBPs mark the hypercatabolic state of critical illness. The origin of these changes appears different during the first hours to days after onset and in the more chronic phase of critical illness. The changes immediately after onset of severe illness or after trauma are low serum concentrations of IGF-I, IGFBP-3, and the ALS in the presence of activated GH secretion, indicating peripheral GH resistance. Reduced GH receptor expression and/or impairment of GH signaling at the intracellular level may play a role. In addition, increased IGFBP-3 protease activity in serum as well as increased circulating levels of IGFBP-1 may alter IGF-I tissue availability. When recovery does not follow within hours to days and critical illness becomes prolonged, GH secretion is no longer elevated and sometimes low, and the GH secretory pattern becomes erratic and almost nonpulsatile. The reduced pulsatile component of GH secretion in this phase appears to contribute to inadequate generation of GH-dependent IGF-I and binding proteins, such as ALS, IGFBP-3, and IGFBP-5, and to impaired anabolism. High IGFBP-1 and low insulin levels predict a fatal outcome for prolonged critical illness, and serum concentrations of IGFBP-2, IGFBP-4, and IGFBP-6 are uniformly elevated. Continuous infusion of GH-secretagogues, either GHRP and/or GHRH, reactivates pulsatile GH secretion in prolonged critical illness and evokes a proportionate rise in the IGF-I and the ternary complex binding proteins IGFBP-3, ALS, and IGFBP-5, indicating recovery of GH responsiveness in this phase of illness. However, only when GH secretagogues are infused together with TRH, whereby the very low circulating levels of thyroid hormones are also normalized, does metabolic improvement ensue. This suggests a form of "IGF-I resistance" that can be resolved by also correcting the concomitant tertiary hypothyroidism. Biphasic changes are also present within the gonadotrope and corticotrope axes. Pulsatile GnRH administration alone is unable to restore the tertiary hypogonadism present in prolonged critical illness. However, when GnRH is administered together with GHRP and TRH infusion, LH secretion can be reamplifed and circulating testosterone levels increased evoking superior endocrine and anabolic effects compared with those obtained by either of the releasing factors separately. These studies indicate a fundamental transition between acute and prolonged critical illness within the IGF system, from acute GH resistance to a state of low (pulsatile) GH (and TSH and LH) secretion but recovered GH responsiveness. Treatment with releasing factors (GH secretagogues, TRH, and GnRH) takes advantage of active feedback inhibition loops and thus prevents overstimulation. Hence, this strategy may not only be a more effective but also a safer one than the administration of high-dose GH *(89)* and/or IGF-I to counter the catabolic state in prolonged critical illness.

ACKNOWLEDGMENTS

Supported by Research grants from the Belgian Fund for Scientific Research (G. 0144.00 and G.3C05.95N), the Research Council of the University of Leuven (OT 99/32), and the Belgian Foundation for Research in Congenital Heart Diseases.

REFERENCES

1. Van den Berghe G. Novel insights into the neuroendocrinology of critical illness. Eur J Endocrinol 2000;143:1–13.
2. Carroll PV. Protein metabolism and the use of growth hormone and insulin-like growth factor-I in the critically ill patient. GH IGF Res 1999;9:400–413.
3. Streat SJ, Beddoe AH, Hill GL. Aggressive nutritional support does not prevent protein loss despite fat gain in septic intensive care patients. J Trauma 1987;27:262–266.
4. Van den Berghe G, Baxter RC, Weekers F, Wouters P, Bowers CY, Veldhuis JD. A paradoxical gender dissociation within the growth hormone / insulin-like growth factor I axis during protracted critical illness. J Clin Endocrinol Metab 2000;85:183–192.
5. Van den Berghe G, Wouters P, Weekers F, Mohan S, Baxter RC, Veldhuis JD, Bowers CY, Bouillon R. Reactivation of pituitary hormone release and metabolic improvement by infusion of growth hormone releasing peptide and thyrotropin-releasing hormone in patients with protracted critical illness. J Clin Endocrinol Metab 1999;84:1311–1323.
6. Van den Berghe G, Weekers F, Baxter RC, Wouters P, Iranmanesh A, Bouillon R, Veldhuis JD. Five days pulsatile GnRH administration unveils combined hypothalamic-pituitary-gonadal defects underlying profound hypoandrogenism in men with prolonged critical illness. J Clin Endocrinol Metab 2001;86:3217–3226
7. Knaus WA, Draper EA, Wagner DP, Zimmerman JE. APACHE II: a severity of disease classification system. Crit Care Med 1985;13:818–829.
8. Le Roith D. Insulin-like growth factors. N Engl J Med 1997;336:633–640.
9. Thorner MO, Vance ML, Laws ER, et al. The anterior pituitary. In: Williams Textbook of Endocrinology. Wilson JD, Foster DW, Kronenberg HM, Larsen PR, (eds.). W.B. Saunders Company, Philadelphia, 1998, pp. 249–340.
10. Van den Berghe G, de Zegher F, Bouillon R. Acute and prolonged critical illness as different neuroendocrine paradigms. J Clin Endocrinol Metab 1998;83:1827–1834.
11. Baxter RC, Hawker FH, To C, Stewart PM, Holman SR. Thirty day monitoring of insulin-like growth factors and their binding proteins in intensive care unit patients. Growth Horm IGF Res 1998;8:455–463.
12. Hermansson M, Wickelgren RB, Hammarqvist F, Bjarnason R, Wennstrom I, Wernerman J, et al. Measurement of human growth hormone receptor messenger ribonucleic acid by a quantitative polymerase chain reaction-based assay: demonstration of reduced expression after elective surgery. J Clin Endocrinol Metab 1997;82:421–428.
13. Mao Y, Ling PR, Fitzgibbons TP, McCowen KC, Frick GP, Bistrian BR, et al. Endotoxin-induced inhibition of growth hormone receptor signaling in rat liver in vivo. Endocrinology 1999;140:5505–5515.

14. Isley WL, Underwood LE, Clemmons DR. Dietary components that regulate serum somatomedin-C concentrations in humans. J Clin Invest 1983:71:175–182.
15. Noel GL, Suh HK, Stone JG, Frantz AG. Human prolactin and growth hormone release during surgery and other conditions of stress. J Clin Endocrinol Metab 1972;35:840–851.
16. Jeffries MK, Vance ML. Growth hormone and cortisol secretion in patients with burn injury. J Burn Care Rehabil 1992;13:391–395.
17. Bowers CY, Momany FA, Reynolds GA, Hong A. On the in vitro and in vivo activity of a new synthetic hexapeptide that acts on the pituitary to specifically release growth hormone. Endocrinology 1984;114:1537–1545.
18. Howard AD, Feighner SD, Cully DF, Arena JP, Liberator PA, Rosenblum CI, et al. A receptor in pituitary and hypothalamus that functions in growth hormone release. Science 1996;273:974–977.
19. Kojima M, Hosoda H, Date Y, Nakazato M, Matsuo H, Kangawa K. Ghrelin is a growth-hormone-releasing acylated peptide from stomach. Nature 1999;402:656–660.
20. Gevers EF, Wit JM, Robinson IC. Growth, growth hormone (GH) binding protein, and GH receptors are differentially regulated by peak and trough components of GH secretory pattern in the rat. Endocrinology 1996;137:1013–1018.
21. Giustina A, Veldhuis JD. Pathophysiology of the neuroregulation of growth hormone secretion in experimental animals and the human. Endocr Rev 1998;19:717–797.
22. Hindmarsh PC, Dennison E, Pincus SM, Cooper C, Fall CH, Matthews DR, et al. A sexually dimorphic pattern of growth hormone secretion in the elderly illness. J Clin Endocrinol Metab 1999;84:2679–2685.
23. Ross R, Miell J, Freeman E, Jones J, Matthews D, Preece M, et al. Critically ill patients have high basal growth hormone levels with attenuated oscillatory activity associated with low levels of insulin-like growth factor-1. Clin Endocrinol 1991;35:47–54.
24. Voerman HJ, Strack van Schijndel RJM, de Boer H, van der Veen EA, Thijs LG. Growth hormone: secretion and administration in catabolic adult patients, with emphasis on the critically ill patient. Neth J Med 1992;41:229–244.
25. Hartman ML, Veldhuis JD, Johnson ML, Lee MM, Alberti KG, Samojlik E, et al. Augmented growth hormone secretory burst frequency and amplitude mediate enhanced GH secretion during a two day fast in normal men. J Clin Endocrinol Metab 1992;74:757–765.
26. Bentham J, Rodriguez-Arnao-J, Ross RJ. Acquired growth hormone resistance in patients with hypercatabolism. Horm Res 1993;40:87–91.
27. Timmins AC, Cotterill AM, Cwyfan Hughes SC, et al. Critical illness is associated with low circulating concentrations of insulin-like growth factors-I and -II, alterations in insulin-like growth factor binding proteins, and induction of an insulin-like growth factor binding protein-3 protease. Crit Care Med 1996;24:1460–1466.
28. Gibson FA, Hinds CJ. Growth hormone and insulin-like growth factors in critical illness. Intensive Care Med 1997;23:369–378.
29. Rodriguez-Arnao J, Yarwood Y, Ferguson C, et al. Reduction in circulating IGF-I and hepatic IGF-I mRNA levels after ceacal ligation and puncture are associated with differential regulation of hepatic IGF-binding protien-1, -2 and -3 mRNA levels. J Endocrinol 1996;151:287–292.
30. Van den Berghe G, de Zegher F, Veldhuis JD, Wouters P, Awouters M, Verbruggen W, et al. The somatotropic axis in critical illness: effect of continuous GHRH and GHRP-2 infusion. J Clin Endocrinol Metab 1997;82:590–599.
31. Van den Berghe G, de Zegher F, Baxter RC, Veldhuis JD, Wouters P, Schetz M, et al. Neuroendocrinology of prolonged critical illness: effect of continuous thyrotropin-releasing hormone infusion and its combination with growth hormone-secretagogues. J Clin Endocrinol Metab 1998;83:309–319.
32. Van den Berghe G, de Zegher F, Lauwers P, Veldhuis JD . Growth hormone secretion in critical illness: effect of dopamine. J Clin Endocrinol Metab 1994;79:1141–1146.
33. Van den Berghe G, de Zegher F. Anterior pituitary function during critical illness and dopamine treatment. Crit Care Med 1996;24:1580–1590.
34. Yeoh SI, Baxter RC. Metabolic regulation of the growth hormone independent insulin-like growth factor binding protein in human plasma. Acta Endocrinol 1988;119:465–473.
35. Lewitt MS, Baxter RC. Regulation of growth hormone-independent insulin-like growth factor-binding protein (BP-28) in cultured human fetal liver explants. J Clin Endocrinol Metab 1989;69:246–252.

36. Lewitt MS, Baxter RC. Inhibitors of glucose uptake stimulate the production of insulin-like growth factor binding protein (IGFBP-1) by human fetal liver. Endocrinology 1990;126:1527–1533.
37. Baxter RC. Circulating binding proteins for the insulin-like growth factors. TEM 1993;4:91–96.
38. Norrelund H, Fisker S, Vahl N, Borglum J, Richelsen B, Christiansen JS, et al. Evidence supporting a direct suppressive effect of growth hormone on serum IGFBP-1 levels, experimental studies in normal, obese and GH-deficient adults. Growth Horm IGF Res 1999;9:52–60.
39. Olivecrona H, Hilding A, Ekström C, et al. Acute and short-term effects of growth hormone on insulin-like growth factors and their binding proteins: serum levels and hepatic messenger ribonucleic acid responses in humans. J Clin Endocrinol Metab 1999;84:553–560.
40. Delhanty PJD, Baxter RC. The regulation of acid-labile subunit gene expression and secretion by cyclic adenosine 3′,5′-monophosphate. Endocrinology 1998;139:260–265.
41. Hu M, Robertson DG, Murphy LJ. Growth hormone modulates insulin regulation of hepatic insulin-like growth factor binding protein-1 transcription. Endocrinology 1996;137:3702–3709.
42. Van den Berghe G, Wouters P, Weekers F, Verwaest C, Bruyninckx F, Schetz M, et al. Intensive insulin therapy in critically ill patients. N Engl J Med 2001;345:1359–1367.
43. Micic D, Popovic V, Doknic M, Macut D, Dieguez C, Casanueva FF. Preserved growth hormone (GH) secretion in aged and very old subjects after testing with the combined stimulus GH-releasing hormone plus GH-releasing hexapeptide-6. J Clin Endocrinol Metab 1998;83:2569–2572.
44. Van den Berghe G, de Zegher F, Bowers CY, Wouters P, Muller P, Soetens F, et al. Pituitary responsiveness to growth hormone (GH) releasing hormone, GH-releasing peptide-2 and thyrotropin releasing hormone in critical illness. Clin Endocrinol 1996;45:341–351.
45. Michalaki M, Vagenakis A, Makri M, Kalfarentoz F, Kyriazopoulou V. Dissociation of the early decline in serum T(3) concentration and serum IL-6 rise and TNFalpha in nonthyroidal illness syndrome induced by abdominal surgery. J Clin Endocrinol Metab. 2001;86:4198–4205.
46. Chopra IJ, Huang TS, Beredo A, Solomon DH, Chua Teco GN, Mead JF. Evidence for an inhibitor of extrathyroidal conversion of thyroxine to 3,5,3′-triiodothyronine in sera of patients with nonthyroidal illness. J Clin Endocrinol Metab 1985;60:666–672.
47. Romijn JA, Wiersinga WM. Decreased nocturnal surge of thyrotropin in nonthyroidal illness. J Clin Endocrinol Metab 1990;70:35–42.
48. Bartalena L, Martino E, Brandi LS, Falcone M, Pacchiarotti A, Ricci C, et al. Lack of nocturnal serum thyrotropin surge after surgery. J Clin Endocrinol Metab 1990;70:293–296.
49. Schlienger JL, Sapin R, Capgras T, Gasser F, Monassier JP, Hauer B, et al. Evaluation of thyroid function after myocardial infarction. Ann d'Endocrinol 1991;52:283–288.
50. Rothwell PM, Lawler PG. Prediction of outcome in intensive care patients using endocrine parameters. Crit Care Med 1995;23:78–83.
51. van der Poll T, van Zee K, Endert E, Coyle S, Stiles D, Prible J, et al. Interleukin-1 receptor blockade does not affect endotoxin-induced changes in plasma thyroid hormone and thyrotropin concentration in man. J Clin Endocrinol Metab 1995;80:1341–1346.
52. Lim CF, Doctor R, Visser TJ, Krenning EP, Bernard B, van Toor H, et al. Inhibition of thyroxine transport into cultured rat hepatocytes by serum of non-uremic critically ill patients: effects of bilirubin and non-esterified fatty acids. J Clin Endocrinol Metab 1993;76:1165–1172.
53. Gardner DF, Kaplan MM, Stanley CA, Utiger RD. Effect of triiodothyronine replacement on the metabolic and pituitary responses to starvation. N Engl J Med 1979;300:579–584.
54. De Groot LJ. Dangerous dogmas in medicine: the non-thyroidal illness syndrome. J Clin Endocrinol Metab 1999;84:151–164.
55. Kemperer JD, Klein I, Gomez M, Helm RE, Ojamaa K, Thomas SJ, et al. Thyroid hormone treatment after coronary bypass surgery. N Engl J Med 1995;333:1522–1527.
56. Mullis-Jansson SL, Argenziano M, Corwin S, Homma S, Weinberg AD, Williams M, et al. A randomized double blind study on the effect of triiodothyronine on cardiac function and morbidity after coronary bypass surgery. J Thoracic Cardiovasc Surg 1999;117:1128–1134.
57. Van den Berghe G, de Zegher F, Veldhuis JD, Wouters P, Gouwy S, Stockman W, et al. Thyrotropin and prolactin release in prolonged critical illness: dynamics of spontaneous secretion and effects of growth hormone secretagogues. Clin Endocrinol 1997;47:599–612.
58. Fliers E, Guldenaar SEF, Wiersinga WM, Swaab DF. Decreased hypothalamic thyrotropin-releasing hormone gene expression in patients with non-thyroidal illness. J Clin Endocrinol Metab 1997;82:4032–4036.

59. Bacci V, Schussler GC, Kaplan TC. The relationship between serum triiodothyronine and thyrotropin during systemic illness. J Clin Endocrinol Metab 1982;54:1229–1235.
60. Damas P, Reuter A, Gysen P, Demonty J, Lamy M, Franchimont P. Tumor necrosis factor and interleukin-1 serum levels during severe sepsis in humans. Crit Care Med 1989;17:975–978.
61. Faglia G, Ferrari C, Beck-Peccoz P, Spada A, Travaglini P, Ambrosi B. Reduced plasma thyrotropin response to thyrotropin releasing hormone after dexamethasone administration in normal humans. Horm Metat Res 1973;5:289–291.
62. Van den Berghe G, de Zegher F, Lauwers P. Dopamine and the sick euthyroid syndrome in critical illness. Clin Endocrinol 1994;41:731–737.
63. Van den Berghe G, Wouters P, Bowers CY, de Zegher F, Bouillon R, Veldhuis JD. Growth hormone releasing peptide-2 infusion synchronizes growth hormone, thyrotropin and prolactin secretion in prolonged critical illness. Eur J Endocrinol 1999;140:17–22.
64. Arem R, Wiener GJ, Kaplan SG, Kim HS, Reichlin S, Kaplan MM. Reduced tissue thyroid hormone levels in fatal illness. Metabolism 1993;42:1102–1108.
65. Vaughan GM, Mason AD, McManus WF, Pruitt BA Jr. Alterations of mental status and thyroid hormones after thermal injury. J Clin Endocrinol Metab 1985;60:1221–1225.
66. Brent GA, Hershman JM. Thyroxine therapy in patients with severe non-thyroidal illnesses and low serum thyroxine concentrations. J Clin Endocrinol Metab 1986;63:1–7.
67. Becker RA, Vaughan GM, Ziegler MG, Seraille LG, Goldfarb IW, Mansour EH, et al. Hypermetabolic low triiodothyronine syndrome in burn injury. Crit Care Med 1982;10:870–875.
68. Bettendorf M, Schmidt KG, Grulich-Henn J, Ulmer HE, Heinrich UE. Triiodothyronine treatment in children after cardiac surgery: a double-blind, randomized, placebo-controlled study. Lancet 2000;356:529–534.
69. Van den Berghe G, Baxter RC, Weekers F, Wouters P, Bowers CY, Iranmanesh A, Veldhuis JD, Bouillon R. The combined administration of GH-releasing peptide-2 (GHRP-2), TRH and GnRH to men with prolonged critical illness evokes superior endocrine and metabolic effects than treatment with GHRP-2 alone. Clin Endocrinol 2002;56:655–669.
70. Belchetz PE, Plant TM, Nakai Y, Keogh EJ, Knobil E. Hypophyseal responses to continuous and intermittent delivery of hypothalamic gonadotropin-releasing hormone. Science 1978;202:631–633.
71. Santoro N, Filicori M, Crowley WF Jr. Hypogonadotropic disorders in men and women: diagnosis and therapy with pulsatile gonadotropin releasing hormone. Endocr Rev 1986;7:11–23.
72. Klibanski A, Beitens IZ, Badger TM, Little R, McArthur J. Reproductive function during fasting in man. J Clin Endocrinol Metab 1981;53:258–266.
73. Veldhuis JD, Iranmanesh A, Evans WS, Lizarralde G, Thorner MO, Vance ML. Amplitude suppression of the pulsatile mode of immunoradiometric LH release in fasting-induced hypoandrogenemia in normal men. J Clin Endocrinol Metab 1993;76:587–593.
74. Wang C, Chan V, Yeung RTT. Effect of surgical stress on pituitary-testicular function. Clin Endocrinol 1978;9:255–266.
75. Wang C, Chan V, Tse TF, Yeung RT. Effect of acute myocardial infarction on pituitary testicular function. Clin Endocrinol 1978;9:249–253.
76. Dong Q, Hawker F, McWilliam D, Bangah M, Burger H, Handelsman DJ. Circulating immunoreactive inhibin and testosterone levels in patients with critical illness. Clin Endocrinol 1992;36:399–404.
77. Vogel AV, Peake GT, Rada RT. Pituitary-testicular axis dysfunction in burned men. J Clin Endocrinol Metab 1985;60:658–665.
78. Lephart ED, Baxter CR, Parker CR jr. Effect of burn trauma on adrenal and testicular steroid hormone production. J Clin Endocrinol Metab 1987;64:842–848.
79. Kreutz LD, Rose RM, Jennings JR. Suppression of plasma testosterone levels and psychological stress: a longitudinal study of young men in officer candidate school. Arch Gen Psych 1972;26:479–482.
80. Aakvaag A, Bentdal O, Quigstad K, Walstad P, Ronningen H, Fonnum F. Testosterone and testosterone binding globulin in young men during prolonged stress. Int J Androl 1978;1:22–31.
81. Van den Berghe G, de Zegher F, Lauwers P, Veldhuis JD. Luteinizing hormone secretion and hypoandrogenemia in critically ill men: effect of dopamine. Clin Endocrinol 1994;41:563–569.
82. Van den Berghe G, Weekers F, Baxter RC, Wouters P, Iranmanesh A, Bouillon R, Veldhuis JD. Five days pulsatile GnRH administration unveils combined hypothalamic-pituitary-gonadal defects under-

lying profound hypoandrogenism in men with prolonged critical illness. J Clin Endocrinol Metab 2001;86:3217–3226.
83. Rivier C, Vale W. In the rat, interleukin 1-a acts at the level of the brain and the gonads to interfere with gonadotropin and sex steroid secretion. Endocrinology 1989;124:2105–210.
84. Guo H, Calkins JH, Sigel MM, Lin T. Interleukin-2 is a potent inhibitor of Leydig cell steroidogenesis. Endocrinology 1990;127:1234–1239.
85. Woolf PD, Hamill RW, McDonald JV, Lee LA, Kelly M. Transient hypogonadotropic hypogonadism caused by critical illness. J Clin Endocrinol Metab 1985;60:444–450.
86. Spratt DI, Cox P, Orav J, Moloney J, Bigos T. Reproductive axis suppression in acute illness is related to disease severity. J Clin Endocrinol Metab 1993;76:1548–1554.
87. Cicero TJ, Bell RD, Wiest WG, Allison JH, Polakoski K, Robins E. Function of the male sex organs in heroin and methadone users. N Engl J Med 1975;292:882–887.
88. Tweedle D, Walton C, Johnston IDA. The effect of an anabolic steroid on postoperative nitrogen balance. Br J Clin Pract 1972;27:130–132.
89. Takala J, Ruokonen E, Webster NR, Nielsen MS, Zandstra DF, Vundelinckx G, Hinds CJ. Increased mortality associated with growth hormone treatment in critically ill adults. N Engl J Med 1999;341:785–792.

17 Mechanisms of Cardiac Hypertrophy and the Development of Heart Failure

Role of Insulin-Like Growth Factor-I and Angiotensin-II

Patrice Delafontaine, Marijke Brink, and Yao-Hua Song

KEY POINTS

- The RAS and the IGF-I system interact at multiple levels to regulate physiological and pathological cardiac growth responses.
- IGF-I promotes growth and survival of cardiac and skeletal muscle which is salutary in heart failure.
- AngII down regulates circulating and skeletal muscle IGF-I and IGF binding proteins, leading to increased myocardial apoptosis and increased skeletal muscle proteolysis.
- Preliminary studies reveal significant alterations in the IGF-I system in heart failure.
- An imbalance between the RAS and the IGF-I system contributes to the progression from compensated to decompensated heart failure.

1. INTRODUCTION

The renin-angiotensin system (RAS) and the insulin growth factor (IGF)-I system interact at multiple levels to regulate both physiological and pathological cardiac growth responses. Through its growth and antiapoptotic effects, IGF-I promotes physiological cardiac growth, whereas chronic angiotensin-II (angII) stimulation promotes left ventricular remodeling and progressive heart failure. Angiotensin-II downregulates circulating and skeletal muscle IGF-I and IGF binding proteins, leading to increased myocardial apoptosis and increased skeletal muscle protein degradation. In addition, angiotensin II interferes with IGF-I receptor signaling. IGF-I, through a variety of mechanisms, including a depressor effect on the cardiac RAS, promotes physiological cardiac growth responses, reduces apoptosis, and has anabolic effects on skeletal muscle, all of which are beneficial in chronic heart failure. Our preliminary studies reveal significant alterations in total IGF-I, free IGF-I, and IGF binding proteins in patients with congestive heart failure, and some of these changes are related to increased angiotensin II. Further elucidation of the crosstalk between the IGF-I system and the

From: *IGF and Nutrition in Health and Disease*
Edited by: M. S. Houston, J. M. P. Holly, and E. L. Feldman © Humana Press Inc., Totowa, NJ

RAS will likely lead to significant advances in the understanding of the cachexia of heart failure and treatment of patients with cardiovascular disease.

2. MECHANISMS OF CARDIAC HYPERTROPHY AND THE DEVELOPMENT OF HEART FAILURE: ROLE OF IGF-I AND ANGII

When stimulated by a variety of neurohumoral factors or when faced with an increase in ventricular-wall tension, cardiomyocytes undergo hypertrophic growth as an adaptive response. However, sustained cardiac hypertrophy is a leading predictor of the subsequent development of heart failure (reviewed by Colucci et al., ref. *1*). A number of neurohumoral factors, including norepinephrine, angII, endothelin, IGF-I and tumor necrosis factor (TNF)-α *(2)*, are potential stimuli for myocyte hypertrophy. However, the contribution of each of these factors in the transition between initial compensated cardiac hypertrophy through decompensated hypertrophy and heart failure are not fully understood. The roles of norepinephrine *(3)*, endothelin *(4)*, and TNF-α *(5–8)* in the development of hypertrophy and progression to heart failure have been reviewed elsewhere. This chapter focuses on the roles of angII and IGF-I.

2.1. AngII and Cardiac Hypertrophy

The RAS is a widely studied hormonal system that comprises substrate-enzyme interactions (reviewed in refs. *9–11*). The kidney produces and releases both renin and its inactive precursor prorenin into the circulation. Liver-derived angiotensinogen is cleaved in the circulating blood by renin to form angI, which is then converted by angiotensin-converting enzyme (ACE), located on the luminal side of the vascular endothelium, into angII. At least two subtypes of angII receptors have been identified: AT1 and AT2 *(9,10)*. The AT1 receptor mediates most of the known actions of angII on blood pressure, cardiac contractility and glomerular filtration, renal tubular sodium reabsorption, and cardiac and vascular hypertrophy. Less is known regarding the function of the AT2 receptor. Evidence suggests that activation of the AT2 receptor inhibits cell proliferation and reverses AT1-induced hypertrophy, although it remains controversial whether AT2 stimulation in the diseased myocardium would actually lead to a net beneficial effect *(11,12)*. AngII type 1A receptor knockout mice display less left ventricular remodeling and improved survival after myocardial infarction *(13)*, indicating that angII plays an important role during the development of heart failure. Agents that interfere with angII formation, the ACE inhibitors in particular, are now widely used for the treatment of hypertension and heart failure (reviewed by Colucci et al. *1*). Both clinical and animal studies indicate that the beneficial effects of ACE inhibitor treatment in heart failure and left ventricular hypertrophy are not solely determined by the effect of ACE inhibition on systemic arterial pressure *(14–20)*.

There is growing evidence to suggest that in cardiac tissue, angII is produced locally and does not originate from circulating angI *(21,22)*. All the components required for angII production are present in the heart. Angiotensinogen and ACE mRNAs have been detected in normal cardiac tissue *(23–26)*. Angiotensinogen mRNA is increased during postinfarction ventricular remodeling in the rat *(24)*, and cardiac ACE mRNA is increased in the setting of pressure overload-induced ventricular hypertrophy in the rat *(25)* and heart failure in humans *(26)*. Increased levels of ACE activity have been found in left ventricular aneurysms of patients after myocardial infarction *(27)*. Thus, cardiac angII formation appears to be regulated independently from the circulating RAS and in animal models and in patients with heart failure, the cardiac RAS is activated and, presumably, local angII formation is enhanced. Historically, angII was only seen as a regulatory hormone that regulated blood pressure, aldosterone release, and sodium reabsorption. Now, it is generally accepted that locally formed angII can regulate the expression of many substances, including growth factors, cytokines, chemokines, and adhesion molecules, which are involved in cell growth, fibrosis, and inflammation *(28–31)*. Interestingly, recent studies have provided evidence that chronically increased angII formation may favor myocyte apoptosis *(32,33)*.

2.2. IGF-I and Cardiac Hypertrophy

IGF-I is a 7.5-kDa protein that is structurally homologous to insulin. IGF-I circulates in blood either free or bound to specific binding proteins *(34,35)*. Six IGF-I binding proteins (IGFBPs) have been identified so far. The circulating IGF-I forms a ternary complex with an acid-labile subunit and the binding proteins. All six IGFBPs are found in the circulation in the free form or in binary complexes with IGFs *(36)*. IGFBP-3 is the most abundant circulating IGFBP; it carries 75% or more of serum IGF-I and IGF-II. IGFBP-5, present at about 10% of the molar concentration of IGFBP-3, can form similar ternary complexes *(36)*. These complexes prolong the half-life of IGF-I in the circulation. Studies using knockout approaches have confirmed that IGF-I in the circulation is primarily produced in the liver, but many cell types can synthesize IGF-I, which can exert autocrine/paracrine effects *(37–42)*. The effects of IGF-I are mediated by the IGF-IR, which is activated by IGF-I and IGF-II, and like the insulin receptor has an $\alpha 2\beta 2$ heterotetrameric structure *(43)*. Once IGF-I binds to the type 1 IGF receptor, it initiates tyrosine autophosphorylation of the receptor and phosphorylation of multiple intermediate substrates, including IRS-1, IRS-2, leading to activation of signaling pathways that include Ras/Raf, phosphatidylinositol 3-kinase (PI3) kinase, and mitogen-activated protein kinase *(43–45)*.

The expression of the various components of the IGF system of ligands (IGF-I/2) and receptors (IGF-IR, IGF-IIR) is ubiquitous throughout intrauterine and postnatal development *(43,46)*. Knockout studies have confirmed that the development of most tissues and organs is regulated to some degree by the IGF system *(47–55)*. Thus, mice lacking either the IGF-I or IGF-II genes exhibited intrauterine growth retardation, and mice lacking a functional IGF-IR gene were born weighing only 45% of normal and died soon after birth from respiratory failure *(47,48,56,57)*. Similarly to its effects in many tissues, IGF-I has multifunctional activities in the heart, including the promotion of cell growth, and thus of DNA, RNA, and protein synthesis; inhibition of apoptosis; and induction of cell differentiation *(58,59)*. In addition, IGF-I promotes myocardial contraction *(60)*, improves hemodynamics and energy metabolism *(61)*, and protects the heart against apoptosis induced by ischemia or oxidative stress *(58,62,63)*.

In a variety of animal models of pressure and volume overload, there is an increase in cardiac IGF-I expression, suggesting that IGF-I promotes the cardiac hypertrophic response *(64–68)*. Our group has shown that angiotensin infusion in rats increases cardiac IGF-I expression concomitantly with the induction of cardiac hypertrophy and that the increase in IGF-I is blocked by hydralazine and thus is likely mediated by a pressor mechanism *(69)*. IGF-I protein was localized to cardiac myocytes. Interestingly, angII infusion also increased cardiac IGF-IR mRNA levels; however, this increase was also seen in sham-infused, pair-fed controls, but not in ad libitum-fed rats, indicating that it was related to the anorexigenic effects of angII and to nutritional intake. IGF-I expression has also been shown to be increased in the human hypertrophic left ventricle *(70)*.

Serneri et al. *(71)* studied cardiac growth factor formation in patients with compensated cardiac hypertrophy defined as end-systolic wall stress (ESS) <90 kdyne/cm^2 or decompensated (ESS >90 kdyne/cm^2) cardiac hypertrophy. Compensated cardiac hypertrophy secondary to aortic regurgitation and aortic stenosis with ESS <90 kdyne/cm^2 was associated with a selective increased formation of IGF-I and mRNA levels for IGF-I were detected mainly in cardiomyocytes. IGF-I formation was closely associated with preserved ventricular contractility. When ESS was >90 kdyne/cm^2, IGF-I synthesis by cardiomyocytes was no longer detectable. In contrast, in these patients with decompensated hypertrophy, there was a significant increase of angII formation, which correlated positively with end-systolic and end-diastolic wall stress. Angiotensinogen mRNA levels were high and were exclusively expressed in the interstitial cells. These data indicated that IGF-I1-induced cardiomyocyte hypertrophy is likely a compensatory response to the increased work load and beneficial to the heart. However, the increase in angII formation in decompensated hypertrophy (which occurs together with a reduction of IGF-I synthesis) could be an important determinant of worsening heart function, potentially via the pro-fibrotic effects of angII *(72)*, which has been demonstrated in several in vitro and in vivo studies *(73,74)*. Indeed, excessive angII formation can produce detrimental effects on overloaded or failing myocytes, including depression of contractility or impaired relaxation *(75)*.

3. APOPTOSIS IN HEART FAILURE: ROLES OF ANGII AND IGF-I

Heart failure results from initial myocardial injury secondary to many causes, such as ischemia, hypertension, myocarditis, toxic causes, for e.g., alcohol, and others (reviewed by Colucci et al., ref. *1*). In response to these conditions, the myocardium initially hypertrophies to compensate for the increased workload. The development of hypertrophy is the result of increased cardiomyocyte size. If the above-mentioned conditions persist, the myocardium will eventually fail to compensate, and patients develop heart failure. During the transition from compensated hypertrophy to decompensated hypertrophy and to heart failure, myocardial cell death occurs. Although some evidence suggests that cardiomyocytes may replicate in vivo *(76)*, these cells are terminally differentiated, and significant replicative repair processes cannot occur. The mechanisms whereby cell death occurs are largely unknown, but emerging evidence indicated that apoptosis might play a major role.

Apoptosis is a highly organized, energy-dependent mechanism whereby a cell commits suicide without causing damage to surrounding tissue and occurs normally during development, tissue turnover, and in the immune system *(77,78)*. In the heart, for instance, apoptosis is involved in postnatal shaping of the right ventricle by eliminating unnecessary cells *(79)*. Morphologically, apoptosis is characterized by cell shrinkage, chromatin condensation, DNA fragmentation, membrane blebbing, and formation of apoptotic bodies. Biochemically, a family of proteases termed caspases play a pivotal role *(80)*. Thus, apoptosis is regulated by the complex interaction of numerous prosurvival and prodeath signals. These include the Bcl-2 family of proteins, which may be antiapoptotic (Bcl-2, Bcl-xL) or proapoptotic (Bax, Bid), and exert their effects primarily at the level of mitochondria *(81–84)*. Other important regulators of apoptosis act at the level of caspases. Such proteins include cellular FADD-like inhibitory protein and the inhibitor of apoptosis family *(85–88)*. Dysregulated apoptosis has been implicated in cardiomyocyte death. Over the past few years, there have been several reports of the occurrence of cardiomyocyte apoptosis during such conditions as cardiomyopathy, myocardial infarction, arrhythmogenic right ventricular dysplasia, hypertrophic cardiomyopathy, ischemia/reperfusion injury *(89–96)*, and heart failure *(97–100)*.

Recent studies indicate that angII plays a major role in cardiomyocyte apoptosis. AngII infusion in the rat induces apoptosis in the heart, which is associated with increased Bax and caspase-3 activity *(101,102)*. The angII effect seems to be mediated via the AT1 receptor because co-infusion of losartan prevents apoptosis and activation of Bax and caspase *(3)*. Formation of angII in the myocardium and stimulation of AT1 receptors causes myocyte apoptosis in a streptozotocin-induced rat diabetes model *(103)*. AngII induces apoptosis in cultured adult rat ventricular myocytes through the activation of AT1 receptors *(33)*. AngII stimulation was associated with translocation of the epsilon and delta isoforms of protein kinase C, which was coupled with an increase in cytosolic Ca^{2+} in the cells *(33)*. Analogous to its effect on blood vessels *(104,105)*, angII induces the formation of reactive oxygen species in neonatal myocytes *(106)*, and these are likely important in angII proapoptotic signaling pathways. Sarcomere stretching is coupled with the synthesis and release of angII *(32,107)* and the transmission of a death signal to myocytes *(32,33,108)*. Stretch-activated apoptosis in myocytes can be inhibited by an AT1 receptor blocker *(109)*.

Contrary to angII, IGF-I is not only an important growth factor for cardiomyocytes, but it also has potent survival effects. Thus, both in vitro and in vivo studies support a role for IGF-I in promoting myocyte survival and improving myocardial function *(58,99,110–112)*. It has been shown that IGF-I protein suppresses apoptosis in cultured cardiomyocytes *(63,113,114)*. IGF-I has also been shown to suppress myocardial apoptosis and improve myocardial function in various models of experimental cardiomyopathy *(111,115–117)*. In a murine model of myocardial ischemia reperfusion, IGF-I administered 1 h before ischemia significantly attenuated myocardial injury via two different mechanisms, inhibition of polymorphonuclear leukocyte-induced cardiac necrosis and inhibition of reperfusion-induced apoptosis of cardiac myocytes *(63,111)*. Normal rats receiving 4 wk of treatment with IGF-I had enhanced ventricular hypertrophy and myocyte function without development of significant fibrosis *(118,119)*. In a coronary occlusion model, left ventricular function was improved by 2 wk of treatment with IGF-I *(119)*. In a canine model of pacing-induced dilated cardiomyopathy, IGF-I treatment improved cardiac output, stroke volume, left-ventricular end-systolic pressure, and left ventricular end-diastolic pressure, and reduced pulmonary wedge pressure and systemic vascular resistance *(115)*.

In addition to the systemic administration of IGF-I protein, transgenic mice overexpressing IGF-I in the myocardium have been generated to study the local effect of IGF-I expression in the heart. Welch et al. *(120)* studied the effect of IGF-I overexpression in a mouse model that mimics the structural and functional characteristics of human dilated cardiomyopathy. These mice were generated by overexpressing tropomodulin (Tmod), an actin filament regulatory protein *(121)*, in the myocardium. Tmod-overexpressing transgenic mice exhibit significant increases in resting levels of Ca^{2+} that precede the expansion in left ventricular volume, consistent with the reported involvement of increased intracellular calcium in apoptotic and necrotic cell death *(122,123)*. The effect of IGF-I was tested by crossbreeding the Tmod-overpressing transgenic line with homozygous transgenic mice overexpressing IGF-I in cardiac myocytes to create *Tmod-IGF-I*-overexpressing mice. The rationale for this strategy was based on the ability of IGF-I to favor the alignment and organization of myofibrils in the cytoplasm *(124)* and to interfere with myocyte apoptosis and necrosis triggered by the formation of oxidative stress *(125)*. Reactive oxygen represents the distal event in Ca^{2+}-mediated cell death *(33,126)*, and IGF-I can attenuate the generation of reactive oxygen species by limiting angII formation *(127)* and, thereby, cytosolic Ca^{2+} *(33)*. The *Tmod-IGF-I*-overexpressing mice showed increased myocyte number, normalization of heart mass, anatomy, hemodynamics, and diminished apoptosis. Cellular analyses revealed that IGF-I inhibited characteristic cardiomyocyte elongation in dilated hearts and restored calcium dynamics comparable to that observed in normal cells.

Other investigators have shown that constitutive overexpression of IGF-I prevented apoptosis in the myocardium after myocardial infarction *(116)*. Overexpression of IGF-I in transgenic mice positively influences the performance of ventricular myocytes by enhancing their shortening velocity and cellular compliance, with consequent improvement of the Frank-Starling relation *(128)*.

4. IGF-I AS A THERAPEUTIC AGENT FOR HEART FAILURE

As noted previously, the systemic administration of IGF-I protein or overexpression of IGF-I in the heart has been shown to increase cardiomyocyte proliferation, reduce apoptosis, and improve cardiac function in animal models of ischemic injury and heart failure *(58,99,110–112,116,129,130)*. Furthermore, IGF-I deficiency in humans has been associated with cardiac atrophy and reduced ventricular function *(131,132)* and it is known that myocytes are able to proliferate postnatally in the presence of elevated IGF-I levels *(129,133)*. These results have led to increased interest in the therapeutic potential of the IGFs. Acute administration of IGF-I has been shown to improve myocardial function in healthy humans as well as in patients with chronic heart failure *(134,135)*. Furthermore, patients with a higher serum level of IGF-I immediately after an acute myocardial infarction had better myocardial remodeling and ventricular function as well as significantly better clinical outcome than patients with lower serum IGF-I levels *(115)*. The effects of growth hormone are mediated in large part via stimulation of autocrine/paracrine IGF-I, and a variety of studies have explored the use of growth hormone in heart failure, but results have been conflicting, potentially because of growth hormone resistance *(136–140)*. Although the data supporting a positive role for IGF-I in the heart are now quite convincing, its therapeutic use is complicated by the finding that circulating IGF-I may also play a role in tumor growth *(141–143)* and proliferative retinopathy *(144)* and be associated with other side effects *(145)*. Although clinical trials that used lower doses of IGF-I to treat younger patients with diabetes reported nearly no adverse reaction *(146)*, chronic treatment with high doses of IGF-I in older patients with diabetes is associated with edema, jaw tenderness, arthralgias, tachycardia, and orthostatic hypotension *(145)*. Systemic delivery of IGFs is further complicated by the presence of multiple IGF binding proteins in serum *(34)*. Thus, a gene therapy-based approach for local overexpression of IGFs in the heart appears to have potential substantial advantages over systemic IGF protein delivery. Tissue-targeted overexpression of IGF-I via gene transfer can augment the local production of IGF-I without increasing the serum levels of IGF-I *(147)*, although spill-over of IGF-I into the circulation can occur *(129)*. For this reason, methods to transiently express IGF-I using plasmid or viral vectors have been tested. Transient expression of IGF-I by intramuscular injection of plasmid in the rat augmented local production of IGF-I but did not increase plasma levels of IGF-I *(147)*. Liposomes containing the IGF-I gene construct proved effective in preventing muscle protein wasting and preserving total body weight after a severe thermal injury in rats *(148)*. A recent study showed that adenoviral vectors expressing IGF-I were able to efficiently transduce cardiomyocytes with consequent IGF expression and secretion *(149)*. This approach effectively protected cardiomyocytes from apoptosis induced by ischemia/reoxygenation, ceramide, and heat shock and enhanced angiogenesis in vivo *(149)*.

5. MECHANISMS OF IGF-I ACTION: ROLE IN CARDIOMYOCYTE GROWTH AND SURVIVAL

IGF-I promotes cellular proliferation and/or differentiation through binding to a specific heterotetrameric receptor with intrinsic tyrosine kinase activity *(150–152)*. The activated IGF-I receptor phosphorylates several adaptor/docking proteins, including the insulin receptor substrates 1 and 2 (IRS-1 and IRS-2), Crk and Shc, leading to signal transduction through multiple downstream signaling proteins, including mitogen-activated protein kinases and PI3K. The regulatory subunit of PI3K contains an SH2 domain that interacts with IRS-1, resulting in PI3K activation *(153)*. PI3K then leads to Akt (protein kinase B) activation, which affects diverse intracellular processes, such as translational regulation and cell survival. Activated Akt kinase plays a central role in suppressing apoptosis by modulating the activities of Bcl-2 family proteins *(154)*, caspase *(9,155)* and Fas ligand *(156)*. Overexpression of an activated form of the PI3K catalytic subunit or Akt in transgenic mice resulted in cardiac hypertrophy with a remarkable increase in cardiac contractility *(157)*. Transfer of mutationally activated PI3 kinase and Akt genes has been shown to prevent apoptosis of cardiac myocytes in vitro *(114)*, and a recent report indicates that an adenoviral vector expressing activated Akt reduces the total number of apoptotic cardiomyocytes and improves regional cardiac function in rat hearts subjected to transient ischemia in vivo *(158)*. Yamashita et al. *(159)* demonstrated that IGF-I ± transgenic mouse hearts are resistant to apoptosis or necrosis in three different models of ischemia, confirming the disease-resistant phenotype of these hearts. The basal level of phosphorylated Akt was increased sixfold as a result of continuous overproduction of IGF-1 in these hearts. Both the induction of phospho-Akt by ischemia/reperfusion and the resistance of the IGF-1 ± hearts to apoptosis were blocked by wortmannin. This confirms the role of PI3 kinase in both responses.

Although the activation of PI3 kinase or Akt alone is sufficient to partially suppress cardiomyocyte apoptosis *(113,160)*, the signals transmitting the anti-apoptotic effect of IGF-I may involve more than one pathway. Thus, Mehrhof et al. *(161)*

showed that IGF-I-stimulation is followed by a PI3K-dependent phosphorylation of Akt and BAD and an MEK1-dependent phosphorylation of extracellular signal-regulated kinase-1 and -2. IGF-I also induced phosphorylation of cyclic AMP response element-binding protein (CREB) in a PI3K- and MEK1-dependent manner. Ectopic overexpression of a dominant-negative mutant of CREB abolished the antiapoptotic effect of IGF-I. Protein levels of the antiapoptotic factor bcl-2 increased after longer periods of IGF-I-stimulation, and this could be reversed by pharmacological inhibition of PI3K as well as MEK1 and also by overexpression of dominant-negative CREB. Therefore, in cardiomyocytes, the antiapoptotic effect of IGF-I requires both PI3K- and MEK1-dependent pathways leading to the activation of the transcription factor CREB, which then induces the expression of the antiapoptotic factor Bcl-2.

6. CACHEXIA ASSOCIATED WITH HEART FAILURE

Chronic heart failure is associated with significant malnutrition, progressive skeletal muscle atrophy, leading to cardiac cachexia. Anker et al. *(162)* have shown that cachexia or wasting is an important predictor of increased mortality in heart failure. Recent evidence suggests that exercise intolerance in heart failure is not simply a result of reduced perfusion of the exercising musculature, rather, it is a result of skeletal muscle dysfunction *(163–165)*. Minotti et al. *(166)* showed that loss of skeletal muscle mass is an important determinant of muscle strength and that muscle wasting occurred in even mild heart failure *(167)*. The causes of muscle atrophy in heart failure are still unknown. It has been hypothesized that loss of anabolic function *(168)* and cytokine activation *(169)* may be of importance.

A recent study by Hambrecht et al. in 47 patients with severe congestive heart failure (left ventricular ejection fraction ≤30%) and 15 age-matched healthy subjects showed that local muscle IGF-I mRNA expression was reduced by 52% in chronic heart failure *(168)*. Local IGF-I expression was significantly correlated with muscle cross-sectional area and growth hormone resistance *(168)*. High tumor necrosis factor-α levels are associated with exercise intolerance and neurohormonal activation in chronic heart failure patients *(170)*. This cytokine is known to produce muscle wasting either by triggering apoptosis or by activating ubiquitin *(171)*.

The potential reduction in IGF-I anabolic effects in skeletal muscle of heart failure patients coupled with the activation of cytokines and angII may induce apoptosis of skeletal muscle cells. Thus, Vescovo et al. *(172)* showed that there was an increased number of TdT-mediated-dUTP nick-end labeling-positive apoptotic myocyte nuclei in biopsies taken from the vastus lateralis muscle of patients with severe chronic heart failure caused by ischemic heart disease. Tissue concentrations of Bcl-2 were decreased, whereas those of caspase-3 and ubiquitin were increased. There was a correlation between the number of apoptotic nuclei and the fiber cross sectional area, but no correlation between myosin heavy chains and the number of apoptotic nuclei. A similar observation has been made by Adams et al. *(173)*, who showed increased levels of skeletal muscle apoptosis in patients with congestive heart failure. Skeletal muscle apoptosis in heart failure is accompanied by higher expression of inducible nitric oxide synthase *(174)*. Muscle wasting has also been demonstrated in animal models of congestive heart failure. Thus, Vescovo et al. have shown that in monocrotaline-induced heart failure in the rat there is a progressive rise in interstitial and myocyte apoptosis in

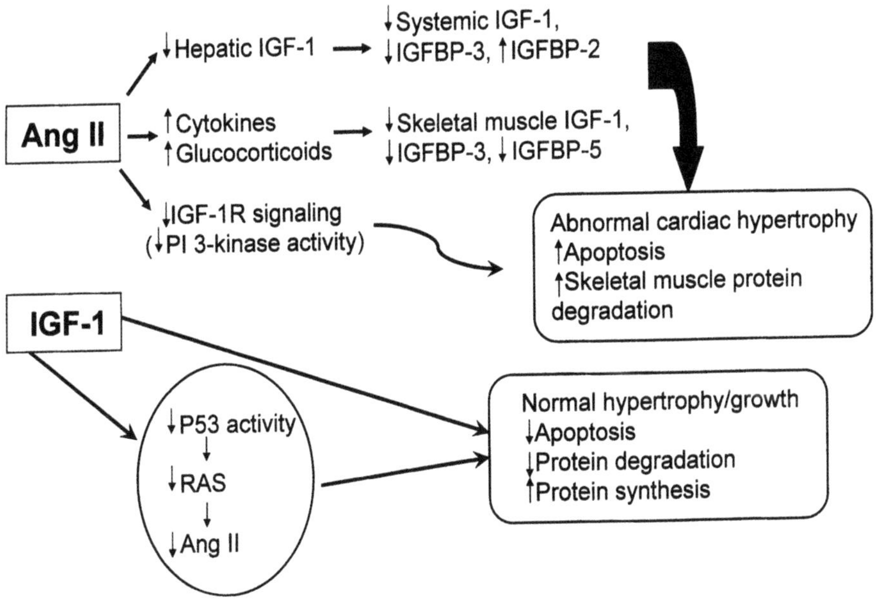

Fig. 1. The interactions between the RAS and the IGF-1 systems mediate beneficial or detrimental effects on cardiac and skeletal muscle function in heart failure.

hind limb skeletal muscle (TdT-mediated-dUTP nick-end labeling-positive cells), accompanied by a drop in fiber cross-sectional area and muscle weight/body weight that was significant at 30 d *(175)*.

Our group has shown that muscle wasting in the rat can be induced by angII infusion, a model that mimics the condition of congestive heart failure, which is characterized by elevated angII levels (Fig. 1). We were the first to show that angII infusion caused a significant reduction of circulating IGF-I levels, concordant with a marked weight loss *(176)*. The weight loss is secondary to both an anorexigenic and catabolic effect of angII. We further showed that these responses are mediated by the AT1 receptor but are independent of pressor responses to angII. We have subsequently explored the mechanisms mediating this catabolic effect of angII *(177)*. AngII did not significantly decrease protein synthesis, but overall protein breakdown was accelerated; inhibiting lysosomal and calcium-activated proteases did not reduce the angII-induced increase in muscle proteolysis, indicating that other systems such as the ubiquitin-proteasome pathway may be involved. In addition to reducing circulating IGF-I (via inhibition of hepatic IGF-I synthesis), angII markedly decreased skeletal muscle IGF-I and IGF binding protein-3 and -5 expression *(177)*. Restoration of normal circulating IGF-I levels did not block angII-induced skeletal muscle weight loss. Our data suggest that angII causes a loss in skeletal muscle mass by enhancing protein degradation probably via its inhibitory effect on the autocrine IGF-I system *(176,177)*. Because skeletal muscle may express low numbers of angII receptors (although this is not a consistent finding; ref. *178*), this catabolic effect could be mediated through intermediate molecules. Possible candidates include glucocorticoids or the proinflammatory cytokine, TNF-α. Indeed, we have shown that cortisol levels are markedly elevated in the angII-infused rat *(177,179)*.

7. IGF-I LEVELS IN HEART FAILURE

Our animal findings provided a link between the RAS and IGF-I and prompted us to conduct a prospective study to determine levels of circulating IGF-I, IGFBP-3, and free IGF-I in patients with congestive heart failure treated with and without ACE inhibitors *(180)*. We found that serum levels of total IGF-I and of its main circulating carrier protein, IGFBP-3, were decreased irrespective of the mechanism and the severity of left ventricular failure. In contrast, free IGF-I was greatly increased. Furthermore, the decrease in total IGF-I was not observed when patients were treated with ACE inhibitors. This was not the case for changes in IGFBP-3 and free IGF-I. Our data suggest that one of the major regulators of circulating IGF-I in heart failure is an increased level of angII *(180)*. This is consistent with a report from Corbalan et al. *(181)* and with our animal data demonstrating that angII infusion reduces hepatic IGF-I synthesis and circulating total IGF-I *(177)*. Reduced circulating IGF-I levels have also been reported in patients with dilated cardiomyopathy and total IGF-I levels correlated positively to systolic function *(182,183)*. Animal data have suggested that an intact GH–IGF-I axis is required for normal myocardial infarction healing. This was demonstrated by Cittadini et al, *(184)* in a coronary ligation model using growth hormone-deficient dwarf rats and in age-matched controls. They found that in dwarf rats, serum IGF-I levels were reduced by 50%, and grow rate was 50% less than normal littermates. The dwarf rats failed to develop compensatory hypertrophy of the noninfarcted posterior wall. Furthermore, the extent of remodeling as assessed by the increase in end-diastolic dimension and depression of function were both greater in the dwarf group. Interestingly, Al-Obaidi et al. have suggested that early heart failure is characterized by an increase in IGF-I, which is then lost as heart failure progresses *(185)*.

8. CROSSTALK BETWEEN IGF-I AND ANGII SIGNALING

As mentioned above, constitutive overexpression of IGF-I in myocytes protects them from apoptosis whereas angII triggers apoptosis of myocytes and promotes cardiac fibrosis. The opposing actions of these two factors have prompted Leri et al. *(127)* to investigate a possible interaction of IGF-I and angII in cardiomyocytes (Fig. 1). The hypothesis was that IGF-I interferes with the activity of p53, depressing the myocyte RAS and the induction of p53-dependent genes such as angiotensinogen (Aogen), AT1 receptor, and Bax. This hypothesis was based on previous findings that the tumor suppressor p53 upregulates the local RAS, leading to the formation of angII *(32,108)*, decreasing the expression of genes opposing cell death, such as Bcl-2 *(108 127,186,187)*, and enhancing genes promoting apoptosis, such as Bax *(188)*. The proto-oncogene mdm2, which possesses in its promoter two perfect consensus sequences for p53 *(189)*, has been shown to decrease the stability of p53 by enhancing the degradation of this protein *(190,191)*. To test the potential interaction between IGF-I and angII, Leri and collaborators generated a transgenic mouse FVB.IGF ± by placing the human IGF-IB cDNA under the control of the rat α-myosin heavy-chain promoter *(129)*. Upregulation of IGF-I in cardiac myocytes from FVB.IGF ± mice was associated with a protein-to-protein interaction between Mdm2 and p53, which attenuated p53 transcriptional activity for Bax, angiotensinogen (Aogen), and AT1 receptor. Similarly, the amount of Bax, Aogen, and AT1 receptor proteins in these cells decreased. The downregulation of Aogen in myocytes from FVB/IGF ± mice was characterized by a reduction in angII. Therefore, these elegant studies established that IGF-I negatively influences the myocyte RAS through the upregulation of Mdm2 and its binding to p53. This may represent an important molecular mechanism responsible for the effects of IGF-I on cell viability and myocyte hypertrophy in the nonpathological and pathological heart in vivo. This model may mimic the early stages of cardiac hypertrophy when IGF-I levels are high. However, when hypertrophy progresses to the decompensated stage, angII effects become dominant *(71)*.

These findings raise the possibility that increased angII in later stages of cardiac hypertrophy might inhibit the synthesis and/or availability of IGF-I. It has been shown previously that angII inhibits insulin and IGF-I signaling systems *(192)*. Using an intact rat heart model, Folli et al. *(193)* demonstrated that angII stimulates tyrosine phosphorylation of the insulin receptor substrates IRS-1 and IRS-2. However, unlike insulin, angII inhibits both basal and insulin/IGF-I-stimulated IRS-1- and IRS-2-associated PI 3-kinase activity. This effect occurs via angII-triggered serine phosphorylation of both the insulin receptor β-subunit and IRS-1, and the p85 regulatory subunit of PI3 kinase and therefore interference with the docking of IRS-1 with the p85 regulatory subunit of PI3 kinase *(192)*.

Our group has shown that angII infusion indeed caused a marked decrease of both circulating and skeletal muscle IGF-I levels in the rat *(176,177)*. In addition, angII infusion reduced skeletal muscle IGFBP-3 and IGFBP-5 expression. Under such circumstances, exogenous introduction of IGF-I may be of therapeutic value. Recombinant adeno-associated virus has been used to overexpress IGF-I in rat skeletal muscle *(194)*. It was shown that increased IGF-I expression promoted an average increase of 15% in muscle mass and a 14% increase in strength in young adult mice and, remarkably, prevented aging-related muscle changes in old adult mice, resulting in a 27% increase in strength as compared with uninjected old muscles. Muscle mass and fiber type distributions were maintained at levels similar to those in young adults *(194)*. These findings have important implications for devising strategies to ameliorate the muscle wasting common in many chronic disease states.

9. SUMMARY AND CONCLUSIONS

The RAS and the IGF-I system are important autocrine/paracrine regulators of cardiac and skeletal muscle growth, differentiation, and survival. Complicated interactions exist between these systems at the levels of regulation of their principal ligands, angII and IGF-I, and at the level of regulation of their receptors and receptor signaling pathways. Both these systems play an important role in the development of cardiac hypertrophy and in the progression from compensated to decompensated heart failure. In addition, these systems play a major role in skeletal muscle homeostasis. Further understanding of the crosstalk between these systems will likely lead to significant advances in the understanding and treatment of patients with cardiovascular disease.

REFERENCES

1. Colucci WS and Braunwald E. Pathophysiology of heart failure. In: Heart Disease: 6th ed. Braunwald E, Zipes DP, and Libby P (eds.). W.B. Saunders, Philadelphia, PA, 2001. p. 503–533.

2. Hefti MA, Harder BA, Eppenberger HM, Schaub MC. Signaling pathways in cardiac myocyte hypertrophy. J Mol Cell Cardiol 1997;29:2873–2892.
3. Sorescu D, Griendling KK. Reactive oxygen species, mitochondria, and NAD(P)H oxidases in the development and progression of heart failure. Congest Heart Fail 2002;8:132–140.
4. Sugden PH. Signalling pathways in cardiac myocyte hypertrophy. Ann Med 2001;33:611–622.
5. Lisman KA, Stetson SJ, Koerner MM, Farmer JA, Torre-Amione G. The role of tumor necrosis factor alpha blockade in the treatment of congestive heart failure. Congest Heart Fail 2002;8:275–279.
6. Sack M. Tumor necrosis factor-alpha in cardiovascular biology and the potential role for anti-tumor necrosis factor-alpha therapy in heart disease. Pharmacol Ther 2002;94:123–135.
7. Grounds MD. Reasons for the degeneration of ageing skeletal muscle: a central role for IGF-1 signalling. Biogerontology 2002;3:19–24.
8. Greenberg B. Treatment of heart failure: state of the art and prospectives. J Cardiovasc Pharmacol 2001;38 Suppl 2:S59–S63.
9. Hollenberg NK. Impact of angiotensin II on the kidney: does an angiotensin II receptor blocker make sense? Am J Kidney Dis 2000;36:S18–S23.
10. Sayeski PP, Ali MS, Semeniuk DJ, Doan TN, Bernstein KE. Angiotensin II signal transduction pathways. Regul Pept 1998;78:19–29.
11. Unger T. The role of the renin-angiotensin system in the development of cardiovascular disease. Am J Cardiol 2002;89:3A–9A; discussion 10A.
12. Opie LH, Sack MN. Enhanced angiotensin II activity in heart failure: reevaluation of the counterregulatory hypothesis of receptor subtypes. Circ Res 2001;88:654–658.
13. Harada K, Sugaya T, Murakami K, Yazaki Y, Komuro I. Angiotensin II type 1A receptor knockout mice display less left ventricular remodeling and improved survival after myocardial infarction. Circulation 1999;100:2093–2099.
14. Latini R, Maggioni AP, Flather M, Sleight P, Tognoni G. ACE inhibitor use in patients with myocardial infarction. Summary of evidence from clinical trials. Circulation 1995;92:3132–3137.
15. Dahlof B. Regression of left ventricular hypertrophy—are there differences between antihypertensive agents? Cardiology 1992;81:307–315.
16. Zuanetti G, Latini R, Maggioni AP, Franzosi M, Santoro L, Tognoni G. Effect of the ACE inhibitor lisinopril on mortality in diabetic patients with acute myocardial infarction: data from the GISSI-3 study. Circulation 1997;96:4239–4245.
17. Nomoto T, Nishina T, Miwa S, et al. Angiotensin-converting enzyme inhibitor helps prevent late remodeling after left ventricular aneurysm repair in rats. Circulation 2002;106:I115–I119.
18. Kanno S, Wu YJ, Lee PC, Billiar TR, Ho C. Angiotensin-converting enzyme inhibitor preserves p21 and endothelial nitric oxide synthase expression in monocrotaline-induced pulmonary arterial hypertension in rats. Circulation 2001;104:945–950.
19. Iwanaga Y, Kihara Y, Inagaki K, et al. Differential effects of angiotensin II versus endothelin-1 inhibitions in hypertrophic left ventricular myocardium during transition to heart failure. Circulation 2001;104:606–612.
20. Givertz MM. Manipulation of the renin-angiotensin system. Circulation 2001;104:E14–E18.
21. Lindpaintner K, Jin MW, Niedermaier N, Wilhelm MJ, Ganten D. Cardiac angiotensinogen and its local activation in the isolated perfused beating heart. Circ Res 1990;67:564–573.
22. Danser AH, van Kats JP, Admiraal PJ, et al. Cardiac renin and angiotensins. Uptake from plasma versus in situ synthesis. Hypertension 1994;24:37–48.
23. Sawa H, Tokuchi F, Mochizuki N, et al. Expression of the angiotensinogen gene and localization of its protein in the human heart. Circulation 1992;86:138–146.
24. Lindpaintner K, Lu W, Neidermajer N, et al. Selective activation of cardiac angiotensinogen gene expression in post- infarction ventricular remodeling in the rat. J Mol Cell Cardiol 1993;25:133–143.
25. Schunkert H, Dzau VJ, Tang SS, Hirsch AT, Apstein CS, Lorell BH. Increased rat cardiac angiotensin converting enzyme activity and mRNA expression in pressure overload left ventricular hypertrophy. Effects on coronary resistance, contractility, and relaxation. J Clin Invest 1990;86:1913–1920.
26. Studer R, Reinecke H, Muller B, Holtz J, Just H, Drexler H. Increased angiotensin-I converting enzyme gene expression in the failing human heart. Quantification by competitive RNA polymerase chain reaction. J Clin Invest 1994;94:301–310.

27. Hokimoto S, Yasue H, Fujimoto K, Sakata R, Miyamoto E. Increased angiotensin converting enzyme activity in left ventricular aneurysm of patients after myocardial infarction. Cardiovasc Res 1995;29:664–669.
28. Egido J. Vasoactive hormones and renal sclerosis. Kidney Int 1996;49:578–597.
29. Mezzano SA, Ruiz-Ortega M, Egido J. Angiotensin II and renal fibrosis. Hypertension 2001;38:635–638.
30. Matsubara H. Pathophysiological role of angiotensin II type 2 receptor in cardiovascular and renal diseases. Circ Res 1998;83:1182–1191.
31. Sadoshima J. Cytokine actions of angiotensin II. Circ Res 2000;86:1187–1189.
32. Leri A, Claudio PP, Li Q, Li P, Cheng W, Meggs LG, et al. Stretch-mediated release of angiotensin II induces myocyte apoptosis by activating p53 that enhances the local renin-angiotensin system and decreases the Bcl-2-to-Bax protein ratio in the cell. J Clin Invest 1998;101:1326–1342.
33. Kajstura J, Cigola E, Malhotra A, Li P, Cheng W, Meggs LG, et al. Angiotensin II induces apoptosis of adult ventricular myocytes in vitro. J Mol Cell Cardiol 1997;29:859–870.
34. Baxter RC. Insulin-like growth factor (IGF)-binding proteins: interactions with IGFs and intrinsic bioactivities. Am J Physiol Endocrinol Metab 2000;278:E967–E976.
35. Binoux M, Hossenlopp P, Hardouin S, Seurin D, Lassarre C, Gourmelen M. Somatomedin (insulin-like growth factors)-binding proteins. Molecular forms and regulation. Horm Res 1986;24:141–151.
36. Firth SM, Baxter RC. Cellular actions of the insulin-like growth factor binding proteins. Endocr Rev 2002;23:824–854.
37. Lund PK, Moats-Staats BM, Hynes MA, et al. Somatomedin-C/insulin-like growth factor-I and insulin-like growth factor-II mRNAs in rat fetal and adult tissues. J Biol Chem 1986;261:14539–14544.
38. Delafontaine P. Insulin-like growth factor I and its binding proteins in the cardiovascular system. Cardiovasc Res 1995;30:825–834.
39. Khorsandi MJ, Fagin JA, Giannella-Neto D, Forrester JS, Cercek B. Regulation of insulin-like growth factor-I and its receptor in rat aorta after balloon denudation. Evidence for local bioactivity. J Clin Invest 1992;90:1926–1931.
40. Lopez-Fernandez J, Sanchez-Franco F, Velasco B, Tolon RM, Pazos F, Cacicedo L. Growth hormone induces somatostatin and insulin-like growth factor I gene expression in the cerebral hemispheres of aging rats. Endocrinology 1996;137:4384–4391.
41. Murphy LJ, Friesen HG. Differential effects of estrogen and growth hormone on uterine and hepatic insulin-like growth factor I gene expression in the ovariectomized hypophysectomized rat. Endocrinology 1988;122:325–232.
42. Yamamoto H, Murphy LJ. Enzymatic conversion of IGF-I to des(1–3)IGF-I in rat serum and tissues: a further potential site of growth hormone regulation of IGF-I action. J Endocrinol 1995;146:141–148.
43. LeRoith D, Werner H, Beitner-Johnson D, Roberts CT, Jr. Molecular and cellular aspects of the insulin-like growth factor I receptor. Endocr Rev 1995;16:143–163.
44. Tseng YH, Ueki K, Kriauciunas KM, Kahn CR. Differential roles of insulin receptor substrates in the anti-apoptotic function of insulin-like growth factor-1 and insulin. J Biol Chem 2002;277:31601–31611.
45. Ueki K, Fruman DA, Brachmann SM, Tseng YH, Cantley LC, Kahn CR. Molecular balance between the regulatory and catalytic subunits of phosphoinositide 3-kinase regulates cell signaling and survival. Mol Cell Biol 2002;22:965–977.
46. Jones JI, Clemmons DR. Insulin-like growth factors and their binding proteins: biological actions. Endocr Rev 1995;16:3–34.
47. Liu JP, Baker J, Perkins AS, Robertson EJ, Efstratiadis A. Mice carrying null mutations of the genes encoding insulin-like growth factor I (Igf-1) and type 1 IGF receptor (Igf1r). Cell 1993;75:59–72.
48. Baker J, Liu JP, Robertson EJ, Efstratiadis A. Role of insulin-like growth factors in embryonic and postnatal growth. Cell 1993;75:73–82.
49. Skrtic S, Wallenius K, Sjogren K, Isaksson OG, Ohlsson C, Jansson JO. Possible roles of insulin-like growth factor in regulation of physiological and pathophysiological liver growth. Horm Res 2001;55(Suppl 1):1–6.
50. Ye P, Li L, Richards RG, DiAugustine RP, D'Ercole AJ. Myelination is altered in insulin-like growth factor-I null mutant mice. J Neurosci 2002;22:6041–6051.

51. Camarero G, Avendano C, Fernandez-Moreno C, et al. Delayed inner ear maturation and neuronal loss in postnatal Igf-1-deficient mice. J Neurosci 2001;21:7630–7641.
52. Kido Y, Nakae J, Hribal ML, Xuan S, Efstratiadis A, Accili D. Effects of mutations in the insulin-like growth factor signaling system on embryonic pancreas development and beta-cell compensation to insulin resistance. J Biol Chem 2002;277:36740–36747.
53. Kadakia R, Arraztoa JA, Bondy C, Zhou J. Granulosa cell proliferation is impaired in the Igf1 null ovary. Growth Horm IGF Res 2001;11:220–224.
54. Liu JL, LeRoith D. Insulin-like growth factor I is essential for postnatal growth in response to growth hormone. Endocrinology 1999;140:5178–5184.
55. Ruan W, Kleinberg DL. Insulin-like growth factor I is essential for terminal end bud formation and ductal morphogenesis during mammary development. Endocrinology 1999;140:5075–5081.
56. DeChiara TM, Efstratiadis A, Robertson EJ. A growth-deficiency phenotype in heterozygous mice carrying an insulin- like growth factor II gene disrupted by targeting. Nature 1990;345:78–80.
57. DeChiara TM, Robertson EJ, Efstratiadis A. Parental imprinting of the mouse insulin-like growth factor II gene. Cell 1991;64:849–859.
58. Ren J, Samson WK, Sowers JR. Insulin-like growth factor I as a cardiac hormone: physiological and pathophysiological implications in heart disease. J Mol Cell Cardiol 1999;31:2049–2061.
59. Khan AS, Sane DC, Wannenburg T, Sonntag WE. Growth hormone, insulin-like growth factor-1 and the aging cardiovascular system. Cardiovasc Res 2002;54:25–35.
60. Norby FL, Wold LE, Duan J, Hintz KK, Ren J. IGF-I attenuates diabetes-induced cardiac contractile dysfunction in ventricular myocytes. Am J Physiol Endocrinol Metab 2002;283:E658–E666.
61. Tivesten A, Caidahl K, Kujacic V, et al. Similar cardiovascular effects of growth hormone and insulin-like growth factor-I in rats after experimental myocardial infarction. Growth Horm IGF Res 2001;11:187–195.
62. Parrizas M, Saltiel AR, LeRoith D. Insulin-like growth factor 1 inhibits apoptosis using the phosphatidylinositol 3'-kinase and mitogen-activated protein kinase pathways. J Biol Chem 1997;272:154–161.
63. Wang L, Ma W, Markovich R, Chen JW, Wang PH. Regulation of cardiomyocyte apoptotic signaling by insulin-like growth factor I. Circ Res 1998;83:516–522.
64. Wahlander H, Isgaard J, Jennische E, Friberg P. Left ventricular insulin-like growth factor I increases in early renal hypertension. Hypertension 1992;19:25–32.
65. Hanson MC, Fath KA, Alexander RW, Delafontaine P. Induction of cardiac insulin-like growth factor I gene expression in pressure overload hypertrophy. Am J Med Sci 1993;306:69–74.
66. Donohue TJ, Dworkin LD, Lango MN, et al. Induction of myocardial insulin-like growth factor-I gene expression in left ventricular hypertrophy. Circulation 1994;89:799–809.
67. Isgaard J, Wahlander H, Adams MA, Friberg P. Increased expression of growth hormone receptor mRNA and insulin-like growth factor-I mRNA in volume-overloaded hearts. Hypertension 1994;23:884–888.
68. Donohue TJ, Dworkin LD, Ma J, Lango MN, Catanese VM. Antihypertensive agents that limit ventricular hypertrophy inhibit cardiac expression of insulin-like growth factor-I. J Invest Med 1997;45:584–591.
69. Brink M, Chrast J, Price SR, Mitch WE, Delafontaine P. Angiotensin II stimulates gene expression of cardiac insulin-like growth factor I and its receptor through effects on blood pressure and food intake. Hypertension 1999;34:1053–1059.
70. Pauliks LB, Cole KE, Mergner WJ. Increased insulin-like growth factor-1 protein in human left ventricular hypertrophy. Exp Mol Pathol 1999;66:53–58.
71. Serneri GG, Modesti PA, Boddi M, et al. Cardiac growth factors in human hypertrophy. Relations with myocardial contractility and wall stress. Circ Res 1999;85:57–67.
72. Kawano H, Do YS, Kawano Y, et al. Angiotensin II has multiple profibrotic effects in human cardiac fibroblasts. Circulation 2000;101:1130–1137.
73. Weber KT. Extracellular matrix remodeling in heart failure: a role for de novo angiotensin II generation. Circulation 1997;96:4065–4082.
74. Schunkert H, Jackson B, Tang SS, et al. Distribution and functional significance of cardiac angiotensin converting enzyme in hypertrophied rat hearts. Circulation 1993;87:1328–1339.
75. Cheng CP, Suzuki M, Ohte N, Ohno M, Wang ZM, Little WC. Altered ventricular and myocyte response to angiotensin II in pacing- induced heart failure. Circ Res 1996;78:880–892.

76. Beltrami AP, Urbanek K, Kajstura J, et al. Evidence that human cardiac myocytes divide after myocardial infarction. N Engl J Med 2001;344:1750–1757.
77. Meier P, Finch A, Evan G. Apoptosis in development. Nature 2000;407:796–801.
78. Krammer PH. CD95's deadly mission in the immune system. Nature 2000;407:789–795.
79. James TN. Apoptosis in cardiac disease. Am J Med 1999;107:606–620.
80. Thornberry NA, Lazebnik Y. Caspases: enemies within. Science 1998;281:1312–1316.
81. Adams JM, Cory S. Life-or-death decisions by the Bcl-2 protein family. Trends Biochem Sci 2001;26:61–66.
82. Adams JM, Cory S. The Bcl-2 protein family: arbiters of cell survival. Science 1998;281:1322–1326.
83. Yin XM, Wang K, Gross A, et al. Bid-deficient mice are resistant to Fas-induced hepatocellular apoptosis. Nature 1999;400:886–891.
84. Shimizu S, Narita M, Tsujimoto Y. Bcl-2 family proteins regulate the release of apoptogenic cytochrome c by the mitochondrial channel VDAC. Nature 1999;399:483–487.
85. Rasper DM, Vaillancourt JP, Hadano S, et al. Cell death attenuation by 'Usurpin', a mammalian DED-caspase homologue that precludes caspase-8 recruitment and activation by the CD-95 (Fas, APO-1) receptor complex. Cell Death Differ 1998;5:271–288.
86. Uren AG, Coulson EJ, Vaux DL. Conservation of baculovirus inhibitor of apoptosis repeat proteins (BIRPs) in viruses, nematodes, vertebrates and yeasts. Trends Biochem Sci 1998;23:159–162.
87. Srinivasula SM, Hegde R, Saleh A, et al. A conserved XIAP-interaction motif in caspase-9 and Smac/DIABLO regulates caspase activity and apoptosis. Nature 2001;410:112–116.
88. Irmler M, Thome M, Hahne M, et al. Inhibition of death receptor signals by cellular FLIP. Nature 1997;388:190–195.
89. Narula J, Haider N, Virmani R, et al. Apoptosis in myocytes in end-stage heart failure. N Engl J Med 1996;335:1182–1189.
90. Olivetti G, Abbi R, Quaini F, et al. Apoptosis in the failing human heart. N Engl J Med 1997;336:1131–1141.
91. Rayment NB, Haven AJ, Madden B, et al. Myocyte loss in chronic heart failure. J Pathol 1999;188:213–219.
92. Kavantzas NG, Lazaris AC, Agapitos EV, Nanas J, Davaris PS. Histological assessment of apoptotic cell death in cardiomyopathies. Pathology 2000;32:176–180.
93. Saraste A, Pulkki K, Kallajoki M, Henriksen K, Parvinen M, Voipio-Pulkki LM. Apoptosis in human acute myocardial infarction. Circulation 1997;95:320–323.
94. Gottlieb RA, Burleson KO, Kloner RA, Babior BM, Engler RL. Reperfusion injury induces apoptosis in rabbit cardiomyocytes. J Clin Invest 1994;94:1621–1628.
95. Guerra S, Leri A, Wang X, et al. Myocyte death in the failing human heart is gender dependent. Circ Res 1999;85:856–866.
96. Mallat Z, Tedgui A, Fontaliran F, Frank R, Durigon M, Fontaine G. Evidence of apoptosis in arrhythmogenic right ventricular dysplasia. N Engl J Med 1996;335:1190–1196.
97. Haunstetter A, Izumo S. Apoptosis: basic mechanisms and implications for cardiovascular disease. Circ Res 1998;82:1111–1129.
98. Kang PM, Izumo S. Apoptosis and heart failure: A critical review of the literature. Circ Res 2000;86:1107–1113.
99. Kotlyar AA, Vered Z, Goldberg I, et al. Insulin-like growth factor I and II preserve myocardial structure in postinfarct swine. Heart 2001;86:693–700.
100. MacLellan WR, Schneider MD. Death by design. Programmed cell death in cardiovascular biology and disease. Circ Res 1997;81:137–144.
101. Diep QN, El Mabrouk M, Yue P, Schiffrin EL. Effect of AT(1) receptor blockade on cardiac apoptosis in angiotensin II-induced hypertension. Am J Physiol Heart Circ Physiol 2002;282:H1635–H1641.
102. De Angelis N, Fiordaliso F, Latini R, et al. Appraisal of the Role of Angiotensin II and Aldosterone in Ventricular Myocyte Apoptosis in Adult Normotensive Rat. J Mol Cell Cardiol 2002;34:1655–1665.
103. Fiordaliso F, Li B, Latini R, et al. Myocyte death in streptozotocin-induced diabetes in rats in angiotensin II- dependent. Lab Invest 2000;80:513–527.
104. Berry C, Hamilton CA, Brosnan MJ, et al. Investigation into the sources of superoxide in human blood vessels: angiotensin II increases superoxide production in human internal mammary arteries. Circulation 2000;101:2206–2212.

105. Rajagopalan S, Kurz S, Munzel T, et al. Angiotensin II-mediated hypertension in the rat increases vascular superoxide production via membrane NADH/NADPH oxidase activation. Contribution to alterations of vasomotor tone. J Clin Invest 1996;97:1916–1923.
106. von Harsdorf R, Li PF, Dietz R. Signaling pathways in reactive oxygen species-induced cardiomyocyte apoptosis. Circulation 1999;99:2934–2941.
107. Sadoshima J, Xu Y, Slayter HS, Izumo S. Autocrine release of angiotensin II mediates stretch-induced hypertrophy of cardiac myocytes in vitro. Cell 1993;75:977–984.
108. Pierzchalski P, Reiss K, Cheng W, et al. p53 Induces myocyte apoptosis via the activation of the renin- angiotensin system. Exp Cell Res 1997;234:57–65.
109. Leri A, Liu Y, Li B, et al. Up-regulation of AT(1) and AT(2) receptors in postinfarcted hypertrophied myocytes and stretch-mediated apoptotic cell death. Am J Pathol 2000;156:1663–1672.
110. Battler A, Hasdai D, Goldberg I, et al. Exogenous insulin-like growth factor II enhances post-infarction regional myocardial function in swine. Eur Heart J 1995;16:1851–1859.
111. Buerke M, Murohara T, Skurk C, Nuss C, Tomaselli K, Lefer AM. Cardioprotective effect of insulin-like growth factor I in myocardial ischemia followed by reperfusion. Proc Natl Acad Sci USA 1995;92:8031–8035.
112. Jin H, Yang R, Gillett N, Clark RG, Ko A, Paoni NF. Beneficial effects of growth hormone and insulin-like growth factor-1 in experimental heart failure in rats treated with chronic ACE inhibition. J Cardiovasc Pharmacol 1995;26:420–425.
113. Fujio Y, Nguyen T, Wencker D, Kitsis RN, Walsh K. Akt promotes survival of cardiomyocytes in vitro and protects against ischemia-reperfusion injury in mouse heart. Circulation 2000;101:660–667.
114. Matsui T, Li L, del Monte F, et al. Adenoviral gene transfer of activated phosphatidylinositol 3'-kinase and Akt inhibits apoptosis of hypoxic cardiomyocytes in vitro. Circulation 1999;100:2373–2379.
115. Lee WL, Chen JW, Ting CT, et al. Insulin-like growth factor I improves cardiovascular function and suppresses apoptosis of cardiomyocytes in dilated cardiomyopathy. Endocrinology 1999;140:4831–4840.
116. Li Q, Li B, Wang X, et al. Overexpression of insulin-like growth factor-1 in mice protects from myocyte death after infarction, attenuating ventricular dilation, wall stress, and cardiac hypertrophy. J Clin Invest 1997;100:1991–1999.
117. Duerr RL, McKirnan MD, Gim RD, Clark RG, Chien KR, Ross J, Jr. Cardiovascular effects of insulin-like growth factor-1 and growth hormone in chronic left ventricular failure in the rat. Circulation 1996;93:2188–2196.
118. Cittadini A, Stromer H, Katz SE, et al. Differential cardiac effects of growth hormone and insulin-like growth factor-1 in the rat. A combined in vivo and in vitro evaluation. Circulation 1996;93:800–809.
119. Duerr RL, Huang S, Miraliakbar HR, Clark R, Chien KR, Ross J, Jr. Insulin-like growth factor-1 enhances ventricular hypertrophy and function during the onset of experimental cardiac failure. J Clin Invest 1995;95:619–627.
120. Welch S, Plank D, Witt S, et al. Cardiac-specific IGF-1 expression attenuates dilated cardiomyopathy in tropomodulin-overexpressing transgenic mice. Circ Res 2002;90:641–648.
121. Weber A, Pennise CR, Babcock GG, Fowler VM. Tropomodulin caps the pointed ends of actin filaments. J Cell Biol 1994;127:1627–1635.
122. Didenko VV, Hornsby PJ. Presence of double-strand breaks with single-base 3' overhangs in cells undergoing apoptosis but not necrosis. J Cell Biol 1996;135:1369–1376.
123. Didenko VV, Tunstead JR, Hornsby PJ. Biotin-labeled hairpin oligonucleotides: probes to detect double-strand breaks in DNA in apoptotic cells. Am J Pathol 1998;152:897–902.
124. Donath MY, Zapf J, Eppenberger-Eberhardt M, Froesch ER, Eppenberger HM. Insulin-like growth factor I stimulates myofibril development and decreases smooth muscle alpha-actin of adult cardiomyocytes. Proc Natl Acad Sci U S A 1994;91:1686–1690.
125. Kajstura J, Fiordaliso F, Andreoli AM, et al. IGF-1 overexpression inhibits the development of diabetic cardiomyopathy and angiotensin II-mediated oxidative stress. Diabetes 2001;50:1414–1424.
126. Nitahara JA, Cheng W, Liu Y, et al. Intracellular calcium, DNase activity and myocyte apoptosis in aging Fischer 344 rats. J Mol Cell Cardiol 1998;30:519–535.
127. Leri A, Liu Y, Wang X, et al. Overexpression of insulin-like growth factor-1 attenuates the myocyte renin-angiotensin system in transgenic mice. Circ Res 1999;84:752–762.

128. Redaelli G, Malhotra A, Li B, et al. Effects of constitutive overexpression of insulin-like growth factor-1 on the mechanical characteristics and molecular properties of ventricular myocytes. Circ Res 1998;82:594–603.
129. Reiss K, Cheng W, Ferber A, et al. Overexpression of insulin-like growth factor-1 in the heart is coupled with myocyte proliferation in transgenic mice. Proc Natl Acad Sci USA 1996;93:8630–8635.
130. Lee WL, Chen JW, Ting CT, Lin SJ, Wang PH. Changes of the insulin-like growth factor I system during acute myocardial infarction: implications on left ventricular remodeling. J Clin Endocrinol Metab 1999;84:1575–1581.
131. Merola B, Cittadini A, Colao A, et al. Cardiac structural and functional abnormalities in adult patients with growth hormone deficiency. J Clin Endocrinol Metab 1993;77:1658–1661.
132. Amato G, Carella C, Fazio S, et al. Body composition, bone metabolism, and heart structure and function in growth hormone (GH)-deficient adults before and after GH replacement therapy at low doses. J Clin Endocrinol Metab 1993;77:1671–1676.
133. Anversa P, Nadal-Ginard B. Myocyte renewal and ventricular remodelling. Nature 2002;415:240–243.
134. Donath MY, Jenni R, Brunner HP, et al. Cardiovascular and metabolic effects of insulin-like growth factor I at rest and during exercise in humans. J Clin Endocrinol Metab 1996;81:4089–4094.
135. Donath MY, Sutsch G, Yan XW, et al. Acute cardiovascular effects of insulin-like growth factor I in patients with chronic heart failure. J Clin Endocrinol Metab 1998;83:3177–3183.
136. Perrot A, Ranke MB, Dietz R, Osterziel KJ. Growth hormone treatment in dilated cardiomyopathy. J Card Surg 2001;16:127–131.
137. Anker SD, Volterrani M, Pflaum CD, et al. Acquired growth hormone resistance in patients with chronic heart failure: implications for therapy with growth hormone. J Am Coll Cardiol 2001;38:443–452.
138. Ross J, Jr., Ryoke T. Effects of growth hormone and insulin-like growth factor I in experimental heart failure. Growth Horm IGF Res 1998;8(Suppl B):159–161.
139. Isgaard J, Bergh CH, Caidahl K, Lomsky M, Hjalmarson A, Bengtsson BA. A placebo-controlled study of growth hormone in patients with congestive heart failure. Eur Heart J 1998;19:1704–1711.
140. Osterziel KJ, Strohm O, Schuler J, et al. Randomised, double-blind, placebo-controlled trial of human recombinant growth hormone in patients with chronic heart failure due to dilated cardiomyopathy. Lancet 1998;351:1233–1237.
141. Baserga R. The IGF-I receptor in cancer research. Exp Cell Res 1999;253:1–6.
142. Ma J, Pollak MN, Giovannucci E, et al. Prospective study of colorectal cancer risk in men and plasma levels of insulin-like growth factor (IGF)-I and IGF-binding protein-3. J Natl Cancer Inst 1999;91:620–625.
143. Wu Y, Yakar S, Zhao L, Hennighausen L, LeRoith D. Circulating insulin-like growth factor-I levels regulate colon cancer growth and metastasis. Cancer Res 2002;62:1030–1035.
144. Smith LE, Shen W, Perruzzi C, Soker S, Kinose F, Xu X, et al. Regulation of vascular endothelial growth factor-dependent retinal neovascularization by insulin-like growth factor-1 receptor. Nat Med 1999;5:1390–1395.
145. Jabri N, Schalch DS, Schwartz SL, et al. Adverse effects of recombinant human insulin-like growth factor I in obese insulin-resistant type II diabetic patients. Diabetes 1994;43:369–374.
146. Acerini CL, Patton CM, Savage MO, Kernell A, Westphal O, Dunger DB. Randomised placebo-controlled trial of human recombinant insulin-like growth factor I plus intensive insulin therapy in adolescents with insulin-dependent diabetes mellitus. Lancet 1997;350:1199–1204.
147. Alila H, Coleman M, Nitta H, et al. Expression of biologically active human insulin-like growth factor-I following intramuscular injection of a formulated plasmid in rats. Hum Gene Ther 1997;8:1785–1795.
148. Jeschke MG, Barrow RE, Hawkins HK, et al. IGF-I gene transfer in thermally injured rats. Gene Ther 1999;6:1015–1020.
149. Su EJ, Cioffi CL, Stefansson S, Mittereder N, Garay M, Hreniuk D, et al. Gene therapy vector-mediated expression of insulin-like growth factors protects cardiomyocytes from apoptosis and enhances neovascularization. Am J Physiol Heart Circ Physiol 2002;284:H1429–H1440.
150. Adams TE, Epa VC, Garrett TP, Ward CW. Structure and function of the type 1 insulin-like growth factor receptor. Cell Mol Life Sci 2000;57:1050–1093.
151. White MF. The IRS-signalling system: a network of docking proteins that mediate insulin action. Mol Cell Biochem 1998;182:3–11.

152. White MF, Kahn CR. The insulin signaling system. J Biol Chem 1994;269:1–4.
153. Dhand R, Hara K, Hiles I, et al. PI 3-kinase: structural and functional analysis of intersubunit interactions. Embo J 1994;13:511–521.
154. Datta SR, Dudek H, Tao X, et al. Akt phosphorylation of BAD couples survival signals to the cell-intrinsic death machinery. Cell 1997;91:231–241.
155. Cardone MH, Roy N, Stennicke HR, et al. Regulation of cell death protease caspase-9 by phosphorylation. Science 1998;282:1318–1321.
156. Brunet A, Bonni A, Zigmond MJ, et al. Akt promotes cell survival by phosphorylating and inhibiting a Forkhead transcription factor. Cell 1999;96:857–868.
157. Condorelli G, Drusco A, Stassi G, et al. Akt induces enhanced myocardial contractility and cell size in vivo in transgenic mice. Proc Natl Acad Sci USA 2002;99:12333–12338.
158. Matsui T, Tao J, del Monte F, et al. Akt activation preserves cardiac function and prevents injury after transient cardiac ischemia in vivo. Circulation 2001;104:330–335.
159. Yamashita K, Kajstura J, Discher DJ, et al. Reperfusion-activated Akt kinase prevents apoptosis in transgenic mouse hearts overexpressing insulin-like growth factor-1. Circ Res 2001;88:609–614.
160. Wu W, Lee WL, Wu YY, et al. Expression of constitutively active phosphatidylinositol 3-kinase inhibits activation of caspase 3 and apoptosis of cardiac muscle cells. J Biol Chem 2000;275:40113–40119.
161. Mehrhof FB, Muller FU, Bergmann MW, et al. In cardiomyocyte hypoxia, insulin-like growth factor-I-induced antiapoptotic signaling requires phosphatidylinositol-3-OH-kinase- dependent and mitogen-activated protein kinase-dependent activation of the transcription factor cAMP response element-binding protein. Circulation 2001;104:2088–2094.
162. Anker SD, Ponikowski P, Varney S, et al. Wasting as independent risk factor for mortality in chronic heart failure. Lancet 1997;349:1050–1053.
163. Fink LI, Wilson JR, Ferraro N. Exercise ventilation and pulmonary artery wedge pressure in chronic stable congestive heart failure. Am J Cardiol 1986;57:249–253.
164. Sullivan MJ, Knight JD, Higginbotham MB, Cobb FR. Relation between central and peripheral hemodynamics during exercise in patients with chronic heart failure. Muscle blood flow is reduced with maintenance of arterial perfusion pressure. Circulation 1989;80:769–781.
165. Wilson JR, Martin JL, Schwartz D, Ferraro N. Exercise intolerance in patients with chronic heart failure: role of impaired nutritive flow to skeletal muscle. Circulation 1984;69:1079–1087.
166. Minotti JR, Pillay P, Oka R, Wells L, Christoph I, Massie BM. Skeletal muscle size: relationship to muscle function in heart failure. J Appl Physiol 1993;75:373–381.
167. Mancini DM, Walter G, Reichek N, et al. Contribution of skeletal muscle atrophy to exercise intolerance and altered muscle metabolism in heart failure. Circulation 1992;85:1364–1373.
168. Hambrecht R, Schulze PC, Gielen S, et al. Reduction of insulin-like growth factor-I expression in the skeletal muscle of noncachectic patients with chronic heart failure. J Am Coll Cardiol 2002;39:1175–1181.
169. McMurray J, Abdullah I, Dargie HJ, Shapiro D. Increased concentrations of tumour necrosis factor in "cachectic" patients with severe chronic heart failure. Br Heart J 1991;66:356–358.
170. Cicoira M, Bolger AP, Doehner W, et al. High tumour necrosis factor-alpha levels are associated with exercise intolerance and neurohormonal activation in chronic heart failure patients. Cytokine 2001;15:80–86.
171. Krown KA, Page MT, Nguyen C, et al. Tumor necrosis factor alpha-induced apoptosis in cardiac myocytes. Involvement of the sphingolipid signaling cascade in cardiac cell death. J Clin Invest 1996;98:2854–2865.
172. Vescovo G, Volterrani M, Zennaro R, et al. Apoptosis in the skeletal muscle of patients with heart failure: investigation of clinical and biochemical changes. Heart 2000;84:431–437.
173. Adams V, Jiang H, Yu J, et al. Apoptosis in skeletal myocytes of patients with chronic heart failure is associated with exercise intolerance. J Am Coll Cardiol 1999;33:959–965.
174. Hambrecht R, Adams V, Gielen S, et al. Exercise intolerance in patients with chronic heart failure and increased expression of inducible nitric oxide synthase in the skeletal muscle. J Am Coll Cardiol 1999;33:174–179.
175. Vescovo G, Zennaro R, Sandri M, et al. Apoptosis of skeletal muscle myofibers and interstitial cells in experimental heart failure. J Mol Cell Cardiol 1998;30:2449–2459.

176. Brink M, Wellen J, Delafontaine P. Angiotensin II causes weight loss and decreases circulating insulin- like growth factor I in rats through a pressor-independent mechanism. J Clin Invest 1996;97:2509–2516.
177. Brink M, Price SR, Chrast J, et al. Angiotensin II induces skeletal muscle wasting through enhanced protein degradation and down-regulates autocrine insulin-like growth factor I. Endocrinology 2001;142:1489–1496.
178. Linderman JR, Greene AS. Distribution of angiotensin II receptor expression in the microcirculation of striated muscle. Microcirculation 2001;8:275–281.
179. Brink M, Anwar A, Delafontaine P. Neurohormonal factors in the development of catabolic/anabolic imbalance and cachexia. Int J Cardiol 2002;85:111–121, discussion 121–124.
180. Anwar A, Gaspoz JM, Pampallona S, et al. Effect of congestive heart failure on the insulin-like growth factor-1 system. Am J Cardiol 2002;90:1402–1405.
181. Corbalan R, Acevedo M, Godoy I, Jalil J, Campusano C, Klassen J. Enalapril restores depressed circulating insulin-like growth factor 1 in patients with chronic heart failure. J Card Fail 1998;4:115–119.
182. Broglio F, Fubini A, Morello M, et al. Activity of GH/IGF-I axis in patients with dilated cardiomyopathy. Clin Endocrinol (Oxf) 1999;50:417–430.
183. Osterziel KJ, Ranke MB, Strohm O, Dietz R. The somatotrophic system in patients with dilated cardiomyopathy: relation of insulin-like growth factor-1 and its alterations during growth hormone therapy to cardiac function. Clin Endocrinol (Oxf) 2000;53:61–68.
184. Cittadini A, Grossman JD, Stromer H, Katz SE, Morgan JP, Douglas PS. Importance of an intact growth hormone/insulin-like growth factor 1 axis for normal post-infarction healing: studies in dwarf rats. Endocrinology 2001;142:332–338.
185. Al-Obaidi MK, Hon JK, Stubbs PJ, et al. Plasma insulin-like growth factor-1 elevated in mild-to-moderate but not severe heart failure. Am Heart J 2001;142:E10.
186. Miyashita T, Krajewski S, Krajewska M, et al. Tumor suppressor p53 is a regulator of bcl-2 and bax gene expression in vitro and in vivo. Oncogene 1994;9:1799–1805.
187. Reed JC. Bcl-2 and the regulation of programmed cell death. J Cell Biol 1994;124:1–6.
188. Miyashita T, Reed JC. Tumor suppressor p53 is a direct transcriptional activator of the human bax gene. Cell 1995;80:293–299.
189. Wu X, Bayle JH, Olson D, Levine AJ. The p53-mdm-2 autoregulatory feedback loop. Genes Dev 1993;7:1126–1132.
190. Haupt Y, Maya R, Kazaz A, Oren M. Mdm2 promotes the rapid degradation of p53. Nature 1997;387:296–299.
191. Kubbutat MH, Jones SN, Vousden KH. Regulation of p53 stability by Mdm2. Nature 1997;387:299–303.
192. Folli F, Kahn CR, Hansen H, Bouchie JL, Feener EP. Angiotensin II inhibits insulin signaling in aortic smooth muscle cells at multiple levels. A potential role for serine phosphorylation in insulin/angiotensin II crosstalk. J Clin Invest 1997;100:2158–2169.
193. Folli F, Saad MJ, Velloso L, et al. Crosstalk between insulin and angiotensin II signalling systems. Exp Clin Endocrinol Diabetes 1999;107:133–139.
194. Barton-Davis ER, Shoturma DI, Musaro A, Rosenthal N, Sweeney HL. Viral mediated expression of insulin-like growth factor I blocks the aging-related loss of skeletal muscle function. Proc Natl Acad Sci U S A 1998;95:15603–15607.

18 Roles of the Insulin-Like Growth Factor System and Nutrition in Cancer

Claire M. Perks and Jeffrey M. P. Holly

KEY POINTS

- Nutrition plays a major role in regulating the IGF axis.
- IGF-I is implicated in mediating the effects of nutrition on somatic growth.
- Nutrition is associated with the incidence of a range of cancers.
- IGF system is implicated in cancer.
- IGF-I may mediate the effects of nutrition on neoplastic growth.

1. INTRODUCTION

Over the last 50 yr, cancer research has predominantly been focused upon identifying and characterizing genes that when mutated may give rise to cancer. This research has fostered huge advances in our understanding of the molecular controls of cell cycle, apoptosis, and cell survival. Within the last decade, however, evidence has accumulated to indicate that the progression of most cancers is dependent more on epigenetic influences than on primary gene mutations *(1)*. For most human cancers, the problem is not that gene mutations occur, but how the body deals with damaged cells. It has been estimated that only about 1% of human cancers can be accounted for by unmistakable hereditary cancer syndromes, only up to 5% can be accounted because of high penetrance single gene mutations, and in total only 5 to 15% of all cancers may have a major genetic component *(2)*. A study of cancers in nearly 45,000 pairs of twins across three Nordic cohorts estimated that genetic factors contributed to between 27 to 42% of cancers of the breast, prostate, and colorectum *(3)* but that most of this was probably the result of relatively common genes that alone would only carry moderate risk, and the influence of many of these may be modified by environmental factors. The predominant contribution to the causation of most sporadic cancers was considered to be environmental factors contributing to between 58 and 82% of different cancers. Despite the lack of direct evidence, the indirect evidence is compelling *(3)*.

The most important environmental factor is undoubtedly nutrition. This chapter summarizes the evidence implicating that the IGF system may mediate, at least in part, the influence of nutrition on cancer.

From: *IGF and Nutrition in Health and Disease*
Edited by: M. S. Houston, J. M. P. Holly, and E. L. Feldman © Humana Press Inc., Totowa, NJ

2. EVIDENCE IMPLICATING THE IGF SYSTEM IN CANCER

2.1. Local IGFs

In addition to being important general tissue growth factors, it is not surprising that the IGFs have also been reported to be potent mitogens for a large number of different human cancer cell lines *(4,5)*. Furthermore, both IGF-I and IGF-II are expressed in many tumors and IGF-II in particular has been observed to be overexpressed in a number of different tumors, including colon *(6)*, liver *(7)*, and in several pediatric cancers *(8)*. Transgenic mice overexpressing GH or IGFs have an increased susceptibility for tumor development in specific tissues *(9)*. Increased expression of either IGF-I *(10)* or IGF-II *(8,11,12)* has been reported to be associated with more aggressive tumor phenotypes. Similarly, increased expression of IGF-II and the IGF-I receptor (IGF-IR) have been associated with a more metastatic phenotype *(13)*.

2.2. Receptors

The mitogenic and survival actions of both IGF-I and IGF-II are primarily mediated via the IGF-IR *(14)*. In contrast, the IGF-II receptor/mannose-6-phosphate receptor is considered to play an important role in the clearance and degradation of IGF-II, although it additionally has an important role in the cellular trafficking of lysosomal enzymes and also acts as a high affinity-binding site for latent transforming growth factor (TGF)-β and retinoids *(15)*. Increased expression of the IGF-IR has been reported in many cancer cell lines and in human tumor biopsies *(16–18)*. The IGF-IR appears to play a critical role in malignant transformation and in the maintenance of a transformed cell phenotype *(19)*. At least partly this is the result of the remarkable efficacy with which the IGF-IR can maintain cell survival and protect cells from apoptosis via multiple signaling pathways *(20)*. Overexpression of the IGF-IR has been reported to be associated with an aggressive phenotype of a variety of tumors *(21,22)*. In a rodent model of prostate cancer progression, however, levels of the IGF-IR were reported to be significantly reduced in advanced disease as androgen independence developed *(23)*.

In addition to the IGF-IR, the insulin receptor (IR) and hybrid IR/IGF-IR may also be present and play a role in mediating the actions of the IGFs in certain tumors *(24,25)*. In contrast to the IGF-I receptor, the IGF-IIR serves to limit IGF-II actions and hence reduce its growth promoting and cell survival potential. A number of gene disruptions resulting in loss of IGF-IIR have been described in various tumor types, including missense mutations, loss of heterozygosity, and microsatellite instability *(26,27)*. Loss of the IGF-IIR has been associated with increased tumor growth potential *(28)*, decreasing IGF-IIR expression has a similar effect *(29)*, whereas introduction of the IGF-IIR into cancer cells reduces growth and increases apoptosis *(30)*.

2.3. Binding Proteins

The six IGF binding proteins (IGFBP-1 to -6) all have greater affinity for binding to the IGFs, than the IGF-IR, and can therefore restrict IGF actions *(4)*. The IGFBPs, however, have the potential to either inhibit or enhance IGF actions in many cell types. Several hypotheses have been proposed to explain enhanced IGF actions, including presentation of IGF to cell surface receptors and preventing receptor down-regulation. To date, most evidence suggests that IGFBPs generally restrict tumor growth and progression by limiting IGF-mitogenic and cell survival actions. The actions of many antiproliferative agents appear to operate, at least in part, via upregulation of endogenous IGFBPs produced by the tumor cells, including TGF-β *(31)*, retinoids *(32)*, vitamin D *(33)*, tamoxifen *(34)*, and butyrate *(35)*. Accumulating evidence indicates that most of the IGFBPs can also act in an intrinsic manner, independent of IGF-binding, affecting various aspects of cell function. Growth inhibition and modulation of apoptosis have been described in a variety of cancer cell lines *(36–40)*.

Prostate cancer cells transfected to overexpress IGFBP-4 have been reported to exhibit higher rates of apoptosis in culture and reduced incidence of tumors when injected into nude mice *(41)*. Altered levels of different IGFBPs have been observed in a variety of different tumors, and some of these perturbations have been proposed as prognostic indicators of disease progression *(42–44)*.

In addition to all the data relating to associations between IGFBP-3 and known tumor cell inhibitors, there have also been suggestions from epidemiology that high serum IGFBP-3 levels (described below) are associated with reduced cancer risk. There have, however, been several reports that would appear to imply conflicting actions. Tumor levels of IGFBP-3 have been found to correlate positively with breast tumor size *(45)* and to be positively associated with poor prognosis *(46)*. The nature of IGFBP actions may well change with advancement of cancer. The change in extracellular pH, proteolysis, and extracellular matrix in addition to changes in tumor cell behavior could all result in a shift in balance between potentiating and inhibiting and between IGF-dependent and independent actions of IGFBPs.

2.4. Binding Protein Proteases

The IGFBPs appear to be particularly susceptible to proteolytic cleavage; in most cases, in vivo cleavage appears to be limited but with a resultant decrease in affinity of IGF-binding *(47)*. The IGFBPs are susceptible to cleavage by a range of proteinases, including metalloproteinases, cathepsins, kallikreins, and plasmin. It has been widely reported that many of these proteinases have increased activity in aggressive and invasive tumors. Indeed breakdown and remodeling of the extracellular matrix is a requirement for tumor progression. This has led to the obvious postulation that tumor associated proteases would be releasing IGFs to support tumor growth and progression. This interpretation is, however, not that straightforward. Studies of IGFBP-proteases in the circulation and in normal extravascular compartments have indicated that although IGFBP proteolysis is normally limited within the circulation because of the presence of inhibitors, in most normal tissues there appears to be high levels of protease activity, and the main carrier protein IGFBP-3 is predominantly in a cleaved form *(47)*. If IGFBP-3 is mainly in a proteolytically cleaved form within normal tissues, the significance of increased proteolysis around tumors is much more difficult to interpret. The realization that proteolysis may also generate bioactive IGFBP fragments that can act in an IGF-independent manner has further complicated this interpretation.

The demonstration that prostate-specific antigen (PSA) could cleave IGFBPs has received particular attention. Proteolysis of IGFBP-3 in vitro by PSA was reported to reduce its growth inhibitory potential *(48)*. There has been much speculation that raised circulating PSA levels in patients with prostate cancer may result in cleavage of circulating IGFBP-3 with a consequent increase in tissue availability of the large pool of IGFs maintained with IGFBP-3. There is, however, no evidence indicating that IGFBP-3 is cleaved by PSA in vivo and it would not be expected for PSA to be active in the circulation. It has also been shown that there are no associations between serum PSA levels and proteolytic cleavage of circulating IGFBP-3 *(48)*. The potential significance of PSA/IGFBP interactions in the local environment of a prostate tumor has yet to be determined.

2.5. Circulating IGFs

The activity of IGFs within any tissue is almost certainly caused by a combination of some locally expressed components together with IGFs and IGFBPs delivered to the tissue from the circulation where high levels are maintained. This provides a mechanism for integrating systemic and local regulation systems. The circulating IGF-system is under the influence of GH, insulin, nutrition and systemic disease status, whereas the locally expressed components are controlled by factors specific to each individual tissue.

There have been many studies documenting changes in circulating levels of IGFs and IGFBPs in patients with different cancers. It is becoming clear that many of the changes reported appear to be part of the general systemic response to serious illness. In the last few years, however, considerable new interest has been generated by results from prospective epidemiology studies linking circulating IGF-I concentrations, measured in samples taken years prior to the onset of disease, with risk of subsequent development of clinical cancer. The strongest associations were reported for individuals with relatively high serum IGF-I levels together with relatively low levels of serum IGFBP-3. Increased relative risks of the order of two- to sevenfold were found for prostate *(49)*, breast *(50)*, and colorectal *(51,52)* cancers. In the subsequent few years there have been many further epidemiological studies reported that generally confirm these disease associations. There have been attempts to group these studies into meta-analyses, although in reality this is probably not appropriate because most of the studies are case-control or studies of screen-detected cancers and there are still relatively few prospective population studies. The case-control studies are very different in that the systemic alterations to the circulating IGF system as a consequence of illness in patients with cancers of varying stages would be expected to confound any analysis of disease risk. Patients with advanced cancer become anorectic and catabolic resulting in suppression of circulating IGF-I and IGFBP-3, this would clearly obscure any investigation of whether raised IGF-I levels increase the risk of developing cancer. Data from most studies do, however, generally appear to be in accordance with the initial prospective studies. Similar risk associations have been reported with childhood leukemia *(53)* and lung cancer *(54)*. There was also a reported interaction between high levels of IGF-I and mutagen sensitivity in the study of lung cancer risk *(54)*, suggesting that IGF-I may act synergistically with other known risk factors. Although the association between relatively high circulating IGF-I level and cancer risk has, to date, proven surprisingly robust, the association between circulating IGFBP-3 levels and cancer risk has been more confused, both positive *(55)* and negative *(51)* associations having been reported.

That circulating levels of IGF-I can impact upon the incidence and growth of tumors has been supported by recent work in laboratory animals. The administration of a well-characterized murine mammary gland carcinogen to transgenic mice overexpressing a GH antagonist resulted in a reduction of tumor incidence of 68% in control mice to just

32% in the transgenic mice *(56)*. This reduction in tumor incidence occurred against a background of a 44% reduction in circulating IGF-I concentration in the transgenic mice. There was, however, a large difference in body size in the transgenic animals considerably confounding interpretation of the mechanism underlying the reduced carcinogenesis. More direct evidence for a role of circulating IGF-I has come from experiments with mice in which the IGF-I gene was disrupted specifically in the liver, resulting in a 75% reduction in serum IGF-I, but without change in IGF-I expression in non-hepatic tissues *(57)*. This large reduction in circulating IGF-I did not have any significant effect on normal growth and development, with no measured difference in body size. When mouse adenocarcinoma tissue fragments were, however, grafted onto the caecum of these mice this resulted in detectable tumors in 31% of animals with disrupted IGF-I expression compared with 57% in control mice *(58)*. Administration of IGF-I to the mice to replace the deficiency of circulating IGF-I resulted in an increase in tumor incidence to 64.5% of animals. There was also a longer latency period before tumor development and fewer hepatic metastases in the IGF-deficient mice. This study indicated that a large difference in circulating IGF-I could have a significant effect on tumor development and metastasis in normal sized mice.

3. GH AND ANTHROPOMETRY

A large body of literature supports the existence of a significant, albeit relatively weak, association between height and cancer risk *(59)*. Together, these reports indicate that taller individuals are at a 20–60% increased risk of a range of cancers. The much fewer studies that have examined components of statural height suggest that the association is largely attributed to variation in leg length *(59)*. There are many potential explanations for these associations. There could be many genes that may impact both upon statural growth and upon cancer risk. Similarly, there are many potential exposures, both prenatal and throughout childhood, that might affect both growth and cancer risk, including nutrition and infections. The well-recognized importance of the IGF system for somatic growth and neoplastic growth suggests, however, that the anthropometric evidence is, at least, compatible with an effect of IGF-I upon risk of cancer.

More circumstantial evidence has arisen from reported associations between circulating growth hormone and cancer risk. Despite the problems of assessing exposure to a hormone secreted in a pulsatile manner, an association between measured circulating GH levels and subsequent cancer has been reported in one prospective study *(60)*. There has also been considerable debate regarding evidence from subjects with acromegaly, who are chronically exposed to pathologically elevated levels of GH. Increased incidence of breast and in particular colorectal cancer has been reported in cohorts of subjects with acromegaly *(61)*. The consequence of elevation of GH status is an increase in circulating levels of both IGF-I and IGFBP-3; whether the increase in IGFBP-3 counter balances any increased risk associated with high IGF-I levels, as suggested by the initial prospective epidemiology, will await clarification when the role of IGFBP-3 is eventually resolved.

4. NUTRITION AND CANCER

The literature linking nutrition with incidence of cancer is far more extensive than that linking anthropometry. The incidence of many different cancers varies hugely between different populations and all of the most common cancers that plague Western societies are rare in populations somewhere in the world. Studies of immigrant populations indicate that within two to three generations cancer, incident rates converge, either up or down, to that of the local population *(62)*. This led to the acceptance that most cancers cannot be attributed to genetic factors within populations but instead must be attributable to lifestyle and environment. Nutrition has been widely regarded as a main contributor to this large effect. The study of associations between diet and cancer is confounded by numerous factors, not least because of the complexity and variety of foods and their multiple constituents. As a result, the evidence linking most single dietary constituents is not unequivocal. There is, however, consensus agreement linking many cancers to a typical Western diet and lifestyle, with a direct relationship between cancer risk and consumption of meat, total animal fat, and simple sugars, as well as with obesity. In contrast, there is an inverse relationship with consumption of fruit and vegetables, whole grains, and fiber, as well as with physical activity *(63,64)*. Experts in both the United States and Europe have concluded that around a third of cancers could be prevented by dietary modifications *(62)* and that between 5 and 10% of cancers are caused by individuals being overweight.

A large number of vitamins and other micronutrients have been linked to various cancers; however, large-scale intervention studies with dietary supplements have to date been disappointing or even harmful *(64)*.

High calorie intake in children has been associated with subsequent increase in cancer incidence later in life *(65)* and in the same cohort there was a significant association between prepubertal leg-length and subsequent incidence of hormone-dependent cancers *(66)*. These studies implied that childhood nutrition may "program" the susceptibility to certain cancers throughout subsequent life.

These population studies were supported by many studies in laboratory rodents indicating overfeeding promotes and diet restriction inhibits the incidence and growth of spontaneous *(67)*, transplanted *(68)*, and hormonally *(69)* or clinically induced *(70)* tumors within a variety of tissues.

5. NUTRITION, IGF-I, AND CANCER

As described throughout this book, nutrition has a major role in regulating the IGF axis, and IGF-I is implicated in mediating the effects of nutrition on somatic growth. It is therefore an attractive extrapolation to suggest that IGF-I may also mediate the effects of nutrition on neoplastic growth. The association of nutrition with incidence of a wide range of different cancers suggests mediation by a common regulatory pathway; IGF-I could readily fulfill such a general effect in many tissues. The beneficial effects of diet restriction in animal models have been associated with the diet-induced changes in circulating IGF-I. The growth of chemically induced liver tumors in mice was reduced by diet restriction, and this was accompanied by a decrease in IGF-I concentration *(70)*. Similarly, in a leukemia cell transplant model in rats, diet restriction decreased the incidence and severity of cancers and increased the latency period, and this was associated with a decrease in IGF-I concentration *(71)*. There was also a decrease in cell proliferation rate and this was restored by infusion of IGF-I. Diet restriction in rats has also been shown to reduce the growth and increase apoptosis of transplanted human prostate cancer cells in association with a decrease in circulating

IGF-I *(68)*. In a model in which p53-deficient mice received a bladder carcinogen, diet restriction was again associated with a reduction in tumor incidence and progression and a decrease in circulating IGF-I *(72)*. Prevention of the decrease in circulating IGF-I by IGF-I infusion negated the benefits of diet restriction, and this was associated with a sixfold increase in cell proliferation and a 10-fold reduction in apoptosis in the hyperplastic foci.

These animal experiments imply that the associations between nutrition and cancer and between circulating IGF-I concentrations and cancer in human populations may be linked, although there is very little direct evidence to date to confirm this linkage. Despite the lack of direct evidence, the indirect evidence is compelling. In a prospective study assessing the risk of colorectal cancer, there was a significant interaction between milk intake and the ratio of circulating IGF-I/IGFBP-3 *(73)*. The protective effect of milk consumption on subsequent development of colorectal cancer was strongest among individuals with high IGF-I/IGFBP-3. Nutrition can clearly affect the systemic IGF-system and interventions, which reduce IGF-I levels, may reduce cancer incidence or progression. Breast cancer risk can be reduced by the prophylactic use of tamoxifen and possibly raloxifene *(74)*, both of which lower circulating IGF-I concentrations *(75,76)*. Octreotide, a more direct intervention that reduces IGF-I levels, may retard growth of a number of tumors *(77)*.

There is a need for much more research to determine the components of human diet that most influence the IGF-system and how this may impact cancer incidence and progression. Most animal and human epidemiological studies to date have examined energy and/or total dietary restriction (partial starvation). Examination of specific nutrients, foods, or bioactive components of foods (nutraceuticals) is a growing area of research. A recent small study has shown a significant inverse association between serum IGF-I and cooked tomato consumption *(78)*; lycopene from cooked tomatoes has been implicated as protective against prostate cancer; but much larger and more extensive studies are required.

6. MECHANISMS UNDERLYING IGF-I –CANCER ASSOCIATIONS

6.1. Mitogenic Effects

There are many potential mechanisms that could underlie the associations between IGF-I and cancer. The simplest explanation for the associations revealed from prospective human epidemiology, would be that in an environment with high IGF-I or high IGF-I/IGFBP-3 any neoplastic lesion progresses more rapidly to clinical presentation. So although more incident cases are observed in subjects with high IGF-I/IGFBP-3 in relatively short follow-ups of 3–10 yr, if the same cohorts are revisited after 20 years, there may be equal incidence of cancers in the subjects with lower IGF-I. The extensive data from animal and cell models suggest that this is not the whole explanation. The simplest mechanism to invoke would be that the mitogenic actions of IGF-I increased epithelial cell number or turnover. The strongest and most consistent associations have been observed for epithelial cancers of the breast, prostate, and colorectum. If there are more epithelial cells or more cells going through the cell cycle, then there are more opportunities for a malignant transformation. There is some evidence for such an effect of systemic IGF-I concentrations on such tissues in non-tumor individuals. A strong association between IGF-I/IGFBP-3 and mammographic breast density has been observed in premenopausal women *(79)*. A high mammographic breast density reflects more glandular epithelial/stromal tissue relative to adipose tissue. Serum IGF-I/IGFBP-3 is associated with increased risk of premenopausal breast cancer *(80)* and high breast density is also strongly associated with increased risk of breast cancer. Subjects with acromegaly have high levels of IGF-I and hyperplasia of the prostate has been reported in young subjects *(81)* and increased epithelial cell proliferation in the colon have been correlated with circulating IGF-I concentration *(82)*.

6.2. Apoptosis

The most fundamental defense against cancer is cellular apoptosis. Damaged cells or cells growing inappropriately should activate apoptosis, the natural mechanism to remove damaged, infected or superfluous cells from the body. A large amount of evidence from cell biology indicates that IGF-I is a very potent cell survival factor and IGFBP-3 not only has an important role in controlling IGF-I availability, but also has intrinsic actions promoting apoptosis *(83)*. Together, this evidence implies that the balance between IGF-I and IGFBP-3 may regulate the threshold for activation of apoptosis. A relatively high IGFBP-3 to IGF-I ratio would promote damaged cells to undergo apoptosis and reduce the risk of cancer whereas a relatively high IGF-I to IGFBP-3, would promote cell survival; if damaged cells survive inappropriately, this might increase the risk of neoplasia.

7. SUMMARY AND CONCLUSIONS

The associations between nutrition, IGF-I, and cancer have many potential implications. The measurement of IGFs may enable identification of high-risk individuals for more intensive screening and for risk reduction strategies. The efficacy of risk reduction strategies has been established by the prophylactic use of tamoxifen in women at high of risk of breast cancer. The nutritional dependence of the IGF system raises the potential for prophylactic risk reduction by dietary manipulations rather than by pharmacological interventions. There are, however, in addition many different pharmaceutical strategies for targeting the IGF-system that are being developed.

Cancer is generally a disease of advancing years. The dramatic increase in survival of individuals into their 80s and 90s in all Western societies suggests that cancer will remain a growing epidemic. In the third world, it is projected that noncommunicable diseases will overtake communicable diseases within the first half of this century. The shift of populations from rural to urban environments is accompanied by a switch from unprocessed agricultural food to a processed Western-style diet. The spread of the cancer epidemic to the third world will necessitate a new approach, as they will not have the economic resource to deal with cancer in the same manner that Western societies have applied to date. The links between nutrition, IGF-I, and the common epithelial cancers suggest further avenues of research that might provide new approaches to prevent the spread of the cancer epidemic.

REFERENCES

1. Folkman J, Hahnfeldt P, Hlatky L. Cancer: looking outside the genome. Nat Rev Mol Cell Biol 2000;1:76–79.

2. Li FP. Identification and management of inherited cancer susceptibility. Environ Health Perspect 1995;103(Suppl 8):297–300.
3. Lichtenstein P, Holm NV, Verkasalo PK, et al. Environmental and heritable factors in the causation of cancer—analyses of cohorts of twins from Sweden, Denmark, and Finland. N Engl J Med 2000;343:78–85.
4. Jones JI, Clemmons DR. Insulin-like growth factors and their binding proteins: biological actions. Endocr Rev 1995;16:3–34.
5. Yu H, Rohan T. Role of the insulin-like growth factor family in cancer development and progression. J Natl Cancer Inst 2000;92:1472–1489.
6. Tricoli JV, Rall LB, Karakousis CP, et al. Enhanced levels of insulin-like growth factor messenger RNA in human colon carcinomas and liposarcomas. Cancer Res 1986;46:6169–6173.
7. Cariani E, Lasserre C, Seurin D, et al. Differential expression of insulin-like growth factor II mRNA in human primary liver cancers, benign liver tumors, and liver cirrhosis. Cancer Res 1988;48:6844–6849.
8. Rogler CE, Yang D, Rossetti L, et al. Altered body composition and increased frequency of diverse malignancies in insulin-like growth factor-II transgenic mice. J Biol Chem 1994;269:13779–13784.
9. Bates P, Fisher R, Ward A, Richardson L, Hill DJ, Graham CF. Mammary cancer in transgenic mice expressing insulin-like growth factor II (IGF-II). Br J Cancer 1995;72:1189–1193.
10. Hirano H, Lopes MB, Laws ER, Jr., et al. Insulin-like growth factor-1 content and pattern of expression correlates with histopathologic grade in diffusely infiltrating astrocytomas. Neuro-oncol 1999;1:109–119.
11. Sohda T, Oka Y, Iwata K, et al. Co-localisation of insulin-like growth factor II and the proliferation marker MIB1 in hepatocellular carcinoma cells. J Clin Pathol 1997;50:135–137.
12. Kawamoto K, Onodera H, Kondo S, et al. Expression of insulin-like growth factor-2 can predict the prognosis of human colorectal cancer patients: correlation with tumor progression, proliferative activity and survival. Oncology 1998;55:242–248.
13. Guerra FK, Eijan AM, Puricelli L, et al. Varying patterns of expression of insulin-like growth factors I and II and their receptors in murine mammary adenocarcinomas of different metastasizing ability. Int J Cancer 1996;65:812–820.
14. LeRoith D, Werner H, Neuenschwander S, Kalebic T, Helman LJ. The role of the insulin-like growth factor-I receptor in cancer. Ann N Y Acad Sci 1995;766:402–408.
15. Braulke T. Type-2 IGF receptor: a multi-ligand binding protein. Horm Metab Res 1999;31:242–246.
16. Papa V, Gliozzo B, Clark GM, et al. Insulin-like growth factor-I receptors are overexpressed and predict a low risk in human breast cancer. Cancer Res 1993;53:3736–3740.
17. Steller MA, Delgado CH, Bartels CJ, Woodworth CD, Zou Z. Overexpression of the insulin-like growth factor-1 receptor and autocrine stimulation in human cervical cancer cells. Cancer Res 1996;56:1761–1765.
18. Jammes H, Peyrat JP, Ban E, et al. Insulin-like growth factor 1 receptors in human breast tumour: localisation and quantification by histo-autoradiographic analysis. Br J Cancer 1992;66:248–253.
19. Valentinis B, Baserga R. IGF-I receptor signalling in transformation and differentiation. Mol Pathol 2001;54:133–137.
20. Peruzzi F, Prisco M, Dews M, et al. Multiple signaling pathways of the insulin-like growth factor 1 receptor in protection from apoptosis. Mol Cell Biol 1999;19:7203–7215.
21. Xie Y, Skytting B, Nilsson G, Brodin B, Larsson O. Expression of insulin-like growth factor-1 receptor in synovial sarcoma: association with an aggressive phenotype. Cancer Res 1999;59:3588–3591.
22. Long L, Rubin R, Brodt P. Enhanced invasion and liver colonization by lung carcinoma cells overexpressing the type 1 insulin-like growth factor receptor. Exp Cell Res 1998;238:116–121.
23. Kaplan PJ, Mohan S, Cohen P, Foster BA, Greenberg NM. The insulin-like growth factor axis and prostate cancer: lessons from the transgenic adenocarcinoma of mouse prostate (TRAMP) model. Cancer Res 1999;59:2203–2209.
24. Sciacca L, Costantino A, Pandini G, et al. Insulin receptor activation by IGF-II in breast cancers: evidence for a new autocrine/paracrine mechanism. Oncogene 1999;18:2471–2479.
25. Pandini G, Vigneri R, Costantino A, et al. Insulin and insulin-like growth factor-I (IGF-I) receptor overexpression in breast cancers leads to insulin/IGF-I hybrid receptor overexpression: evidence for a second mechanism of IGF-I signaling. Clin Cancer Res 1999;5:1935–1944.
26. Oates AJ, Schumaker LM, Jenkins SB, et al. The mannose 6-phosphate/insulin-like growth factor 2 receptor (M6P/IGF2R), a putative breast tumor suppressor gene. Breast Cancer Res Treat 1998;47:269–281.

27. De Souza AT, Hankins GR, Washington MK, Orton TC, Jirtle RL. M6P/IGF2R gene is mutated in human hepatocellular carcinomas with loss of heterozygosity. Nat Genet 1995;11:447–449.
28. Byrd JC, Devi GR, de Souza AT, Jirtle RL, MacDonald RG. Disruption of ligand binding to the insulin-like growth factor II/mannose 6-phosphate receptor by cancer-associated missense mutations. J Biol Chem 1999;274:24408–24416.
29. O'Gorman DB, Costello M, Weiss J, Firth SM, Scott CD. Decreased insulin-like growth factor-II/mannose 6-phosphate receptor expression enhances tumorigenicity in JEG-3 cells. Cancer Res 1999;59:5692–5694.
30. Souza RF, Wang S, Thakar M, et al. Expression of the wild-type insulin-like growth factor II receptor gene suppresses growth and causes death in colorectal carcinoma cells. Oncogene 1999;18:4063–4068.
31. Oh Y, Muller HL, Ng L, Rosenfeld RG. Transforming growth factor-beta-induced cell growth inhibition in human breast cancer cells is mediated through insulin-like growth factor-binding protein-3 action. J Biol Chem 1995;270:13589–13592.
32. Shemer J, Yaron A, Werner H, et al. Regulation of insulin-like growth factor (IGF) binding protein-5 in the T47D human breast carcinoma cell line by IGF-I and retinoic acid. J Clin Endocrinol Metab 1993;77:1246–1250.
33. Colston KW, Perks CM, Xie SP, Holly JM. Growth inhibition of both MCF-7 and Hs578T human breast cancer cell lines by vitamin D analogues is associated with increased expression of insulin-like growth factor binding protein-3. J Mol Endocrinol 1998;20:157–162.
34. Karas M, Kleinman D, Danilenko M, et al. Components of the IGF system mediate the opposing effects of tamoxifen on endometrial and breast cancer cell growth. Prog Growth Factor Res 1995;6:513–520.
35. Nishimura A, Fujimoto M, Oguchi S, Fusunyan RD, MacDermott RP, Sanderson IR. Short-chain fatty acids regulate IGF-binding protein secretion by intestinal epithelial cells. Am J Physiol 1998;275:E55–E63.
36. Oh Y, Muller HL, Lamson G, Rosenfeld RG. Insulin-like growth factor (IGF)-independent action of IGF-binding protein-3 in Hs578T human breast cancer cells. Cell surface binding and growth inhibition. J Biol Chem 1993;268:14964–14971.
37. Hollowood AD, Lai T, Perks CM, Newcomb PV, Alderson D, Holly JM. IGFBP-3 prolongs the p53 response and enhances apoptosis following UV irradiation. Int J Cancer 2000;88:336–341.
38. Perks CM, Bowen S, Gill ZP, Newcomb PV, Holly JM. Differential IGF-independent effects of insulin-like growth factor binding proteins (1–6) on apoptosis of breast epithelial cells. J Cell Biochem 1999;75:652–664.
39. Gill ZP, Perks CM, Newcomb PV, Holly JM. Insulin-like growth factor-binding protein (IGFBP-3) predisposes breast cancer cells to programmed cell death in a non-IGF-dependent manner. J Biol Chem 1997;272:25602–607.
40. Williams AC, Collard TJ, Perks CM, et al. Increased p53-dependent apoptosis by the insulin-like growth factor binding protein IGFBP-3 in human colonic adenoma-derived cells. Cancer Res 2000;60:22–27.
41. Damon SE, Haugk KL, Birnbaum RS, Quinn LS. Retrovirally mediated overexpression of insulin-like growth factor binding protein 4: evidence that insulin-like growth factor is required for skeletal muscle differentiation. J Cell Physiol 1998;175:109–120.
42. Zumkeller W, Schwander J, Mitchell CD, Morrell DJ, Schofield PN, Preece MA. Insulin-like growth factor (IGF)-I, -II and IGF binding protein-2 (IGFBP-2) in the plasma of children with Wilms' tumour. Eur J Cancer 1993;14:1973–1977.
43. Rutanen EM, Wahlstrom T, Koistinen R, Sipponen P, Jalanko H, Seppala M. Placental protein 12 (PP12) in primary liver cancer and cirrhosis. Tumour Biol 1984;5:95–102.
44. Renehan AG, Jones J, Potten CS, Shalet SM, O'Dwyer ST. Elevated serum insulin-like growth factor (IGF)-II and IGF binding protein-2 in patients with colorectal cancer. Br J Cancer 2000;83:1344–1350.
45. Rocha RL, Hilsenbeck SG, Jackson JG, et al. Insulin-like growth factor binding protein-3 and insulin receptor substrate-1 in breast cancer: correlation with clinical parameters and disease-free survival. Clin Cancer Res 1997;3:103–109.
46. Rocha RL, Hilsenbeck SG, Jackson JG, Lee AV, Figueroa JA, Yee D. Correlation of insulin-like growth factor-binding protein-3 messenger RNA with protein expression in primary breast cancer tissues:

detection of higher levels in tumors with poor prognostic features. J Natl Cancer Inst 1996;88:601–606.
47. Maile LA, Holly JM. Insulin-like growth factor binding protein (IGFBP) proteolysis: occurrence, identification, role and regulation. Growth Horm IGF Res 1999;9:85–95.
48. Koistinen H, Paju A, Koistinen R, et al. Prostate-specific antigen and other prostate-derived proteases cleave IGFBP-3, but prostate cancer is not associated with proteolytically cleaved circulating IGFBP-3. Prostate 2002;50:112–118.
49. Chan JM, Stampfer MJ, Giovannucci E, et al. Plasma insulin-like growth factor-I and prostate cancer risk: a prospective study. Science 1998;279:563–566.
50. Hankinson SE, Willett WC, Colditz GA, et al. Circulating concentrations of insulin-like growth factor-I and risk of breast cancer. Lancet 1998;351:1393–1396.
51. Ma J, Pollak MN, Giovannucci E, et al. Prospective study of colorectal cancer risk in men and plasma levels of insulin-like growth factor (IGF)-I and IGF-binding protein-3. J Natl Cancer Inst 1999;91:620–625.
52. Giovannucci E, Pollak MN, Platz EA, et al. A prospective study of plasma insulin-like growth factor-1 and binding protein-3 and risk of colorectal neoplasia in women. Cancer Epidemiol Biomarkers Prev 2000;9:345–349.
53. Petridou E, Dessypris N, Spanos E, et al. Insulin-like growth factor-I and binding protein-3 in relation to childhood leukaemia. Int J Cancer 1999;80:494–496.
54. Wu X, Yu H, Amos CI, Hong WK, Spitz MR. Joint effect of insulin-like growth factors and mutagen sensitivity in lung cancer risk. Growth Horm IGF Res 2000;10(Suppl A):S26–S27.
55. Shi R, Berkel HJ, Yu H. Insulin-like growth factor-I and prostate cancer: a meta-analysis. Br J Cancer 2001;85:991–996.
56. Pollak M, Blouin MJ, Zhang JC, Kopchick JJ. Reduced mammary gland carcinogenesis in transgenic mice expressing a growth hormone antagonist. Br J Cancer 2001;85:428–430.
57. Yakar S, Liu JL, Stannard B, et al. Normal growth and development in the absence of hepatic insulin-like growth factor I. Proc Natl Acad Sci USA 1999;96:7324–7329.
58. Wu Y, Yakar S, Zhao L, Hennighausen L, LeRoith D. Circulating insulin-like growth factor-I levels regulate colon cancer growth and metastasis. Cancer Res 2002;62:1030–1035.
59. Gunnell D. Commentary: Early insights into height, leg length, proportionate growth and health. Int J Epidemiol 2001;30:221–222.
60. Maison P, Balkau B, Simon D, Chanson P, Rosselin G, Eschwege E. Growth hormone as a risk for premature mortality in healthy subjects: data from the Paris prospective study. Bmj 1998;316:1132–1133.
61. Jenkins PJ, Fairclough PD, Richards T, et al. Acromegaly, colonic polyps and carcinoma. Clin Endocrinol (Oxf) 1997;47:17–22.
62. Peto J. Cancer epidemiology in the last century and the next decade. Nature 2001;411:390–395.
63. Riboli E, Norat T. Cancer prevention and diet: opportunities in Europe. Public Health Nutr 2001;4:475–484.
64. Greenwald P, Clifford CK, Milner JA. Diet and cancer prevention. Eur J Cancer 2001;37:948–965.
65. Frankel S, Gunnell DJ, Peters TJ, Maynard M, Davey Smith G. Childhood energy intake and adult mortality from cancer: the Boyd Orr Cohort Study. BMJ 1998;316:499–504.
66. Gunnell DJ, Davey Smith G, Frankel S, et al. Childhood leg length and adult mortality: follow up of the Carnegie (Boyd Orr) Survey of Diet and Health in Pre-war Britain. J Epidemiol Community Health 1998;52:142–152.
67. Hursting SD, Perkins SN, Phang JM. Calorie restriction delays spontaneous tumorigenesis in p53-knockout transgenic mice. Proc Natl Acad Sci USA 1994;91:7036–7040.
68. Mukherjee P, Sotnikov AV, Mangian HJ, Zhou JR, Visek WJ, Clinton SK. Energy intake and prostate tumor growth, angiogenesis, and vascular endothelial growth factor expression. J Natl Cancer Inst 1999;91:512–523.
69. Spady TJ, Lemus-Wilson AM, Pennington KL, et al. Dietary energy restriction abolishes development of prolactin-producing pituitary tumors in Fischer 344 rats treated with 17beta-estradiol. Mol Carcinog 1998;23:86–95.
70. Lagopoulos L, Sunahara GI, Wurzner H, Dombrowsky I, Stalder R. The effects of alternating dietary restriction and ad libitum feeding of mice on the development of diethylnitrosamine-induced liver tumours and its correlation to insulinaemia. Carcinogenesis 1991;12:311–315.

71. Hursting SD, Switzer BR, French JE, Kari FW. The growth hormone: insulin-like growth factor 1 axis is a mediator of diet restriction-induced inhibition of mononuclear cell leukemia in Fischer rats. Cancer Res 1993;53:2750–2757.
72. Dunn SE, Kari FW, French J, et al. Dietary restriction reduces insulin-like growth factor I levels, which modulates apoptosis, cell proliferation, and tumor progression in p53-deficient mice. Cancer Res 1997;57:4667–72.
73. Ma J, Giovannucci E, Pollak M, et al. Milk intake, circulating levels of insulin-like growth factor-I, and risk of colorectal cancer in men. J Natl Cancer Inst 2001;93:1330–1336.
74. Chlebowski RT. Breast cancer risk reduction: strategies for women at increased risk. Annu Rev Med 2002;53:519–540.
75. Helle SI, Holly JM, Tally M, Hall K, Vander Stappen J, Lonning PE. Influence of treatment with tamoxifen and change in tumor burden on the IGF-system in breast cancer patients. Int J Cancer 1996;69:335–339.
76. Torrisi R, Baglietto L, Johansson H, et al. Effect of raloxifene on IGF-I and IGFBP-3 in postmenopausal women with breast cancer. Br J Cancer 2001;85:1838–1841.
77. Pollak MN, Polychronakos C, Guyda H. Somatostatin analogue SMS 201–995 reduces serum IGF-I levels in patients with neoplasms potentially dependent on IGF-I. Anticancer Res 1989;9:889–891.
78. Mucci LA, Tamimi R, Lagiou P, et al. Are dietary influences on the risk of prostate cancer mediated through the insulin-like growth factor system? BJU Int 2001;87:814–820.
79. Byrne C, Colditz GA, Willett WC, Speizer FE, Pollak M, Hankinson SE. Plasma insulin-like growth factor (IGF) I, IGF-binding protein 3, and mammographic density. Cancer Res 2000;60:3744–3748.
80. Hankinson SE, Willett WC, Colditz GA, et al. Circulating concentrations of insulin-like growth factor-I and risk of breast cancer. Lancet 1998;351:1393–1396.
81. Colao A, Marzullo P, Ferone D, et al. Prostatic hyperplasia: an unknown feature of acromegaly. J Clin Endocrinol Metab 1998;83:775–779.
82. Cats A, Dullaart RP, Kleibeuker JH, et al. Increased epithelial cell proliferation in the colon of patients with acromegaly. Cancer Res 1996;56:523–526.
83. Holly JM, Gunnell DJ, Davey Smith G. Growth hormone, IGF-I and cancer. Less intervention to avoid cancer? More intervention to prevent cancer? J Endocrinol 1999;162:321–330.

APPENDIX

A Reviews and Background

The Insulin-Like Growth Factors

1. Rosenfeld RG and Roberts CT (eds.) 1999. The IGF system. molecularbiology, bhysiology, and clinical applications. Totowa, NJ: Humana Press.
2. LeRoith D, Zumkeller W, and Baxter RC. (eds.) 2003. Insulin-like growth factors. New York : Kluwer Academic/Plenum Publishers.
3. International Symposium on Insulin-like Growth Factors (4th) (1998): Tokyo, Japan. Amsterdam, New York: Elsevier.
4. Muller EE (ed.) 1998. IGFs in the nervous system. Milano; New York; Springer.
5. Simpson HL, Umpleby AM, and Russell-Jones DL. Insulin-like growth factor-I and diabetes. A review. Growth Horm IGF Res 1998;8:83–95.
6. Baxter RC.Insulin-like growth factor (IGF)-binding proteins: interactions with IGFs and intrinsic bioactivities. Am J Physiol Endocrinol Metab 2000;278:E967–E976.
7. Jones JI and Clemmons DR. Insulin-like growth factors and their binding proteins: biological actions. Endocr Rev 1995;16:3–34.
8. Rajaram S, Baylink DJ, and Mohan S. Insulin-like growth factor-binding proteins in serum and other biological fluids: regulation and functions. Endocr Rev 1997;18:801–831.
9. Rosenbloom AL. IGF-I treatment of diabetes. Pediatr Diabetes 2001;2:123–130.
10. LeRoith D and Roberts CT, Jr. The insulin-like growth factor system and cancer. Cancer Lett 2003;195:127–137.
11. LeRoith D and Helman L. The new kid on the block(ade) of the IGF-1 receptor. Cancer Cell 2004;5:201–202.
12. Holly JM, Perks CM, and Stewart CE. Overview of insulin-like growth factor physiology. Growth Horm IGF Res 2000;10 Suppl A:S8–S9.
13. Thissen JP, Ketelslegers, JM, and Underwood LE. Nutritional regulation of the insulin-like growth factors. Endocr Rev 1994;15:80–101.
14. Le Roith, D, Bondy C, Yakar S, Liu J, and Butler A. The somatomedin hypothesis: 2001 Endocr. Rev 2001;22: 53–74.
15. Jerome L, Shiry L, Leyland-Jones B. Anti-insulin-like growth factor strategies in breast cancer. Seminars in Oncology 2004;31:54–63.
16. Daughaday WH, Hall Kl, Raben MS, Salmon WD, Jr., Van Den Brande J., and Van Wyk JJ. Somatomedin: proposed designation for sulphation factor. Nature 1972;235:107.
17. Salmon WD, Jr. and Daughaday WH. A hormonally controlled serum factor which stimulates sulfate incorporation by cartilage in vitro. J Lab Clin Med 1957;49:825–836.

From: *IGF and Nutrition in Health and Disease*
Edited by: M. S. Houston, J. M. P. Holly, and E. L. Feldman © Humana Press Inc., Totowa, NJ

APPENDIX

B Related Professional Organizations and Journals

PROFESSIONAL SOCIETIES AND ORGANIZATIONS

http://www.igf-society.org/h/join_igfs.html

With close to 1000 members from dozens of countries, the **International Society for IGF Research** is a unique organization devoted to basic and applied research on a network of molecules called insulin-like growth factors (IGFs), their receptors, and their binding proteins (IGFBPs). Together, these scientists, educators, clinicians, and students who make up the organization's membership represent the spectrum of interests in IGF research from molecular biology to clinical applications. Since its inception, the IGF Society has worked to promote excellence and interest in research and education on the role of these molecules in the etiology, pathogenesis, and treatment of diseases such as cancer, diabetes, growth disorders, heart disease, and neurological illnesses.

http://www.asns.org/

The American Society for Nutritional Sciences (3500+ members) is the premier research society dedicated to improving the quality of life through the science of nutrition. The society fulfills its mission by: fostering and enhancing research in animal and human nutrition; providing opportunities for sharing, disseminating, and archiving peer-reviewed nutrition research results (at its annual meeting and in its official publication, the *Journal of Nutrition*): fostering quality education and training in nutrition; upholding standards for ethical behavior in research, the protection of human subjects, and the care and treatment of research animals; providing opportunities for fellowship and support among nutritionists; and bringing scientific knowledge to bear on nutrition issues through communication and influence in the public domain. The clinical division is the **American Society of Clinical Nutrition** (http://www.ascn.org/). The official publication is *The American Journal of Clinical Nutrition*, which focuses on basic and clinical studies relevant to human nutrition.

http://www.endo-society.org/

The Endocrine Society is the world's largest and most active professional organization of endocrinologists in the world. Founded in 1916, the society is internationally

From: *IGF, Nutrition, and Health*
Edited by: S. M. Houston, J. M. P. Holly, and E. L. Feldman © Humana Press Inc., Totowa, NJ

known as the leading source of state-of-the-art research and clinical advancements in endocrinology and metabolism. The Endocrine Society is dedicated to promoting excellence in research, education, and clinical practice in the field of endocrinology. The Endocrine Society is an international body with more than 11,000 members from more than 80 countries. The diverse membership represents medicine, molecular and cellular biology, biochemistry, physiology, genetics, immunology, education, industry, and allied health.

http://www.clinnutr.org/

The American Society for Parenteral and Enteral Nutrition promotes professional communication among and within professional disciplines in the broad field of clinical nutrition including parenteral and enteral nutrition through national and regional meetings, local seminars, scientific, and clinical and educational exhibits and publications. The society promotes proper application of clinical and research experience to the practice of nutritionally sound medicine.

http://www.nih.gov

Founded in 1887, the **National Institutes of Health** (NIH) today is one of the world's foremost medical research centers, and the Federal focal point for medical research in the United States. The NIH, comprising 27 separate institutes and centers, is one of eight health agencies of the Public Health Service which, in turn, is part of the US Department of Health and Human Services. Simply described, the goal of NIH research is to acquire new knowledge to help prevent, detect, diagnose, and treat disease and disability from the rarest genetic disorder to the common cold. NIH works toward that mission by: conducting research in its own laboratories; supporting the research of non-federal scientists in universities, medical schools, hospitals, and research institutions throughout the country and abroad; helping in the training of research investigators; and fostering communication of medical and health sciences information.

http://www.nsf.gov/

The National Science Foundation (NSF) is an independent agency of the US Government, established by the National Science Foundation Act of 1950. NSF's mission is to promote the progress of science, to advance the national health, prosperity, and welfare, and to secure the national defense.

http://www.ilsi.org/

Founded in 1978, the **International Life Sciences Institute** (ILSI) is a nonprofit, worldwide foundation that seeks to improve the well-being of the general public through the pursuit of balanced science. Its goal is to further the understanding of scientific issues relating to nutrition, food safety, toxicology, risk assessment, and the environment by bringing together scientists from academia, government, and industry.

http://www.eatright.org/

The American Dietetic Association is the largest group of food and nutrition professionals in the United States, members are primarily registered dietitians and dietetic technicians, registered. Programs and services include promoting nutrition information for the public; sponsoring national events, media and marketing programs, and publications (*The Journal of the American Dietetic Association*), and lobbying for federal legislation. Also available through the web site are member services, nutrition resources, news, classifieds, and government affairs. Assistance in finding a dietitian, marketplace news, and links to related sites also can be found.

http://www.faseb.org

The **Federation of American Societies for Experimental Biology** (FASEB) is a coalition of member societies with the purpose of enhancing the profession of biomedical and life scientists, emphasizing public policy issues. FASEB offers logistical and operational support as well as sponsoring scientific conferences and publications (*The FASEB Journal*).

http://www.usda.gov

The **United States Department of Agriculture** (USDA) provides a broad scope of service to the nation's farmers and ranchers. In addition, the USDA ensures open markets for agricultural products, food safety, environmental protection, conservation of forests and rural land, and the research of human nutrition. The Food and Nutrition Service administers the USDA's 15 food assistance programs for children and needy families with the mission to reduce hunger and food insecurity. http://www.fns.usda.gov/fns/

http://www.who.int/nut/

The **World Health Organization** has regarded nutrition to be of fundamental importance for overall health and sustainable development. The global priority of nutritional issues, activities, mandates, resources, and research are presented in detail.

http://www.diabetes.org

American Diabetes Association

http://www.aace.com

American Society of Clinical Endocrinologists

http://www.amcollnutr.org/

American College of Nutrition

http://www.asbmr.org/

American Society for Bone and Mineral Research

http://wwww.jdf.org
Juvenile Diabetes Research Foundation

http://www.nmss.org
National Multiple Sclerosis Society

http://www.neuropathy.org
The Neuropathy Association

http://www.asas.org/
American Society of Animal Science

http://www.bsped.org.uk
British Society for Paediatric Endocrinology and Diabetes

http://www.hgfound.org/
Human Growth Foundation

http://www.ghresearchsociety.org/bin/Default.asp
Growth Hormone Research Society

http://www.endocrinology.org/default.htm
Society for Endocrinology

http://www.the-aps.org/about/index.htm
American Physiological Society

http://www.aacr.org/
American Association of Cancer Research

http://www.asbmb.org/ASBMB/
American Society for Biochemistry and Molecular Biology

http://www.ascb.org/
American Society for Cell Biology

http://www.ama-assn.org/
American Medical Association

http://www.ibmsonline.org/
International Bone and Mineral Society

http://www.nof.org/
National Osteoporosis Foundation

JOURNALS

http://www.harcourt-international.com/journals/ghir/
Growth Hormone and IGF Research

http://www.nutrition.org/
Journal of Nutrition

http://www.ajcn.org/
American Journal of Clinical Nutrition

http://jcem.endojournals.org/
Journal of Endocrinology and Metabolism

http://endo.endojournals.org/
Endocrinology

http://mend.endojournals.org/
Molecular Endocrinology

http://journals.endocrinology.org/JME/jme.htm
Journal of Molecular Endocrinology

http://edrv.endojournals.org/
Endocrine Reviews

http://www.blackwellpublishing.com/
Clinical Endocrinology

http://journals.endocrinology.org/JOE/joe.htm
Journal of Endocrinology

http://www.elsevier.com/
Trends in Endocrinology and Metabolism

http://www.the-aps.org/publications/ajpendo/index.htm
American Journal of Physiology – Endocrinology and Metabolism

http://www.the-aps.org/publications/ajpendo/index.htm
American Journal of Physiology – Cell Physiology

http://rphr.endojournals.org/
Recent Progress in Hormone Research

http://www.sciencemag.org/
Science

http://www.nature.com/
Nature

http://www.cellpress.com/
Cell; Molecular Cell; Neuron; Cancer Cell; Immunity
Chemistry and Biology; Developmental Cell

http://annurev.org/
Annual Review of Nutrition

http://www.ilsi.org/
Nutrition Reviews

http://www.clinnutr.org
Journal of Parenteral and Enteral Nutrition

http://www.nature.com/ejcn
European Journal of Clinical Nutrition

http://www.eatright.org/journaltoc.html
Journal of the American Dietetic Association

http://www.ingenta.com/journals/browse/els/09552863
Journal of Nutritional Biochemistry

http://www.thieme.com/SID1990087552676/journals/pubid-388413336.html
Hormone and Metabolic Research

http://www.jbc.org/
Journal of Biological Chemistry

http://bmj.bmjjournals.com/
British Medical Journal

http://embojournal.npgjournals.com/
EMBO Journal

http://www.pnas.org/
Proceeding of the National Academy of Sciences

http://content.nejm.org/
New England Journal of Medicine

http://bmj.bmjjournals.com/
British Medical Journal

http://www.aacc.org/ccj/
Clinical Chemistry

http://www.currentopinion.com/
Current Opinion Series

http://www.elsevier.com/
Cytokine and Growth Factor Reviews

http://www.cabi-publishing.org/Journals.asp?SubjectArea=&PID=63
British Journal of Nutrition

http://journals.endocrinology.org/ERC/erc.htm
Endocrine Related Cancer

http://jas.fass.org/
Journal of Animal Science

http://www.thelancet.com/
The Lancet

http://www.annals.org/
Annals of Internal Medicine

http://diabetes.diabetesjournals.org
Diabetes

http://www.harcourt-international.com/journals/cale
Cancer Letters

http://www.jci.org
Journal of Clinical Investigation

http://www.jbc.org
Journal of Biological Chemistry

http://cancerres.aacrjournals.org
Cancer Research

http://content.karger.com
Hormone Research

http://www.elsevier.com
Biochemical Biophysical Research Communications

Index

About the Editors

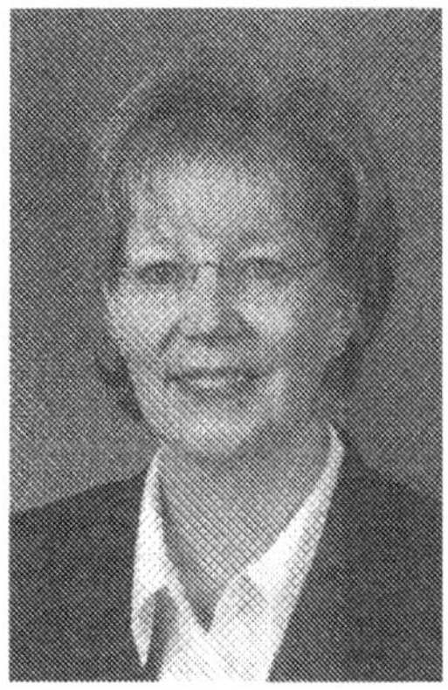

M. Sue Houston, PhD, RD is Associate Professor in the Food and Nutrition Program, School of Family and Consumer Sciences, and Graduate Faculty in the Department of Biological Sciences and Center for Biomolecular Sciences at Bowling Green State University, Bowling Green, Ohio. Dr. Houston completed graduate degrees in nutritional sciences at The Pennsylvania State University and Kansas State University. As a faculty member at The Ohio State University and Bowling Green State University, she has been involved in developing and teaching undergraduate, graduate, and clinical internship programs in nutrition. Dr. Houston initiated her studies on the insulin-like growth factors in doctoral work examining the effects of specific nutrients on somatomedin bioactivity. Research on the interrelationship of nutrition and the IGF proteins has continued using a variety of approaches including basic animal and in vitro models to human clinical studies. Her current research focuses on the interaction of nutrient and bioactive components of food on the IGF proteins and cancer.

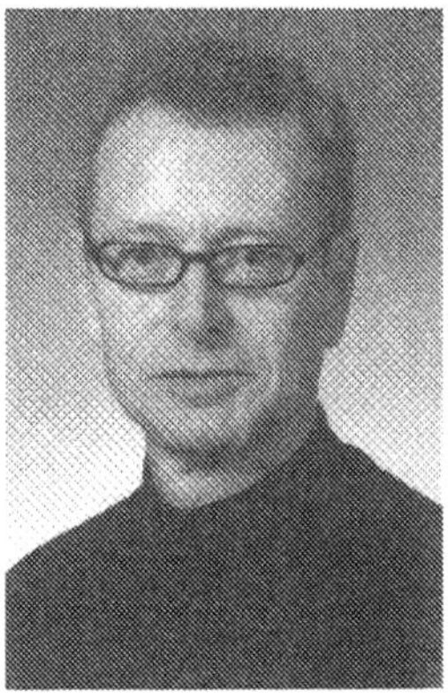

Jeff Holly is Professor of Clinical Science and Director of Research of the Academic Unit of Surgery at the University of Bristol in the United Kingdom. He is Vice-President of the International Society for IGF Research. He has published more than 200 articles on the physiology of the growth hormone-IGF system in relation to a variety of human pathologies. He is editor-in-chief of the journal *Best Practice and Research in Clinical Endocrinology and Metabolism* and on the editorial board of a number of other journals.

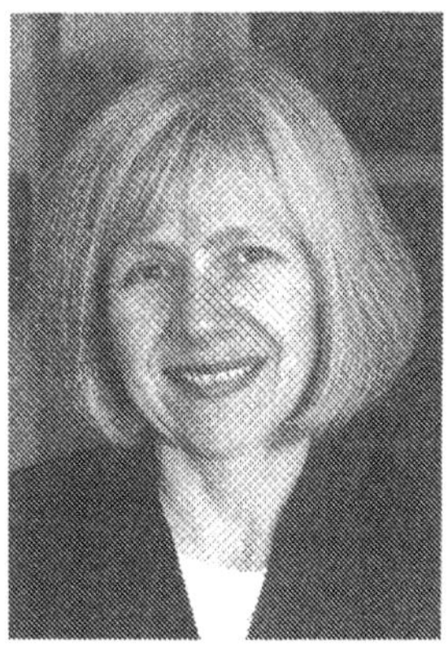

Eva Feldman received her PhD in Neuroscience and her MD at the University of Michigan. She performed her residency in Neurology at The Johns Hopkins Hospital. She returned to the University of Michigan and is currently a Professor of Neurology and Director of the Juvenile Diabetes Research Foundation (JDRF) Center on the Complications of Diabetes. She is recognized as a leading expert in the field of insulin-like growth factors and their role in the pathogenesis and treatment of neurological diseases and diabetes. She has published more than 120 papers and 40 book chapters in the area of insulin-like growth factor and neurologic diseases. Dr. Feldman's research is funded by the National Institutes of Health, the JDRF, and the Program for Understanding Neurological Diseases.

GPSR Compliance
The European Union's (EU) General Product Safety Regulation (GPSR) is a set of rules that requires consumer products to be safe and our obligations to ensure this.

If you have any concerns about our products, you can contact us on

ProductSafety@springernature.com

In case Publisher is established outside the EU, the EU authorized representative is:

Springer Nature Customer Service Center GmbH
Europaplatz 3
69115 Heidelberg, Germany

www.ingramcontent.com/pod-product-compliance
Ingram Content Group UK Ltd.
Pitfield, Milton Keynes, MK11 3LW, UK
UKHW050227160926
475607UK00005B/116
* 9 7 8 1 5 8 8 2 9 1 9 0 5 *